Portia M. Frederick, CMA—AC

Coordinator, Medical Assisting Program
West Valley College
Saratoga, California

Mary E. Kinn, CPS, CMA—A

Instructor in Health Technologies
Long Beach City College
Long Beach, California

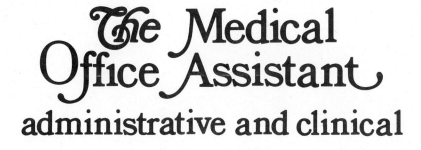

# The Medical Office Assistant

## administrative and clinical

FOURTH EDITION

W. B. SAUNDERS COMPANY
Philadelphia, London, Toronto

W. B. Saunders Company: West Washington Square
Philadelphia, PA 19105

1 St. Anne's Road
Eastbourne, East Sussex BN21 3UN, England

1 Goldthorne Avenue
Toronto, Ontario M8Z 5T9, Canada

The Medical Office Assistant
Administrative and Clinical

ISBN 0-7216-3862-7

Print No.:     9

# CONTRIBUTORS

LEE WELLER CALLAWAY, R.D., M.P.H., Ph.D.

Instructor, Food Service and Restaurant Management Department, West Valley College. Therapeutic dietitian, St. Rose Hospital, Hayward, California

MARY W. FALCONER, R.N., M.A.

Formerly Instructor of Pharmacology, O'Connor Hospital School of Nursing, San Jose, California

RHODA G. FINNERON

Chairman, Department of Secretarial Science and Law, Centennial College of Applied Arts and Technology, Scarborough, Ontario, Canada

# FOREWORD

Time was—and it wasn't long ago—when the majority of physicians worked alone. I don't mean that few doctors were in partnership; I mean they worked *alone.*

They peeked down throats, pounded torsos, doled out pills, sharpened needles, made change, answered the phone, and even popped their heads into their waiting rooms and grunted: "Next, please!" I know they did these things because I used to watch them do it.

That's all changed now. Pick any ten U.S. private practitioners at random and you'll find that five of them have at least two aides apiece. Three of the five will have three aides each, and two of these last three will have four each.

In fact, it's now worth my while to travel a hundred miles to watch a do-it-all-yourself doctor at work—and write an article about him. That's exactly what I did a few years ago. Sure enough, I found him swabbing out the sink in his examining room.

The modern doctor doesn't hire an aide just to swab out sinks, of course. He knows better than that. He knows that a skilled aide can do more for him than anything but his own eyes, ears, and fingers. He's proud of his motorized examining table, but he knows it won't drape a female patient for a pelvic examination. He's sold on disposable syringes, but he knows the syringe hasn't been made that knows where to jab. And although he's expecting a lot from computers in the next few years, he won't be looking for one that's programed to undress a baby or explain to a persistent caller that the doctor can't come to the phone.

Don't get me wrong. I'm not knocking the mechanical marvels. My point is simply that, knowing upwards of 3000 private practitioners, being familiar with what goes on in more than 1000 medical offices, and having watched at least 5000 aides on the job, I've yet to see any hardware that's as useful to a physician as a trained, experienced medical assistant—except two of the same.

Doctors agree with me. At last count (a *Medical Economics* Survey), 49.5 per cent of all U.S. self-employed physicians employed more than one aide. Why? That's easy. Because with the extra help they can see more patients in less time. You might think that's short-changing the patients. Not a bit of it; the opposite is true. The patients of a physician with plenty of help get a better deal all round.

Ever heard the old advice that a shoemaker should stick to his last? It goes for physicians as well as shoemakers. Doctors are at their best when they're doctoring. The fewer their nonmedical chores, the more mileage they get out of their professional skills. So the medical assistant doesn't only step up the physician's productivity; she helps him keep up the quality of his care.

There's a joker in the deck, though. These results aren't achieved simply by hiring a female to hand him things and tell patients where the toilet is. They're achieved only when the medical assistant is as expert in her work as the doctor is in his. It takes more than a sweet disposition — though that's indispensable — to cope simultaneously with a shrilling phone, a bawling tot, an irritable hypertensive patient, and a neurotic dowager who's positive her bill is wrong. It takes intelligence, training, experience, a flair for organization, and the patience of Job.

That's why this book, co-authored by two people who themselves measure up to this specification, fills a gap. It tells the girl who wants to help a doctor how to equip herself for the task. It does more. It tells girls who are already helping doctors how to help them more. And as if these two considerable feats weren't enough, there's a bonus: This book will help any doctor who snitches it from his aide's desk and takes it home for quiet reading. After all, if he doesn't know what expertise his office assistant is supposed to have, how can he know if she's got it?

It isn't my job to tell you what's in the book. You can discover that in the simplest manner imaginable: Read it. But if you're a medical assistant, don't be content with that. Keep on reading it. Study it. Refer to it. It won't hurt you to memorize great chunks of it. Not that it was written to be memorized; what the co-authors desperately want is that it shall be *understood*.

Myself, I think they've achieved their aim. I even understand it myself. And that's pretty good for a man who's never answered a doctor's phone, filed a chart, written a line in a daybook, or calmed down an indignant debtor. As a matter of fact, until I saw the manuscript of this book, I thought Trendelenburg was a place east of the Berlin wall.

Now settle down and find out what *you* don't know.

HORACE COTTON

# PREFACE

This is the fourth edition of a book originally published in 1956 under the title *The Office Assistant in Medical or Dental Practice.* That first edition of 350 pages met a long-felt need for a volume that was at once a handbook for the experienced office assistant, a text for the aspiring assistant, and a guide for the doctor attempting to teach a new employee. It was the forerunner of what is now a rapidly expanding field of education. With each revision the authors have attempted to keep pace with the increasing duties and responsibilities of the medical assistant by adding new material, deleting those portions that no longer seemed applicable, and updating all information.

The present volume exceeds 700 pages. An entirely new format has been developed and a slight change made in the title to introduce the contents more precisely. Each chapter begins with an outline and behavioral objectives as an aid to instructors as well as to students. New material has been added on applying for a position, the history of medicine, letter writing, payroll duties, nutrition and diet therapy, microbiology and the need for sterilization, diagnostic laboratory procedures, and assisting in the medical and surgical specialties. Many new illustrations have been included. New appendices include a color atlas of human anatomy, a compilation of frequently encountered combining forms in medical terminology, and the Canadian aspects of medicolegal and insurance matters. An instructor's guide is available to schools and colleges that adopt the book. The authors express their appreciation to Mary Falconer, R.N., for her invaluable assistance in preparing this guide. Both authors were first medical assistants, then educators; both appreciate the value of the kind of assistance offered in the Instructor's Guide.

This book is designed essentially as a teaching aid in training programs for medical assistants. However, many who are employed as doctors' assistants have had no opportunity for formal training in their field; they have learned their duties on the job and have supplemented their education by reading articles in medical journals and studying books on office assisting and office management. This book will serve as a handy reference manual for all assistants in medical offices. In addition to offering suggestions for the most efficient ways to complete routine tasks, the book may provide those already working in the medical field with a new perspective of their responsibilities. Actually, the objectives of the book may be summed up by quoting the first paragraph of the objectives of the American Association of Medical Assistants: "To inspire its members to render honest, loyal, and more efficient service to the profession and to the public which they serve."

The experienced medical assistant who plans to take the national examination for Certified Medical Assistant will find this book useful in reviewing her knowledge in the areas covered by the examination. However, the book has not been sponsored or officially approved by the American Association of Medical Assistants or its Certifying Board.

The authors wish to express their sincere thanks to the American Medical Association, the American Association of Medical Assistants, and to the many individuals with whom they have counseled and from whom they have received guidance and encouragement in the preparation of this book. Special recognition is given to the assistance of W. J. Baumgardner, Aetna Life & Casualty Insurance Company; Dr. Lee Weller Callaway for her chapter on Nutrition and Diet Therapy; Lewis E. Cook, Ritter Company, for assistance with the materials on electrosurgery; Rhoda Finneron, who provided the appendix on Law and Insurance for the Canadian Medical Secretary; Fredrick B. Mears, M.D.: Alan R. Senac; officials of the Union Bank; Isadore Pitesky, M.D., for material he contributed for the chapter on allergies; and the editorial staff of the W. B. Saunders Company.

Appreciation is also due the many supply companies, pharmaceutical firms, professional organizations, and publishers who have shared their wealth of materials and illustrations. Appropriate recognition is given throughout the book.

The countless students and medical assistants with whom the authors have associated over a span of many years in the profession, the doctors for and with whom they have worked, and the authors of various books in allied fields, have all, directly or indirectly, contributed to the knowledge and personal experience contained in this volume. The authors have benefited appreciably from the comments of other instructors who have reviewed previous editions and offered constructive criticism and suggestions. It is the authors' hope that documenting this information will inspire and aid the professional growth of all medical assistants, both present and future.

The authors feel fortunate in having a Foreword to their work by Mr. Horace Cotton, a person whose name is well known to medical assistants and physicians alike for his contributions as a management consultant to the profession and author of many articles in professional journals as well as *Aid for the Doctor's Aide* and *Medical Practice Management.* Mr. Cotton is not one to write the usual stuffy prolegomenon, to use a stuffy term, or to praise when no praise is meant. His sprightly and kind words are especially appreciated since he knows so well the field of which he speaks.

PORTIA M. FREDERICK, CMA — AC
MARY E. KINN, CPS, CMA — A

# CONTENTS

**Section Three**
**THE CLINICAL ASSISTANT**

# Section One

# Being
# a Member
# of a Service
# Profession

# Chapter 1

**BEHAVIORAL OBJECTIVES**

*The medical office assistant should be able to:*

Explore a variety of job possibilities that require knowledge of medical assisting.

List the expected qualifications of a medical office assistant.

Compare the duties of an administrative assistant with those of a clinical assistant.

State the possible avenues for acquiring necessary and approved training.

# A Career as an Office Assistant

There's a career in the medical field tailor-made for the girl with an interest in medicine and in people. It's a career as assistant to a physician.

Though doctors have employed women in their offices for many years, the role of medical assistant has become more than just a job—it is a career. As the qualifications for the office assistant have become more clearly defined, formal training programs have been established to train competent assistants. Medical office assisting has developed into an important allied health profession.

Women have proved that they are particularly suited to medical and health careers. Thousands of girls today become nurses, laboratory and x-ray technicians, physical or occupational therapists, speech pathologists, medical technologists, medical record administrators, or serve in other capacities in the health field. Employment opportunities abound in the health field and are increasing every day because of the growing concern for health protection for every individual in the nation. It is estimated that for every physician there are 12 persons engaged in an allied health career. Presently there is a shortage of adequately trained people to fill these challenging positions.

The advantages of a career in medicine rarely need to be "sold" by enumerating specific benefits. Medicine is of great interest to everyone; it is front-page news. Most Americans are better informed on health and medical subjects than ever before. New discoveries push back the frontiers of medical science so rapidly that a new drug may be obsolete before druggists get it on their shelves. The continuing battle of medical men, researchers, and allied health personnel to defeat illness and prolong life is a never-ending, exciting one.

Helen B. Shaffer, in an Editorial Research Report on Medical Ethics, published in 1972 by Congressional Quarterly, Inc., states:

> Major new developments in the biological and medical sciences call for moral and ethical decisions for which there are few precedents. They include fertilization of human egg cells in the laboratory; determination of certain genetic characteristics, including the sex, of the human embryo; modification of genetic traits by tampering with egg cells; modification of behavior and mood by chemical and neurological means; transplantation of vital organs from one person to another; and prolongation of life.

When Dr. Christiaan N. Barnard of Cape Town, South Africa, performed the first human heart transplantation on December 3, 1967, he became the center of world attention. Although the high mortality rate suffered by early re-

3

cipients of heart transplants was somewhat disillusioning, still it was a major breakthrough, and work is continuing in the development of an artificial heart.

In 1952, before the introduction of the Salk and Sabin polio vaccines, there were 21,300 cases of paralytic polio and 1400 deaths from polio in the United States. In 1969 no person in the United States died of polio. The Salk Institute in California was established on proceeds from the polio vaccine discovered by Dr. Jonas Salk. It is one of the nation's major centers for biologic research.

Exciting new treatments for diabetes, Parkinson's disease, and cancers are emerging. These are but a few of the dramatic medical events which those who travel the medical progress road have witnessed. Medical horizons are constantly changing, each one more promising than the last.

These are the spectacular dramas of medicine. Those who work beside the doctor in his office each day know the satisfaction of less dramatic but no less rewarding experiences. A woman who has worked in a physician's office for more than ten years wrote: "I get a wonderful sense of satisfaction from my work. It's still a thrill to share the joy of the girl who finds she's going to have a baby—or share the victory of the young man over a serious disease. I see quiet bravery every day. We do our best to make people well and cheer them up a little in the process. I know that even the little things I do in the office are worthwhile, and it's a real joy to know you are helping others."

In the medical field the accent is on youth. Many health careers are comparatively young occupations. Manpower and womanpower get top priority in the health field today, and there is no end in sight to the demand.

A girl who trains to be a medical assistant equips herself with a flexible, adaptable career. The skills she acquires she can carry with her all through her life. She can readily find work anywhere in the world that medicine is practiced.

The girl who thinks she would like the career of medical office assistant must realize at the onset that, in medicine, fame is incidental. In a booklet on medical careers entitled *Partners for Health,* published by the National Health Council, it is pointed out that:

"Those whose one end and aim is to get rich quick, to make a big splash, or to take it easy will find no place here. They will have small use for a health career, and the field of health will have even smaller use for them."

## JOB POSSIBILITIES

Opportunities for the girl who trains as a doctor's assistant are extremely varied. She can work as a medical assistant, a medical secretary, a medical or hospital receptionist, a psychiatric aide, or a hospital admitting officer. She may choose to work for a physician in private practice or for several physicians in a clinic. She may work with a general practitioner or with a specialist in one of the many recognized fields of medical specialties, which include surgery, internal medicine, dermatology, obstetrics, pediatrics, psychiatry, radiology, and many others.

There are career opportunities for her in public health work, in hospitals, laboratories, medical schools, research institutions, colleges, or with voluntary health agencies or medical firms of all kinds. There are also opportunities for work with such federal agencies as the Veterans Administration, the United States Health Service, or Armed Forces clinics or hospitals.

Although her training may equip her for work in the fields described above, this book is designed primarily for the girl who wishes to become a medical office assistant and for the girl already employed as a medical office assistant.

In medicine, a new concept of office assistant is emerging. Not many years ago, the administrative duties in a physician's office were relatively simple. This has been rapidly changing, and the medical assistant today requires training in office management, as well as an understanding of clinical procedures. The physician must concentrate his efforts toward caring for the patient and keeping up with new developments in medicine, leaving the business and administrative responsibilities in the hands of a competent office force. Few physicians in private practice attempt to get along without at least one assistant. The great majority have at least two, and many have five or more.

Whether a physician employs only one assistant or a half dozen, one assistant must be in charge of the administrative and business aspects of the office. It is her responsibility to keep up to date on the newest equipment, to purchase supplies, keep records, schedule appointments carefully to conserve the physician's time, and supervise the ever-increasing volume of paper work. Such a position requires training in secretarial, administrative, and medically oriented skills.

While the career of medical office assistant is more challenging than it may have been in years past, it also offers more opportunities for advancement. In the larger medical office, the medical assistant's job will most likely be specialized in either the administrative or clinical responsibilities, but in the "one-girl office" the office assistant will be expected to have some degree of familiarity with all the duties which the job encompasses.

The job turnover among medical assistants is surprisingly low, a fact which may indicate that girls who work in doctors' offices derive a high degree of satisfaction from their work. Many cases have been reported of women who were hired when a physician started practice and remained with him until his retirement.

What kind of earnings can the medical assistant expect? As in any other field of work, salaries vary in different parts of the country. There is also usually some difference between earnings in rural and in urban areas. However, the office assistant generally gets a satisfactory return on her investment in training, experience, and skill. Medical organizations encourage physicians to pay better-than-average salaries to their office assistants, and most medical men have come to realize that a good office assistant is worth a good salary. Many have learned through bitter experience that cheap, untrained help is often the most expensive help in the long run.

## QUALIFICATIONS FOR OFFICE ASSISTANT

**Skills.** Every profession has its nomenclature, and medical terminology must be learned by anyone who expects to work in a physician's office. To qualify for secretarial duties, the medical assistant must be a good typist and have basic skills in English and mathematics. Shorthand is helpful, but in many medical offices today the dictation-transcription machine has become standard equipment. Just as the private secretary needs a basic knowledge of business law, the assistant in a physician's office should be familiar with the law as it affects medical practice.

The clinical assistant must be skilled in certain nursing arts and must have training necessary to do some routine medical tests.

**Personal Assets.** The services performed by a medical assistant are extremely personal. For this reason, her personality can actually affect the health and welfare of the patient. Physicians rank intelligence, dependability, and personality as top qualifications for the ideal office assistant.

The American Medical Association, in a public relations booklet for physicians' assistants entitled *Winning Ways with Patients,* compares the duties of the doctor's assistant with those of the airline stewardess, who greets passengers in a friendly, tactful manner and cares for their needs during flight. The booklet contains this little personality test for the office assistant:

1. Do you like people?
2. Do you enjoy helping people?
3. Are you cheerful?
4. Are you friendly?
5. Are you polite?
6. Do you try to be tactful in every situation?
7. Are you kind and sympathetic toward the doctor's patients?

The key to a good office personality is consideration, human kindness, and sympathy. The good assistant learns to view a situation from the patients' standpoint and to give her attention to their problems, no matter how insignificant they may seem.

A pleasant, friendly disposition is as necessary in the medical office assistant as secretarial or medical skills. She must combine sympathy, friendliness, and graciousness with calm efficiency.

She must be neat, accurate, dependable, and have a good head for details. Because the assistant often must assume charge of the office when the doctor is out, she must not hesitate to accept responsibility. Should an emergency arise, she must be able to meet it with composure. Discretion and good judgment also are important requirements for the girl who works in a doctor's office.

**Public Relations Responsibilities.** Every assistant, even though she may not serve as office receptionist, comes into daily contact with the doctor's patients. For this reason she is of tremendous importance in helping him create either favorable or unfavorable personal public relations. The kind of impression which the assistant makes upon patients often affects their opinions of the doctor himself. An assistant can attract or repel patients by her very personality. She is the front door to the physician's practice — his office hostess and, often, his receptionist.

A public relations manual published by the American Medical Association points up the public relations importance of the medical assistant in these words:

> If you employ an assistant. . ., she is a key person in determining what people think of you and your office. Into her hands you entrust the good will of your patients.
>
> A neat, attractive assistant is "good medicine" for any patient. As your goodwill ambassador she should have a nice personality, combining friendliness, courtesy, graciousness and sympathy. A girl who dislikes or becomes impatient with people should not work in a doctor's office. A sad-faced gal with a mournful mien, a bored miss with a perpetual sneer, or a dragon who strikes terror into the hearts of

patients is no asset to a physician. His assistant should be cheerful, tactful and efficient, prepared to meet any emergency with cool-headed composure.

The medical assistant is ladylike. This is evidenced in her good grooming, proper dress (be it a uniform or appropriate street clothes), respect for the feelings of others, and deportment with both her employer and his patients. The physician may address his assistant by her first name, but she does not reply in kind. Patients are inclined to look with suspicion on any such informality in the professional office.

She will be very cautious, too, about any laughter or frivolity with other members of the office staff in situations where the cause of the laughter is not entirely evident to waiting patients. A person who is not well, or who has any obvious personal defect, could quite easily get the idea that the laughter is about him. The medical assistant will observe this caution out of respect for the patients.

## DUTIES OF THE OFFICE ASSISTANT

The duties of the office assistant will vary in every medical office, since the schedule must be geared to the working habits and type of practice of the individual physician. In a one-girl office she may divide her time between administrative and clinical duties. In an office where a nurse also is employed, her duties of a clinical nature may be simpler or may be limited to those periods when the nurse is not on duty.

**Administrative Duties.**   The administrative duties of the medical office assistant will be similar to those of any responsible secretary to a top executive, but will have specific medical aspects. She will answer telephones, schedule appointments, interview new patients to complete a registration form, screen non-patient visitors and salesmen requesting to see the doctor, explain the doctor's fees to patients, open and sort mail, answer routine correspondence, pull medical charts for scheduled appointments and file reports and correspondence in patients' charts. She may make arrangements for patient admission to a hospital and instruct the patient regarding admission.

She will make financial arrangements with patients, complete insurance claim forms, maintain the financial records and files, prepare and mail statements, prepare checks for doctor's signature, maintain a file of paid and unpaid invoices, prepare and maintain employees' payroll records or submit payroll information to an outside accountant.

Sometimes she serves as an informal editorial secretary to the doctor, helping him in the preparation of manuscripts or speeches or clipping professional journals and assisting him with the maintenance of his personal medical library (see Chapter 12).

The secretary-assistant in the professional office probably will assume more responsibilities than other secretaries in the business world, since the busy doctor depends upon her to manage his everyday affairs and also requires her assistance with certain professional duties as well.

**Clinical Duties.**   The clinical duties of the medical office assistant will also vary. Generally speaking, she helps patients prepare for examinations and other office procedures, stands by to assist the doctor when he requests her to do so, cleans and sterilizes instruments and equipment, and keeps the supply cabinets well-stocked. She may collect specimens from patients and either send them to a laboratory or perform certain diagnostic tests for which she has been adequately trained. She may assist with EKGs and x-rays, take and record the patient's temperature, pulse, and respiration, prepare treatment trays, and assist with minor surgery. She may be called upon to administer emergency first aid.

**Task Analysis.** In 1971 the Division of Vocational Education of the University of California at Los Angeles, under a grant from the U.S. Department of Health, Education, and Welfare, concluded a three-year research and demonstration project instituted to develop curricula and instructional materials in the allied health occupations. The medical office assistant occupation was included in this study. The task inventory developed for this project encompassed 122 tasks related to clerical, secretarial, office management and business functions, and 108 tasks classified as clinical and technical tasks. The task inventory was arranged in four major groupings with 22 subclassifications:

1. Clerical, Secretarial, and Management
    (a) Reception of Patients and Visitors
    (b) Public Relations
    (c) Secretarial
    (d) Scheduling Patients
    (e) Medical Records
    (f) Office Management and Housekeeping
2. Business Office
    (a) Billing and Bookkeeping
    (b) Cashiering and Banking
    (c) Credits and Collection
    (d) Payment of Vendors' Bills
    (e) Payroll
3. Diagnostic Tests and Procedures
    (a) Specimens: Obtaining and Handling
    (b) Urinalysis
    (c) Hematology
    (d) Microbiology, Pathology, and Sterilization
    (e) Electrocardiograms
    (f) X-ray Procedures
4. Examination and Treatment Room Procedures
    (a) Preparation of Patient and Assistance to Doctor
    (b) Injections
    (c) Physical Therapy
    (d) First Aid and Emergency
    (e) Specialty Practice Procedures

The 210 respondents whose questionnaires were used reported 45 different occupational titles. These 45 titles were consolidated into five categories:

> Registered Nurse – RN
> Licensed Professional or Vocational Nurse – LPN
> Medical Office Assistant (technical) – MOA-T
> Medical Office Assistant (generalist) – MOA-G
> Administrative and Clerical – ADM-CL

With the exception of hematology, x-ray and physical therapy, all of the 22 subclassifications of duties were performed by more than 25 per cent of the MOA-G group, the audience for which this text is designed.

## TRAINING

**Getting Started.**   How does a girl who wants to become a medical office assistant train for the job? At one time, about one-fourth of the women hired by physicians were registered nurses, about one-fourth had taken business training, and a small percentage were laboratory or x-ray technicians. The majority were girls with no special training who learned their duties in an actual office apprenticeship.

There are few instances today in which an untrained girl can step into a job as a physician's office assistant and expect on-the-job training by the doctor. *Horizons Unlimited,* a handbook published by the American Medical Association in 1966, states:

> The minimum education requirement for medical assistants is four years of high school, with studies emphasizing secretarial training, English and the biological sciences. In actual practice, however, many medical assistants have qualified for their positions by completing from one to four years of college. Physicians today generally prefer to hire individuals having some college or special training, or business experience.

Many two-year colleges today are offering vocational courses for medical assistants, leading to the Associate of Arts or Associate in Science degree. These schools are combining medical secretarial training with special courses in office assisting and basic laboratory skills. Medical assistants already employed in the field were among the first to recognize the need for more trained personnel for doctors' offices. Through chapters of the American Association of Medical Assistants, aided by medical societies, they have been instrumental in rapidly accelerating the development of such training programs. Courses include medical terminology, accounting practices, medical shorthand, typing and transcription, business English, anatomy, biology, psychology, human relations, nutrition, first aid, medical laboratory procedures, and elementary nursing arts. Many of the college courses include in-service training in the offices of local physicians. Instructors for these courses have been drawn from the ranks of those with practical experience in the field.

**Continuing Education Through A.A.M.A.**   The medical assistant on the job must continue her education, just as her employer does. For the assistant this can best be done through membership and participation in her local, state, and national medical assistants' groups.

Although random organizations of medical assistants have been in existence since the 1930s, it was not until the founding of the American Association of Medical Assistants in 1956 that these groups became a real force in the education of the medical office assistant.

At regular meetings, medical assistants' groups hear speakers on a variety of educational topics related to medicine and their work in the doctor's office. Many times these speakers are physicians. Through bulletins, conventions, symposia, workshops, and other media, the members of medical assistants' groups exchange ideas on more efficient ways to perform office responsibilities and keep abreast of the nonscientific subjects of interest to their employers.

Physician advisers to these groups, as well as the American Medical Association, have commended their aims, which are to inspire the assistant to render more loyal, efficient service to the medical profession and to educate their members. The American Medical Association, in encouraging such groups to continue their educational programs, said:

"The medical assistant is not only the doctor's ally in bringing the people of the community better medical care, but is tremendously important in the over-all medical public relations picture."

Every chapter of the American Association of Medical Assistants has an advisory board of physicians. Several past presidents of the American Medical Association have served as advisers to the national group. At its clinical meeting in November, 1962, the A.M.A. House of Delegates passed the following resolution:

*Whereas,* The American Association of Medical Assistants has as its objectives basically the same purposes as the American Medical Association; and

*Whereas,* The American Association of Medical Assistants has, in its short span of six years' growth, rendered inestimable services not only to the people of America but also to the medical profession; and

*Whereas,* The potential for growth and service of the American Association of Medical Assistants is recognized by the American Medical Association; therefore be it

*Resolved,* That the American Medical Association express to the American Association of Medical Assistants its sincere appreciation for the dedicated and unselfish assistance and work in the combined goal of the two organizations in continually striving to improve the character of medical standards; and be it further

*Resolved,* That the American Medical Association wholeheartedly endorse the program and functions of the American Association of Medical Assistants and encourage every physician who has in his employ or under his supervision medical assistants who are eligible for membership in the American Association of Medical Assistants to urge all these assistants not only to join the American Association of Medical Assistants but to actively participate in their programs.

**Importance of Professional Organization.** In 1959 the American Association of Medical Assistants established an executive office in Chicago, Illinois, with only one employee. Since that time the activities and responsibilities of this professional organization of medical assistants have continued to expand year after year. In only 15 years the headquarters office has thrice outgrown its space, and the number of employees increased to eight and then to ten individuals. Its bimonthly publication, *The Professional Medical Assistant,* is one that the members can be proud to receive. The PMA keeps the members abreast of current developments in medical office practices, offers useful hints for increasing the assistant's efficiency and includes original articles by experts in the fields of health insurance, medical law, clinical procedures, and a wide range of activities of interest to the medical assistant. At present, the American Association of Medical Assistants has over 15,000 members, with chapters in 46 states and the District of Columbia. In the fall of each year, the national organization holds a convention where members can participate in workshops, learn of educational advances in the field, hear renowned speakers on medical and management problems, and perhaps most importantly of all, develop personal friendships with medical assistants throughout the nation.

In 1962, after a three-year study, the A.A.M.A. established a Certifying Board to encourage and assist in the postgraduate education of the medical assistant. An annual examination is offered on the fourth Friday in June, at various test centers throughout the United States. Those who meet the qualifications for testing, and who are successful in passing the examination, are awarded a certificate and recognition as a Certified Medical Assistant (C.M.A.). The examination is offered in two categories, Administrative and Clinical, and the candidate for certification may be certified in the area in which her special interest lies; a number have been successful in obtaining both certificates. The examination is not restricted to members of A.A.M.A.

While the A.A.M.A. encourages its members to enroll in formal courses of study for the examination and, through its education committee, assists schools in setting up such courses, it also furnishes a study outline for the individual medical assistant to use in guiding her own study program.

To help girls who wish to train for a career as a medical assistant, the A.A.M.A. maintains a scholarship loan program, which was established in honor of Miss Maxine Williams, the Association's first president. The scholarship program is supported entirely by contributions. High school graduates who indicate an interest in becoming a certified medical assistant, and who are of good moral character and are willing to repay the loan, are eligible to apply for this assistance.

Other association plans include guided study programs, and specialty certification.

The American Medical Association Council on Medical Education, in collaboration with A.A.M.A., established the essentials of an approved educational program for medical assistants. Those schools with medical assisting training courses who wish to apply for accreditation by the A.M.A. may request an application from

Department of Allied Medical
Professions and Services
Division of Medical Education
American Medical Association
535 North Dearborn Street
Chicago, Illinois 60610

Certification and career inquiries should be directed to

American Association of Medical Assistants
One East Wacker Drive, Suite 1510
Chicago, Illinois 60601

Medical assisting has come a long way since the first edition of this book and the organizational meeting of A.A.M.A., both of which occurred in the year 1956.

## REWARDS OF A HEALTH CAREER

There are rewards above and beyond those of salary and job security for the office assistant. There is the stimulation of growing with the job, and there is a justifiable pride and humility which result from participation in the professional partnership. The role of assistant is a demanding but rewarding one. It is stated in *Partners for Health* that:

> Compared job for job with like occupations in other fields, health occupations are generally above average so far as surroundings and working conditions are concerned. But as far as time and energy, alertness and dependability, patience and determination, skill and accuracy, responsibility and integrity, courage and character are concerned—for all of these qualities, there is no denying that health careers make demands beyond the call of duty.
>
> Choosing a health career is a big decision because working for health is more than just a job. It is a point of view, a way of looking at life—your own life and the lives of the people you see and serve and work with every day.

Anyone who decides to become a medical office assistant makes that important decision. It's one which few women ever regret having made—and a decision which thousands will make in the future as the career of medical office assistant is more widely publicized and its rewards cited.

## MEMBERS OF THE TEAM

The girl who seeks employment in a medical office must be prepared to function as a member of a team. A solo practitioner may hire only one assistant, the "Girl Friday," in which case the team will be only the assistant and the doctor. The trend, however, is toward a multiple number of employees, even in those offices where there is only one physician. There is a strong possibility, too, that the assistant will be employed in a group practice or clinic where there are many members of the team.

The medical office assistant needs some acquaintance with the scope of duties and the training required of other paramedical employees. These may include a nurse, an x-ray technologist, inhalation therapist, EKG technician, EEG technician, medical transcriber, insurance clerk, bookkeeper, and office manager, as well as others.

A licensed practical nurse or, in some states, *licensed vocational nurse*, is prepared to work in almost all fields of nursing. She works under the direct supervision of the physician or a registered nurse. Since the LPN/LVN is licensed, she legally may be capable of performing some clinical duties in the doctor's office that may not be performed by the unlicensed medical assistant. The *registered nurse* (associate degree or baccalaureate degree) is more likely to be found in the hospital situation rather than a physician's office.

The medical profession is making more and more use of x-rays and other sources of radioactive energy. Therefore, the *radiologic technologist* may be found in the physician's office. The x-ray technologist works under the direct supervision of the physician in taking the films that are required for radiographic examination of disease and injury. The technologist has usually completed at least 24 months of specialized education and experience in a hospital, followed by successful completion of the certifying examination conducted by the American Registry of Radiologic Technologists.

Medical Technologists are allied health professionals, and are often referred to as the detectives of the health care team. Usually they work in a medical laboratory, helping to determine the nature and causes of disease, but group practices often employ an MT on the team. With the help of microscopes and precision instruments they examine and analyze samples of tissues and body fluids to assist in the diagnosis of disease. MT's bring important skills and knowledge of chemistry, physics, and biology to the health care team.

*Inhalation therapy* is an allied health specialty in the treatment, management, control, and care of patients with difficulties and abnormalities associated with the process of breathing. It is used primarily in the treatment of heart and lung ailments, such as cardiac failure, asthma, pulmonary edema, emphysema, cerebral thrombosis, hemorrhaging, and shock. The therapist must be fully capable, under medical supervision, of operating inhalation therapy equipment, and administering to patients the therapeutic and diagnostic procedures of inhalation therapy.

The electrocardiograph is an instrument which records a patient's heart action. An *EKG technician* is employed in the offices of many physicians, especially cardiologists and internists. The technician prepares the patient and makes the recording of the patient's heart action. The tracings are then "read" and interpreted by the physician.

The electroencephalograph is an instrument which records brain waves. The *EEG technician* might be employed in the office of a neurologist.

A *medical transcriber* may be employed by a physician who dictates a great deal of correspondence, reports, records, and so forth. The transcriber has a thorough knowledge of medical terminology, is a good typist, and must be familiar with the use of dictating equipment.

Most multiple-doctor practices will employ someone specialized in processing insurance claim forms. The *insurance clerk* may have had on-the-job training or she may have attended special classes to familiarize herself with local insurance plans. She needs an understanding of medical diagnoses and procedures, as well as the numerous insurance plans and requirements.

Larger practices will probably employ a full-time *bookkeeper* with advanced training and experience in accounting practices.

In the one-doctor, one-assistant office, delegation of duties and responsibilities goes hand in hand. When there is more than one employee there usually must be one individual designated as *office manager,* on whom final responsibility must fall for the smooth operation of the office. When there are many employees, the managerial responsibility becomes greater, and someone specially trained in management techniques may be needed for this position.

Large or small, the medical facility must function as a unit with each person assuming full responsibility for her own duties, but with an awareness that the cooperation of every member of the team is vital to the best care of the patient.

## REFERENCES

American Medical Association, *Winning Ways with Patients,* Chicago, American Medical Association, 1966

DiCicco, O., and B. S. Earl, *Occupational Analysis, Medical Office Assistant,* University of California, Los Angeles, Division of Vocational Education, Allied Health Professions Project, December 1971

National Health Council, *Partners for Health*

*New York Times Encyclopedic Almanac,* 1971, New York Times

Shaffer, H. B., *Medical Ethics: Editorial Research Reports on Medical Issues,* Washington, D.C., Congressional Quarterly, Inc., 1972

# Chapter 2

**BEHAVIORAL OBJECTIVES**

*The medical office assistant should be able to:*

Plan the appropriate strategy for applying for a job as a medical office assistant.

Prepare an effective personal data sheet and letter requesting an interview.

Assist her employer in screening applicants for a job.

Assist her employer in evaluating a new employee.

# Applying For a Job

## THE MEDICAL ASSISTANT AS AN APPLICANT

After the medical office assistant has been trained for employment in a doctor's office, the next step is to match her capabilities with the requirements of a physician who is seeking an employee. It may be the assistant's first job, she may be returning to the field after an absence of several years, or an employed assistant may be planning to change employers. The essential steps in applying for a job will be similar in all of these situations:

Step One:     Preparation for Job Hunting
Step Two:     Locating Prospective Employers
Step Three:   The Job Interview

**Looking for a Job?**   Prepare yourself for job hunting by first taking a personal inventory:

What type of work do you really want?
Do you prefer clinical or administrative duty?
Do you prefer to work in a solo practice or in a large medical group?
Do you prefer general practice or a specialty?
How important to you are salary, hours, and location?

You may not get exactly what you want, and if you have very definite answers to all of these questions, you may be too inflexible to find suitable employment in medical assisting. On the other hand, if you are absolutely certain of something that would make you unhappy, that is a different matter. Remember, though, that your attitude can also alert an interviewer to whether you are favorably motivated, or to the likelihood that you are just looking for a paycheck.

**Preparation for Job Hunting.**   The most important thing you can do to prepare yourself for an interview is to make a personal data sheet. It can be innovative in style (Figs. 2–1 and 2–2), but the data sheet must be typewritten, preferably on one sheet of paper, and as attractively as possible. There must be absolutely no errors or misspelled words. The examples shown contain the basic information a prospective employer will need to know.

**15**

PERSONAL DATA SHEET

Personal

Name:                                          Date of Birth:
Address:                                       Birthplace:
                                               Nationality:
Telephone:                                     Height:
Age:                                           Weight:
Marital Status:                                Physical Condition:

Education

College:

High School:

Awards

Extracurricular Activities

College:

High School:

Other:

Skills and Abilities

(List those that would be useful to the kind of employment you are seeking)

Work Experience

References

(List 3 to 5 — may include former employers, teachers, associates on former jobs, local business owners, or professional persons; do not use names of relatives)

**Figure 2–1**

PERSONAL RESUMÉ

NAME:                                                    DATE:

ADDRESS AND TELEPHONE:

## PERSONAL DATA

Age:                                    Height:
Date of Birth:                          Weight:
Birthplace:                             Physical Condition:
Marital Status:                         Social Security No.:

## EDUCATION

College:

High School:

Major Courses:

Extracurricular Activities:

Skills:

## EXPERIENCE

(List chronologically, latest first. Include name and address of employer, name of immediate superior, telephone number, position held, general scope of duties, beginning and ending dates of employment. Include part-time and volunteer services)

## REFERENCES

Furnished upon request.

**Figure 2-2**

**Locating Prospective Employers.** If you are a student in an accredited school, your instructor or the school may be able to give you names of prospective employers. Other good sources of job leads are the local medical society, other medical office assistants, and branches of the United States Employment Service and state-operated employment offices. You may also wish to check the classified advertisements in your local newspaper, or place your name with an employment agency. Private employment agencies generally charge a fee equivalent to two to four weeks' salary to successful applicants.

**Requesting an Interview.** You may either telephone an employer asking for an interview, or write a letter requesting an interview (Fig. 2–3). Send your personal data sheet along with the letter. Each interviewer is to be given a copy of the data sheet. This should be either an original or a good quality copy. Do not use carbon copies or poor photocopies. Never ask the interviewer to return the copy of your data sheet.

**Day of the Interview.** Appearance is extremely important, whether you are wearing street clothes or a uniform. Your hair should be neat, and worn in a professional looking style. Makeup should be carefully applied and in good taste. Do not go to an interview with bare legs or wearing an extreme shoe or dress style. Carry a modest purse that is not bulging with unnecessary items. Take a critical look at yourself in the mirror before leaving home. An employer may attach importance to some careless detail. Your appearance at the time of the interview is his only way of judging how you will look as an employee.

*Arrive promptly* for the interview. Under no circumstances should you be even so much as a minute late and then have to make a weak excuse. *Go alone.* You may want moral support, but you will be more relaxed if there is no one waiting for you. *Enter the office confidently,* without appearing rushed. Introduce yourself to the receptionist, then thank her when she asks you to be seated. If you must wait, relax but maintain a ladylike posture. *Do not smoke or chew gum!*

When you are ushered into the interviewer's room, wait to be seated until you are invited to do so. Let the interviewer lead the conversation. Be prepared to answer such questions as "Tell me about yourself," and "Why do you want to work here?" Remember, the interviewer will be observing your manners, poise, speech, alertness, and ability to give direct answers. Your sense of humor may be

At the suggestion of Miss _____, my medical assisting instructor at _____ College, I am writing to inquire whether you have an opening for a medical assistant on your staff.

In a few weeks I will be graduating with an A.S. Degree and a certificate in medical assisting. As you will see from the enclosed resumé, my training has included both the administrative and the clinical skills necessary for employment in a physician's office. If you will require a replacement or addition to your staff in the near future, may I be considered as an applicant for this job?

Please call me at 123-4567 and suggest a time when I may come to your office for an interview.

Sincerely yours,

**Figure 2–3** Letter Requesting an Interview.

tested as well, and questions may be directed to you that will test your common sense and frankness. You can promote yourself honestly and graciously by showing that you enjoy others, are willing to work and accept responsibility, and that you have an open mind about the job and are willing to learn.

At the end of the interview, if the interviewer has not mentioned hours and salary, you may properly inquire at this time. If you are not really interested in the job, do not bother to ask, but if the job sounds satisfactory and is one that you would like to accept, you may then ask if the interviewer wishes to discuss the salary. This should be enough of a lead, since it was probably an oversight on the interviewer's part. If the interviewer seems reluctant to discuss it, though, do not press the issue since he may not be interested in your qualifications and does not wish to pursue the interview further.

If you have been given a tour of the office, you may make some pleasant observations and comments, but do not be falsely overenthusiastic. When you are introduced to the staff be gracious and friendly. Try to remember their names so that you can thank them later. Show enthusiasm, but do not overdo it because it may appear to others that you are "putting on an act."

**Closing the Interview.**   The interviewer will usually take the initiative in closing the interview. He may slide back his chair and ask if you have further questions about the job. Do not show disappointment if the job is not offered to you at the time of the interview. The interviewer may have other applicants to see, or he may wish to check your references before making a commitment. Thank him for the interview as you leave. Remember, too, to thank the receptionist and say a friendly goodbye.

**Follow-up Activities.**   A brief, well-worded letter of thanks sent to the interviewer immediately after the interview makes a good impression. After a few days you may call the office and ask if the position has been filled, and tell them you are interested because you enjoyed your interview and the office. If the job is still open, and if it is one you really want, then inquire again in a few days. Always be brief, and thank the person with whom you speak. Even if you do not get the job, you should never feel that an interview is a waste of time. You learn from each experience, and with experience you are better able to promote your qualifications in future interviews.

**Survey of Desirable Qualities.**   An extensive survey* conducted by several college students in January, 1972, reported maturity, compatibility, and personality as highly rated qualities. Ambition and initiative were also mentioned by all employers. This survey found the following qualities to be the ones most widely looked for by employers:

1. Appearance.
2. Common sense.
3. Ability to think.
4. Ability to take criticism.
5. Interest in job (and company).
6. Pleasing personality.

---

*Qualities of the Industrial Office Worker, National Business Education Association, November 1972, Volume 27, No. 2.

Most surveys have shown that many people fail to get or keep jobs because of personality problems. Technical skills are usually considered less important than the ability to work amicably with others.

Also listed here are some "pet peeves" of employers. Read them carefully so that you will not be guilty of similar actions:

1. Lack of eye contact during interview.
2. Came on too strong.
3. Talked of salary and hours immediately.
4. Wiggled in chair and fidgeted with hands.
5. Had to dig too hard for information.
6. Used poor grammar or too much slang.
7. Was chewing gum.
8. Too much makeup and perfume.
9. Was late.
10. Too much chatter, tried too hard to explain.
11. Was too aggressive or too blasé.
12. Answers were unclear, tried to hide something.
13. No enthusiasm.
14. Poor data sheet.
15. Poor grooming, showed lack of respect for interview.

## THE MEDICAL ASSISTANT AS AN INTERVIEWER

**Looking for a Medical Assistant?**  Many times a physician will ask his experienced medical assistant to aid in finding someone to fill a job opening to either increase the staff or to replace someone who is retiring or moving away. The assistant who is given this responsibility must use great care and judgment, and remain objective in her search for a prospective employee. If an applicant for the position is a friend or former classmate, she must still meet the qualifications set by office needs. The individual you recommend to the doctor may be working with you and the other members of the staff for a long while.

**Preliminary Steps.**  First, ask the doctor to state (a) what personal qualifications the applicant should have, (b) what her duties will be, (c) what salary he is willing to pay, and (d) how soon he expects the job to start. Next, add your own suggestions to the list. Then, set forth these requirements in an outline to guide you in selecting prospective applicants. Here are some suggested guidelines:

1. What age range would blend best with present office personnel?

2. Is the applicant's appearance satisfactory? Is weight an important consideration? Is personal grooming up to expectations?

3. Work experience: Has she had previous employment? What were her duties on her last job? In what skills is she proficient? How long was she on her last job? Did she enjoy her work? Does she accept and enjoy responsibility?

4. Why did she leave her last job? The manner in which she describes her last employer and the office staff may provide a clue to her general attitude or disposition.

5. Educational background: What has been her formal education? Is she a

Certified Medical Assistant? If not, is she planning to take the certifying examination? Does she attend medical assisting workshops? Is she a member of the local chapter of the A.A.M.A.? An assistant who thinks she knows all there is to running an office may be less satisfactory than one who is inexperienced but willing to learn.

6. What are her family responsibilities? Is she married or single? If she has young children, has she made adequate child care arrangements?

7. Check the applicant's references. Can she give the names of responsible persons? References from close friends or neighbors are virtually useless. Has she provided full name, title, address, and telephone number so that you can easily check with these individuals?

**Arranging the Personal Interview.**   If the applicant sent a letter asking for an interview, you probably noted whether the letter was correctly typed, included the essential information, and enclosed a personal data sheet. You cannot be certain that the applicant personally prepared the letter and data sheet; ask her at the time of the interview. Forget the applicant who sends a letter handwritten with pencil!

If the applicant telephoned for an interview appointment, then you had the opportunity to hear her telephone voice. If her telephone voice is poor, you may not wish to consider her further.

Set a time for the personal interview when you most likely will be able to give the applicant your undivided attention. However, the applicant should have an opportunity to see your office when there is a fairly normal amount of activity. The prospective employee who is interviewed in a peaceful, quiet office on the doctor's day out may have a rude awakening when she appears for work on a normal day.

**The Day of the Interview.**   You may have an application form you wish completed. This could serve as a check of the applicant's penmanship and neatness, as well as of her memory. She should be meticulous about following instructions and filling in *all* the blanks. As you speak with the applicant, make a mental note of these observations: Does she converse easily? Is she a good listener? Is she free of annoying mannerisms? Does she have a ready smile? Is she interested enough to ask, as well as to answer questions? Does she appear interested in the office and the doctor's specialty?

An interview should not be a one-way flow of information from applicant to interviewer. If the applicant appears to be one who will receive serious consideration, you have the responsibility of telling her what will be expected of her in the way of duties; office policies regarding appearance, working hours, overtime, time off, and vacations; what initial salary is offered, any fringe benefits, and the office policy on increases. Oftentimes the interviewer fails to mention these items, and the applicant may be too timid to inquire.

**Follow-up Activities.**   When the interview is over, take a few moments to immediately rate the applicant on your check list. Jot down some notes to refresh your memory when you refer this applicant to the doctor for the final interview. Do not trust to memory, especially if several applicants will be interviewed. At the top of the following page is a suggested checklist which may be modified to suit your own circumstances.

| Name _____ | | Date _____ | | Time _____ | |
| | Superior | Above Average | Average | Poor | Remarks |
| Appearance and grooming | | | | | |
| General health | | | | | |
| Voice and diction | | | | | |
| Mannerisms | | | | | |
| Poise | | | | | |
| Friendliness | | | | | |
| Interest in work | | | | | |
| Did applicant ask questions? | | | | | |
| Overall impression | | | | | |

If your employer is a member of a credit bureau, it may be advisable to check the applicant's credit rating, especially if she will be expected to handle the office finances. It can be safely assumed that one who is unable to handle her own financial affairs will be a poor risk in handling office finances. The ability to handle one's financial affairs may also be considered a mark of maturity.

If you had no telephone contact with the applicant, find a reason to call her on the telephone. You might ask a question about her data sheet or application form; you may call to say you are still interviewing and wondered if she were still available; or you may be completely candid and say you wanted to hear her telephone voice.

**Checking References.**   It is always advisable to carefully check all references, and follow through on any leads for information. Sometimes certain names have been omitted, and this could be important. It is best to use the telephone in checking references, because people are sometimes less than candid in a letter; furthermore, letter writing is time-consuming and you may not get a reply. Prepare a check list before you place the call, and then when you talk with the person called be sure to "listen between the lines." Note the tone of the replies to your questions. Here are some questions you might ask in your inquiry:

Applicant's name _____

**Name of Reference Called** _____ **Telephone No.** _____

1. When did _____ work for you? How long?
2. What were her duties? Did she seem to enjoy the work?
3. Why did she leave? (listen carefully)
4. Would you rehire her under the right circumstances?
5. Was she frequently absent or late?
6. Was she in good health?
7. Did she assume responsibility well?
8. How was her rapport with other staff members?
9. Does the previous employer have any suggestions or advice about hiring this person?

Do not recommend an applicant to the doctor for his final approval and interview until you have completed your share of the investigation and have prepared a report for him. This preliminary screening may save an embarrassment for the doctor and for you as well. It may also prevent having to start the process all over again within a few months.

**The Other Applicants.**    When a decision has been reached to hire someone, remember to notify others who have applied. They may have hesitated to accept other interviews in hope of hearing from you. It is unfair to keep individuals who are seeking employment "on the string." Good etiquette requires that you drop them a note or call by telephone, and say the position is filled. Thank the individual for applying, and say that you will keep her application on file.

**Evaluating the New Employee.**    A new employee should be given a 60- to 90-day probationary period. A definite date for a performance review at the end of this period should be set at the time of employment. This review should not be squeezed in between patient visits, or be given a token few minutes at the end of a day. There should be ample time to relax and talk. At this time the new employee is told how well she has met expectations and whether there are any deficiencies in her work. She should be given the opportunity to ask questions. Sometimes an employee does not perform as expected because she was never told what she was supposed to do.

If, at the time of the performance review, her work has not been satisfactory and there is little hope that she will work out, her employment should be terminated then and there. In all fairness, an individual should be told why the employment is ended, and not be given weak excuses or untruths that do not give her the opportunity to correct her deficiencies. Many times an employee never knows the true reason for termination, and does not know whether the employer can be used as a future job reference.

Although 60 to 90 days does not allow time to fully train an individual for a specific office, it is fair to assume that her potential for being a satisfactory employee can be judged at this time. Now is the time to talk out any problems and make suggestions for improvement. The assistant who is doing fine should be told so, then a raise and a welcome to the staff will do wonders for her and the office. It is encouraging to any employee, but especially so for the new employee, to hear "You are doing great and we are glad to have you with us."

# Chapter 3

**BEHAVIORAL OBJECTIVES**

*The medical office assistant should be able to:*

Identify the contributions to medicine
    made by important historical
    figures.

Modern medicine reflects its history in the names given to anatomy, physiology, medications, diagnoses, instruments, and so on. The latest medical discoveries often have names drawn from the ancients. It is impossible to live in the world of medicine and to talk its language without being constantly touched by this fascinating past. Medicine has a rich cultural heritage to draw upon, one filled with hardships and disappointments that were pushed aside so that determined men and women could pursue their dreams and goals.

It may seem strange for modern medicine to borrow so liberally from ancient mythology, and to use so actively the classical languages that most men abandoned centuries ago. Yet today's medicine uses words whose origins stem from the romance and fantasy of this long "dead" world. Anatomy, especially,

24

# A Brief History of Medicine

seems to reach back to the dawn of history and, although some terms are today erroneous when translated literally because the ancients did not correctly understand body functions, many early anatomical terms have reached modern times almost unchanged.

## MEDICINE AND MYTHOLOGY

Greek and Roman mythology has contributed a major portion of our medical terms, but we have also borrowed liberally from Arabic, Anglo-Saxon, and German sources, with a heavy dash of the Bible added. Here are a few of the many examples using this classical past: the anatomical name for the first cervical vertebra upon which the head rests is aptly named Atlas, the famous Greek Titan, who, according to mythology, was condemned by Zeus to bear the heavens on his shoulders. The tendon of Achilles reminds us of the story of the youth whose mother held him by the heel and dipped him into the river Styx to make him invulnerable. This particular tendon was not immersed and later a mortal wound was inflicted in Achilles' heel. The dubious honors given in medicine to Venus, the Roman Goddess of Love, are paid to her not so much as the goddess of love but of lust. She has a portion of the female anatomy, the mons veneris, dedicated to her memory. She is also remembered, and again doubtfully honored, by having venereal diseases named after her. Aphrodite, the Greek Goddess of Love and Beauty, gave her name to the sex-exciting drugs known as aphrodisiacs.

Aesculapius, the son of Apollo, was revered as the God of Medicine. His daughters were Hygeia, Goddess of Health, and Panacea, Goddess of All Heal and Restorer of Health. These two names are prominent in our language today. The early Greeks followed the teachings of Aesculapius and built many temples in his honor.

## MEN OF MEDICINE

There is evidence that from 5000 to 2000 B.C. drugs, surgery, and other treatments were used by the Babylonians and Assyrians. The rules of health which Moses incorporated into the Hebrew religion in order to help his people are evident. Moses (c. 1250 B.C.) was the first advocate of preventive medicine. It has been said that he was also the first "public health officer." Moses knew that some animal diseases may be passed on to man and that contamination may

**25**

linger on unclean dishes. Thus, it became a religious law that no one was permitted to eat animals that were not freshly slaughtered or to eat or drink from dirty dishes, lest they become defiled and lose their souls.

Hippocrates (460–377 B.C.) is the most famous of the ancient Greek physicians and is known as the "Father of Medicine." He did much to separate medicine from mysticism and gave it the scientific basis of today. He is best remembered for the "Hippocratic Oath," which was administered to ancient physicians and is still used after more than 2000 years. Hippocrates' astute clinical descriptions of diseases and his voluminous writings on epidemics, fevers, epilepsy, fractures, and instruments were studied for centuries. He believed that the body tends to heal itself and it is the physician's responsibility to help nature.

There were many Greek physicians who practiced, studied, and taught in Rome in the time after Hippocrates. Rome had few physicians of her own since most were Greco-Roman, as was Galen (131–201 A.D.), who came to Rome in 162 A.D. and was known as the "Prince of Physicians." Galen is said to have written five hundred treatises on medicine. He was also appointed physician to the Emperor Marcus Aurelius. He wrote an excellent summary of anatomy as it was known at that time, and is considered to be the father of experimental physiology. Galen had profound influence on medicine and his works were recognized as authoritative until the 16th century, when Andreas Vesalius (1514–1564) corrected some of Galen's errors.

Vesalius was a Belgian anatomist. He is known as the *Father of Modern Anatomy*, and at the age of 29 he published his great *De Corporis Humani Fabrica*. He served as professor of anatomy and court physician to Phillip II of Spain. While in Spain he performed a post-mortem examination on a Spanish nobleman who was not quite dead. To atone for this error, he went on a pilgrimage to the Holy Land but died on the return journey. Vesalius introduced many new anatomical terms but, despite his great contributions to the science of anatomy, his name does not appear with any important anatomical structures. A student of Vesalius', Gabriele Fallopius, gave his name to the oviducts known as the fallopian tubes. He also gave the vagina and the placenta their present names. He was an accurate and detailed dissector and described and named many parts of the anatomy.

In 1628 William Harvey (1578–1657) made his great pronouncement on the circulation of the blood. The work of this English physician was not fully recognized until 1827, when the full importance of his work was substantiated. Harvey's writings were recognized in Germany before the English permitted their publication at home. Modern England now considers Harvey to be its "medical Shakespeare."

Great advances in medicine were somewhat stilled for a century or so, but the unseen world of microorganisms was opened as Anton van Leeuwenhoek (1632–1723) pursued his hobby of grinding lenses. Leeuwenhoek was a Dutch draper and custodian of the city hall of Leyden and, although an amateur scientist, his work was not conducted according to the strictest of scientific plans. His writings on his discoveries and theories were rambling and not accepted by the learned men of his time, nor was he very willing to share the viewing of his "tiny little beasties," as he called the microorganisms. Leeuwenhoek was considered to be rather temperamental and eccentric. In grinding lenses, Leeuwenhoek discovered how to make use of a simple biconvex lens to magnify the minute world of organisms and structures never seen before. In 1677 he described his findings to the Royal Society in London, but there was considerable variation in acceptance of his report.

A few years after Leeuwenhoek's death, a famous English surgeon and anatomist, John Hunter (1728–1793), was born. Hunter has been given the title of *Founder of Scientific Surgery* because his surgical procedures were based on sound pathological reasons. He was the first to classify teeth in a scientific manner. In 1778 he introduced artificial feeding by means of a flexible tube passed into the stomach. His description of the syphilitic chancre is classic, and the lesion is sometimes called the "Hunterian chancre." In an unsuccessful attempt to differentiate gonorrhea from syphilis, Hunter inoculated himself with what he thought was gonorrhea, but acquired syphilis. His great collection of anatomical and animal specimens formed the basis for the museum of the Royal College of Surgeons. He was also a member of the Royal Society of Medicine and the Royal Academy of Surgery at Paris. Hunter wrote many papers on anatomy and physiology; he was a brilliant lecturer and teacher. Among his many students was one who would become famous and well-loved — Edward Jenner.

Edward Jenner (1749–1823) was a country physician in Dorsetshire, England. He is listed among the immortals of preventive medicine for his discovery of the smallpox vaccine. The story goes that one day, while Jenner was serving as an apprentice in the office of Daniel Ludlow, his preceptor, a dairy maid was being given treatment. Smallpox was mentioned, and she said, "I cannot take that disease, for I have had cowpox." Smallpox at that time was the deadliest of pandemics. Jenner observed that farmers and dairy maids who once had cowpox never contracted smallpox. Later, as a practicing physician, Jenner continued investigating the relationship between cowpox and smallpox, to the extent that other medical society members felt bored and threatened to expel him from their ranks.

On May 14, 1796, Dr. Jenner took some purulent matter from a pustule on the hand of Sarah Nelmes, a dairy maid, and inserted it through two small superficial incisions into the arm of James Phipps, a healthy boy of eight. This was the first vaccination. Later, on July 1, a virulent dose of smallpox matter was given to young Phipps in the same arm. It had no effect: Phipps had been vaccinated and was safe from the dreaded disease. Edward Jenner's method of vaccination spread throughout the world to all people. The results of his methods and experiments were published in 1798. He called this method of protection "vaccination" because the latin word *vacca* means cow. Cowpox was called "vaccinia." Pasteur applied the term "vaccine" to suspensions of dead bacteria or attenuated bacteria; unfortunately, this term has since been used in reference to other immunizing antigens not derived from cows.

Victor Robinson, in *Pathfinders in Medicine*, said of Dr. Jenner, "He died where an intellectual man should die — in his library. The village which gave him birth received his illustrious ashes. When his worn out body was laid to rest, it would not be surprising if some humble woman, whose child he had saved from smallpox, imagined that Edward Jenner had gone to heaven — to vaccinate the angels."

In the early 1800s there were several men who are remembered for their fight against puerperal fever and for their concern for women. Puerperal fever, an infectious disease of childbirth, is also known as puerperal sepsis or childbed fever. This term is from *puerpera,* denoting a woman in childbed, from the Latin *puer,* a child, and pario, to bring forth. The word "puerperium" now designates the period from delivery to the time the uterus returns to normal size.

The best known of these men is Ignaz Philipp Semmelweis (1818–1865). History has called him the "Savior of Mothers." His fight against puerperal fever is a sad story of hardships and resistance, especially from his instructor, Professor Klein. Semmelweis noted the terrible results of puerperal fever in lying-in hospitals and observed that it occurred with special frequency in cases delivered by medical students who came directly from the autopsy or dissecting room. Semmelweis directed that in his wards the students were to wash and disinfect their hands with a solution of chloride of lime after leaving the dissection room and before going to the wards to examine a woman and deliver her child. This brought about a marked reduction of cases of childbed fever on his ward, but violent opposition was given by the hospital's medical men, and especially by Dr. Klein. As his theories were proven correct, Semmelweis began to feel the horror of the deaths he had caused in the past. He related this to James Young Simpson, a Scottish obstetrician, who was the first to use chloroform as an anesthetic in 1847. (A type of obstetrical forcep bears Simpson's name.)

At the age of 47 Semmelweis died, ironically from the infection he had fought, brought on by a cut in his finger while he was doing an autopsy. His grave had hardly been closed when Pasteur and Lister began to reveal the secrets that had caused this deadly disease. A monument to Semmelweis in Budapest is given great care and it has been said that if people had been as tender to the man as they are to his statue, his career would have been happier.

A man with the same concerns as Semmelweis and Simpson was James Marion Sims (1813–1883). Dr. Sims was the genius of American gynecology. He was the designer of the duck-billed vaginal speculum and he introduced the Sims' position. Dr. Sims traveled to Edinburgh to see Dr. Simpson, whose theories and surgical techniques he had closely followed. Both men, however, had their share of mortality statistics before surgical techniques became more perfected.

With Doctors Sims, Simpson and Semmelweis was another pioneer, Oliver Wendell Holmes (1809–1894). Dr. Holmes presents many different pictures to his admirers. To us he was a physician, to others a poet and essayist. To all he was a Boston "personality." Some history books do not mention his role as a physician, only his brilliant writings, or the fact that he was the father of Chief Justice Oliver Wendell Holmes. Dr. Holmes is credited with coining the word "anesthesia," which became the accepted term of today. Even before Holmes knew of Semmelweis' work, he had gotten together facts showing that puerperal fever was contagious, and in 1843 he wrote *The Contagiousness of Puerperal Fever.* He was professor of anatomy at Harvard Medical School and a delight to his students.

Much time is spent with honoring great men in medical history, but women have also played important roles which during those times was not an easy thing to do. Two famous women, in particular, are Florence Nightingale (1820–1910), and Clara Barton (1821–1912). If you will notice, these careers overlap almost to the year.

Florence Nightingale has been honored and known far and wide as "The Lady with the Lamp" and is immortalized as the founder of nursing. She was of noble birth, and somewhat late in life she sought nurse's training in both England and Europe. By the time of the Crimean War in 1854 she already had a reputation for her work in hospital organization. She was invited by the Secretary of War to visit the Crimea to correct the terrible conditions that existed in caring for the wounded. She created the Woman's Nursing Service at Scutari and Balaklava. The doctors at Scutari regarded Florence Nightingale as a troublesome female intruder and treated her and her nurses quite shabbily. Only a crisis that brought thousands of wounded and sick soldiers to army hospitals persuaded the doctors to accept help from her and her nurses.

Miss Nightingale ruled her nurses with an iron hand. Aside from the practical work she did, it was she who insisted the nursing profession get public recognition, and that nursing required special training and experience. From donated funds she organized a school of nursing that bears her name. The modern conception of nursing is based largely on the foundations she laid.

The American counterpart to Florence Nightingale's story is the one of Clara Barton. She was a nurse and philanthropist whose work during the American Civil War led her to recognize that very poor records, if any at all, were kept in Washington to aid in the search for missing men wounded or killed in combat. This led to the formation of the Bureau of Records. Clara Barton's fame spread as a result of her organization and recruitment of supplies for the wounded. In 1870 she observed the work of the Red Cross in the Franco-Prussian War, and in 1881 she organized a Red Cross Committee in Washington, forming the American Red Cross, of which she served as the first president from 1881 to 1904.

Surely Semmelweis' death was just a matter of tragic timing, for the year of his death was to introduce the great works of Pasteur and a physician in Edinburgh and Glasgow named Joseph Lister.

This era of history was truly the golden era for medicine, because in 1822 one of the most famous men in medical history was born, Louis Pasteur. Pasteur was a French chemist who achieved fame in bacteriology. His work as a chemist was brilliant but it was his studies in bacteriology that earned him the title "Father of Bacteriology"; he has also been given the honor of being called the "Father of Preventative Medicine" (although historians differ somewhat upon this last title). His skills and studies reached far beyond the outermost boundaries of the knowledge of the time. He pursued everything with the fire of genius. The statement, "Genius does what it must, and talent does what it can," may be applied to Pasteur and his forceful quest for more knowledge.

His adventures included studying the maladies of wine. He saved the most important industry of France at that time from disaster by a process now called pasteurization. By this process wine was prevented from turning into vinegar. This made great improvements in spirit and malt liquors. The French people called on Pasteur again to help the ailing silkworm industry. The silkworm epidemic in the south of France had reached such proportions that whole plantations were ruined. For five years Pasteur devoted himself to this cause before conquering the two diseases that infected the silkworm. His work was interrupted only when he was stricken with hemiplegia. But after a long, difficult recovery time, when his mind was always fully active, he continued his work with a stiff hand and a limping foot.

With the conviction that the "infinitely small" world of bacteria had the key to the secrets of contagious diseases, he again left chemistry, this time to become a medical man. Many renowned scientists denied the germ theory of disease and devoted themselves to degrading Pasteur. In the midst of all this "denying-the-germ" battle he became involved in the prevention of anthrax, which threatened the health of the cattle and sheep of France, as well as of the world. Pasteur's work with anthrax overlapped that of Robert Koch, who was also investigating the disease. Koch and Pasteur were often working on the same problem, but there was ill-concealed animosity between the two; their goals were the same but their paths were not together.

Pasteur's name was also honored for work on many other diseases, such as rabies, chicken cholera, and swine erysipelas. Pasteur and Joseph Lister met at the Sorbonne after years of great mutual admiration. The meeting was filled with emotion and Robinson, in *Pathfinders in Medicine*, has said that "a new star should have appeared in the heavens to commemorate the event. Only a small percentage of the human race entertains any adequate realization of how much we really owe to the combined labors of Louis Pasteur and Joseph Lister."

Pasteur died in 1895, with his family at his bedside. His last words were said to be "There is still a great deal to do."

Joseph Lister (1827–1912) was to revolutionize surgery through the application of Pasteur's discoveries. He saw the similarity between the infections that were taking place in post-surgical wounds and the processes of putrefaction which Pasteur had proven were caused by microorganisms. Before this time surgeons accepted infection in surgical wounds as inevitable. Lister reasoned that microorganisms must be the cause of infection and must, therefore, be kept out of wounds. His own colleagues were quite indifferent to Lister's theories since they felt infections were God-given and natural. Lister had once seen pain quelled by the administration of an anesthetic, and pain had been thought to be God-given and inevitable also. He developed antiseptic methods by using carbolic acid for sterilization. By spraying the room with a fine mist of the acid, by soaking the instruments and ligatures, and by washing his hands in carbolic solutions, Lister proved his theory. He is honored with the title of "Father of Sterile Surgery."

The name Robert Koch (1843–1910) is familiar to all bacteriologists, for the first law learned as a neophyte in this microscopic world is Koch's Postulates, which state rules that must be followed before an organism can be accepted as the causative agent in a given disease.

Robert Koch was a German physician who truly earned great honors in bacteriology and public health. He gave the bacteriology laboratory many of its "tools," such as the culture-plate method for isolation of bacteria. He discovered the cause of cholera and demonstrated its transmission by food and water. This discovery completely transformed health departments and proved the importance of bacteriology. It also established a place of great respect for Koch in the scientific world. A great disappointment in Koch's career was his discovery of tuberculin while working with tuberculosis. This was not the cure for tuberculosis that he hoped to find, but a diagnostic aid; however, as modern medicine knows, this discovery has proven of immense value.

Koch's work took him throughout the world. He traveled to America, Africa, Bombay, Italy and anywhere nations sought his help in ridding themselves of feared diseases. In 1885 the University of Berlin created the Chair of

Hygiene and Bacteriology in his honor. He became the Nobel Laureate in 1905. In 1910 he died in his sleep while on a holiday to Baden-Baden.

While Robert Koch's brilliant career was nearing an end because of age and illnesses, the work of Paul Ehrlich (1854–1915) was reaching its zenith. Ehrlich had been greatly honored when Koch had invited him to work in his laboratory. Koch had known Ehrlich well, since he had been a distinguished student of his and had already made a place for himself in scientific circles.

Ehrlich was a German physician, and one of the pioneers in the fields of bacteriology, immunology, and especially chemotherapy, a fairly new science. He was only 28 years old when he wrote his first paper on typhoid, but his greatest gift to mankind was to be called his "magic bullet," or "606," and was designed to fight the terrible disease, syphilis. Only three years before, Bordet and Wasserman had identified the organism and devised a test that would smoke it out of hiding. With the offending germ identified, Ehrlich set out to find a chemical that would destroy the organism but not harm the germ's host, the human body. The search was long and tedious, and history tells us it was the 606th drug which Ehrlich tried that finally did the healing. He called the drug salvarsan because he felt it offered mankind salvation from this disease. This also was the beginning of injecting chemicals into the body to destroy a specific organism.

Later, in 1912, Ehrlich discovered a less toxic drug, called neosalvarsan, to replace the original 606. The new drug bore the number 914. In 1908 Ehrlich shared the Nobel prize with Eli Metchinkoff, who is remembered for his theory of phagocytosis and immunology.

There are so many to whom we owe so much, that one chapter cannot do justice to these dedicated persons. Their names may just be names to those who may owe them the most. Patients who have received radium therapy should know the long struggle of Marie and Pierre Curie. Diabetics should give thanks to Frederick Banting, the Canadian physician who discovered insulin in 1922. Anyone who has ever been spared the pain of surgery through the sleep of an anesthetic can give thanks to the memory of three men: two dentists, Dr. Horace Wells and Dr. William T. G. Morton; and a physician from Danielsville, Georgia, Dr. Crawford Williamson Long. There has been considerable controversy as to whom should be given final credit for the actual discovery of anesthesia, but it now seems to be established that Dr. Long (1815–1878) was the first to employ ether as an anesthetic agent. Early in 1842, after lectures on chemistry, a group of students would have a social gathering and inhale ether as a form of amusement. At one of these so-called "ether frolics" Dr. Long observed that people under the influence of ether did not seem to feel pain. After considerable thought, Dr. Long decided to use ether for a surgical operation. On March 30, 1842, he removed a tumor from the neck of James M. Venable after placing him under the influence of ether. Long did not report this operation or his discovery until 1848. Wells reported his discovery in 1844, and Morton his in 1846, when he extracted a tooth after the patient had been given ether, and he also used it at Massachusetts General Hospital for a surgical procedure.

## REFERENCES

Robinson, V., *Pathfinders in Medicine*. Medical Life Press, New York, 1929
Thorwald, J., *The Century of the Surgeon*. Thames and Hudson, London, 1957

# Chapter 4

**BEHAVIORAL OBJECTIVES**

*The medical office assistant should be able to:*

Define medical ethics.
Trace the evolution of the modern
    code of medical ethics.

Apply the code as set forth in the
    Principles of Medical Ethics of the
    American Medical Association.

# Medical Ethics

For centuries the medical profession has set for itself a rigid standard of ethical conduct toward patients and colleagues. Because each physician pledges himself to put the welfare of the patient before his own interests, the medical profession has achieved a position of great respect.

Hippocrates, the Greek physician known as the father of medicine, spelled out one of the first statements of medical ethics some 400 years before the birth of Christ.

## The Oath of Hippocrates

I swear by Apollo, the physician, and Aesculapius, and Health, and Allheal, and all the gods and goddesses, that, according to my ability and judgment, I will keep this oath and stipulation, to reckon him who taught me this art equally dear to me as my parents, to share my substance with him and relieve his necessities if required; to regard his offspring as on the same footing with my own brothers, and to teach them this art if they should wish to learn it, without fee or stipulation, and that by precept, lecture and every other mode of instruction, I will impart a knowledge of the art to my own sons and to those of my teachers, and to disciples bound by a stipulation and oath, according to the law of medicine, but to none others.

I will follow that method of treatment which, according to my ability and judgment, I consider for the benefit of my patients, and abstain from whatever is deleterious and mischievous. I will give no deadly medicine to anyone if asked, nor suggest any such counsel; furthermore, I will not give to a woman an instrument to produce abortion.

With purity and holiness I will pass my life and practice my art. I will not cut a person who is suffering with a stone, but will leave this to be done by practitioners of this work. Into whatever houses I enter I will go into them for the benefit of the sick and will abstain from every voluntary act of mischief and corruption; and further from the seduction of females or males, bond or free.

Whatever, in connection with my professional practice, or not in connection with it, I may see or hear in the lives of men which ought not to be spoken abroad, I will not divulge, as reckoning that all such should be kept secret.

While I continue to keep this oath unviolated, may it be granted to me to enjoy life and the practice of the art, respected by all men at all times, but should I trespass and violate this oath, may the reverse be my lot.

## MODERN CODES

The practice of medicine today is guided by a more modern code, known as the Principles of Medical Ethics, which contains the same underlying philosophy

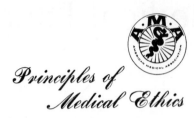

### Principles of Medical Ethics

**Preamble:** These principles are intended to aid physicians individually and collectively in maintaining a high level of ethical conduct. They are not laws but standards by which a physician may determine the propriety of his conduct in his relationship with patients, with colleagues, with members of allied professions, and with the public.

**Section 1**—The principal objective of the medical profession is to render service to humanity with full respect for the dignity of man. Physicians should merit the confidence of patients entrusted to their care, rendering to each a full measure of service and devotion.

**Section 2**—Physicians should strive continually to improve medical knowledge and skill, and should make available to their patients and colleagues the benefits of their professional attainments.

**Section 3**—A physician should practice a method of healing founded on a scientific basis; and he should not voluntarily associate professionally with anyone who violates this principle.

**Section 4**—The medical profession should safeguard the public and itself against physicians deficient in moral character or professional competence. Physicians should observe all laws, uphold the dignity and honor of the profession and accept its self-imposed disciplines. They should expose, without hesitation, illegal or unethical conduct of fellow members of the profession.

**Section 5**—A physician may choose whom he will serve. In an emergency, however, he should render service to the best of his ability. Having undertaken the care of a patient, he may not neglect him; and unless he has been discharged he may discontinue his services only after giving adequate notice. He should not solicit patients.

**Section 6**—A physician should not dispose of his services under terms or conditions which tend to interfere with or impair the free and complete exercise of his medical judgment and skill or tend to cause a deterioration of the quality of medical care.

**Section 7**—In the practice of medicine a physician should limit the source of his professional income to medical services actually rendered by him, or under his supervision, to his patients. His fee should be commensurate with the services rendered and the patient's ability to pay. He should neither pay nor receive a commission for referral of patients. Drugs, remedies or appliances may be dispensed or supplied by the physician provided it is in the best interests of the patient.

**Section 8**—A physician should seek consultation upon request; in doubtful or difficult cases; or whenever it appears that the quality of medical service may be enhanced thereby.

**Section 9**—A physician may not reveal the confidences entrusted to him in the course of medical attendance, or the deficiencies he may observe in the character of patients, unless he is required to do so by law or unless it becomes necessary in order to protect the welfare of the individual or of the community.

**Section 10**—The honored ideals of the medical profession imply that the responsibilities of the physician extend not only to the individual, but also to society where these responsibilities deserve his interest and participation in activities which have the purpose of improving both the health and the well-being of the individual and the community.

**Figure 4–1**  A.M.A. Principles of Medical Ethics. (Reprinted with permission of American Medical Association.)

as the oath of Hippocrates. An English physician, Sir Thomas Percival, wrote the first Principles of Ethics in 1803 to provide a model statement of what a doctor should be. In 1847 the newly organized American Medical Association patterned its code of ethics upon Percival's *Code of Medical Ethics*. The A.M.A. Principles of Medical Ethics has been revised at least six times since 1900 to keep it consistent with the times, but there has never been a change in its moral intent or over-all idealism. In 1957, the Principles of Medical Ethics of the American Medical Association was condensed to a preamble and ten sections (see Fig. 4–1). The Judicial Council of the A.M.A. is charged with interpreting the Principles of Medical Ethics as adopted by the House of Delegates of the American Medical Association.

# WHAT IS ETHICS?

Medical ethics should not be confused with medical etiquette. According to Webster's Dictionary, ethics is "broadly speaking, the science of the ideal human character and the ideal ends of human action—the chief problem with which ethics deals concerns the nature of the summum bonum or highest good—the origin and validity of the sense of duty and the character and authority of moral obligation." Etiquette deals with courtesy, customs, and manners; ethics concerns itself with the underlying philosophies in the ideal relationships of men.

In the Preamble to the Principles of Medical Ethics it is pointed out that "These principles are intended to aid physicians individually and collectively in maintaining a high level of ethical conduct. They are not laws but standards by which a physician may determine the propriety of his conduct in his relationship with patients, with colleagues, with members of allied professions, and with the public."

*They are not laws but standards* . . . Laws vary from state to state, from community to community. Ethical standards do not. The Judicial Council of the A.M.A. emphasizes that "there is but one code of ethics for all, be they group, clinic or individual and be they great and prominent or small and unknown." Ethical standards are never less than the standards required by law; frequently they may be higher. Violation of the ethical standards of an association or society may result in expulsion or suspension of membership. Violation of a law followed by conviction may result in punishment by fine, imprisonment, or revocation of license.

The medical assistant has more than an historical interest in the Principles of Medical Ethics. As a member of the team in the medical field of endeavor, she must in effect also pledge herself to abide by these Principles; they will be her professional conscience, just as they are her employer's standard of ethical conduct.

Let's examine some of the principles, as set down, and see how they affect the medical assistant.

# PRINCIPLES OF MEDICAL ETHICS

**Principle of Service.** Section One states: "The principal objective of the medical profession is to render service to humanity with full respect for the dignity of man. Physicians should merit the confidence of patients entrusted to their care, rendering to each a full measure of service and devotion."

Section One encompasses the principle that reward or financial gain is a subordinate consideration, and that service should be available to all the people whether they are able to pay or not. Free choice of physician, optician, pharmacist, and so on is encouraged. It is stressed throughout the Code that the patient is entitled to the best treatment possible and that pecuniary gain must not interfere with this purpose, including the physician's selection of a consultant.

Professional courtesy is also discussed. The 1972 Judicial Council Opinions and Reports state "Where professional courtesy is offered by a physician but the recipient of services insists upon payment, the physician need not be embarrassed to accept a fee for his services." Further, "If a physician or his dependents have insurance providing benefits for medical or surgical care, a physician who renders such service may accept the insurance benefits without violating the traditional ethical practice of physicians caring for the medical needs of colleagues and their dependents without charge."

The medical office assistant also embraces the concept of *service* and *devotion*. At times this will be at the expense of her own convenience or personal wishes, but it is basic in the fulfillment of her obligation. She should "merit the confidence of patients." Only with a full knowledge of her responsibilities, and being ever mindful of details, is she worthy of such confidence.

**Improving Knowledge and Skill.** Section Two states: "Physicians should strive continually to improve medical knowledge and skill, and should make available to their patients and colleagues the benefits of their professional attainments." Guidelines are offered in regard to experimentation with either new drugs or procedures. Three requirements must be satisfied in connection with the use of experimental drugs or procedures:

(1) the voluntary consent of the person on whom the experiment is to be performed should be obtained;

(2) the danger of each experiment must be previously investigated by animal experimentation; and

(3) the experiment must be performed under proper medical protection and management.

The Principles of Medical Ethics does not prohibit a physician from patenting a surgical or diagnostic instrument he has discovered or developed, but it is stated that should a physician use such a patent for his own financial interest to the detriment of the profession or the public he would be acting unethically.

The medical office assistant, too, assumes the obligation of continually improving her knowledge and skill. This may be accomplished through reading, participation in special classes or study groups, and through observation of her employer and trained paramedical colleagues.

**Method of Healing Founded on a Scientific Basis.** Section Three states that the physician should not voluntarily associate professionally with sectarians or cultists, and defines some of those areas, for instance, chiropractic. Podiatry and optometry are *not* cults. The policy toward doctors of osteopathy is in transition, and the A.M.A. position is that the policy "should now be applied individually at state level according to the facts as they exist," instead of collectively at the national level as it has been in the past.

**Dignity and Honor.** Section Four includes these words: "Physicians should observe all laws, uphold the dignity and honor of the profession and accept its self-imposed disciplines." Some aspects of medical law will be dealt with in more detail later, but the medical assistant must keep in mind at all times that she is acting as the physician's agent and should be aware of the legal implications involved.

The medical office assistant must uphold the dignity and honor of the profession of medicine. Medicine has been likened to the ministry in the eyes of the public. While the employee in a business or commercial enterprise may be entitled to believe that her personal life is of no concern to others, the medical assistant does not enjoy this immunity. She is a member of the medical team, and her private life is subject to the same scrutiny as that of her employer. Particularly when she is attending a meeting or convention of her professional organization, her behavior must be above reproach, for to her observers she represents the medical profession and she must accept its self-imposed disciplines.

The physician is encouraged to "affiliate with medical societies and contribute his time, energy and means so that these societies may represent the ideals of the profession." Many medical office assistants have followed this tenet through their affiliation with the American Association of Medical Assistants and other professional organizations.

**Patient Cannot be Neglected.**    Section Five of the Principles states: "A physician may choose whom he will serve. In an emergency, however, he should render service to the best of his ability. Having undertaken the care of a patient, he may not neglect him; and unless he has been discharged he may discontinue his services only after giving adequate notice."

This would indicate that although a physician is free to choose whom he will serve, once he initiates care of a patient, he must do so to the best of his ability. If a doctor-patient relationship is established, he cannot withdraw from the case without giving notice to the patient (see sample letter below), his relatives, or his responsible friends sufficiently in advance to allow them to secure another

---

## Form A-1

## LETTER OF WITHDRAWAL FROM CASE

Dear Mr._____:

    I find it necessary to inform you that I am withdrawing from further professional attendance upon you for the reason that you have persisted in refusing to follow my medical advice and treatment. Since your condition requires medical attention, I suggest that you place yourself under the care of another physician without delay. If you so desire, I shall be available to attend you for a reasonable time after you have received this letter, but in no event for more than five days.

    This should give you ample time to select a physician of your choice from the many competent practitioners in this city. With your approval, I will make available to this physician your case history and information regarding the diagnosis and treatment which you have received from me.

Very truly yours,

_____, M.D.

**Figure 4–2**    (From *Medicolegal Forms with Legal Analysis. 3rd Ed.* Office of the General Counsel, 1973, p. 3. Copyright © 1973. American Medical Association.)

physician. For this reason it is important that each physician provide round-the-clock coverage of his practice. Also, if he withdraws from a case a form letter, such as the one shown, should be sent to the patient and a carbon filed. The office assistant who is able to remind the physician of these responsibilities can be worth her weight in gold.

ADVERTISING. Ethical physicians may not advertise for patients. This principle protects the public from the medical care salesman by making it easy to determine the distinction between an ethical and an unethical physician. A good doctor does not need to advertise; he soon builds a reputation for professional ability and fidelity. On opening an office or on removing an office, "a physician may properly send announcements to his colleagues, to his intimate personal friends not in the medical profession, and to those persons in allied fields with whom it may reasonably be expected he will associate." Insertion of simple notices in the local newspaper that a physician is opening practice, returning from service, or moving his office is considered ethical. Because local custom varies, it is best for the physician or his medical assistant, if she is charged with this responsibility, to check with the local medical society regarding practices in the community.

**Terms and Conditions of Services Must Not Impair Exercise of Medical Judgment and Skill.** Section Six sets forth principles regarding contract practice, lay corporations, professional corporations, physician-hospital relations, physicians' relations with psychiatrists and psychologists, and so forth. In essence, that "it is within the limits of ethical propriety for physicians to join together as partnerships, associations or other lawful groups provided that the ownership and management of the affairs thereof remain in the hands of licensed physicians."

**Fee Commensurate with Services Rendered and Patient's Ability to Pay.** The tone of Section Seven is set by these words from the 1972 Judicial Council Opinions and Reports: "The ethical physician, engaged in the practice of medicine, limits the sources of his income received from professional activities to services rendered the patient."

The medical office assistant is clearly concerned with the billing and collection of fees for professional services and will be interested in the provision that the physician's "fee should be commensurate with the services rendered and the patient's ability to pay." Many potential fee complaints can be eliminated by advance discussion with patients, particularly when a sizable fee is to be expected, for instance in major surgery or long-term medical care.

With the passing of time we are now confronted with the ethic of billing for the completion of health insurance claim forms, charging for broken appointments, billing for outside respiratory and laboratory services, the use of bank cards, and the charging of interest or a penalty on delinquent accounts, as well as a multitude of other problems.

The Principles state that the attending physician should complete without charge one simplified form, such as the Health Insurance Council form, but that there is nothing improper in charging for additional forms if the patient has been informed in advance.

Charging for missed or uncanceled appointments should be resorted to infrequently, and only after consideration of the circumstances. The use of bank cards is not encouraged; physicians should consult with their county medical society before participating in their use.

It is not ethical for a physician to bill a patient for respiratory services provided by a lay organization. In some cases the physician can bill for outside laboratory services since the practice of pathology is an integral part of the practice of medicine.

"When two or more physicians actually and in person render service to one patient, they should render separate bills." An awareness of this principle will aid the medical office assistant in her explanations to patients who inquire about the bill for services of an anesthesiologist, an assistant surgeon, a consultant, or a pathology laboratory.

Occasionally the question arises as to whether a patient should be additionally assessed in some manner on a delinquent account. The A.M.A. Judicial Council (1972) states:

> It is not in the best interest of the public or the profession to charge interest on an unpaid bill or note or to charge a penalty on fees for professional services not paid within a prescribed period of time nor is it proper to charge a patient a flat collection fee if it becomes necessary to refer the account to an agency for collection.

**Requests for Consultation.**   Section Eight reads: "A physician should seek consultation upon request; in doubtful or difficult cases; or whenever it appears that the quality of medical service may be enhanced thereby."

It is never the medical assistant's responsibility to determine *when* consultation is desirable. However, it is nearly certain that at some time she will be confronted with an inquiry from a patient under the care of another physician, asking for a consultation with her employer. Her handling of this situation is a delicate one and may permanently affect the relationship between her employer and his colleagues. The assistant should, at the outset of her employment, have a definite understanding with her employer on the procedure to be followed in such instances. Two points of general interest can be set forth here:

> When a physician has acted as consultant in an illness, he should not become the physician in charge in the course of that illness, except with the consent of the physician who was in charge at the time of the consultation.
>
> As soon as possible after the consulting physician has seen the patient he should address the physician in charge and advise him of the results of his investigation.

**Confidential Matters.**   Of particular importance is Section Nine, regarding confidential information received by the doctor or his assistants from patients: "A physician may not reveal the confidences entrusted to him in the course of medical attendance, or the deficiencies he may observe in the character of patients, unless he is required to do so by law or unless it becomes necessary in order to protect the welfare of the individual or of the community."

This means that the assistant in a doctor's office must be able to keep a secret, since she is entrusted with many of them each day. Confidences about patients, their illnesses, or their personal lives that she learns through her work should never be repeated. She must avoid mentioning the names of patients, for sometimes the doctor's specialty reveals the patient's reason for consulting him.

In *Winning Ways with Patients* the A.M.A. tells doctors' assistants: "Curious patients will often ask you personal questions about other patients, you, or the doctor. You must firmly refuse information without giving offense. A tactful, courteous refusal will discourage further questioning. Then change the subject. Some patients will query you about their own case. Refer them to the doctor for such information."

Confidential papers, case histories, and even the appointment book should be kept out of reach of curious eyes — to protect the patient, as well as the doctor and his assistants. Violation of the confidential doctor-patient relationship is considered highly unethical. There are certain times, however, when the doctor justifiably must break confidences. One such instance is that of discovery of a contagious disease. The doctor must report the disease in order that healthy persons who might be exposed to it can be protected.

LEGAL DISCLOSURES. According to state laws, which vary somewhat throughout the country, certain disclosures must be made. Births and deaths must be reported. Births out of wedlock must be reported on special forms in some states; others require detailed information about stillbirths. A physician is required to report cases he treats which he thinks may have been a result of violence, such as gunshot wounds, knifings, or poisonings. He also must report deaths from accidental or unexplained causes. In some states occupational diseases which he diagnoses must be reported within ten days or two weeks. He must report any cases of contagious, infectious, or communicable diseases. Venereal diseases are reportable in every state. He also must file reports of find-

---

## Form D-7

## AUTHORIZATION TO FURNISH INFORMATION

Date_____Time_____
A.M.
P.M.

I authorize and request the _____ Hospital, and the physicians who attended me while I was a patient in said hos-

pital during the approximate period from _____, 19____ to

_____, 19____, to furnish to _____ all information concerning my case history and the treatment, examinations or hospitalization which I received, including copies of hospital and medical records.

Signed_____

Witness_____

**Figure 4–3** (From *Medicolegal Forms with Legal Analysis. 3rd Ed.* Office of the General Counsel, 1973, p. 11. Copyright © 1973. American Medical Association.)

```
┌─────────────────────────────────────────────────────────────┐
│                         Form D-5                              │
│                                                               │
│           AUTHORIZATION FOR EXAMINATION OF                    │
│                  PHYSICIAN'S RECORDS                          │
│                                                               │
│   To Dr. _____:                                    │
│                                                               │
│     I authorize you to furnish a copy of the medical records of│
│                                                               │
│   _____, covering the period from  │
│     (state name of patient or "myself")                       │
│                                                               │
│   _____, 19____ to _____, 19____ or to allow those│
│                                                               │
│   records to be inspected or copied by _____. I release│
│   you from all legal responsibility or liability that may arise from│
│   this authorization.                                         │
│                                       Signed_____      │
│                                                               │
│                                       Date_____        │
│   Witness_____                                         │
│                                                               │
└─────────────────────────────────────────────────────────────┘
```

**Figure 4–4** (From *Medicolegal Forms with Legal Analysis. 3rd Ed.* Office of the General Counsel, 1973, p. 11. Copyright © 1973. American Medical Association.)

ings in premarital examinations. It should be remembered that a disclosure of information that is required by law does not violate the Principles of Medical Ethics.

WAIVER OF PRIVILEGE. The privilege of maintaining a confidential doctor-patient relationship is the patient's. If a patient takes the witness stand in court, for example, and testifies about matters within the privilege, he waives the privilege and the doctor then can testify about matters that are otherwise confidential.

AUTHORIZATION FOR DISCLOSURE OF INFORMATION. When neither a basis for legal disclosure nor a waiver of privilege exists, care must be taken to obtain the written consent of the patient before divulging information to a third party. Printed forms, such as the following, are often used to secure the patient's waiver.

OWNERSHIP OF THE MEDICAL RECORD. There is a common misconception on the part of the patient that the medical record belongs to him "because he paid for it." The medical office assistant must not only be aware that the record belongs to the *physician*; she must also understand *why*, because this is a question

---

## Form D-1

### AUTHORIZATION FOR DISCLOSURE OF INFORMATION BY PATIENT'S PHYSICIAN

1. I authorize Dr. _____ to disclose complete

information to _____ concerning his medical findings

and treatment of the undersigned from on or about _____

19____ until date of the conclusion of such treatment.

 2. Further, I authorize him to testify, without limitation, as to all of his medical findings and the treatment administered to the undersigned, in any legal action, suit, or proceedings to which I am, or may become, a party; and I waive on behalf of myself and any persons who may have an interest in the matter, all provisions of law relating to the disclosure of confidential medical information.

Signed_____

Place_____

Date_____

Witness_____

---

**Figure 4–5**   (From *Medicolegal Forms with Legal Analysis. 3rd Ed.* Office of the General Counsel, 1973, p. 9. Copyright © 1973. American Medical Association.)

which will be frequently encountered. As stated by the A.M.A. Judicial Council (1972):

> These records are primarily the physician's own notes compiled during the course of diagnosis and treatment so that he may review and study the course of the illness and his treatment. The records are medical and technical, personal and often informal. Standing alone they are meaningless to the patient but of value to the physician and perhaps to a succeeding physician. The patient, however, or one responsible for him, is entitled to know the nature of the illness and the general course or regimen of therapy employed by his physician.

How does this apply to the record of the patient who has neglected or refused to pay his bill for services? The author has on more than one occasion heard the question raised by a medical assistant, "If a patient moves away without paying his bill, and subsequently requests that his record be forwarded to his new physician, is it all right to demand that he pay his bill before forwarding the record?" Section Nine of the Principles clearly states:

> It is unethical for a physician who formerly treated a patient, to refuse for any reason to make his records of that patient promptly available on request to another physician presently treating the patient.

**Responsibilities of the Physician Extend Not only to the Individual but also to Society: Section Ten.**   The duties of the physician to the public are also outlined. Physicians, as good citizens, are urged to advise concerning the health of their communities and to help enforce those laws and sustain the institutions which advance the interest of humanity.

The standards of the medical profession forbid that physicians exploit their ability or achievements to the laity. However, they are encouraged to cooperate with medical society requests to write, act or speak for general readers or audiences.

The medical assistant often will aid her employer in carrying out his civic responsibilities. Sometimes it will be her job to accept or tactfully decline a committee appointment, to keep meeting notes, or to handle mail or make telephone calls related to these activities. But the medical assistant, like her physician employer, has a certain civic responsibility of her own that she is discharging partially when performing these tasks.

In the medical profession, as in any other field of endeavor, one hears little of the individuals who go about their duties each day in accordance with the accepted standards. It is the deviate who gains attention. And thus sometimes the sense of loyalty is strained. A study of the entire Code of Ethics will bring to the medical office assistant not only a better understanding of her physician-employer's obligations and limitations. It will be a sustaining inspiration throughout her career as a member of the medical team.

## REFERENCES

American Medical Association, *Judicial Council Opinions and Reports,* Chicago, American Medical Association, 1972

American Medical Association, *Medicolegal Forms with Legal Analysis,* Chicago, American Medical Association, 1973

American Medical Association, *Winning Ways with Patients,* Chicago, American Medical Association, 1966

# Chapter 5

**BEHAVIORAL OBJECTIVES**

*The medical office assistant should be able to:*

State the requirements for licensure of
   physicians.
State the possible reasons for
   revocation or suspension of
   license.
Define professional liability in
   medicine.

Recognize the legal responsibilities of
   the medical assistant in the
   performance of her professional
   duties.
Recall and recognize the definitions of
   legal terms included in the
   Chapter Glossary.

# Medicine and the Law

Closely allied with medical ethics are certain medicolegal principles which must be considered in the daily operation of the doctor's office.

What is the "practice of medicine"? A book of this nature can touch only the surface of such a complex subject.

## Medical Practice Acts

Although medical practice acts existed as early as colonial days, these were later repealed, and in the mid-nineteenth century practically none of the states had laws governing the practice of medicine. As might be expected, there was a rapid decline in professional standards. The general welfare of the people was endangered by medical quackery and inadequate care. By the beginning of this century, however, medical practice acts were again in effect in every state.

Medical practice acts are state statutes. They define what is included in the practice of medicine within that state and govern the methods and requirements of licensure and the grounds for suspension or revocation of license. With but a few exceptions, a physician must be licensed by the state in which he practices.

**Licensing.** The license to practice medicine is granted by a state licensing board, known as the Board of Medical Examiners. License may be by *examination*, by *reciprocity*, or by *endorsement*. State examinations are prepared and graded by physicians. Some states grant a license to practice medicine by *reciprocity*; that is, they recognize that the requirements of another state in which the physician is already licensed meet or surpass their own requirements. If an applicant has passed the examination of the National Board of Medical Examiners, he may be granted a license by *endorsement*, although this is not obligatory upon the state.

The applicant for a license to practice medicine must meet other requirements, which vary from state to state. Forty-seven states require either United States citizenship or the declared intention to become a citizen. There are also requirements as to age, moral character, formal training, and residence. After license is granted, periodic re-registration is necessary, either annually or biennially. This is accomplished by payment of a registration fee upon notification by the Board of Medical Examiners.

The medical assistant must remember that the practice of medicine by an unlicensed person is a criminal offense.

**Revocation or Suspension.** Under certain conditions the license to practice medicine may be revoked or suspended. Stetler and Moritz, in *Doctor and Patient* *and the Law*, group the grounds for revocation or suspension of a medical license under three headings: (1) conviction of a crime; (2) unprofessional conduct; and (3) personal or professional incapacity.

## Professional Liability

**Definition.** The term "medical professional liability" encompasses all possible civil liability which a physician can incur as a result of any of his professional acts. It is preferred over the term "medical malpractice" because the latter carries some disreputable overtones. Medical professional liability is more easily prevented than defended.

**Assistant's Role in Claims Prevention.** The competent medical assistant, with empathy for the patient's problems, has an important role in claims prevention. For instance, a patient who is kept waiting for what he considers an inexcusably long time, without explanation or reassurance, has developed some feeling of hostility before he ever sees the doctor. A few words from the receptionist at the proper time may forestall hostility and promote understanding. Any time a medical assistant has reason to believe that a patient is dissatisfied, it is her duty to pass along such information to her employer.

**Malpractice and Negligence.** Negligence, when applied to the medical profession, is called malpractice. It is generally defined as the "doing of some act which a reasonable and prudent physician would not do, or the failure to do some act which such a person should or would do. The standard of prudent conduct is not defined by law but is left to the determination of a judge or jury." This definition is taken from *The Law of Hospital, Physician and Patient*, by Hayt, Hayt and Groeschel, Hospital Textbook Company, New York, 1952.

When injury results to a patient through a doctor's negligence, the patient can legally initiate a malpractice suit to recover financial damages. Experience has shown, however, that the incidence of malpractice claims is directly related to the *personal relationship* existing between the physician and the patient. A person seldom sues someone whom he regards as a true friend.

A physician who performs an operation carelessly or contrary to accepted standards, for example, is guilty of negligence or malpractice. If the state prescribes by law that drops be placed in the eyes of all newborn infants and a physician does not do it, he is guilty of statutory negligence. If an illegal abortion is performed, the physician is guilty of criminal negligence and is also liable for prosecution under the penal statutes. A nurse is guilty of negligence if she fails "to exercise reasonable and ordinary care and the application of her knowledge and exert her best judgment" in the care and treatment of the patient.

If a physician were held legally responsible for every unsuccessful result occurring in treatment, no man would undertake the responsibility of practicing medicine. The courts hold that a physician must use reasonable care, attention, and diligence in the performance of his professional services, follow his best judgment in treating his patients, and possess and exercise the skill and care that are commonly possessed and exercised by other reputable physicians in the same or a similar locality. If he calls himself a specialist, he must meet the standards of practice of his specialty. Whether or not he has met these requirements in treating a particular case is generally a matter for the court to decide upon the basis of expert testimony provided by another physician. *Negligence is not presumed; it must be proved.*

No doctor is required to possess extraordinary learning and skill. But he must keep abreast with medical developments and techniques and he cannot experiment. He also is bound to advise his patients if he discovers that the condition is one beyond his knowledge or technical skill.

## THE FOUR D'S OF NEGLIGENCE

The Committee on Medicolegal Problems, American Medical Association, states in a 1963 report that

> To obtain a judgment against a physician for negligence, the patient must present evidence of what have been referred to as the "Four D's." He must show: (1) that the physician owed a *duty* to the patient, (2) that the physician was *derelict* and breached that duty by failing to act as the ordinary, competent physician in the same community would have acted under the same or similar circumstances, (3) that such failure or breach was the *direct cause* of the patient's injuries, and (4) that *damages* to the patient resulted therefrom.

**Duty** exists when the physician-patient relationship has been established. That is, the patient has sought the assistance of the physician and the physician has knowingly undertaken to provide the needed medical service.

**Derelict** (neglectful of obligation). Proof of dereliction, or proof of negligence of an obligation, must be shown in obtaining a judgment for malpractice.

**Direct cause.** "There must be a proof of a direct and uninterrupted chain of causation from the wrongful act or omission of the physician to the injury suffered by the patient. There must be no independent intervening cause capable of producing the injury."

**Damages.** There are three kinds of damages recognized by the law: (1) nominal, (2) compensatory or actual, and (3) punitive or exemplary. It is the compensatory or actual damages which are most frequently involved in professional liability cases. Compensatory damages may be *general* or *special*.

Compensation for injuries or losses which are the natural and necessary consequences of the physician's negligent act or omission is called "general damages." General damages include compensation for pain and suffering, for loss of a bodily member or faculty, for disfigurement, and other similar direct losses or injuries. The *fact* of the losses must be proved—the *monetary value* need not be proved.

Special damages are those injuries or losses which are not a necessary consequence of the physician's negligent act or omission. This may include the costs of medical and hospital care, loss of earnings, cost of travel, and so forth. *Both* the fact of these injuries or losses and the monetary value must be proved.

The Committee on Professional Liability of the California Medical Association in 1971 called these same four elements the "A B C D's" of negligence in medical practice:

A    Acceptance of a person as a patient.

B    Breach of the physician's duty of skill or care.

C    Causal connection between the breach by the physician and the damage to the patient.
D    Damage of foreseeable nature—that is, injury, pain, loss of earnings, and so on, which could reasonably have been foreseen to result.

## Law of Contracts

Although we do not give it much thought, the law of contracts touches us in many ways, practically every day of our lives. For instance, when you order medications or supplies for the office, you have entered into a contract. In fact, your employment is in itself a contract, though not necessarily in writing.

A contract, to be valid, must have these four basic requisites: (1) manifestation of assent (an offer and an acceptance), (2) legal subject matter, (3) parties must have legal capacity to contract, and (4) consideration.

A contract may be written or oral, express or implied. The party making the offer is known as the *offeror* and the party to whom the offer is made is the *offeree*. Let us illustrate how this would apply to the doctor-patient relationship, which is generally held by the courts to be a contractual relationship. When the doctor "hangs out his shingle" he is inviting an offer. The patient, in presenting himself for treatment, is making an offer. The doctor accepts the offer when he undertakes treatment of the patient.

Until he accepts the offer, the doctor is under no obligation, and no contract exists. Once he has accepted the patient, however, an implied contract does exist that he will treat the patient, using reasonable care, and that he possesses the degree of knowledge, skill, and judgment which might be expected of another physician in the same locality and under similar circumstantes. It is extremely important that no *express* promise of a cure be made, for this then becomes a part of the contract.

The patient's part of the agreement includes the liability for payment for services and a willingness to follow the advice of the doctor.

## Statute of Frauds

Some contracts, in order to be enforceable, must be in writing. One of these is the promise to pay the debts of another. Thus, if a third party, not legally responsible, agrees to pay a patient's medical bills, the agreement cannot be enforced unless it is in writing. Any agreement which cannot be completed within one year from the date of the contract must be in writing.

## Good Samaritan Acts

The physician is sometimes reluctant to fulfill his ethical obligation to render aid in an emergency to someone who is not his patient, for fear he may later be charged with negligence or abandonment by a total stranger. In 1959, California passed the first Good Samaritan Act, and many other states have followed suit. Although there are minor variations in the state statutes, their purpose is to protect the physician from liability for any civil damages as a result of rendering emergency care, provided such care is given in good faith and with due care under the circumstances. In some states the law applies to nurses as well as to physicians. In at least two states, Texas and Wyoming, the statute extends to all persons. There is no creation of a contract in giving emergency care.

## Controlled Substances Act of 1970

Prior to April, 1968, physicians practiced their professions primarily under the Narcotic Acts and the Drug Abuse Control Amendments. Under the Harrison Narcotic Act, physicians registered with the Internal Revenue Service, which issued narcotic stamps with the physician's registration number and also issued the order form books to physicians.

On April 8, 1968, the Federal Bureau of Narcotics in the Treasury Department and the Bureau of Drug Abuse Control in the Food and Drug Administration merged into a new agency known as the Bureau of Narcotics and Dangerous Drugs (BNDD), located in the Department of Justice. From April, 1968, to May, 1971, the new Bureau operated under the laws and regulations of the two former agencies.

On May 1, 1971, the new Controlled Substances Act of 1970 became fully effective, replacing the former Narcotic Acts and the Drug Abuse Control Amendments. In October, 1973, the regulatory agency became known as the Drug Enforcement Administration. The Internal Revenue Service no longer registers physicians, nor do they issue order forms. Both of these functions are now carried out by the Drug Enforcement Administration (DEA). Physicians are required to register with the Registration Branch, Drug Enforcement Administration, P. O. Box 28083, Central Station, Washington, D.C. 20005, or the nearest regional office. If a physician has more than one office in which he administers and/or dispenses any of the drugs listed in the five Schedules, he is required to register at each office. However, if he only administers or dispenses at his principal office and only writes prescriptions at the other office or offices, he then is only required to register at his principal office where he administers or dispenses. (NOTE: The word "physician," as used in this Act, means any physician, dentist, veterinarian, or other practitioner authorized to administer, dispense, and prescribe controlled substances.)

Under the Controlled Substances Act, drugs are categorized into Schedules I, II, III, IV, and V. Schedule I drugs are those that have *no* accepted medical use in treatment in the United States. A physician will have no concern with Schedule I unless he is involved in conducting research with such drugs. Regulations regarding the writing, telephoning, and refilling of prescriptions vary according to which Schedule is involved. The physician and his assistant must keep abreast of regulations as they are issued.

### RECORDS UNDER THE ACT

**Narcotic Drugs.** A physician who *prescribes* and/or *administers* narcotic drugs in the course of his professional practice *is not* required to keep records of those transactions. If a physician *dispenses* a narcotic drug to a patient, he *is* required to keep a record of such dispensing.

**Non-Narcotic Drugs.** A physician who regularly engages in dispensing any of the non-narcotic drugs listed in the Schedules to his patients as a regular part of his professional practice, and for which he charges his patients either separately or together with other professional services, must keep records of all such drugs received and dispensed. The records must be kept for a period of two years and are subject to inspection by the D.E.A.

If the physician only occasionally dispenses a non-narcotic controlled drug to a patient (such as a physician's sample) he is not required to maintain a record of such dispensing.

**Inventory.** A physician who is required to keep records as stated above must take an inventory every two years of all stocks of controlled drugs on hand. The first inventory was required on May 1, 1971. A physician who registered after May 1, 1971 should take the initial inventory when he first engages in dispensing. He must keep this record for two years; he is *not* required to submit a copy to the D.E.A.

**Order Forms.** A physician who has need for controlled drugs in Schedule II for use in his office or medical bag must obtain these drugs by the use of a triplicate order form. Order forms are obtained from the D.E.A. at no charge to the physician. The Federal Triplicate Order Forms should not be confused with the triplicate prescription blanks that are required by some states.

**Security.** A physician who has controlled substances stored in his office or clinic must keep these drugs in a locked cabinet or safe. Any loss of controlled drugs by theft must be reported to the regional office of the D.E.A. at the time the theft is discovered. The local police department should also be notified.

**Discontinuance of Practice.** A physician who discontinues his practice must return his Registration Certificate and any unused order forms to the nearest office of the D.E.A. The regional office of the D.E.A. in his area will advise him on how to dispose of any controlled drugs still in his possession.

## Uniform Anatomical Gift Act

A Uniform Anatomical Gift Act was approved by the National Conference of Commissioners on Uniform State Laws on July 30, 1968. Although many states had passed laws prior to this time that permitted a living person to make a gift of his body or portions of it after death, the laws were so different from state to state that arrangements for a donation in one state might not be recognized in another.

By 1970, at least 44 states had enacted laws that were reasonably similar and followed the model act in all major respects. Essentially, the model law for donation states that: (1) any person of sound mind and 18 years of age or over may give all or any part of his body after death for research, transplantation, or placement in a tissue bank; (2) a donor's valid statement of gift is paramount to the rights of others except where a state autopsy law may prevail; (3) if a donor has not acted during his lifetime, his survivors, in a specified order of priority, may do so; (4) physicians who accept organs or tissues, relying in good faith on the documents, are protected from law suits. The physician attending at the time of

## UNIFORM DONOR CARD

OF_____
Print or type name of donor

In the hope that I may help others, I hereby make this anatomical gift, if medically acceptable, to take effect upon my death. The words and marks below indicate my desires.

I give:  (a) _____ any needed organs or parts

(b) _____ only the following organs or parts

_____
Specify the organ(s) or part(s)

for the purposes of transplantation, therapy, medical research or education;

(c) _____ my body for anatomical study if needed.

Limitations or
special wishes, if any :_____

Signed by the donor and the following two witnesses in the presence of each other:

_____     _____
Signature of Donor                            Date of Birth of Donor

_____     _____
Date Signed                                         City & State

_____     _____
Witness                                               Witness

This is a legal document under the Uniform Anatomical Gift Act or similar laws.

**Figure 5–1**

death, if acquainted with the donor's wishes, may dispose of the body under the Uniform Anatomical Gift Act; (5) the time of death must be determined by a physician who is not involved in the transplantation, and the attending physician cannot be a member of the transplant team; (6) the donor may revoke the gift or the gift may be rejected. The most important clause permits the donation to be made by a will (without waiting for probate) or by other written or witnessed documents, such as a card designed to be carried on the person (Fig. 5–1).

The provisions of the Uniform Anatomical Gift Act are so designed that the offer is exercised only after death. Therefore, the donor should reveal his intentions to as many of his relatives and friends as possible, including his physician. Also, since the human body or its parts are not commodities in commerce, no money can be exchanged in making an anatomical donation. Additional details about organ and tissue donations and donor cards may be obtained from the National Kidney Foundation, 315 Park Avenue South, New York 10010.

## Securing Patient's Consent

A physician must have consent to treat a patient, even though this consent is usually implied by virtue of the fact that the patient chooses a particular physician to treat him. Consent may be express or implied, oral or written.

In *Medicolegal Forms with Legal Analysis,* the American Medical Association explains some of the implications of consent in this way:

> Usually authority to treat or operate arises from the valid consent of the patient or someone authorized to act in his behalf. A statute in Georgia (Georgia Code, Chapter 88–29), enumerates those who may consent to treatment for themselves or for others. The consent given may be either express or implied and, if express, it may either be written or oral. The consent given must be an informed consent with an understanding of what is to be done and of the risks involved. The procedure involved and its attendant risks should be explained to the patient in understandable nontechnical terms. The consent given may be invalid (a) because the act consented to is unlawful, (b) because the consent was given by one who had no legal right to give it, or (c) because it was obtained by misrepresentation or fraud.

Sometimes, if a physician fails to secure some formal expression of consent, he can be charged with trespass or assault and battery. The American Medical Association's Law Division states that "a prudent physician will demand a written consent or authorization with respect to any operation which involves an element of recognized danger to the patient or which requires hospitalization." This is desirable in order to avoid misunderstandings which can lead to lawsuits; it also facilitates proof when necessary.

Forms on which a patient can grant written consent for operations or other procedures are kept in most physicians' offices. Figures 5–2 and 5–3 illustrate a general form of consent to operation.

(*Text continued on page 56.*)

---

### Form P-1

### CONSENT TO OPERATION, ANESTHETICS, AND OTHER MEDICAL SERVICES[9]

Date_____Time_____ A.M.
P.M.

1. I authorize the performance upon _____
                                      (*myself or name of patient*)

of the following operation _____
                           (*state nature and extent of operation*)

to be performed by or under the direction of Dr._____.

---

Figure 5–2

(*Illustration continued on opposite page.*)

2. I consent to the performance of operations and procedures in addition to or different from those now contemplated, whether or not arising from presently unforeseen conditions, which the above-named doctor or his associates or assistants may consider necessary or advisable in the course of the operation.

3. I consent to the administration of such anesthetics as may be considered necessary or advisable by the physician responsi-

ble for this service, with the exception of _____
*(state "none," "spinal anesthesia," etc.)*

4. The nature and purpose of the operation, possible alternative methods of treatment, the risks involved, the possible consequences, and the possibility of complications have been ex-

plained to me by Dr._____ and by_____.

5. I acknowledge that no guarantee or assurance has been given by anyone as to the results that may be obtained.

6. I consent to the photographing or televising of the operations or procedures to be performed, including appropriate portions of my body, for medical, scientific or educational purposes, provided my identity is not revealed by the pictures or by descriptive texts accompanying them.

7. For the purpose of advancing medical education, I consent to the admittance of observers to the operating room.

8. I consent to the disposal by hospital authorities of any tissues or body parts which may be removed.

9. I am aware that sterility may result from this operation. I know that a sterile person is incapable of becoming a parent.

10. I acknowledge that all blank spaces on this document have been either completed or crossed off prior to my signing.

**(CROSS OUT ANY PARAGRAPHS ABOVE
WHICH DO NOT APPLY)**

Signed _____
*(Patient or person authorized
to consent for patient)*

Witness_____

**Figure 5–2** *Continued.* (From *Medicolegal Forms with Legal Analysis. 3rd Ed.* Office of the General Counsel, 1973, p. 57. Copyright © 1973. American Medical Association.)

## Form P-2

## CONSENT TO OPERATION, ANESTHETICS, AND OTHER MEDICAL SERVICES (ALTERNATE FORM)[10]

A.M.

Date_____Time_____P.M.

1. I authorize the performance upon _____
   *(myself or name of patient)*

of the following operation _____
   *(state name of operation)*

to be performed under the direction of Dr. _____.

2. The following have been explained to me by Dr._____:

   A. The nature of the operation _____
      *(describe the operation)*

   _____

   _____

   B. The purpose of the operation_____
      *(describe the purpose)*

   _____

   C. The possible alternative methods of treatment _____

   _____

   *(describe the alternative methods)*

Figure 5-3

*(Illustration continued on opposite page.)*

D. The possible consequences of the operation _____

_____
*(describe the possible consequences)*


E. The risks involved _____
*(describe the risks involved)*

_____


F. The possibility of complications _____

_____
*(describe the possible complications)*

3. I have been advised of the serious nature of the operation and have been advised that if I desire a further and more detailed explanation of any of the foregoing or further information about the possible risks or complications of the above listed operation it will be given to me.

4. I do not request a further and more detailed listing and explanation of any of the items listed in paragraph 2.

Signed _____
*(Patient or person authorized*
*to consent for patient)*

Witness_____

**Figure 5–3** *Continued.* (From *Medicolegal Forms with Legal Analysis. 3rd Ed.* Office of the General Counsel, 1973, p. 59. Copyright © 1973. American Medical Association.)

A patient must be of legal age and be in full possession of his faculties to give consent for an operation. The legal age will vary from state to state; sometimes a girl of eighteen who is married is considered legally of age, for example. If the patient is a minor, the consent of a parent or the acting guardian is necessary, except in the case of an emancipated minor.

No consent is necessary if a person is dangerously ill and unconscious and his life is in danger. The physician can use his best judgment in proceeding with treatment. However, consultation is advisable in such cases.

Voluntary non-therapeutic surgical sterilization is lawful in some states, and such operations are permissible for the purpose of family limitation motivated solely by personal or socioeconomic consideration. It is recommended that for every such procedure the physician should obtain from the patient and the spouse, if any, a signed, written informed consent. See Figure 5–4.

---

## Form P-17

## REQUEST FOR STERILIZATION[15]

A.M.
Date_____ Time_____P.M.

We, the undersigned husband and wife, each being more than twenty-one years of age and of sound mind, request Dr.

_____, and assistants of his choice, to perform upon

_____, the following operation: _____.
(name of patient)        (state nature and extent of operation)

It has been explained to us that this operation is intended to result in sterility although this result has not been guaranteed. We understand that a sterile person is NOT capable of becoming a parent.

We voluntarily request the operation and understand that if it proves successful the results will be permanent and it will thereafter be physically impossible for the patient to inseminate, or to conceive or bear children.

Signed_____
(Husband)

Signed_____[16]
(Wife)

Witness_____

---

**Figure 5–4**  (From *Medicolegal Forms with Legal Analysis. 3rd Ed.* Office of the General Counsel, 1973, p. 69. Copyright © 1973. American Medical Association.)

## Keeping Complete Records

To protect the doctor from malpractice actions, it is important to keep ideal medical records which could be taken to court if necessary to show that the care and treatment given fully met standards of law and medical practice. For this reason details should be fairly complete on medical records and dates upon which treatment was given indicated. Sometimes it is necessary to make a correction or change in a record. This should be done by lightly crossing out the part to be changed and inserting the correction. If any patient fails to keep an appointment, discontinues treatment before he should, or fails to follow advice, the medical record should show this information. The doctor should write to these patients, advising of the importance of continued medical treatment, and include copies of all such letters in the patient's record. Samples of these letters are reproduced in Figures 5–5, 5–6, and 5–7.

## Legal Responsibility of the Medical Assistant

What is the responsibility of the medical assistant for any acts which she performs while working for a physician? This is a question of vital importance to anyone who is employed in a doctor's office.

**Agent of Employer.**   The medical assistant, while acting within the scope of her employment, is considered an "agent" of her employer. If she would say to a

---

### Form B-1

### LETTER TO CONFIRM DISCHARGE BY PATIENT

Dear Mr. _____:

This will confirm our telephone conversation of today in which you discharged me from attending you as your physician in your present illness. In my opinion your condition requires continued medical treatment by a physician. If you have not already done so, I suggest that you employ another physician without delay. You may be assured that, at your request, I will furnish him with information regarding the diagnosis and treatment which you have received from me.

Very truly yours,

_____, M.D.

**Figure 5–5**   (From *Medicolegal Forms with Legal Analysis. 3rd Ed.* Office of the General Counsel, 1973, p. 5. Copyright © 1973. American Medical Association.)

---

## Form B-3

## STATEMENT OF PATIENT LEAVING
## HOSPITAL AGAINST ADVICE

This is to certify that I am leaving _____ Hospital at my own insistence and against the advice of the hospital authorities and my attending physician. I have been informed by them of the dangers of my leaving the hospital at this time. I release the hospital, its employees and officers, and my attending physician from all liability for any adverse results caused by my leaving the hospital prematurely.

Signed_____ [2]

I agree to hold harmless the _____ Hospital, its employees and officers, and the attending physician from all liability, with reference to the discharge of the patient named above.

_____
*(Husband, wife, parent, etc.)*

Date _____

Witness_____

---

**Figure 5–6** (From *Medicolegal Forms with Legal Analysis. 3rd Ed.* Office of the General Counsel, 1973, p. 6. Copyright © 1973. American Medical Association.)

patient, "Go right to the hospital; Dr. White will see you there," then Dr. White is bound by contract to do so.

Generally, the law holds that every person is liable for the consequences of his own negligence when another person is injured as a result. In some situations this liability also extends to the employer. Physicians may be held responsible for the mistakes of those who work in their offices and sometimes must respond in damages for their negligent acts.

The physician is legally responsible for the acts of his assistants or employees when they are acting within the scope of their duties or employment. He is also responsible for the acts of those who assist him, even though they are not directly employed by him, if they commit acts of negligence while under his immediate supervision and in his presence. For example, a nurse who is a hospital employee makes an error in a procedure while acting under a physician's direction. The court may determine that she came so completely under the direction and supervision of the physician that the physician is liable for her negligence. This is known as the doctrine of *respondeat superior* (let the master answer). When doctors practice as partners, each partner is liable not only for his own acts and those

## Form B-5

### LETTER TO PATIENT WHO
### FAILS TO KEEP APPOINTMENT

Dear Mr. _____:

   On _____, 19____, you failed to keep your appointment at my office. In my opinion your condition requires continued medical treatment. If you so desire, you may telephone me for another appointment, but if you prefer to have another physician attend you, I suggest that you arrange to do so without delay. You may be assured that, at your request, I am entirely willing to make available my knowledge of your case to the physician of your choice.
   I trust that you will understand that my purpose in writing this letter is out of concern for your health and well-being.

Very truly yours,

_____, M.D.

## Form B-7

### LETTER TO PATIENT WHO FAILS TO FOLLOW ADVICE

Dear Mr. _____:

   At the time that you brought your son, William, to me for examination this afternoon, I informed you that I was unable to determine without X-ray pictures whether a fracture existed in his injured right arm. I strongly urge you to permit me or some other physician of your choice to make this X-ray examination without further delay.
   Your neglect in not permitting a proper X-ray examination to be made of William's arm may result in serious consequences if in fact a fracture does exist.

Very truly yours,

_____, M.D.

**Figure 5–7**   (From *Medicolegal Forms with Legal Analysis. 3rd Ed.* Office of the General Counsel, 1973, p. 7. Copyright © 1973. American Medical Association.)

of his partner but also for the negligent acts of any agent or employee of the partnership.

American Medical Association attorney George Hall has written, "The things a medical technician does in the employ of a hospital or laboratory are really acts of the hospital or laboratory and as such the hospital or laboratory is liable for any damages caused by the technician during the performance of regular duties." According to Hall, this liability works no injustice on the employer. It is based upon the policy of protection of the third person. After all, the employer made it possible for the employee to cause the injury in the first place. The employer holds out his employees as competent and, in effect, warrants their conduct in all matters within the scope of employment.

**Need for Extreme Care.**   A medical assistant who is guilty of negligence is liable for her own actions, but the injured party generally sues the physician since there is a better chance of collecting from him. However, even if the assistant has no money, she can still be liable for her actions. This fact should indicate the continuing importance of exercising extreme care in performing all duties in the professional office. While working under pressure there is always the danger she may interchange blood, serum, or medications, or mix names or improperly prepare labels. Never proceed with administration of a medication or treatment without checking all details at least twice, and preferably three times.

**Rechecking Equipment.**   The doctor and his staff should frequently check the condition of all office equipment and make use of every available safety installation to prevent accidents to patients. Each assistant should be alert for potential hazards, such as slipping rugs, exposed telephone and light cords, highly waxed floors, and protruding objects, since patients who are harmed as a result of these things can sue for damages.

**Illegal Practice of Medicine.**   There are certain other medicolegal aspects of her work which the assistant must understand. The doctor goes to school many years to learn his profession; he is licensed by his state to practice medicine. *The assistant is not licensed to practice medicine.* She must never prescribe, even though she feels she knows what the doctor would order. This is unlawful. She must never try to diagnose a patient's ailment. This, too, is the illegal practice of medicine. As a result, it is not good policy for the assistant to discuss patients' ailments with them. Patients tend to identify the assistant's every remark with the doctor himself.

**Instructions to Patient.**   Both the doctor and his staff must be extremely careful in giving instructions to patients. If the patient misunderstands the instructions, the physician may have a malpractice suit on his hands. When written instructions can be provided, this should be done.

**Examinations of Women.**   Except in an actual emergency, the physician should not examine a female patient unless a third person is present. The charge of undue familiarity against a doctor is very damaging. That is why the assistant generally will stand by when the doctor performs such examinations.

**Emergency Aid.**   The question sometimes arises: should the assistant give emergency care to a patient brought into the office while the doctor is away? The assistant, as any other layman, in a medical emergency may do whatever is reasonably necessary provided that the action taken is within her skill and competence. The physician should instruct his assistant regarding what course of action he wishes her to take in such instances. She must immediately get in touch with the doctor or another physician to care for the patient, once she has performed any emergency measures.

**Claims Prevention.** It is not expected that the medical assistant will know all the legal ramifications of the practice of medicine; nor should she develop an attitude of skepticism. The majority of patients never entertain the thought of legal action against their physicians. She should be aware, however, of her role in "claims prevention."

The American Medical Association Committee on Medicolegal Problems in 1963 set forth 21 prevention "commandments." Many of these commandments require the active cooperation of the medical office assistant. They are set forth here for your study and frequent review:

1. The physician must care for every patient with scrupulous attention given to the requirements of good medical practice.

2. The physician must know and exercise his legal duty to the patient.

3. The physician must avoid destructive and unethical criticism of the work of other physicians.

4. The physician must keep records which clearly show what was done and when it was done, which clearly indicate that nothing was neglected, and which demonstrate that the care given met fully the standards demanded by the law. If any patient discontinues treatment before he should, or fails to follow instructions, the records should show it; a good method is to preserve a carbon copy of the physician's letter advising the patient against an unwise course.

5. The physician must avoid making any statement which constitutes, or might be construed as constituting, an admission of fault on his part. He should instruct employees to make no such statements.

6. The physician must exercise tact as well as professional ability in handling his patients and should insist on a professional consultation if the patient is not doing well, if the patient is unhappy and complaining, or if the family's attitude indicates dissatisfaction.

7. The physician must refrain from overly optimistic prognoses.

8. The physician must advise his patients of any intended absences from practice and recommend, or make available, a qualified substitute. The patient must not be abandoned.

9. The physician must unfailingly secure an "informed" consent (preferably in writing) for medical and surgical procedures and for autopsy.

10. The physician must carefully select and supervise assistants and employees and take great care in delegating duties to them.

11. The physician must keep abreast of general medical and scientific progress.

12. The physician should limit his practice to those fields which are well within his qualifications.

13. The physician must frequently check the condition of his equipment and make use of every available safety installation.

14. The physician should make every effort to reach an understanding with his patient in the matter of fees, preferably in advance of treatment.

15. The physician must realize that it is dangerous to diagnose or prescribe by telephone.

16. The physician should not sterilize a patient solely for the patient's convenience, except after a reasonably complete explanation of the procedure, its risks and possible complications, and after obtaining a signed consent from the patient and the patient's spouse, if the patient is married. Such sterilization is a crime in Connecticut, Kansas, and Utah, and should not be performed in those states. Eugenic sterilization should be performed only in conformity with the law of the state, if any exists. Sterilization for therapeutic purposes may lawfully be performed with the informed consent of the patient and preferably with the informed consent of the patient's spouse, if the patient is married.

17. Except in an actual emergency situation which makes it impossible to avoid doing so, a male physician should not examine a female patient unless an assistant or nurse, or a member of the patient's family, is present.

18. The physician should exhaust all reasonable methods of securing a diagnosis before embarking upon a therapeutic course.

19. The physician should use conservative and less dangerous methods of diagnosis and treatment whenever possible, in preference to highly toxic agents or dangerous surgical procedures.

20. The physician should read the manufacturer's brochure accompanying a toxic agent to be used for diagnostic or therapeutic purposes, and, in addition, should ascertain the customary dosage or usage in his area.

21. The physician should be aware of all the known toxic reactions to any drug he uses, together with the proper methods for treating such reactions.

## REFERENCES

American Medical Association, *Professional Liability and the Physician*, Chicago, American Medical Association, 1963

American Medical Association, *Medicolegal Forms with Legal Analysis*, Chicago, American Medical Association, 1973

Black's Law Dictionary, Revised 4th Edition, 1968

California Medical Association, *Professional Liability*, San Francisco, California Medical Association, 1971

Hayt, E., Hayt, J., and A. H. Groeschel, *The Law of Hospital, Physician and Patient*, New York, Hospital Textbook Co., 1952

Regan, L. J., and A. R. Moritz, *Handbook of Legal Medicine*, St. Louis, C. V. Mosby Company, 1956

Stetler, J. and A. R. Moritz, *Doctor and Patient and the Law* (4th Ed.) St. Louis, C. V. Mosby Company, 1962

U.S. Dept. of Justice, Bureau of Narcotics and Dangerous Drugs: *Practitioners Informational Outline of the Controlled Substances Act of 1970*, 1972

# GLOSSARY OF LEGAL TERMS

**Administer**        To instill a drug into the body of a patient.

**Agent**        A person authorized by another to act for him; one entrusted with another's business.

**Assault**        An intentional, unlawful attempt of corporal injury to another by force.

**Battery**        A willful and unlawful use of force or violence upon the person of another.

A surgical operation is a technical "battery" regardless of its result, and is excusable only where there is express or implied consent by the patient.

**Breach**        The breaking or violating of a law, right, or duty, either by commission or omission.

**Breach of Duty**        In a general sense, any violation or omission of a legal or moral duty.

**Burden of Proof**        The necessity or duty of affirmatively proving a fact or facts in dispute on an issue raised between the parties in a cause.

**Civil Law**        That division of municipal law which is occupied with the exposition and enforcement of civil rights as distinguished from criminal law.

**Contributory Negligence**        The act or omission amounting to want of ordinary care on the part of the patient, which, concurring with defendant's negligence, is proximate cause of injury.

**Criminal Case**        An action suit, or cause instituted to punish an infraction of the criminal laws.

**Defendant**        The person defending or denying; the party against whom relief or recovery is sought in an action or suit.

**Deposition**        Sometimes used as synonymous with oath, but the term is specifically applicable to the testimony of a witness taken in writing, under oath or affirmation, before a judicial officer, in answer to oral or written interrogatories.

| | |
|---|---|
| **Dispense** | The giving of drugs, in some type of bottle, box or other container, to the patient (under the Controlled Substances Act of 1970, the definition of "dispense" also includes the administering of Controlled Substances). |
| **Emancipation** | A term principally used with reference to the emancipation of a minor child by its parents, which involves an entire surrender of the right to the care, custody, and earnings of such child, as well as a renunciation of parental duties. |
| **Ethics** | That branch of moral science which treats of the duties a member of a profession owes to the public, to his colleagues, and to his patient or client. |
| **Expert Testimony** | Testimony given in relation to some scientific, technical, or professional matter by experts, i.e., persons qualified to speak authoritatively by reason of their special training, skill, or familiarity with the subject. |
| **Feasance** | The doing of an act; a performing or performance. |
| | *Malfeasance.* The doing of an act which is wholly wrongful and unlawful. |
| | *Misfeasance.* The improper performance of some act which a man may lawfully do. |
| | *Nonfeasance.* The omission of an act which a person ought to do. |
| **Felony** | A crime of a graver or more atrocious nature than those designated as misdemeanors. Generally, an offense punishable by imprisonment in a penitentiary. |
| **Grievance Committee** | A committee established by a local medical society to hear and investigate the complaints of patients respecting professional care rendered by an attending physician or allegedly excessive fees charged by him. |
| **Invasion of Privacy** | The right of privacy is the right to be "left alone" to live in seclusion without being subjected to unwarranted or undesired publicity. Thus, without the knowledge and authorization of the patient, there should be no publication of his medical case record and no showing of a photograph or motion picture from which the identity of the patient is determinable. |

**Judgment** The official decision of a court of justice upon the respective rights and claims of the parties to an action or suit therein litigated and submitted to its determination.

**Judicial** Relating to or connected with the administration of justice.

**Jurisprudence** The philosophy of law, or the science which treats of the principles of positive law and legal relations.

**Liable** Bound or obliged in law or equity; responsible; chargeable; answerable; compellable to make satisfaction, compensation, or restitution.

**Litigation** Contest in a court of justice for the purpose of enforcing a right.

**Locum Tenens** "Holding the place." A deputy, substitute, lieutenant, or representative.

**Negligence** The omission to do something which a reasonable man, guided by those considerations which ordinarily regulate human affairs, would do, or the doing of something which a reasonable and prudent man would not do.

**Non Compos Mentis** Not sound of mind; insane. This is a very general term, embracing all varieties of mental derangement.

**Plaintiff** The person who brings an action; the party who complains or sues in a personal action and is so named in the record.

**Prescribe** To issue a prescription for the patient. To direct, designate, or order use of a remedy.

**Proximate Cause** That which, in a natural and continuous sequence, unbroken by any efficient intervening cause, produces the injury, and without which the result would not have occurred.

**Prudence** Carefulness, precaution, attentiveness, and good judgment, as applied to action or conduct. That degree of care required by the exigencies or circumstances under which it is to be exercised.

**Qui Facit per Alium Facit per se** "He who acts through another acts himself."

**Res Gestae**          "Things done." Res gestae is considered as an exception to the hearsay rule. In its operation it renders acts and declarations which constitute a part of the things done and said admissible in evidence, even though they would otherwise come within the rule excluding hearsay evidence or self-serving declarations.

**Res Ipsa Loquitur**   "The thing speaks for itself."

**Res Judicata**        A matter adjudged; a thing judicially acted upon or decided; a thing or matter settled by judgment.

**Respondeat Superior** "Let the master answer." This maxim means that a master is liable in certain cases for the wrongful acts of his servant, and a principal for those of his agent.

**Statute**             An act of the legislature declaring, commanding, or prohibiting something. This word is used to designate the written law, in contradistinction to the unwritten law.

**Statutory**           Relating to a statute; conforming to a statute.

**Subpoena**            A writ or order directed to a person and requiring his attendance at a particular time and place to testify. It may also require him to bring with him any books, documents, or other things under his control which he is bound by law to produce in evidence (subpoena duces tecum).

**Suit**                A generic term, of comprehensive signification, applicable to any proceeding by one person or persons against another or others in a court of justice, in which the plaintiff pursues, in such court, the remedy which the law affords him for the redress of an injury or the enforcement of a right, whether at law or in equity. The term is seldom applied to a criminal prosecution.

**Suspend**             To interrupt; to discontinue temporarily, but with an expectation or purpose of resumption.

**Tort**                A private or civil wrong or injury.

Section Two

# The Administrative Assistant

# Chapter 6

**CHAPTER OUTLINE**
Introduction
A Sample Day
Office Procedure Manual

**BEHAVIORAL OBJECTIVES**

*The medical office assistant should be able to:*

Describe a sample day in a physician's
office.
Develop a plan for a procedure
manual for a physician's office.

# Planning Your Work

A smoothly run office is a well-planned office in which work and time are organized. There's a recurrent success formula, heard at sales meetings, which applies no less to the medical assistant. *Plan your work; then work your plan!*

The busy medical assistant must budget her on-the-job time, not only to make the most of every minute but to make her work pleasant and conserve energy. Wasted motion is wasted effort. The best way to get more hours — productive hours — in your day, without actually staying overtime, is to have your office arranged efficiently, your day well planned, and each individual task simplified as much as possible. This is not to say that your day can be arranged to the last detail. This would be dull, indeed. But a well-organized medical assistant can handle the unexpected without going into a tailspin, because she moves easily from one task to another without wasting energy.

## A SAMPLE DAY

First, let us examine a hypothetical average day in a professional office. Because offices vary greatly, and duties differ with each individual office, it is not possible to set a hard and fast pattern for all to follow.

Be prompt in arriving at the office, at least ten minutes before the actual time you are to start. A nine o'clock job does not mean you arrive at nine sharp and then change into your uniform and take care of your make-up. It means that by nine o'clock you are neatly dressed, the office is well aired, the sterilizers turned on, and a quick check has been given the reception room. Don't forget to unlock the front door if you have entered by another entrance.

Call the telephone exchange service and ask about the calls that have been handled by them. Make the necessary notes on these calls to provide to the doctor.

You may now open the mail and sort it as instructed in the chapter on how to handle mail. This is also a good time to organize your records and correspondence. Most medical offices are fairly quiet in the morning while the doctor is making hospital and home calls, so you may do the bookkeeping without too many interruptions.

After you have finished the daily books you can make out the bank deposit slips and check the previous day's cash. The mornings are also a good time to do as much typing as possible if your desk is located in the reception room. Also, collection telephone calls can be made while the office is empty. Try each day to have completed the previous day's business before your employer arrives and the reception room is full of patients. This way you will be able to give your doctor and his patients your full attention and assistance.

Just before your boss arrives check his office for any last-minute attention. Have the mail well organized on his desk; messages should be neat and easily understood and typed if possible. An outline of the appointments and the patients' case histories may be placed in their proper position on his desk. Work with your doctor in organizing a system to start the day, then follow it carefully. Variations are good in vacations, but not in a pattern of daily office routine.

Remember to take a recheck of the reception room and also your personal appearance before patients begin to arrive.

After the doctor arrives take a few moments to list the patients who have been seen outside the office since the previous day. Go over the list of messages with him and get your instructions.

Now it is time to concentrate on the patients. Usher in the first patient and start whatever preparations are necessary. The rules of organization and planning are extremely important in running the "back office." Remember to check each room after a patient leaves and tidy it up. The sterilizer should be checked about four times a day for water. Stop occasionally and consider the room temperatures and the freshness of the air.

Usually the back office duties keep the afternoon well filled. You should never find idle time on your hands. Routine bookkeeping that does not require too extensive concentration may be left for the quiet moments in the afternoon.

After the last patient has gone, take a few minutes to go over the events of the day with your boss. He may wish to dictate some case histories, sign some letters, or give you special instructions regarding the next day's work. Before you leave the office make certain all the doors and windows are carefully locked. The cash box should be placed safely away and the case histories should also be stored out of sight. Go from room to room with a watchful eye. Turn off the sterilizers and open them. Close drawers and cupboards. Clear table tops of unnecessary equipment. Turn off any electrical equipment. Very often a physician is called upon to return to his office outside of regular hours, and he should find it neat and clean with the equipment ready for use.

The efficient medical assistant will develop her own system and daily schedule of duties suited to the peculiarities of her own office and employer. The mark of a good employee is to have her work so well organized that the office will continue to run smoothly during her absence, not fall apart because one individual is gone a few days.

## THE OFFICE PROCEDURE MANUAL

Ideally, every office should have a written procedure manual. Such a guide will not only make the medical assistant's own work easier but will be invaluable during vacation periods or unexpected absences, as well as for the new employee. If your office does not have such a manual, suggest that one be prepared for approval by your employer.

You can develop your own procedure manual as you gain experience in your office. What should your manual contain? It starts with a "job description"—a detailed account of just what is expected of you on your job. It might be divided into three categories: administrative, clinical, and general duties. After the *what* part of the job description has been outlined, you should detail the *how* of each duty. For instance, if the job description lists the duty "Process Incoming Mail," you may expand this into:

Sort incoming mail by class: third and second class, money receipts, first class, personal mail.

Open all mail except letters marked "personal."

Set aside cash receipts for processing.

Arrange mail with second and third class on bottom, then first class, with any personal mail on top.

Place entire stack on right-hand side of doctor's desk.

And don't forget the *when* part of the instructions. Instead of a simple statement such as "deposit receipts at bank," be more explicit:

Deposits are made every day (twice a week; every Friday) at First Citizens Bank, Tenth and Broadway.

The doctor permits extending your lunch period 15 minutes on banking days.

The procedure manual should include a chapter on general office policies, such as the doctor's office hours, the assistant's office hours, lunch period and break time, holidays observed, vacation policy, sick leave, and salary increments.

Preferred office procedures, both front and back, should be spelled out in detail. How are records prepared and filed? A description of the filing system may save the day if a temporary employee must find something for the doctor during your absence. What kind of setup does the doctor prefer for various office surgeries or treatments? Is there a card index showing these setups? If so, where is it kept?

How is the telephone to be answered? Which calls are put through to the doctor immediately, and which may the assistant handle? How much time is allotted for new patients? Old patients? Postoperative patients?

Have a page explaining where and how supplies are ordered, and where they're stored. The name, address, and telephone number of each supplier should be included. List the major pieces of equipment with their serial numbers, where purchased, and whom to call for servicing.

Explain your billing and collection procedures. Is billing done weekly, twice monthly, monthly? Are the statements individually typed? Do you use a collection agency? Which one?

Keep a record of any personal duties the doctor expects of his assistant: organizational activities, travel arrangements, shopping for gifts. Professional information regarding your employer's education and specialty boards, his membership in professional societies, his state license number, and his narcotic registry number belongs in the manual. Remember, the new employee or the temporary help will not know these things.

A check list for daily, weekly, monthly, quarterly, and yearly duties, such as the one illustrated, can be an invaluable aid to the old-timer as well as the new employee.

**Dr.** _____ **Day** _____ **Date** _____

### ACTIVITIES

**DAILY DUTIES:**

TO DO                    SEQUENCE   DONE

PATIENTS TO WORK INTO TODAY'S
APPOINTMENT SCHEDULE IF POSSIBLE

- OPEN AND HANDLE INCOMING MAIL
- TIDY THE OFFICE
- CHECK SUPPLIES & LAUNDRY
- STERILIZE INSTRUMENTS
- PREPARE DAILY ROSTER OF PATS.
- CK. LAB & X-R CASES FOR TODAY
- ARRANGE HOSPITAL ADMISSIONS
- PREPARE REPORTS FOR REF. DRS.
- TYPE CORRESPONDENCE
- MAKE TELEPHONE CALLS TO:
- _____
- _____
- POST YESTERDAY'S CHARGES & PAYMENTS
- REFILE YESTERDAY'S CHARTS
- PULL CHARTS FOR TOMORROW
- CHECK BUDGETS DUE YESTERDAY
- PREPARE BANK DEPOSIT SLIP

NAME                 TELEPHONE

**WEEKLY DUTIES:**
- PREPARE SALARY CHECKS
- POST RCPTS. & DISBMTS. TO LEDGER

**MONTHLY DUTIES:**
- RECONCILE CKBK. TO BANK STATE.
- FOLLOW-UP ON DELINQUENT ACCTS.
- PREPARE PROFIT & LOSS STATE.
- PREPARE & SEND STATEMENTS
- SEND AUDIT NOTICES OR COLLN. LETTERS
- PAY CURRENT BILLS BEFORE 10TH OF MO.
- TALK WITH MGT. CONS. OR ACCT. ON NEXT VISIT HERE
- _____
- _____

TODAY'S PATIENTS TO CALENDAR
FOR FUTURE APPOINTMENTS

NAME                 APPT. DATE

**QUARTERLY DUTIES:**
- PREPARE QUARTERLY SS & WT FORMS
- PREPARE UNEMP. & DISAB. INS. FORMS
- AGE THE OUTSTANDING ACCTS.
- FOLLOW-UP ON LIAB., WK. COMP. & INS. FORMS
- TALK WITH MGT. CONS. OR ACCT. ON NEXT VISIT HERE
- _____
- _____

**YEARLY DUTIES:**
- PICK UP YEARLY TAX ITEMS NOT IN CKBK.
- CK. WITH DR. RE VACATION PERIODS
- PREPARE XMAS CARD LIST & SEND CARDS
- SEE THAT #1040 TAX FORMS, ETC., IN MAIL
- SHOP FOR PROFESSIONAL XMAS GIFTS
- GO THROUGH FILES AND FINALIZE OLD MATERIAL

**STAT DUTIES:**
- CHECK LAUNDRY SUPPLY
- ORDER FOLLOWING OFFICE SUPPLIES:
- _____
- _____
- ORDER FOLLOWING PROF. SUPPLIES:
- _____
- CHECK MIMEOGRAPH FORMS
- CALL HOSPITAL RE.
- _____
- CALL EMPLOYMENT AGENCY RE:
- CALL FOLLOWING PATIENTS CANCLG. APPTS. (OR WORK FOLLOWING PATIENTS IN TO APPT. SCHED.)
- _____
- _____
- _____
- _____
- _____

| | TODAY | YEAR TO DATE |
|---|---|---|
| No. Patients Seen | | |
| Total Charges | | |
| Total Pymts. Rcvd. | | |
| No. Lab Tests | | |
| Charges, Lab. | | |
| No. X-Rays | | |
| Charges, X-Ray | | |
| No. New Patients | | |
| (Add'l Stat. Inform.) | | |

**Figure 6-1** Activities sheet for a one-girl office.

In offices with more than one assistant, a procedure manual will clearly define the responsibilities of each. There will be times when one assistant is too busy to take care of all her responsibilities and another will wish to help out. A well-planned office guide will make this easier and help to create a more harmonious office, with all working toward the common good.

It is not possible in one brief chapter to provide a complete guide for your office manual. These few suggestions will give you an idea of how to start. Each is an individual production, but the medical assistant, as a faithful employee, has a responsibility to share the experience she gains on the job with other present or future employees of her doctor.

# Chapter 7

**BEHAVIORAL OBJECTIVES**

*The medical office assistant should be able to:*

Compare the utilization of time in offices using (a) scheduled appointments and (b) no scheduled appointments.

Choose an appropriate appointment book for a particular office.

Apply efficient guidelines for scheduling appointments.

Adjust a schedule interrupted by an emergency or delay.

Determine appropriate procedures for handling callers who do not have appointments.

Schedule appointments for procedures required outside the office.

# Scheduling Appointments

One of the most important duties which the doctor delegates to his assistant is the scheduling of appointments. In most offices, the appointment book is the hub around which all activity revolves. Properly controlled, the appointment book can be a highly useful device for running the office smoothly. Improperly controlled, it can become either an overly stern taskmaster, or an ineffectual mechanism of little or no consequence in the operation of the office. The effectiveness of the appointment book is determined by (a) the skill the medical assistant develops in using it and (b) the effort the doctor himself exerts in abiding by the schedule.

## IMPORTANCE OF TIME MANAGEMENT

When the physician delegates responsibility for the appointment book to his assistant, he is in effect saying, "Here, manage my time, a most precious commodity which must be used well but never wasted."

Management of the schedule is a two-pronged responsibility: first, arranging the schedule; second, keeping the schedule operating smoothly. The first part will be dealt with in this chapter; the second in Chapter 8 on reception techniques.

There are two opposing views among physicians on the utilization of office time—*open office hours* with no appointments vs. *scheduled appointments.*

**Open Office Hours.**   A minority of physicians prefer to keep open office hours rather than schedule appointments. This tendency is more common in rural areas where the general population, although consisting of busy people, is not governed so much by the clock as by the sun and the weather. It is made generally known that the doctor is in his office at given hours of the day. He most probably "schedules" his patients by saying something like "come back in a couple of weeks." On a day convenient for the patient, he comes in and waits his turn to see the doctor. The patient knows ahead of time that he may have a considerable wait and takes it in his stride. Physicians who use this method say that it eliminates the annoyance of broken appointments and "running late." The assistant in this kind of office need not worry much about how much time to allow per individual patient.

**Scheduled Appointments.**   Studies have shown that physicians are able to see more patients with less pressure when they schedule appointments. It does have its hazards, however. The patient who is given an appointment may feel that if only a few minutes were needed for the examination or treatment, he is entitled to the "rest of the time allotted to him," regardless of the number of people waiting in the reception room. Some patients need *more* time than was planned. They may have told the assistant of one complaint when making the appointment, but "discover" additional complaints when they are being examined by the doctor. Judicious scheduling will keep most of the inherent hazards to a minimum.

## THE APPOINTMENT BOOK

**Choose the Right Kind.**　Planning the schedule must start with an appointment book that suits the practice. Appointments for the solo practitioner who sees a very limited number of patients per day may be entered on an ordinary desk calendar; appointments for a busy, multiple-doctor practice cannot. So choose the book carefully. There are standard styles designed for physicians readily available. It is also fairly simple to get an individualized design for a specific practice. But in either case there are certain features to watch for. The appointment book should

1. Conform to the size of desk space available
2. Be large enough to accommodate the practice
3. Open flat
4. Allow space for *when, who,* and *why*

A looseleaf, undated appointment book has many advantages. It can easily be tailored to a specific practice and it permits smooth transition to the next month or year.

**Establish the Matrix.**　Each page in the book should have three columns, one each for *when, who,* and *why.* Block off in advance, in pencil, those periods when the doctor is routinely not available to see patients (days off, holidays, hospital rounds, lunch, meetings, and so forth). Use the *who* or *memo* column to show the reason for blocking out these spaces. Always try to account for every time period in each day.

If your doctor keeps you informed of his social engagements, write them at the bottom of the appointment sheet. If his wife is giving a dinner party, or has tickets for a theatre engagement, she'll appreciate your getting him out of the office on time that day.

## GUIDELINES FOR SCHEDULING

There can be no hard and fast rules for scheduling appointments efficiently. The system to be used must be individualized to the specific office, and the doctor's own preferences and habits. There are, however, certain general basic considerations to be observed in every practice: patient need, doctor's preferences, and available facilities.

**Patient Need.**    Time must be allotted to patients on the basis of each one's particular needs. What is the purpose of the visit? What is the age of the patient? A teenager will probably not require as much time as his grandparent will. Will the patient require the *doctor's* time for the entire visit or will another member of the staff be performing part or all of the service? Is the patient the mother of several schoolchildren who likes to schedule her appointments during the school hours? If an attempt is made to make the appointment suit the convenience of the patient, one possible cause for complaint is eliminated.

**Doctor's Preferences.**    Is the doctor methodical and careful about being in the office when patient appointments are scheduled to begin? Or must you allow for his being late? Does he move easily from one patient to the next or must you allow a "break" time for him? If he would rather see fewer patients and spend more time with each one, then that is his prerogative — but it must be taken into account in the scheduling. Some doctors become restless if the reception room isn't packed with waiting patients; others worry if one patient is kept waiting. All these personal preferences and habits become an integral part of the scheduling problem.

**Available Facilities.**    There's no point in getting a patient into the office at a time when no facilities are available for the service he needs. For instance, suppose in a two-physician office that there is only one room which can be used for minor surgery. You wouldn't schedule two patients requiring minor surgery to come in at the same time, even though both doctors could be available. If there is only one sigmoidoscope, the intelligent medical assistant will not book a second sigmoidoscopy immediately following a similar examination. She will provide time for cleaning and sterilization procedures, and for readying the examination room. With some knowledge of the patients' needs, the medical office assistant attempts to pair those needs with the available facilities in an open time slot.

**Double Booking.**    The office assistant who books two patients concurrently, both of whom are to be seen by the doctor, is fooling only herself. Of course, if each is expected to take only five minutes or so, there is no harm in telling both to come at two o-clock, and reserve a 15-minute period for the two. But if each one will require 15 minutes, two will require 30 minutes no matter how their names are written in the book. The average patient who has an appointment, say at three o'clock, does not like to discover another patient in the reception room who also has an appointment at three o'clock.

It is not "double booking" if a patient comes to the office for a treatment or injection from the nurse. In a case such as this, the office assistant should briefly say, when she calls this patient in from the reception room, "You may come in now; the nurse can take care of you," or "You were not to see the doctor today; the nurse will take care of you." A comment such as this reveals no medical information about the patient but does let the waiting patients know that this patient is not being shown preference in seeing the doctor.

**Advance Booking.**    When booking appointments weeks or months ahead, make it a policy to leave some open time during each day's schedule. Then, if a patient calls with a somewhat acute problem which is not an immediate emergency, you won't have to tell him, "We don't have any time open until next month." The busy doctor will always be able to fill these appointments, and no

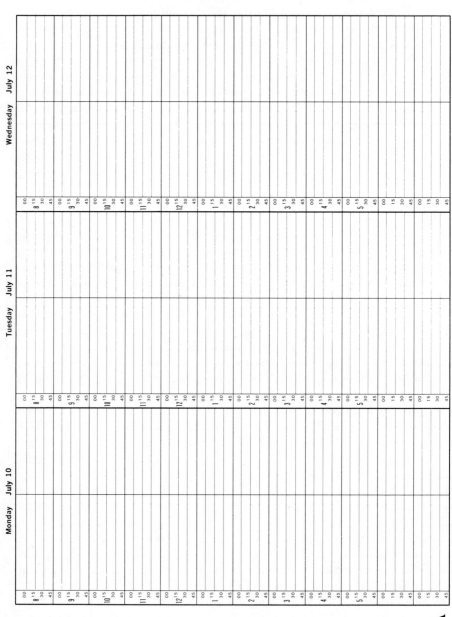

**Figure 7-1** Styles of appointment books. **A,** for a two-doctor practice; **B,** for a three-doctor practice. (Courtesy of the Colwell Co., Champaign, Ill.)

(Illustration continued on opposite page.)

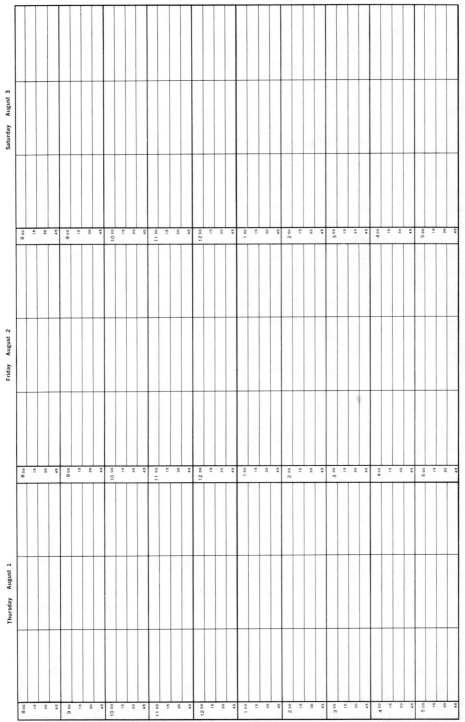

**Figure 7-1** *Continued.*

time will be lost, but his patients will appreciate that it is possible to see their doctor within a reasonable time when the circumstances warrant.

It may be a good idea, if possible, to set time aside in the morning and afternoon for a breather. Even 15 or 20 minutes will give the doctor an opportunity to return calls from patients, O.K. prescription calls, or answer questions you may have that were not an emergency; this is especially necessary in pediatrics and obstetrics.

## EXCEPTIONS TO APPOINTMENT SYSTEM

The day that goes along according to schedule, without having to make any adjustments in the plan, is the exception in some offices rather than the rule. The medical office assistant realizes there are certain situations that will require an immediate adjustment in the schedule.

**Emergency Patients.**   If someone telephones to report an emergency that can be seen or treated in the office, the medical office assistant will have no hesitancy in having the patient come immediately. However, she must be sure it really is an emergency, and not just a patient who has suddenly decided this is the day he wants to see a doctor. Before such a situation arises, the assistant should have reached some agreement with her doctor on what kinds of emergencies he will see in the office, his criteria for determining whether it is an emergency, and what steps the assistant should take. Until you have had a chance to discuss this with your doctor here are some questions you might ask:

Is there bleeding?
Where is the blood coming from?
What is the patient's temperature?
Are there chills?
Is there nausea or vomiting?
If there is pain, is it steady or intermittent?
Is it severe? sharp? dull?
How long have the symptoms been present?

The application of first aid and emergency care for cases that present in the office is discussed in Chapter 33. Here we are concerned mainly with the telephone caller who reports an emergency and requests to be seen.

**Acutely Ill Patients.**   Patients can't always give advance notice of when they will need a doctor. There is a fine line that can be drawn between an emergency patient and the acutely ill patient, but the latter should be seen as soon as possible. At the very least, let the physician decide whether the patient should be seen immediately or whether he can safely wait. The 15- to 20-minute breather time you saved in the middle of the morning and afternoon may save your schedule.

**Physician Referrals.**   If another physician telephones and requests that a patient be seen by your doctor today, this is another exception you will have to make. Most physicians recognize the importance of keeping a schedule and will not be inconsiderate in this respect (you'll soon learn to recognize the few who are).

## HANDLING CANCELLATIONS AND DELAYS

**When the Patient Cancels.** If the patient cancels an appointment on a day that is heavily booked and you're already behind schedule, you'll probably just feel grateful. But suppose it's a fairly light day and you don't want to let that time be wasted. If you've formed the habit of keeping a list of patients with advance appointments who wanted to come in sooner, get busy on the telephone and try to get one of them in to fill that available time.

**When the Doctor is Delayed.** Inevitably, there are days when the doctor is delayed in reaching the office. If you have advance notice of this you can start calling those patients with early appointments and suggest they come later. If some have already arrived before you learn of the delay, you will have to explain that an emergency has prevented the doctor from getting in. You must show concern for the patient, but avoid being over-apologetic. This would imply some degree of guilt feeling. Most patients realize that a doctor has certain priorities, and that the patient who is able to be in the office may be inconvenienced but it is not a life-and-death matter. If this kind of situation occurs frequently, though, you may have to devise a different scheduling system or have a talk with your doctor about it.

**When the Doctor is Called Out on Emergencies.** All physicians are conscious of their responsibilities for responding to medical emergencies. Most patients will be sympathetic to such occurrences if the assistant will take time to explain what has happened. You can say something like this: "Dr. Wright has been called away to answer an emergency. He asked me to tell you he is very sorry to keep you waiting. He will be gone at least an hour. Do you wish to wait? If it is inconvenient, I'll be glad to give you another appointment that will be more convenient. Or perhaps you'd like to have some coffee or do some shopping and return in an hour."

In the meantime, head off patients scheduled for a later hour. In many offices, especially those of obstetricians, surgeons, and general practitioners, it is sometimes necessary to cancel a whole day's appointments. For this reason it is particularly important that you have the telephone number of each patient available so that you can cancel the appointment and make a new one. If it is at all possible, cancel appointments before the patients arrive in the office to find that the doctor is not in.

**The Doctor is Ill or is Called Out of Town.** Although it comes as a shock to most patients, physicians do get ill, too. The patients who are scheduled to be seen during the course of the doctor's expected absence must be informed of this. They need not be told the nature of his illness. It is customary to provide the patient with the name of another physician, or possibly a choice of several, who will take care of the doctor's patients during his absence. The physician may be called out of town for personal or professional reasons, and his appointments will have to be canceled.

## FAILED APPOINTMENTS

Some patients are forgetful about appointments. If you detect this tendency in a patient, form the habit of telephoning him the day before his appointment to remind him, or send a postcard timed to arrive a day or two in advance of his appointment. If your office consistently runs behind schedule, with patients being kept waiting for an hour or two, the patient whose own time is well planned may simply decide he doesn't have time today to come and sit in your office. Perhaps you gave him an appointment at a time that really was not agreeable to him. Or if you have been pressing a patient for payment he may stay away because he is unable to pay on that day. Try to determine the reason for failed appointments and do what you can to remedy it. Anyone can forget an appointment once, but if broken appointments occur frequently, you will be wise to reexamine your appointment system to see where the problem lies.

Legally, a patient may be charged for an uncanceled appointment which he has not kept. However, few doctors attempt to collect for such occasions. The risk of poor public relations such a procedure engenders is too great; it generally results in a lost patient. Some other way must be found to handle failed appointments if they become a problem.

A notation should be made in the patient's record if an appointment is not kept and the patient is seriously ill. The doctor should also be told of this unkept appointment. This may be a legal consideration at some later date. In some cases it may be necessary for the doctor or the assistant to call and remind the patient that an unkept appointment may have serious results on the patient's health.

## MAKING THE APPOINTMENT

Many return appointments are arranged while a patient is in the office. The patient's first appointment, though, was probably made by telephone, as are more than 50 per cent of all appointments. Pleasantness on the part of the assistant who sets up the appointment is extremely important, whether the encounter is in person or by telephone.

**In Person.** As the patient is leaving the office, the physician will probably ask him to stop by the desk and make his next appointment. While you reach for your pencil and the appointment book, *look* at the patient and say something like this: "Will next Thursday, the 8th, at ten o'clock be satisfactory?" Avoid asking the question, "When would you like to come in?" Chances are this will only open up a debate and the patient will finally decide on a time that you don't have available anyway. Write his name in the book, in pencil, followed by his telephone number, and hand the patient a completed appointment card (after you have double checked the date and time with your book), along with your best smile.

**By Telephone.** It is as important for the assistant to express pleasantness and her desire to be helpful when she uses the telephone as it is when she meets patients face to face. This is particularly essential in the arranging of appointments, since it is often the manner in which the booking is made rather than the actual time of the appointment which is important to the patient.

Study the principles of telephone technique as set forth in Chapter 9, Effective Telephone Practices. Be especially considerate if you must refuse an appointment for the time requested. Explain why and offer a substitute time and date. Comply with the patient's desires as much as possible and do not show impatience if a few patients are not understanding of the problems involved in scheduling appointments. Most people do appreciate the need for a well-managed office and are willing to cooperate. End the conversation pleasantly with something like this: "Thank you for calling, Mrs. Albright. Dr. Wright will see you next Wednesday, the 18th, at two-thirty. Goodbye." This little courtesy adds to the patient's feeling of esteem, along with reinforcing the time of the appointment. While you are saying this, you should be rechecking your appointment page to be certain you have written it in the right time slot on the right day.

**Appointments for New Patients.** Arranging the first appointment for a new patient requires a bit more time and attention to detail. Check carefully the correct spelling of the name by repeating or spelling it back. Obtain the address, the telephone number where the patient can be reached, the patient's age, and the name of the referring doctor or individual. If possible, determine the nature of the visit so that the proper amount of time can be allotted on the appointment book.

If another physician has referred the patient, the assistant may need to call his office and obtain additional information for her employer. This information should be typed and given to the doctor in advance of the patient's arrival.

**Special Problems.** Probably every doctor has a few patients who are habitually late for appointments. This seems to be a congenital problem for which no cure has yet been found; consequently, you must find a way of booking this patient without disrupting your entire schedule. One way of handling this is to book the patient as the last appointment of the day. Then if closing time arrives before he does, you need feel no obligation to wait for him. Some assistants simply tell the patient to come in a half hour earlier than the time they actually write in the book. The point to remember is that you must learn to work around this patient, with the realization that in all likelihood he is not going to change.

When a former patient returns after a lengthy absence, the medical assistant should recheck the address, telephone number, and employment information. If the appointment is made by telephone, be sure to ask for the patient's telephone number. You may need to call him, and you cannot safely assume that he still has the same number. You should also inquire into the nature of the current complaint.

## MECHANICS OF THE APPOINTMENT BOOK

Use a pencil for making entries in the appointment book. Trying to change an entry made in ink is difficult and messy. At the end of the day the names may be written over in ink for a permanent record, if desired.

Always write the patient's name *in full*, last name first, together with the reason for the appointment, *immediately*. DO NOT TRUST TO MEMORY. Be sure to cross off sufficient time for the appointment. It's a good idea to write the patient's telephone number after every entry in the appointment book. You may have to cancel or rearrange that day's schedule in a hurry, and many precious minutes can be saved if you don't have to look up each patient's telephone number.

Sometimes changes must be made in the appointment schedule. For instance, the patient who has a three o'clock appointment next Monday calls and asks to have this changed to one week later. You find an opening at three o'clock on the following Monday and write in the patient's name, but in your haste you fail to cross out the first appointment. Someone else looking at the appointment book (or possibly even yourself a couple of days later) will either expect the patient on both days or be unable to determine *which* day she is expected. Avoid this embarrassing situation by making it a habit to cross out or erase the first appointment *before* writing in the new one.

You may have a patient who requires a series of appointments, say at weekly intervals. Try to set up the appointments on the same day of each week, at the same time of day if possible. This considerably reduces the risk of a forgotten appointment. A calendar that shows the dates several months in advance at a glance is useful to have on or near the appointment desk.

## APPOINTMENT CARDS AND REMINDERS

Most offices use appointment cards to remind patients of appointments, as well as to eliminate misunderstandings about dates and times. There are many styles of such cards. Samples of appointment cards are shown in Figure 7–2.

Make a habit of reaching for an appointment card while making an entry in the appointment book. After you have written the date and time on the appointment card, double check with the book to see that the entries agree. Some offices mail cards to patients who have made appointments several weeks in advance. Patients who telephone for appointments also can be sent reminder cards.

Some patients like to be sent reminders of when they are to return to see the doctor. A simple way of handling this is to have a supply of postal cards on hand; while he is still in the office, have the patient write his name and address on one; then file it in your tickler under the date it is to be mailed.

## PATIENTS WITHOUT APPOINTMENTS

The assistant often is faced with this question: What shall I do about patients who arrive without an appointment? There are a number of suggested procedures, but the policy in your office must be agreed upon by the doctor and then carried out by the assistant.

If the patient requires immediate attention, he must be fitted into the schedule somehow. If his case does not need immediate care, he can be given a short visit with the doctor and asked to schedule an appointment at a time when the doctor can devote more attention to his complaints.

The assistant should always make it clear, even when sending patients without appointments in to see the doctor, that the office runs on an appointment basis. She can say, for example:

"The doctor will be able to see you now, but we would appreciate it very much if you would make an appointment for your next visit." Or,

"The doctor can see you now. I'm sorry you had to wait so long. Perhaps it will be possible for you to make an appointment the next time."

Patients should be told as gently as possible that appointments save not only the doctor's time but theirs as well. Emphasize to these patients that the doctor will be able to give them his full attention and more time on the next visit if an advance appointment is made.

It is important to remember one thing, however. Don't play favorites in sending patients in to see the doctor. If you're "found out" by the other waiting patients, their esteem for the doctor, as well as for you, will decline rapidly.

## OTHER CALLERS

**Pharmaceutical Representatives.**  Also known as "detail men," representatives from leading pharmaceutical houses are frequent visitors to physicians' offices and are generally welcomed by the doctor if his schedule permits. They are well trained and bring the doctor valuable information on new drugs. The assistant is often able to screen such visitors and turn away those who would have nothing to offer her employer. If the assistant does not know the caller, she may ask for his card, then check with the doctor and let him decide whether or not he wishes to see the caller.

If the doctor is in a specialty practice or limits his callers to a few selected pharmaceutical houses, the medical assistant can ask him to help her prepare a list of the representatives whom he will see, time permitting. Then, when a detail man arrives at the office, she can quickly tell, by consulting her list, whether she should try to work him in. The detail man who knows he is not on the list for a particular doctor will also appreciate the saving in time for him. Most representatives say they would rather be told outright if the doctor does not wish to see them rather than be given some evasive reply.

The pharmaceutical representative is willing to wait patiently a long while for just a brief visit with the doctor. The assistant can tell him whether or not the doctor can see him that day, give him an idea of how long he will have to wait, or suggest a later time at which he can return. He can then make his own decision as to whether he wishes to wait or return later. The pharmaceutical representative is usually quite understanding and cooperative. The assistant should in turn treat him with courtesy and give him as much cooperation as possible. In some cases, she herself can accept the literature or materials for the doctor and make sure he receives it.

**Physicians.**  When another physician calls at your doctor's office, he should be ushered in to see the doctor as soon as possible. He should not be kept waiting, regardless of your previous appointment schedule. If the physician arrives when your doctor is seeing a patient, explain this to him and, if possible, take him into an inside room so that the doctor can see him as soon as he is finished with the patient. If this is not convenient for the visiting doctor, make arrangements for him to see the doctor at an acceptable time. When another doctor has been ushered into an inside room or is waiting in the reception room, tell your employer at once. The visits of other physicians are usually brief, since these men have heavy schedules of their own to maintain.

APPOINTMENT

FOR M_____

_____AT_____O'CLOCK

LEONARD S. TAYLOR, M.D.

2100 WEST PARK AVENUE          TELEPHONE
CHAMPAIGN, ILLINOIS  61822          367-6671

PLEASE LEAVE THIS SLIP WITH RECEPTIONIST

DATE_____

PATIENT_____

OFFICE CALL . . . . _____

HOUSE CALL . . . . . _____

SURGERY . . . . . _____

INJECTION . . . . . _____

DRUGS . . . . . . _____

LABORATORY . . . . _____

TOTAL . . . _____

NEXT APPOINTMENT _____

. . . . . . . . . . . . . . . . . . . . . . . . . . . . . . . . . . . . . . . . . . .

FRANK F. LEONE, M.D.
1025 PARK AVENUE
UTICA, NEW YORK  13501

DATE_____

REC'D
OF_____

_____DOLLARS

PER_____

**Figure 7-2**  Styles of appointment cards. (All cards courtesy of the Colwell Co., Champaign, Ill.)

(*Illustration continued on opposite page.*)

M_____

HAS AN APPOINTMENT WITH

LEONARD S. TAYLOR, M.D.
2100 WEST PARK AVENUE
CHAMPAIGN, ILLINOIS 61822
———
TELEPHONE 367-6671

FOR

MON._____AT_____

TUES._____AT_____

WED._____AT_____

THURS._____AT_____

FRI._____AT_____

SAT._____AT_____

IF UNABLE TO KEEP THIS APPOINT-
MENT KINDLY GIVE 24 HOURS
NOTICE.

# COMBINATION CARDS

TELEPHONE 367-6671

LEONARD S. TAYLOR, M.D.

**FRONT**

OFFICE HOURS          2100 WEST PARK AVENUE
BY APPOINTMENT          CHAMPAIGN, ILLINOIS 61822

**BACK**

APPOINTMENT

FOR M_____

_____AT_____O'CLOCK

IF UNABLE TO KEEP THIS APPOINTMENT KINDLY GIVE 24 HOURS NOTICE.

**Figure 7-2** *Continued.*

**Salesmen.** Salesmen from medical and surgical supply houses call regularly at physicians' offices. Sometimes they will want to see the doctor, but if the assistant is in charge of ordering supplies she may be able to handle this herself. Unwelcome salesmen sometimes constitute a problem in the professional office. If the physician does not wish to see such a caller, the assistant must firmly but tactfully send him away. She can suggest that such callers leave their literature and cards for the doctor to study and say that the doctor will contact them if he desires further information. Persistent salesmen can be dispatched with alacrity if they ignore a polite "no" merely by suggesting that perhaps they would like to schedule an appointment — at the doctor's customary fee!

**Miscellaneous.** From time to time, other callers appear in the doctor's office. Some are civic leaders seeking the doctor's aid in community projects. Others may be ministers, insurance men, solicitors for fund drives, and so forth. Most doctors inform their assistants of their general policy in regard to seeing such callers. Check with your employer in advance on procedure to follow in such instances.

Civic leaders should be treated with courtesy and consideration when they telephone or enter the office. Every doctor has a real responsibility to take an active part in community affairs. However, no doctor can participate in *all* activities. Often, he delegates to his assistant the responsibility for accepting or refusing such community appointments for him. In this event, she must use discretion and exercise complete tact and courtesy. Disgruntled community leaders who are turned away with a terse refusal do not help create good medical public relations. If it is necessary to refuse such callers, be sure to explain that the doctor would be happy to cooperate but that he is already participating in such community projects as the Boy Scouts, Kiwanis, and the Health Council, and his schedule does not permit him to accept additional responsibilities. The same rule regarding the exercise of tact, courtesy, and consideration should always apply to every caller in a doctor's office.

## APPOINTMENTS OUTSIDE THE OFFICE

There are other appointments that the assistant will make, and which will appear on the appointment book, such as scheduled surgery at the hospital, consultations at the hospital or at another physician's office, house calls at extended care facilities or in the home. The doctor must have time to get from one place to another, so be sure to allow for traveling time when arranging these appointments.

**Scheduling Surgeries.** You may be responsible for scheduling surgeries. In most hospitals you should call the secretary in surgery *first* when your doctor plans an operation. Give the surgical secretary the date and time the doctor prefers, the type of surgery to be performed, and the approximate time he will require. After the date and hour have been established, give the patient's full name, sex, age, and telephone number; also any special requests the doctor may have, such as the amount of blood to have available. Be sure you have all this information at hand before placing the call. It may also be the responsibility of the assistant to arrange for the surgical assistant, the anesthesiologist, and the bed reservation.

Procedures vary in different areas and different hospitals, but the assistant will soon learn how her doctor's surgeries are to be handled. Some hospitals request the patient to complete a preadmittance form so that all records can be processed before the patient is admitted. Be sure the patient receives adequate admitting instructions.

**House Calls.** If your doctor regularly makes house calls you probably set aside a special block of time for this on your appointment schedule. If it's only an occasional event, though, be sure to check with the doctor before committing him to make the call. He may decide after learning all the details that the patient can come into the office, or that the patient should go to the hospital. In speaking with the patient be sure to get all the pertinent details — name and address of patient, telephone number, best way to reach the home, nearest cross street, and name of person making the request. Again, traveling time must be allowed for.

**Outside Appointments for Patients.** Your doctor may ask you to arrange laboratory or x-ray appointments for patients. Before calling the laboratory or x-ray facility, determine from the physician the exact procedure he wants done, whether expediency is a factor, and whether he wants a stat report. Also ask the patient if there is any time he *cannot* have the procedure done. With this information before you, you can set up the appointment with confidence. When you inform the patient of the time, you can also give him any special instructions that may be necessary. Then be sure to note these arrangements on the patient's chart, and place a follow up reminder on your tickler or desk calendar.

## REFERENCES

American Medical Association, *Winning Ways with Patients,* Chicago, Illinois, American Medical Association, 1966

Cotton, H., *Aid for the Doctor's Aide,* Oradell, New Jersey, Medical Economics Book Division, Inc., 1963

# Chapter 8

**BEHAVIORAL OBJECTIVES**

*The medical office assistant should be able to:*

Create an attractive personal appearance through good grooming habits.

Create and maintain a reception room that will appear attractive and cheerful to the patients.

Manage effectively patient flow in the physicians's office.

Direct the smooth operation of an appointment schedule.

Control interpersonal relations in the reception area.

# Your Role as Receptionist

Appearances and first impressions mean a great deal in any situation. This is especially true in the physician's office, where an atmosphere of cleanliness and order must prevail. The kind of impression that the doctor's assistant makes upon his patients often colors their impressions about the doctor himself or his office. If the patient feels friendly toward the assistant, he'll probably feel friendly toward the doctor.

## FIRST IMPRESSIONS

**The Assistant.**  A neat, attractive assistant has a good psychologic effect upon patients. The three most essential aspects of an attractive appearance are:

1. Good health
2. Good grooming
3. Good taste

Good health means getting plenty of sleep, eating balanced meals, and getting sufficient exercise to keep fit. No crash diets or all-night orgies for the medical assistant, just a sensible regimen of healthful living and a regular checkup at least once each year.

The medical assistant usually wears a uniform. This gives her a fresh, professional look and identifies her as a member of the team. She is no longer limited to the traditional white, however. Modern fabrics and styling in uniforms have made it possible for the office assistant to be attractive, as well as practical. Her "uniform" may be a pantsuit, in white or color, or perhaps with contrasting top and pant. She may wear a two-piece dress-type uniform in white or color, or she may choose an attractive design in the traditional white dress uniform. Some physicians, particularly pediatricians, often prefer that their assistants wear pastels. Today's fabrics are so easy to care for, there should be no temptation to wear a uniform a second day without laundering. Even spills and spots which occur during the course of the working day can usually be washed out immediately.

Whatever style of uniform the assistant chooses, it should be one that is becoming to her personally, and should be worn over the proper "underpinnings," without extraneous ornamentation. Keep jewelry to a minimum—only an engagement ring, wedding band, and professional pin—no fluffy handkerchiefs or other adornments.

If there is more than one assistant in the office, name pins worn by everyone in the office help the patient to identify each assistant by name. There are commercial organizations that sell so-called professional pins for medical assistants and grant meaningless certificates of competence. It is best to check with your medical society or the American Medical Association before investing in such items. At present the American Association of Medical Assistants is the only professionally recognized group of medical assistants (see Chapter 1).

Some girls employed in doctors' offices like to wear a white cap. Unless an assistant is a registered nurse or is entitled by graduation from a medical assisting school to wear a special assistant's cap, she should not violate professional etiquette by wearing a cap outside the office.

The shoes she wears should be appropriate for a uniform, spotlessly clean, and comfortable! White shoes worn in the professional office must be *kept* white by daily cleaning. A damp sponge and Ivory soap will take care of quick cleanups during the working day; when you give them a thorough cleaning at night, don't forget that shoestrings need cleaning, too, if you wear a tie shoe.

In some offices the physician prefers that his assistant not wear a uniform. Some psychiatrists, for example, feel that the clinical appearance of a uniform may have an adverse effect upon patients. If you do not wear a uniform, you should still follow the dictates of good taste and appropriateness in choosing your office wardrobe. The high style dress that looked great at last week's party will do nothing to enhance the appearance of the medical assistant at work. The garments worn on the job must be comfortable, becoming, allow easy movement, and still look good at the end of a busy day.

The medical assistant's makeup should be carefully selected and applied. There's no need for the assistant to appear drab just because she is in uniform, but harsh or exaggerated makeup is definitely out of place in the professional office. Subtle eye makeup and discreet shades of nail polish enhance the assistant's appearance; the boldly artificial distracts. The hair should be clean, neatly styled, and off the collar; never allow it to fall untidily around the shoulders.

Good grooming is little more than attention to the details of personal appearance. Personal cleanliness, which includes the daily bath, a good deodorant, and oral hygiene, is vital. A girl who is well groomed looks her best from top to toe: her shoes are polished; stockings are of neutral shade or white; her hemline is even; the costume is well chosen and in good condition; nails are clean; makeup is carefully applied; and her hair is attractively arranged. The personal drawer in her desk should hold extra hose, a clothes brush, spot remover, and a small mirror for checking her appearance occasionally. The assistant who will take that extra few minutes each day to attend to the details of her appearance will make a better impression upon the people with whom she comes in contact.

**The Reception Room.**   Take an objective look around the reception room in your doctor's office every once in a while. Could it use a little brightening or freshening up? It is so easy not to see what we've become accustomed to. The American Medical Association, in its publication *Winning Ways with Patients*, points out that no one who is sick wants to go into depressing surroundings for relief. "Every patient needs the assurance that he is a special important individual. That's why the doctor's reception room should be as comfortable, tidy, attractive and cheerful as you can make it. It should be planned for the patient's comfort and enjoyment while waiting."

Elaborate furnishings, expensive carpeting or draperies are not necessary to achieve the desired effect. Fresh harmonious colors and cleanliness are the basis of an attractive room. Add comfortable furniture, adequate to accommodate the peak load of patients seen each day, and arrange it in conversational groupings rather than around the room so that nervous patients must either stare into one another's faces or keep their eyes on the floor. Then provide good lighting, ventilation, and a regulated temperature for additional comfort, and you have the essentials of an attractive reception room that tells the patient you care. A place to hang coats, rainwear, and umbrellas will help reduce reception room clutter. The over-all effect should be bright and cheerful, or subdued and restful, but never gaudy or depressing.

Plants, pictures, travel posters, and bulletin board displays can add charm and individuality to a reception room. Indoor plants are suitable but fresh flowers may cause allergic reactions. Artificial flower arrangements and plants are now so attractive and realistic it seems impractical to spend time in the care of fresh ones. In some areas, a rental service will provide a new flower arrangement every week or two. One word of caution is in order — don't allow those artificial arrangements to collect dust. Either wipe them off regularly or take time to "dunk" them occasionally.

Most physicians' offices are well supplied with recent magazines in washable plastic covers. Many patients, especially women, like to clip or copy recipes from magazines. Try placing an exotic cookbook or two in the reception area (well identified with your doctor's name) and be sure you have some 3 by 5 cards handy. Another popular diversion is the pictorial travel book. Patients seem to enjoy looking at pictures rather than at something that requires concentrated reading. The reception room, incidentally, is not the proper place for the professional journals your doctor receives.

Some doctors place writing desks and writing paper in the room for the convenience of patients; others play restful music over a concealed speaker. In practices with a large number of children as patients, a children's corner, equipped with small-scale furniture and some playthings, is a good idea. It helps keep youngsters occupied who might otherwise get into mischief. Toys should be easily cleanable; plastic washable ones are especially good. Be scrupulously careful that the toy has no sharp corners that could injure a child, or small parts that could be swallowed. Also, in selecting toys, make sure they will not stimulate the child to make loud noises or create an uproar in the office. And no rubber balls.

Even such additions as a television set, a lighted aquarium, or an educational display of some sort enhance the attractiveness and individuality of the "front door to the doctor's practice."

The assistant is at least partly responsible for the appearance of the reception room. She sometimes has to exert her efforts or enlist the help of the doctor's wife to make reception room improvements that add to the patients' comfort and enjoyment. It is her duty to make sure that the room remains neat and orderly throughout the day. A quick check at intervals during the day and a minute or two devoted to putting the room back to rights help keep it looking its best.

If the assistant's desk is in the reception room or in open view of patients, she should keep it free of clutter. In particular, patients' charts or financial cards should not be in sight. Personal articles, coffee cups, and ashtrays should not be on the receptionist's desk.

## BEFORE THE PATIENT ARRIVES

When the patients start arriving, you want to have everything ready for the day so that you and the doctor can give undivided attention to their needs. If the previous day was a busy one, the supplies in the treatment rooms may have been depleted and instruments may need sterilizing. Your doctor may have had to return to the office to care for a patient during the evening. Check the rooms to make certain that everything is clean, the cabinets well stocked, and everything ready for the first patient of the day. If reserve supplies are kept in another room, you may wish to obtain a hand basket or a cart on wheels so that everything can be carried at one time rather than having to make numerous trips to and fro.

Supplies at your desk should also be checked periodically. Stationery, appointment cards, charge slips, sharpened pencils, and any items you are likely to use during the day should be on hand to avoid needless trips to the supply closet.

If the appointment list was typed before you left last evening, refresh your memory of the patients' names by going over the list now, and place a duplicate copy on your doctor's desk. On this schedule, special notations should be made concerning new patients, special examinations, and so forth. Pull the charts for the patients to be seen that day, noting any special instructions, and place them in the order they are expected to be seen. Laboratory reports, x-ray readings, and any other data concerning the patient's records should also be placed with the history. The assistant should check each history before the physician sees it to make certain that all information has been correctly entered and is up to date. The physician may want the charts placed on his desk, or he may expect the assistant to hand the chart to him as the patient arrives.

This advance preparation will make your day go more smoothly, and contribute toward a more relaxed atmosphere for all who enter.

## ENTER THE PATIENT

Every patient has a right to expect courteous treatment in the doctor's office. No matter what his economic status, each individual who enters the reception room should receive a cordial, friendly greeting.

The assistant can do a great deal to give each patient assurance and a feeling of importance by the manner in which she receives him. Contrast the closed opaque window over a sign that reads "Ring Bell and Be Seated" with the friendly greeting of the assistant: "Good morning, Mr. Barker. I see you are right on time! The doctor will see you in just a few minutes. Won't you sit down? There are some new magazines on the table."

Ideally, the assistant's desk is placed so that she can see all visitors who come into the office. In a one-girl office it is sometimes impossible for the assistant to be on hand to welcome personally each new caller. In this event some announcement system must be worked out. The patient who enters an empty reception room doesn't know whether to sit down or to try to announce his presence in some way. Sometimes a register is placed in the reception room with a sign above it reading: "Please sign the register when you arrive. Doctor will see you shortly." This is a makeshift arrangement, as is the bell advising the patient to ring and be seated. Either of these arrangements is better than no reception at all, but cannot compare with the personal greeting of the assistant.

The importance of the personal touch in receiving patients should not be overlooked. A good receptionist cultivates the habit of greeting each patient in a friendly, self-assured manner. Yet she guards against appearing too effusive, since this sometimes implies insincerity or overfamiliarity. She can introduce herself if the patient is new or greet him with friendliness, calling him by name, if he is a patient she has met before. She tries to become acquainted with each patient by name and to remember something personal about each one, so that on his return visit she can inquire about his garden or the activities of his children. She is careful to learn how to pronounce each patient's name correctly, since incorrect pronunciations offend and irritate people. If the name is unusual it is a good idea to write the phonetic spelling on the history card. This may save embarrassment at future visits.

It isn't wise to appear over-curious about patients' personal lives, but each individual appreciates the interest of the doctor and his staff in his family, hobbies, or work. Sometimes the assistant can jot down key words on the patient's history card that provide her and the doctor with subjects for future conversations. She can get other valuable "conversation pieces" from the pages of the local newspaper.

## PATIENT FLOW

The patient's first question, once he has been received, almost always is "When can I see the doctor?" The assistant should get the patient in to see the doctor as near his appointment time as possible or explain why he must wait. It is her responsibility to convey both her own and the doctor's concern if there will be a delay. The major point to remember is that the patients' time is valuable, too.

It is said that in a well-managed, busy office there are never more than three to five patients in the reception room. When long waits in the doctor's office are eliminated, one of the major sources of complaints by the public about doctors is also eliminated. "Too long a wait in the doctor's office" is one of the most frequently heard condemnations of the medical profession. When a patient complains about medical fees or care he may really be complaining about the long wait or discourteous service.

The claim that a crowded waiting room is an indication of a doctor's popularity may not be true. It may reveal, instead, that the doctor or his assistant is inefficient in scheduling patients. In some rare instance it is a haughty disregard for the patient. Patients don't seem to mind waiting 20 to 30 minutes to see the doctor, but they do consider a wait of more than a half hour excessive.

The experienced medical assistant will keep the appointment schedule operating smoothly by tidying each examining room immediately and moving the next patient in so that the doctor need have no idle moments waiting for a patient to be prepared. It is very inconsiderate, however, to place a patient in an examining room just to get him out of the reception area, and then keep him waiting a long time. Avoid placing a patient on a table, draped in an uncomfortable position, only to be "forgotten" for an hour while the doctor is doing something else. If you think there might be some delay, suggest that the patient take along a magazine or something to occupy his time during the additional wait. Avoid an assembly line atmosphere.

When you do direct a patient to an examining room, take him at least to the door if you can. If the patient is to disrobe, be specific about how much clothing to remove and where to hang it.

You may have to rescue your doctor sometimes from an over-talkative patient. This should be done with the greatest possible tact, by reminding the doctor that his "three o'clock appointment is here now" or his "next patient must leave in half an hour to meet another appointment." Once you learn the patients who take extra time, then you can book them for the end of the day or simply allow more time for them.

## SOOTHE THE WAITING PATIENT

When prolonged waiting is unavoidable, the assistant can help the patients pass the time as pleasantly as possible. This is something of a challenge since most people do not like to wait. Businessmen, for example, who are in the habit of making the most of their time, are particularly resentful at what may appear to them to be inefficient scheduling of appointments.

The assistant can often suggest a particularly good story or article in a magazine to a patient who wants to read. She sometimes can chat briefly with a restless patient. It should, however, be the patient's decision in regard to whether or not he wants to talk. Select conversational subjects which interest the patient—his hobbies, family, business, profession, or recreational interests—and steer clear of controversial subjects such as religion and politics.

The assistant can sometimes increase patients' esteem for the physician by mentioning his hobby or telling about his forthcoming trip to a medical meeting to present a scientific paper. She should also be well versed on such subjects as health insurance, new medical discoveries, local health agencies, and other topics pertaining to medical care which patients may raise during conversation. She can often distribute literature on these subjects from medical organizations to answer patients' questions. Active members of medical assistants' groups keep well informed on such subjects by attending local meetings regularly.

Some personal attention, such as offering a drink of water, presentation of a new magazine, or a brief conversation, sometimes will quiet a patient who is becoming visibly irritated at waiting. If possible, he should be taken into an inner office. Usually one patient can be placed in an examining room and another in a treatment room, while the doctor talks to a third in his office.

Because most patients are fearful and tense, a good assistant tries to divert their attention to reading material or conversation during their wait to see the doctor. She can often put patients in a better frame of mind merely by a friendly smile and show of concern.

## PROBLEM PATIENTS

**The Talker.** There are certain "problem patients" in any professional office. The talker, for example, takes up far more of the doctor's time than is justified. An alert assistant can usually spot these individuals during her initial visit with them. She can check such a patient's card with a symbol to alert the doctor.

A prearranged agreement to buzz the doctor on the intercom at the end of the appointment time, telling him his next patient has arrived, gives him an opportunity to conclude the interview.

**Children.**   Children sometimes present special management problems. It is often advisable for young patients to come into the treatment room without their parents. This, of course, should be at the discretion of the physician.

While this technique of separating children from their parents to treat their needs is not always feasible in every professional office, it sometimes can be applied with great success. In some offices a token of the doctor's friendship such as a trinket or toy, is given the child at the completion of his visit.

**The Angry Patient.**   Every office assistant at some time is confronted with the angry patient. The anger may be simply a reflection of the patient's pain or his fear of what the doctor may discover on his examination. It is usually best to let him talk out his anger. A calm attitude on the part of the medical assistant, with a few remarks interjected in a low voice, will often quiet the patient. Under no circumstances should the assistant return the anger or become argumentative.

**The Patient's Relatives.**   A patient will sometimes be accompanied by a relative or well-meaning friend who may become restless while waiting for the patient and attempt to discuss the patient's illness. The tactful assistant should side-step any discussion that borders on gossip. She should also avoid a too-casual attitude, such as, "I'm sure there's nothing to worry about." A show of moderate concern, offering reassurance that "the patient is in good hands," will usually take care of the situation.

## FRIENDLY FAREWELL

The assistant should be ready to take over the patient as soon as the physician has finished. She can assist the patient in dressing, if necessary, or show her to the powder room. Ask the patient whether she is to have another appointment and, if so, be sure the appointment time is arranged before the patient leaves the office.

If a patient seems hesitant to leave, there may be some problem still on her mind. A friendly offer on the part of the assistant to help or explain a problem will often relieve anxiety and save a telephone call later. The assistant can help convey the impression of friendliness by speeding patients on their way with the same cordiality she would use with guests in her own home. If she has time, she can walk to the door with the patient. She should make certain there are no unanswered questions. If the patient is returning for another visit, the assistant can say, "See you next week." If it is the patient's last visit, say something like "I certainly hope you'll be feeling fine from now on." The assistant may want to tell a patient on his last visit that he has been a fine patient and that it has been a pleasure to serve him. Whatever words of goodbye she chooses, each patient or caller should leave the doctor's office feeling that he or she has received top quality care and has been treated with friendliness and courtesy.

## REFERENCE

American Medical Association, *Winning Ways with Patients,* Chicago, Illinois, American Medical Association, 1966

# Chapter 9

**BEHAVIORAL OBJECTIVES**

*The medical office assistant should be able to:*

Utilize the principles of good telephone etiquette.

Receive, transmit, and record telephone messages.

Recognize the kinds of telephone calls the assistant can appropriately handle.

Recognize the kinds of calls requiring the attention of the physician.

Describe available kinds of telephone answering services.

Plan and place outgoing telephone calls.

List the major features of special telephone equipment.

List the classes of available telegrams and related services.

# Effective Telephone Practices

The telephone is a powerful public relations instrument. Its *proper* use can build a beginning medical practice; its *improper* use can do much to destroy a flourishing one. The physician's office without one or more telephones is difficult to imagine, and the assistant who regards the telephone as a nuisance has no place in the doctor's office.

To the seasoned medical assistant, the ringing telephone is not an unwelcome interruption — it is the lifeline of the office. A patient previously treated may be calling for an appointment or to seek advice; another may be reporting an emergency; a physician may be calling to make a referral; the laboratory may be reporting vital information regarding one of the doctor's patients; a new patient may be making his first contact.

The telephone responsibilities of the medical assistant CANNOT BE OVEREMPHASIZED.

## YOUR TELEPHONE PERSONALITY

To a telephone caller, your voice constitutes your entire personality. He can't see you, your smile, or your facial expression. His impressions of you and the office you represent will be formed only from your voice. What impression *will* you create with your telephone personality? If your voice is warm and friendly, if it sounds confident, if your conversation is courteous and tactful, you will be practicing good public relations and creating a favorable impression with each telephone call you handle. Try to visualize the person to whom you are talking. A small mirror, placed near the telephone, will remind you to smile. Now pretend that each caller is a new patient meeting you for the first time.

Every caller should be made to feel that you have time to attend to his wishes, regardless of how tedious some telephone requests may be. If you are rushed when you pick up the receiver, wait a few seconds until you are able to answer graciously. The person calling does not know you were assisting the doctor or at work in the laboratory; he only infers from your impatient, breathless tone that you resent being bothered by his call.

The assistant should always remember that the office telephone is for business use only and not for her personal use. If a friend calls, it is best to take down the number and graciously say that you will return the call in the evening from your own home. The privilege of monopolizing the office telephone with personal calls does not apply even during lunch hours. The lines to the doctor's office should be clear to receive emergency calls and other calls from patients.

## INCOMING CALLS

### Receiving Calls

You will be receiving many calls during the course of a single day. Each one deserves your most competent attention. Here are a few guidelines to follow in answering all telephone calls.

**Answer Promptly.**   Always answer the telephone promptly, on the first ring if possible. An answer on the first ring helps create an image of efficiency. If you are unable to complete the conversation when you first answer the telephone, you might say, "Will you please hold the line for one moment and I will be with you." Do not pick up the receiver and snap, "Just a minute!" or "Doctor's office, hold please!" When you return to the telephone, make certain you thank the caller for waiting. Of course you would not delay completing a call unless it were absolutely necessary.

**Hold the Instrument Correctly.**   Hold the headset around the middle, with the mouthpiece about one inch from the lips, and directly in front of the teeth. Never hold it under your chin. You can check the proper distance by taking your first two fingers and passing them through sideways in the space between your lips and the mouthpiece. If your fingers just squeeze through, your lips are the correct distance from the telephone and your voice will go over the wires as close to its natural tone as possible. Speak directly into the telephone immediately after removing it from the cradle. If you turn to face a window or another part of the room, make sure the telephone transmitter moves too, or your voice will be lost.

**Develop a Pleasing Telephone Voice.**   What are the qualities of a good telephone voice? And how do you cultivate good voice quality? Here are some tips from the Bell Telephone system:

(1) STAY ALERT.   Give the impression you are wide-awake and alert, interested in the calling person. Let him know he has your full attention.

(2) BE PLEASANT.   Build a pleasant, friendly image for you and your office. Be the "voice with a smile."

(3) TALK NATURALLY. BE YOURSELF.   Use your own words and expressions. Avoid repetition of mechanical words or phrases. Do not use slang. Avoid the temptation to use those impressive medical terms you've recently learned.

(4) SPEAK DISTINCTLY.   Clear, distinct pronunciation and enunciation is vital. Move the lips, tongue, and jaw freely. Talk directly into the transmitter. Never answer the telephone when you are eating or chewing gum.

(5) BE EXPRESSIVE.   A well-modulated voice carries best. Use a normal tone of voice, neither too loud nor too soft. Talk at a moderate rate, neither too fast nor too slow. Vary your tone. It will bring out the meaning of sentences and add color and vitality to what you say.

To develop a good voice, your facial muscles must be trained. These muscles should not be tense, nor should they sag. Do not set your teeth or jaws. The lips should move freely. Proper breathing also contributes to a good voice and helps in enunciation.

Everyone should have the experience of hearing his own voice; it reveals immediately the importance of careful diction. Try putting your voice on tape and listening to a playback. Each word and each sound must be given individual attention in order to achieve clarity. Slurring your words or dropping your voice too much at the end of a sentence can place a strain on your listener. Try to avoid the habit of allowing "ers," "uhs," and long pauses in your conversation. Remember, though, it is seldom necessary to *raise* the pitch of your voice in order to be heard. If a person has trouble being heard, it is generally because he speaks too fast, does not enunciate clearly, or does not speak into the transmitter.

## GUIDES TO GOOD DICTION

| NUMERAL OR LETTER | SOUNDED AS | PRINCIPAL SOUNDS |
|---|---|---|
| 0 | oh | Round and long O |
| 1 | wun | Strong W and N |
| 2 | too | Strong T and long OO |
| 3 | th-r-ee | A single roll of the R and long EE |
| 4 | fo-er | Strong F, long O, and strong final R |
| 5 | fi-iv | I changing from long to short, strong V |
| 6 | siks | Strong S and KS |
| 7 | sev-en | Strong S and V, well-sounded EN |
| 8 | ate | Long A and strong T |
| 9 | ni-en | Strong N, long I, well-sounded EN |
| 10 | ten | Strong T and N |
| J | jay | Strong J and long AY |
| R | ahr | Strong R |
| M | em | Short E and strong M |
| W | dubble-yoo | Full value given to every syllable |
| F | ef | Short E and strong F |

Do not over-accentuate; it causes you to sound artificial. Use a friendly natural style. Few words need to be spelled over the telephone if a person speaks slowly and clearly. Below are key words you can use when it is necessary to verify letters in spelling back over the telephone:

| | | |
|---|---|---|
| A as in Adams | J as in John | S as in Samuel |
| B as in Boston | K as in Katie | T as in Thomas |
| C as in Charles | L as in Lewis | U as in Utah |
| D as in David | M as in Mary | V as in Victor |
| E as in Edward | N as in Nellie | W as in William |
| F as in Frank | O as in Oliver | X as in X-ray |
| G as in George | P as in Peter | Y as in Young |
| H as in Henry | Q as in Queen | Z as in Zebra |
| I as in Ida | R as in Robert | |

A telephone conversation necessarily involves two persons. We put a great deal of stress upon rules for speaking, but we often neglect the importance of good listening. The same attention should be given a telephone conversation that would be given a face-to-face conversation. Concentration is not always easy; it must be practiced. It is annoying to a caller to have to repeat himself because the assistant did not listen closely to his original statement.

**Identify Yourself.** The telephone should never be answered with just "Hello." Your response should identify first the office, and then yourself. There are several variations of telephone greetings that can be used, which you will probably wish to discuss with the doctor, but your response might be something like this: "Doctor Black's office—Miss Anderson." If the doctor's surname is fairly common to your area, you may wish to use his given name also to provide further identification, saying, "Dr. Sherman Black's office—Miss Anderson."

The use of salutations in telephone identifications is optional. Sometimes the addition of "Good morning" or "Good afternoon" to the identification is awkward. A rising inflection or a questioning tone in your voice will indicate interest and a willingness to assist, and eliminate the need for an additional greeting.

If there are two doctors in the office, both names should be included in the identification. Say "Doctors Smith and Taylor," or "Doctors Taylor and Smith's office." Some names will not blend smoothly; then you must modify the identification so that it will be easy to say and easy to understand. Keep in mind the reason for answering the phone by using the doctor's name. You are telling the caller he has reached the correct number. If callers frequently ask you to repeat, you must analyze the failure to communicate and modify your response in some way. Some authorities suggest preceding the identification with the words "This is ... " by saying "This is Dr. Black's office," theorizing that the first two words are probably lost on the listener, and he will only begin to hear you when you have reached "... Dr. Black's office."

Answering an office telephone merely by repeating the telephone number is even less desirable than saying "Hello." The caller will invariably ask, "Is this Doctor Black's office?" Rarely can a person immediately recall the number he has just dialed. Time is wasted, the caller is psychologically rebuffed, and you have lost another opportunity to create a favorable impression of your office.

There are some legal regulations which apply to the manner of identification to use when answering the telephone of a medical corporation. If yours is a corporate practice, check with the physician's attorney for clarification.

When you have decided upon the greeting to be used, practice it until you can say it easily and smoothly without thinking about what you are saying.

**Identify the Caller.** If the caller does not identify himself, you must always ask to whom you are speaking. It is a good idea to repeat the name by using it in the conversation as soon as possible, *unless* there are other patients within the range of your voice and the caller's privacy should be respected.

**Offer Assistance.** Always offer assistance, both in the tone of your voice and in your conversation. The phrase "May I help you?" or "How may I help you?"

helps start the conversation and assures the caller you are both willing and capable of being of service.

**Screen Incoming Calls.** Most employers expect the assistant to screen all telephone calls. Good judgment in deciding whether or not to put calls through to the doctor comes only with experience.

Put through calls from other physicians at once. If your doctor is busy and cannot possibly come to the telephone, explain this briefly and politely and say that you will have him return the call the moment he is free. Make sure he does.

Most callers will ask, "Is the doctor in?" You should never answer the question with a simple "Yes" or "No" or respond with the question, "Who is calling, please?" If the doctor is *not* in, say so before asking the identity of the caller. Otherwise the person calling may suspect the doctor is simply not willing to talk to him.

If the doctor is not in the office, the rule of offering assistance still holds. You can say, "No, I am sorry, Doctor Black is not in. May I take a message?" or "No, I am sorry, but Doctor Black will be at the hospital most of the morning. May I ask him to return your call after 12 o'clock?"

If the doctor *is* in, and available for the telephone, a typical response would be, "Yes, Doctor Black is in; may I tell him who is calling, please?" If your doctor prefers to keep his calls to a minimum, you might say, "Yes, Doctor Black is here, but I'm not sure he's free to come to the phone. May I tell him who is calling, please?" That way, if it's someone he does not wish to speak with, you have given him an out.

If the doctor is with a patient, he probably will not wish to be disturbed for a routine call. In this case, you might say, "Yes, Doctor Black is in, but he is with a patient right now. May I help you?" or "Yes, Doctor Black is in but he is with a patient right now. Is there anything you want me to ask him?"

You must guard against being overprotective. A patient has a right to talk with his doctor; however, unless it is an emergency, he is probably willing to do so at the doctor's convenience. Don't let it be said of your doctor, "He's a good doctor, but you can never get to talk to him." The assistant who answers the telephone should act as a screen—not as an impenetrable wall.

Find out exactly how your doctor wishes calls to be handled when he is out of the office and under what circumstances he is willing to be interrupted when he is in the office; be firm in your commitment to his preferences; and cultivate a reputation for being helpful and reliable. You will save the doctor many trips to the telephone if patients develop confidence in your ability to help them, and have faith in your promise to take their messages and deliver them properly.

**Minimize Waiting Time.** If a caller asks to speak with the doctor when he is talking on another line, or if it will take a few minutes for him to accept the call, ask, "Will you wait, or shall I call you back when he is free?"

If the caller elects to wait, remember that waiting with a silent telephone can be irritating. The waiting time, no matter how brief, always seems long. Let no more than one minute pass without breaking in with some reassuring comment, for instance, "I'm sorry, Doctor Black is still busy."

Sometimes if the waiting is longer than expected, the caller will want to reconsider and call back another time or have the call returned, but he wants you to know this. By going back on the line at frequent intervals, you give the caller an opportunity to express his wishes. In fact, you may ask him if he wishes to continue waiting. Say something like this: "I'm sorry to keep you waiting so long, Mr. Hughes. Would you prefer to have me return your call when Doctor Black is free?" Try to give the caller some estimate of when he may expect the return call. In any event, irritation can be lessened by your consideration in saying, "Thank you for waiting, Mr. Hughes."

Sometimes it is necessary for you to leave the telephone to obtain information. Ask the caller, "Will you please wait while I get the information?" and then *wait for a reply*. When you return to the telephone, thank the caller for waiting. If it will take longer than a few seconds to get the information, give some estimate of the time required and offer to call back.

**Transferring a Call.** Always identify the caller when transferring a call to the doctor. Any person who refuses to give his name should not be put through unless your doctor instructs you otherwise.

If it is a patient calling, the doctor will presumably want the patient's history in front of him when he is talking. If there is no concern about others hearing your conversation, you can announce the caller's name on the intercom and tell the doctor you will bring the history. If there are other persons within hearing, you might simply take the history to the doctor and say, "Doctor Black, this party is waiting on the telephone to speak with you." In this way, the patient's right to privacy is protected even in regard to his telephone calls.

**Answering a Second Call.** If your office has several incoming lines, or more than one telephone, it will sometimes be necessary for you to interrupt a conversation to answer another ring. Excuse yourself by saying, "Pardon me just a moment, the other line is ringing." Answer the second call, determine who is calling, and ask that person to hold while you complete the first call. Return to your first call as soon as possible, and apologize briefly for the interruption.

Do not make the mistake of continuing with the second call while the first one waits. Think what you would do if this were a face-to-face conversation. You would not allow a second person to just interrupt a conversation and then ignore the one you were speaking with first.

If the second call is an emergency, you can still take a moment to return to the first line and alert the caller that you will have to keep him waiting or call back. NEVER answer a call by saying, "Hold the line, please," without first finding out who is calling. It could be an emergency. It takes only a moment to be courteous—and this courtesy could save a life.

**Ending a Call.** When a caller's requests have been satisfied, do not encourage needless chatting or permit him to monopolize your time unnecessarily. The telephone lines should be cleared for other calls.

End the call pleasantly. It is considered good telephone etiquette to allow the person who placed the call to hang up first. Replace the telephone on the cradle, as gently as if you were closing a door in the office; do not slam it. It is a gracious gesture to thank a person for calling. Always close the conversation with some form of goodbye; do not just hang up abruptly.

## Summary of Office Telephone Rules

1. Answer promptly
2. Visualize the person to whom you are talking
3. Hold the instrument correctly
4. Develop a pleasing telephone voice
5. Identify your office and yourself
6. Identify the caller
7. Offer assistance
8. Screen incoming calls
9. Minimize waiting time
10. Identify the caller when transferring a call
11. When answering a second call, identify the caller, then return to first call
12. End each call pleasantly and graciously
13. wait for caller to hang up first.

## The Telephone Message

**Be Prepared.**   NEVER answer the telephone without a pen or pencil in your hand and a message pad nearby. You may be answering several calls before you have an opportunity to relay a message or carry out a promise of action. Therefore, the *written* message is vital.

What kind of message pad will you use? Probably the most satisfactory is an ordinary spiral-bound stenographer's notebook. It is inexpensive, sturdy, well-proportioned, will lie flat on your desk, and can be filed for future reference if desired. Do not be guilty of using small scraps of paper for messages. They are too easily lost. Date the bottom of the first blank page in your notebook at the beginning of each day. You will then have a permanent record which can be referred to later if the need arises. If you will draw a half-inch column down one side of each page, you can use this area to check off each message as it is delivered or taken care of. This is a good reminder system for yourself.

**Minimum Information Required.**   The minimum information you will need from each call includes:

(1) the caller's name
(2) his telephone number
(3) the reason for the call
(4) the action to be taken

**Transmitting and Recording the Message.**   Messages which are to be transmitted to another person may be rewritten on individual slips and delivered or posted on a message board later. The nature of the message will determine whether you must report it immediately or not. Special message pads that provide for a carbon copy of each page are good insurance that no message has been forgotten. It is also possible to get message forms with a self-adhesive back that can be placed permanently in the patient's case history (Fig. 9–1). If the call

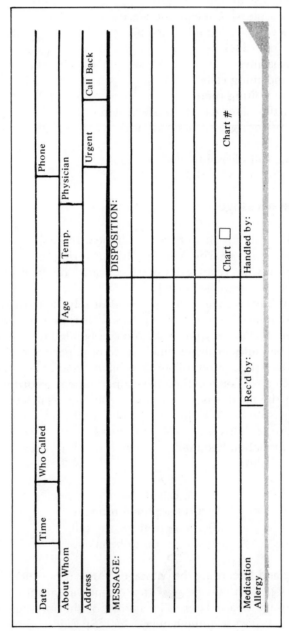

**Figure 9–1** (© 1971 Patient Care Systems, Inc.)

is from a patient, and relates in any way to his medical history, or if any instructions were given, or queries answered, this information should be recorded in the patient's chart.

**Taking Action.** The message procedure is not complete until the necessary action has been taken. Notations on the memo pad should be carried over to the following day if they have not been attended to. Just place an X in front of the item and move it onto the next page. Sometimes a notation will be carried over for several days until action can be completed. Do not trust to memory in regard to messages unattended to from previous days; always carry them forward in writing.

Make brief notations of patients' reactions while you are talking to them on the telephone. The doctor does not require a character study, but it certainly is helpful to him if he learns from his assistant that a patient revealed extreme fear, apprehension, or nervousness. If a patient shows such symptoms, it may be wise to transfer the call to the doctor himself.

When your employer is talking to another physician in regard to a referral, he sometimes may ask you to take down a brief outline of the patient's case history by listening on the extension telephone. This information can be typed and placed on the doctor's desk just before the patient arrives in the office.

## INCOMING CALLS THE ASSISTANT CAN HANDLE

One reason for having the office assistant answer the incoming calls is to spare the physician unnecessary interruptions during his time with patients. Additonally, many calls relate to the administrative aspects of the office and can actually be better handled by the assistant. The doctor's policy regarding how calls are to be handled by the assistant should be set forth in the office procedure manual. Figure 9–2 shows how the instruction page might be arranged in the manual. Listed below are some kinds of calls that can be handled by the assistant in most offices.

**Appointments for New Patients.** As mentioned in Chapter 7, Scheduling Appointments, over 50 per cent of the patient appointments are made by telephone. The assistant who is in charge of scheduling appointments should handle these calls. It is well to remember that you are in a sense "opening the door." The patient will form a first impression of the office, of you, and of the doctor from his first telephone contact. Follow all the prescribed rules of telephone courtesy in offering your friendly assistance.

Take the patient's full name, age, complete address and telephone number, name of person who referred him, and the general type of examination required. This helps decide how much time to allot the patient on the appointment schedule. Your doctor also may ask you to give general instructions to patients seeking care for specific complaints; for example, to request the patient to bring in a urine specimen.

When you have recorded the necessary data, you may ask the patient, "Do you prefer morning or afternoon?" and then offer the first available date. Make certain the patient knows where the office is located and, if necessary, how to get there. If there are special parking conveniences, tell the patient. Before hanging

STANDARD PROCEDURE FOR TELEPHONE CALLS IN THE OFFICE OF

_____ :

CALLS THE ASSISTANT CAN HANDLE:

    Appointments for New Patients _____

    Office Administration Problems _____

    _____

    _____

    _____

    _____

    _____

    _____

    _____

CALLS TO BE PUT THROUGH IMMEDIATELY:

    Calls from Other Physicians _____

    Emergency Calls _____

    _____

    _____

CALLS TO BE REFERRED TO PHYSICIAN:

    Unsatisfactory Progress Reports _____

    Third Party Requests for Information _____

    _____

    _____

    _____

    _____

**Figure 9–2**

up, repeat the appointment date and time agreed upon and thank the person for calling.

**Return Appointments.**    Usually it will only be necessary to determine when the patient was expected to return, then find a suitable time on the schedule. It will not be necessary to give extensive explanations about the location of the office and parking facilities. However, if it has been some time since he has been in the office, it is advisable to ask whether his address and telephone number remain the same. You may also wish to inquire whether the patient wants to see the doctor about a condition similar to his former one. He may have a different complaint which might require a longer or shorter visit than previously.

**Inquiries about Bills.**    A patient may telephone and say he has received a bill and wants to talk to the doctor about it. The assistant may ask the caller to "Hold" for a moment while she pulls the ledger. If she finds nothing irregular noted on the ledger, she can return to the telephone and say, "I have your account in front of me now. Perhaps I can answer your inquiry." The chances are the patient will have some simple inquiry such as "Is that my total bill?" "Has my insurance paid anything?" or "May I wait until next month to make a payment?" Not all patients realize that it is the assistant who usually takes charge of these matters.

**Requests for Insurance Assistance.**    Again, it is the office assistant who is in a better position to answer inquiries about insurance. Oftentimes patients find insurance claims very confusing and think they must answer questions with precise medical terminology. A simple statement to "just put it in your own words" may take care of this kind of inquiry. It is best to steer clear of interpreting insurance coverage by telephone. If the patient has a complicated problem that will tie up the telephone for a long while, the assistant can ask him to mail in the pages so that she can review them.

**Receiving X-ray and Laboratory Reports.**    Many physicians have x-ray and laboratory reports telephoned to their offices on the day the test is completed. The assistant can take these reports. Her task will be greatly simplified if she has blank forms on which she can just fill in the results rather than having to write down the names of all the tests, particularly on laboratory reports. If it is impossible to get blank forms from the laboratory, she can type up her own and run it through the copy machine. By typing four or six to a page, the expense of duplication will be cut considerably. They can then be cut to size.

**Satisfactory Progress Reports from Patients.**    Doctors sometimes ask a patient to "phone and let me know how you're feeling in a few days." The assistant can take this call and relay the information to the doctor if it is a satisfactory report. Say something to the patient that will assure him that you will inform the doctor about the call; for example, "I'll give this information to the doctor as soon as he arrives in the office."

**Routine Reports from Hospitals and Other Sources.**    There may be routine calls from the hospital and other sources reporting a patient's progress. If it is only a reporting procedure, take the message carefully, make sure that the doctor sees it, and then place it in the patient's history.

**Office Administration Matters.**    Not all calls concern patients. There may be calls from the accountant or auditor, or calls regarding banking procedures, office supplies, office maintenance, and so forth, all of which the assistant can either handle immediately or get the necessary information and call back.

**Requests for Referrals.**   Doctors who are liked and respected by their patients frequently receive requests from patients for referrals to other specialists, for themselves or for friends. If the physician has furnished the assistant with a list of doctors to whom he usually refers certain types of cases, she can handle these inquiries without referring them to the physician. She should, however, tell the physician about the calls.

**Prescription Refills.**   If the physician has placed a note upon the patient's chart indicating that a prescription may be filled a certain number of times, the assistant can give an O.K. to the pharmacist after double-checking with him on the number of times it has already been filled. This information should appear on the patient's chart, but it is always well to double-check. If there is any question, tell the pharmacist you will have to check with the doctor and call back.

## Calls that Require Transfer to the Doctor or Call Back

**Calls from Other Physicians.**   As stated earlier, calls from other physicians should be put through immediately. If it is impossible for the doctor to take the call at once, be sure to offer to call back as soon as possible.

**Patients Who Will Not Reveal Symptoms.**   Sometimes a patient will call and wish to talk with the doctor about symptoms which he is reluctant to discuss with an assistant. Do not make the mistake of pressing for details. Even though you may not be embarrassed, the patient has the right to some privacy. Put these calls through to the doctor or offer to have him call back.

**Unsatisfactory Progress Reports.**   If the patient reports that he "still is not feeling well," or the "prescription the doctor gave me makes me feel sick," do not try to practice medicine by telling the patient "this is to be expected." Even if you think the doctor will say the same thing, the patient should hear it from the doctor himself for reassurance.

**Requests for Test Results.**   When the physician orders special tests for the patient, he may tell him to call the office in a couple of days for the results. Be sure the physician has seen the results and has given you permission to tell the patient before giving out any information. Particularly if the result is unfavorable, the physician should be the one to inform the patient and give him further instructions. This call must be handled tactfully; otherwise, the patient may get the feeling that you are hiding something from him. Some patients do not understand that the assistant does not have the privilege of giving out information without permission of the physician. You might answer the inquiry like this: "The doctor has not seen the report yet; will you please call back after two o'clock? I will try to have the information for you then." Or offer to call the patient as soon as you have the necessary information.

**Third Party Requests for Information.**   Remember, if there is no legal requirement for disclosure of information, you must have the written permission of the patient before giving information to third-party callers. This includes insurance companies, attorneys, relatives, neighbors, employers, or any other third party.

**Complaints About Care or Fees.**    You may be able to offer a satisfactory explanation to a patient who complains about the care he received or the fee charged. If the patient is angry when he calls, you may tell him it will take a few moments to pull his chart, and offer to call him back. This reassures him that someone is willing to talk to him about his problem, and also gives him a chance to "cool off." If you are unable to appease the patient easily, though, your doctor would probably prefer to talk to the patient himself.

## Special Telephone Problems

**Unidentified Callers.**    Although it will happen rarely, you will sometimes encounter an individual who refuses to give you his name or business but is rudely insistent upon speaking to the doctor. Such callers usually are sales persons who are fully aware that if their identity is revealed they will never get the opportunity to speak to the doctor. Your own course in such instances is to say firmly, "Doctor Jones is very busy with a patient and has asked me to take all messages. If you will not give me a message, I suggest you write the doctor a letter. I'm sure he will give it his immediate attention."

**Calls from Family and Friends.**    Every doctor receives a certain number of personal calls at his office from his family and friends. As you become acquainted with the doctor and his practice, you will soon know how to handle these calls. However, some persons abuse the telephone privilege. If a friend of the doctor calls too often and the doctor does not wish to speak with him, the assistant must deal politely with him. She can say, "Doctor Wilson is with a patient now and I cannot disturb him. He is booked rather heavily this afternoon, and you may have more time to talk with him if you call him at home this evening. His home telephone number is . . . ."

**Angry Callers.**    No matter how efficient you are at the telephone or how beloved your employer may be, now and then you will find an angry caller on the other end of the line. He may have a legitimate reason for his anger, or it may have resulted from a misunderstanding. Here is a suggestion which appeared in the August, 1960, *Public Relations Journal* by Dr. A. Westley Rowland on how to handle such calls:

> It is a real challenge to handle the angry person who is calling. The best bit of advice is to avoid getting angry yourself. Try to find out what the problem is and provide the answers if possible. If answers are not readily available, assure the caller you will find the answer and will call him back immediately.
>
> A friendly, sincere, unaffected voice that is well modulated makes the caller feel that the person at the other end of the line is efficient and likeable. Good enunciation and good grammer, concise, to-the-point statements lead to effective telephone communications.

In other words, listen and let the caller talk, express interest and understanding, do not "pass the buck," take careful notes, maintain your own poise, and then take the required action, even if it is to say that you will take the matter up with your employer as soon as possible and call back later.

**Monitoring Calls.**    Occasionally you may be asked by your employer to monitor a telephone call. You will be expected to listen from an extension phone and take notes on the conversation. It is possible to record both sides of a telephone call by placing a dictating machine close to the telephone receiver. However, you should be aware that this is illegal unless the other person is told that his conversation is being recorded.

**Requests for House Calls.**    Scheduling house calls was discussed briefly in Chapter 7. In response to a telephone request for a home visit, be sure to inquire the nature of the illness. There are certain conditions that are impossible to treat at home, and time will be saved if the patient is sent directly to the hospital, where the doctor can meet him. Or urge the patient to come to the office. It can be pointed out that facilities for giving the best medical treatment are available there and office calls are more economical. This also conserves the doctor's time.

Consult the doctor, if possible, before obligating him to a house call. In most cases you can explain to the patient that you will check with the doctor and call back immediately. If he cannot visit the patient, you must see that another doctor is sent out. It is easier for you to call another physician than it is for the distraught patient. One of the most common complaints about the medical profession is that you cannot get a doctor in an emergency. It is particularly difficult for newcomers to get a doctor to make a house call. Your medical society may operate an emergency answering panel which can be of service in such cases.

If your doctor agrees to make a house call and the area is unfamiliar to him, it is a good idea to have a local map on which you can pinpoint the location of the house for him. This is a little extra service that your doctor will greatly appreciate, since it may save him precious moments he might spend uselessly hunting for the house.

## Routine but Troublesome Calls

Many of the so-called "routine calls" coming into the physician's office will be difficult for a new assistant to handle. Though no stock answer can be phrased for these calls, a gracious and prompt answer paves the way for a quicker handling of the call, since it tells the patient the assistant is capable, pleasant, and willing to offer assistance.

Here are a few typical calls that any medical assistant may receive:

|   |   |
|---|---|
| 1. The Call | "I have an appointment with the doctor this morning and cannot keep it. May I come in this afternoon instead?" |
| The Answer | Even though this type of call throws the appointment book into confusion, showing irritation with the patient won't help the situation. Make a sincere effort to help the caller make a new appointment. Explain that appointments are made in order that the doctor can give the very best care without rushing his patients and that consequently keeping appointments is to each patient's personal benefit. |
| 2. The Call | "I received my statement this morning and I don't understand why it is so high." |
| The Answer | When this type of call comes in, politely ask the patient to hold the line while you pull the financial card. When you return to the line, thank the patient for waiting and explain the charges carefully. If there is an error, apologize |

and say a corrected statement will be sent out at once. Thank the patient for calling. If patients are properly advised about charges at the time services are rendered, the number of these calls will be considerably reduced.

3. The Call "Last time I had an office call, Doctor gave me a prescription for some sleeping tablets. I want you to call the druggist and okay a refill."

The Answer Remember that the medical assistant is *not* licensed to practice medicine. Ask the patient for the prescription number, the date, the name, address and telephone number of the druggist, and obtain the patient's phone number. Explain that you will give the message to the doctor as soon as he returns to the office. At this point it may be advisable to pull the patient's history card and have it ready with the message when the doctor comes in. If he okays the refill, he may ask the assistant to phone the patient with the information.

4. The Call "Does the doctor treat stomach trouble?"

The Answer It depends upon the doctor's field of practice. Many people don't understand the various medical specialties, and this call may come from a person referred to the doctor by a friend who didn't explain that the doctor is a specialist. If your doctor is unable to handle the case, you may have to refer the patient to another doctor. Always give the patient the names of at least three physicians when possible; these should only be names which your employer has had you place on the referral list. Never presume to make a diagnosis when a patient calls in with bizarre complaints; transfer the call to the doctor himself or take the caller's name and number and have the doctor return the call later.

5. The Call "My next door neighbor is a patient of the doctor and I am quite concerned about her. Could you tell me what is wrong with her?"

The Answer Professional ethics is involved here. It is not the role of the medical assistant to give out any information about a patient's condition, except that information the physician has specifically okayed for "release." The caller in this case may be merely curious, or may actually be a kindly neighbor who wishes to help her friend. Generally, refer such calls to the doctor.

## Telephone Answering Services

Because a physician's telephone is an all-important tool of his practice, it must be constantly "covered"—that is, there must be someone to answer it at all times—day and night, Sundays and holidays. This presents no problem during weekdays, but nights and weekends present special problems. Most doctors subscribe to telephone answering services which assume around-the-clock coverage. Some telephone answering services are privately owned; others are owned and operated by the local medical society. Or the doctor may own an automatic answering device.

**Operator-Answered Services.** There are two types of operator-answered services: (1) doctor-subscribers leave messages with, or obtain patients' messages from, a service whose number appears in the local telephone directory in this way: "After_____p.m., call_____(number)," or "If no answer, call_____(number)." Such listings are found immediately following the doctor's own telephone number. This form of service offers some inconvenience for the patient but is far better than no coverage at all. (2) The answering service has a direct connection with the office telephone. When the telephone rings in the physician's office or at home, it also signals on the switchboard of the answering service. As long as the telephone is ringing, it will continue to signal at the answering service. If the doctor or someone in his office or home does not answer within a certain agreed upon number of rings, the answering service operator takes the call. This method provides constant telephone coverage.

Even during the day, such an answering service can function effectively. There may be times when you are assisting the doctor and it is impossible for you or anyone else to answer the telephone. An unanswered telephone is extremely poor policy; but, if you have an agreement with the answering service, its operators will accept calls for you in such situations. With this direct-wire answering method, the operator answers the telephone in your employer's name, as you would in the office, explaining, "This is Dr. Wilson's exchange. May I take a message?" The operators on the exchange switchboards are usually exceptionally well trained, especially if the service is owned by the medical society.

The answering service will greatly appreciate your cooperation if you call them every evening before leaving the office, telling them where the doctor will be during the evening or giving them other special messages. Then, in the morning when you return to the office, call the exchange and ask for any messages they may have. Invariably, there will be messages from patients who called during the night but whose calls were not important enough to merit an emergency call to the doctor. An exchange can act as a buffer for your doctor and help eliminate too frequent, unnecessary calls during the night. Here's how the system works.

During the night and on weekends and holidays, the exchange will answer the doctor's office telephone, take a message, and immediately relay it to the doctor. If the doctor feels it is necessary, he will then return the call to the patient; if not, the exchange will call the patient and explain that the doctor will call first thing in the morning. Of course, the exchange does not tell the patient about its recent conversation with the doctor but reports he is not available. Emergency calls, however, are immediately put through by the exchange to the doctor.

Occasionally, it is a good idea to check up on your answering service by placing a few test calls at various hours. It may be that now and then the service does not answer the call or the response is gruff and rude, offering absolutely no cooperation to the "patient." Such poor service can deal a bad blow to a doctor's reputation.

**Automatic Answering Devices.** Many doctors use an automatic answering device after office hours. Callers who dial the office hear a recorded message either telling them how to reach the doctor (or a colleague who may be covering the practice for him) or inviting the caller to leave a message. The caller's message is recorded for later checking by the doctor or his staff.

One type of telephone-answering device is equipped with a remote control with which the doctor can call his office from any telephone and, by simply holding the remote control near the mouthpiece of the telephone he is calling from, receive the messages which have been recorded during his absence.

The automatic telephone-answering devices are particularly useful in areas where no competent answering service is available.

## OUTGOING CALLS

### Organizing Telephone Numbers

Organize your telephone numbers in an indexed 3 by 5 inch desktop file or a rotary file. Emergency numbers might be typed on a colored card or flagged with a color tab. Your procedure manual should include lists of

1. specialists to whom your employer sometimes refers patients
2. physicians who will take house calls if your doctor does not find it possible to accept them or is unable to make such calls on a particular day
3. professional facilities, such as hospitals, the poison control center, pharmacies, ambulance companies, laboratories
4. special duty nurses—registered, practical, and general duty—along with their ages, specialties, and other information
5. administrative contacts, such as stationers, equipment dealers and repair services, laundry and maintenance services, surgical supply houses
6. personal numbers, such as doctor's family, special friends, his insurance agent, stock broker, accountant, lawyer

**Pre-Planning the Call.**    Before placing a call, make certain you have the correct telephone number. If you are not absolutely sure about it, look it up in the directory. Have the information you will need during the call at your fingertips. If you are reporting a patient's history, have the complete record before you, including all the latest laboratory and x-ray reports. If you are placing a call to order supplies, have the catalog in front of you with any previous order sheets or invoices. Also have a list of the items desired, the specifications for them, and any questions you may have regarding them. Apply this rule to every call you make. The called party will be impressed with your competence, and you will save a great deal of time.

**Placing the Call.**    Lift the receiver, listen for the dial tone, then start dialing your number. It sometimes happens that just as you pick up the telephone to place a call, an incoming call has reached your line but you lifted the receiver before the telephone had a chance to ring. If you start dialing without listening for the dial tone, you will not only fail to reach your number, you will have offended the ear of the party trying to reach you. Use the index finger or a special dialing instrument for dialing your call. Do not use the eraser end of a pencil and do not let your finger remain in the dial openings on the return of the dial. It is the return of the dial that determines the number you reach, and if it is not allowed to return freely you may reach a wrong number.

**Calling Etiquette.**    When placing a call to another doctor or to a patient at the doctor's request, your employer should be ready to receive the call. Doctors, because of their busy schedules, sometimes are negligent in this respect. The telephone company's courtesy rule is that the person placing the call should be on the wire ready to speak when the called party answers. You may have to ask your doctor when he requests you to place a call for him if he is ready to answer the telephone while you are putting through the call. Promptness is one of the first rules of telephone etiquette.

If you are calling a patient to change an appointment, be ready to offer a new appointment time. Also, give the patient a logical reason for the inconvenience of having to change his original appointment. This change may cause considerable disruption in his plans, and he is fully entitled to an explanation. Your employer may ask you to call a patient and change a medication instruction. Or it may be your duty to call a patient and instruct him to go to the hospital or laboratory for a special test or x-ray. Make certain you have the correct instructions written down carefully and that you have checked these instructions. This is of particular importance when you are changing medication instructions. Remember that if your telephone is within hearing distance of office patients you should be careful in mentioning names or diagnoses.

**Long Distance Calls.**    Long distance calls are no longer reserved for special occasions. The calls are simple to place and not exorbitant in cost. It is certainly much easier to telephone to obtain information than it is to wait for an exchange of letters.

Before placing a long distance call, have the correct number ready. This number often may be obtained from a letterhead or from other records. The telephone company also has a collection of major city telephone directories in every town. If you do not have the number, you can dial the area code, then 555-1212 for information service. There is no charge for calls to information.

It is important to keep in mind the different time zones when you are calling long distance. The Continental United States is divided into four standard time zones: Pacific, Mountain, Central, and Eastern. When it is 12 noon Pacific time, it is 3 p.m. Eastern time. If you are calling from Los Angeles to New York, you will probably want to make the call no later than 2 p.m. if you are calling a business or professional office, because it will already be 5 p.m. on the East coast.

There are two types of long distance calls: (1) person-to-person service, in which a call is placed to a particular individual; and (2) station-to-station service, in which the person calling does not ask the operator to reach any particular person or extension but will talk to anyone who answers the telephone at that number. Station-to-station rates are cheaper but the calls are often more expensive in the long run because of the occasional delay in reaching a special person or in obtaining certain information from various departments.

Person-to-person or collect calls require an operator. In placing the call, state the area code and the seven digit telephone number. In the case of a person-to-person call, follow this information with the name of the individual to be reached.

DIRECT DISTANCE DIALING (DDD).    In most parts of the nation, direct distance dialing is now possible. By combining the proper three-digit area code with the seven-digit telephone number, you can dial direct to points far distant. Consequently, your area code is as important a part of your telephone number as the Zip code assigned to you by the post office to get mail to you quickly. Area codes for many principal cities throughout the nation appear in the front of your telephone directory. For area codes not listed, contact your own operator or give her the name of the city and state you are calling, then be sure to write down the area code that she gives you.

**Wrong Numbers.** One slip in direct distance dialing can give you Los Angeles instead of Dallas. If you reach a wrong number when dialing long distance, be sure to obtain the name of the city, state, and central office you have reached. By reporting this information promptly to the operator in your own city, you will not be charged for this wrong number. If you are cut off before terminating your call, this too should be reported to the operator, who will either reconnect your call or make an adjustment of the charge.

**Conference Calls.** Conference telephone service is of great value to the medical profession. This service is used in special postgraduate course presentations, in consultations, and in notifying and explaining to a family how a patient is progressing. This service may connect from 3 to 14 long distance points for a two-way conference. Each person can hear or talk to all others participating. Up to 49 points can be connected for a one-way conference call in which only the voice of the caller is heard. This service is available through the long distance operator; call her and ask for the conference operator. The charges are based on person-to-person rates to the two farthest points, plus a lower rate for each additional telephone used in the conference. This service has exceptional value in family conferences requiring a quick decision by the entire family in regard to a patient's condition.

By following these suggested techniques the assistant will be able to use the telephone wisely and efficiently. Correct use of the telephone really is an art which can be developed only through actual practice. It is one of the most important skills the medical assistant should possess.

## Special Equipment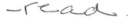

In many medical offices, in addition to the usual desk or wall telephone, you may need to become acquainted with more complex equipment—telephones with several buttons, which permit you to hold one call while answering another or allow you to hold a call while using an intercom to speak with someone in the office. Extensions to save steps are now common in many rooms of a medical office. With the addition of a device called an *exclusion button,* all other extensions on the line may be closed off, ensuring the privacy of the call.

You may be asked to operate a small switchboard through which incoming and outgoing calls are routed. However, though the range of services today in the telephone field is greater, operation of such equipment is usually quite simple. Here are just a few of the types of equipment you may encounter.

**Six-Button Key Set.** Quite common is the telephone with six buttons, which can have several outside lines, can hold calls, and can be used as an intercom or for signaling. Lights within the buttons flash for incoming calls and wink rapidly to remind you of calls being held. A steady light indicates that the line is in use. This is the basic instrument in the small business or professional office.

**Speakerphone.** Some doctors like the Speakerphone, a small receiver-transmitter which sits on the desk and picks up and amplifies normal conversation, freeing the hands for note-taking. This same device can be very useful to the secretary or receptionist who may receive frequent calls which require her to leave her desk to refer to charts or financial records. With the Speakerphone there is no break in communication while she goes to the files for information. The Speakerphone is convertible; at the touch of a button it changes from a regular telephone to a hands-free communications system.

**Rapidial.**\*   This is a piece of equipment tied in with the telephone which permits prerecording of up to 290 telephone numbers for speedy, accurate, and convenient automatic dialing.

**Call-Director or Call-Commander Telephone.**   This piece of equipment is compact and versatile, serving as a regular office telephone but also permitting use of lines with dial intercom, allowing calls to be held, and also providing means for setting up conference calls or adding other extensions to incoming calls. This equipment is most likely to be found in offices where one receptionist answers calls for three or more doctors.

**Card-Dialer Telephone.**   Some offices use a card-dialer telephone, a device which permits automatic dialing of numbers frequently called via punched cards with prerecorded numbers.

**Touch-Tone Telephones.**   Though still only available in selected areas, the touch-tone telephone greatly speeds and simplifies placing outside calls. Instead of a dial, the set has ten buttons, one for each digit 0 to 9. Much like touching the keys of an adding machine, and just as rapid, a button is pressed in proper sequence for each digit of the telephone number.

**Mobile Telephones.**   To guarantee continual availability to patients, some doctors utilize telephones in their automobiles. Others use a pocket radio receiver which signals with a tone that he is to call his office or the hospital.

**Telephone Dictation.**   In hospitals, dial dictation and recording services are quite common. A doctor can dictate a case history or report by telephone into a centrally located recording machine. His report can then be transcribed by typists at the central location. In a group practice, the recording machine may be in the doctor's office, where the office personnel will do the typing.

## Telegraph Services

Although most long distance communications from the physician's office will be via the telephone, there are instances in which the telegraph message is the one of choice. The projected delivery time and the urgency of the message would determine the type of service to be used. There are two basic classes of domestic telegraph service: the *regular telegram* and the more economical *overnight telegram.*

**Regular Telegram.**   The regular telegram is accepted at any time and transmitted immediately. Usually delivery may be expected within two hours. The minimum charge is based on 15 words, and an extra charge is made for each additional word.

**Overnight Telegram.**   The overnight telegram may be sent up until midnight for delivery the next morning. The minimum charge is based on 100 words, and an extra charge is made for each additional word.

---

\*Registered trademark, McGraw-Edison Company.

**Mailgram.**  The mailgram is a variation of the overnight telegram. It is wired to the office of the U.S. Postal Service nearest the recipient, where it is placed in a special Mailgram envelope and delivered by the regular letter carrier.

The secretary should be familiar with the methods used in counting the chargeable words and characters. One address and one signature are free. Punctuation marks are not charged for; however, if such words as *stop, period,* or *quote* are used, they are considered chargeable words. Three of the characters on your typewriter cannot be transmitted and must be written as words in a telegram: these are ¢, @, and ° (for degree).

Telegrams may be telephoned to the telegraph company and charged on your telephone bill. However, before telephoning, the message should be carefully composed and a copy typed for the office files, including the date and time sent. Telegrams may be addressed to airports, to sailing or arriving ships, to ships at sea, and even to isolated places if there is a telephone there.

**Types of Equipment.**  The private practitioner will ordinarily have no need for telegraph transmitting equipment in his office. However, with the growing tendency toward more complex practices, in clinical group practice and hospitals, the medical assistant should familiarize herself with the more commonly used equipment: Desk-fax, Intrafax, Wirefax, Telex Service, and Tieline.

**Other Services from Western Union.**  Your Western Union office will make and confirm hotel or motel reservations. They will sometimes call as many as eight hotels or motels in the same city in order to get the accommodations you wish.

It is possible to send money by telegraph and cable to all parts of the world. Payments in foreign countries are made in the currency of that country. In addition to the amount of money being wired, you must pay for the cost of a 15-word telegram or a 100-word overnight telegram, plus a service charge based on the amount of money to be sent.

Western Union offers many additional services, although there would be little need for most of them in the average doctor's office.

## REFERENCES

*What Every Telephone User Should Know,* General Telephone System
*Your Telephone Personality,* Bell Telephone System
*Your Voice is You,* Bell Telephone System

# Chapter 10

**BEHAVIORAL OBJECTIVES**

*The medical office assistant should be able to:*

Apply time and motion-saving principles to processing incoming mail.

Describe the various classifications of mail and their uses.

Select appropriate special postal services when required.

Prepare outgoing mail for efficient handling by postal service.

Plan appropriate procedure for handling vacation mail during the doctor's absence.

# Processing the Mail

Probably no other business or professional person receives more mail than a physician. Into his office each day flows a variety of mail: letters from patients and other physicians, payments for services, bills for office purchases, laboratory reports, hospital reports, medical society mailings, flashy promotional pieces and samples from drug houses, advertisements from equipment houses, requests for contributions, professional periodicals, and other personal mail.

In large clinics the mail is opened by a person specially delegated in some central department to speed up this daily task. But in the average professional office, the assistant or secretary opens the mail, using the tried and true letter-opener method.

## INCOMING MAIL

### Procedure for Handling

Before opening any mail, a new girl in a doctor's office should ask her employer what procedure she should follow in regard to incoming mail. In other words, what letters should the assistant open and what pieces does the doctor prefer to open himself? If there is any doubt in the assistant's mind in regard to opening a letter, the best rule to follow is, Don't! Treat your doctor's mail with the same consideration you expect others to exercise toward your own. Assuming you have been instructed to sort and open all except personal items, here are some suggestions for proceeding efficiently.

**Sorting.** When mail arrives, usually early in the morning, it should be separated according to importance and urgency. Before settling down to this daily task, assemble the tools and supplies you will need: a letter opener, paper clips, stapler, mending tape, and date stamp. Here is a rule-of-thumb sorting guide:

1. Telegrams or special delivery letters
2. Air mail
3. Receipts from patients
4. Doctor's personal mail
5. Ordinary first class mail
6. Periodicals and newspapers
7. All other classes, including drug samples

**Opening.** Even such a simple procedure as opening the day's mail can be done with more efficiency if a good system is adopted. Since the letterknife is the most generally used opener for mail in the average office, its use will be described. Have a clear working space on your desk or counter. Then, keeping the mail in the sorted groups, open the letters along the top edges for easiest removal of contents. Proceed in this fashion:

1. Place your stack of envelopes to the left, flap side up, and top edges to the right
2. Holding the envelope in the left hand and the opener in the right hand, slip the opener under the flap and open the edge with one stroke
3. Lay the opened letter down in a second pile to the left, still keeping the cut edge to the right
4. Pick up the next envelope and repeat the process for the entire stack without putting down the letter opener

When all the envelopes have been opened, start removing the contents. With envelopes still in a pile near the left hand, pull out the letter with the right hand, hold the envelope up to the light with the left hand, checking to see that nothing remains inside, then lay it in a separate pile to the far left. Use both hands to flatten the letter and attach any enclosures. Do not take time to read the letter at this time, but do glance to see if there is a return address on the letter. If not, retrieve the envelope and attach it to the letter. If there is an enclosure notation at the bottom of the letter, check to be sure the enclosure was included. Should the enclosure be missing, indicate this on the notation by writing the word "no" and circling it.

After all of the envelopes have been emptied, you will have a neat stack of mail near your right hand and only empty envelopes at the left. Now, date stamp each letter or write the date in pencil at the top. Sometimes the letter bears no date, or possibly one which does not correspond closely to the current date. Also, the date of receipt appearing on a letter oftentimes provides the necessary incentive to get it answered more quickly.

**Annotating.** It may be that this is as far as your employer will want you to proceed with handling the mail. You can be of far greater service, though, if you are permitted to read each letter through, underlining the significant words and phrases, and noting in the margin (annotating) any action required. If it is a letter that needs no reply, you can code it for filing at this time. A non-print pencil that does not photocopy may be used for the annotating if desired.

When mail refers to previous correspondence, secure this from the file and attach it. Or if a patient's chart is needed in replying to an inquiry, pull the chart and place it with the letter.

In some offices the doctor and his secretary go over the pieces of mail together. As you gain confidence, you will find that you can draft a reply to some inquiries. Most doctors are very pleased to relinquish this responsibility, especially on matters that do not relate to patient care.

Letters of referral from other physicians should be carefully noted so that an answer may be sent after the doctor has seen the patient and can give a report. If considerable time may pass before such information can be sent, it is a nice policy to write a note to the referring physician thanking him and advising him that a detailed letter will follow. Some physicians send printed cards expressing thanks for referrals; others prefer to write thank-you letters to professional colleagues.

## Mail the Assistant Can Handle

**Cash Receipts and Insurance Forms.** There will be some mail that the assistant can handle alone; for instance, payments from patients and insurance forms to be completed. All cash and checks should be separated and recorded immediately in the day's receipts. Insurance forms should be placed with the patient's history on your desk for attention at a time during the day when it is convenient for you to handle them. Do not place them where they may be covered with other papers, and misplaced or forgotten; have a specific place where you will keep insurance forms.

**Samples.** Almost every mail brings in samples and related literature. The assistant should learn from her doctor what types of literature and samples he wishes to have placed on his desk for review. For example, a psychiatrist probably would not be greatly interested in a new vitamin preparation for expectant mothers. Most physicians keep pertinent new samples in their desks, along with the accompanying literature for immediate reference. Other samples are placed in the sample cabinet in their respective categories. Many offices maintain a "catch-all" box for samples that are of no interest. Contents of these boxes are generally given to a medical charity clinic or a medical missionary. In some areas the women's auxiliary to the medical association makes this their project. Samples should never be tossed into the trash. Too many people who are in need of care can make use of these valuable preparations. There is also the danger that youngsters may find the discarded samples and experiment with them; the result could be disastrous.

A definite place should be agreed upon for placing the opened mail for your doctor's perusal. This will probably be some spot on his desk. When you have completed the sorting, opening, and annotating of mail, place those items that the doctor will wish to see in the established place, with the most important mail on top. Personal mail, of course, is unopened. Should you in error open a piece of personal mail addressed to your employer, fold and replace it inside the envelope, and write across the outside "Opened in error," followed by your initials. Use the same procedure with a piece of mail addressed to another office that may have been opened in error. In that case, reseal the envelope with transparent tape, and hand it to your carrier.

These are the general directions for handling incoming mail that will help eliminate some of the assistant's confusion. With thought and organization she can make the work easier for herself and her doctor-employer. She should keep in mind her purpose for being there—performing all tasks within her capabilities that save time and effort for the doctor.

## OUTGOING MAIL

Mail also flows out from the professional office. The mailing costs for even a small office are a sizable item in the annual budget. The greater the assistant's knowledge of the U.S. Postal Service, the more the doctor will get for his postage dollar. In addition to saving postage dollars, the knowledgeable assistant can utilize many special postal services. But first she must be aware of what services are available, what type of service best fits each situation, and how to handle unusual postal problems. *The Postal Manual* may be purchased from the Superintendent of Documents, U.S. Government Printing Office, Washington, D.C. 20402. Smaller publications which contain basic postal information are available without charge from local post offices. A summary of the most common services are described in this chapter.

## Classifications of Mail

Mail is classified according to type, weight, and destination. The ounce and pound are the units of measurement. Here are types of mail commonly handled in a medical office.

**First Class Mail.**   Sealed or unsealed handwritten or typed material, such as letters, postal cards, post cards, and business reply mail.

**Second Class Mail.**   Newspaper and periodical publications. Publishers who mail in bulk lots, and who have been granted second class mail privileges, pay a special second class rate. Copies mailed unsealed by the public go by *transient rate,* six cents for the first two ounces and two cents for each additional ounce, or the fourth class rate, whichever is lower.

**Third Class Mail.**   Printed matter or merchandise weighing up to but not including 16 ounces not included in first or second class. Third class mail includes such things as catalogues, circulars, books, photographs, and other printed matter, and even seeds, bulbs, keys, and so forth. Pieces should be sealed or secured so that they can be handled by machine but must be clearly marked with the two words "Third Class." Mailing of sealed articles at the third class rate carries the implied consent of the mailer to postal inspection of the contents.

**Fourth Class Mail (Parcel Post).**   Merchandise, books, printed matter, and so forth not included in first or second class, and weighing 16 ounces or more but not exceeding 70 pounds. There are also size limitations on fourth class mail; check with your post office regarding regulations on very large parcels. Rates are determined on the basis of weight and destination. Such mail may be sealed or unsealed.

**Combination Mailing.**   A first class letter may be sent along with a parcel, either by placing the letter in an envelope and attaching it to the outside of the package or by enclosing it within the parcel and writing on the outside, just below the space for postage, "Letter Enclosed." In either case, separate postage is paid for the letter. This method is often used in the physician's office when mailing x-rays and an accompanying letter.

**Educational Materials.**    A special rate, lower than regular fourth class, is applicable for educational materials. This includes bound books of 24 or more pages, manuscripts for books, sound recordings and films, and printed tests. The package must be marked "Educational Materials." This was formerly called the *book rate.*

## Postal Services

**Air Mail.**    This is used for more rapid delivery, particularly when mailing pieces to a destination more than 150 miles away. Air mail is limited to 70 pounds. Anything over 8 ounces travels at air parcel post rates, which vary depending upon the zone to which the piece is being sent, and should be mailed at post offices. Air mail weighing eight ounces or less may be deposited in mailboxes. Air mail should always be clearly marked as such; merely placing an air mail stamp on the envelope is not enough. Red "Air Mail" stickers are available at local stationers; a blue "Par Avion" (by air mail) can be secured for overseas air mail. Special air mail stationery, especially envelopes, is also popular. This lightweight stationery does not require special air mail stickers, since "Air Mail" is clearly imprinted on the envelope. Regular stamps may be used on air mail, but air mail stamps may not be used on ordinary mail. Call the local post office to secure air mail rates to various destinations or to check on whether there is air service into a particular area.

**Certificates of Mailing.**    If a sender needs proof of mailing but is not especially concerned with proof of receipt of an item, the most economical method is to obtain a Certificate of Mailing. Fill in the required information, attach a five-cent stamp, and hand it to the postal clerk along with the piece of mail. The clerk will postmark the receipt, initial it, and hand it back as acknowledgment of having received the piece of mail at the post office. This is sometimes used when mailing income tax reports or other items which must be posted by a certain date.

**Certified Mail.**    This provides the sender of domestic mail with a receipt of delivery if requested and fee paid. A record of delivery is kept at the post office of delivery for two years. However, no record is kept at the post office at which it is mailed, and this type of mail does not provide insurance coverage. Anything you wish to mail (which has no intrinsic value) on which postage is paid at the first class rate will be accepted as certified mail. Such things as contracts, deeds, mortgages, bank books, checks, passports, insurance policies, money orders, and birth certificates, which are not valuable intrinsically but would be hard to duplicate if lost, should be certified. Certified mail can be sent special delivery if the prescribed additional fees are paid. The secretary should keep a supply of certified mail forms and return receipts on hand. These may be obtained at any post office. The current fee for certified mail, in addition to regular postage, is 30 cents. If a return receipt is desired, an additional fee of 15 cents is payable.

Full instructions are included on the forms. Fees and postage may be paid by ordinary postage stamps, meter stamps, or permit imprint. Certified mail can be mailed at any post office, station, or branch, or can be deposited in mail drops or in street letter boxes if you follow specific directions. Certified mail is often used as an aid in collections.

**Express Mail Service.**   This service is based on a high-speed delivery network linking more than 50 major cities in the United States. One of its features is a Downtown-to-Downtown service which guarantees that if you mail by 5 p.m. at the designated window, your urgent communication or parcel will be ready for pickup at the receiving post office at 10 a.m. the next business day — or your money back. Five other service options are available on a contract basis under Express Mail: 1. Door to door; 2. Your door to a destination airport; 3. Originating airport to addressee; 4. Airport to airport; and 5. United States to England. Check with your local post office for the availability of this service in your area.

**Insured Mail.**   Third or fourth class mail which has been insured against loss. All packages valued at more than 25 dollars and not registered should be insured. Parcel post packages may be registered with postage paid at the first class rate, but generally they are insured instead of registered. Indemnity on insured mail is limited to 200 dollars.

**International Mail.**   Sending mail to distant points of the globe has become quite commonplace. In almost all cases, letters will be sent air mail and can be expected to reach their destination within a very few days. First class mail to Canada and Mexico travels at the same rate as within the United States. A table of international rates can be obtained from your local post office. The rate of international mail is based on one-half ounce. Aerogrammes, a thin air mail–weight sheet of paper which can be folded for mailing and which does not require an envelope, can be purchased at the post office (currently for 15 cents) and used for sending messages anywhere in the world. In some cases this is a considerable saving. Writing can be on only one side and no enclosures are permitted. Aerogrammes are convenient, as well as inexpensive.

**Mailgram.**   A popular new service offered jointly by the Postal Service and Western Union. Described in the previous chapter under Telegraph Services.

**Postal Money Orders.**   Prior to October, 1973, postal money orders were limited to amounts up to $100. The limit has been increased to $300. To the purchaser of a $300 money order, the new system represents a two-thirds savings in fees. For up to $10 the fee is 25 cents; from $10.01 to $50 the fee is 35 cents; and from $50.01 to $300 the buyer will pay only one fee of 40 cents. Under the old system, the buyer would have had to pay a 40-cent fee for each of three money orders in the amount of $100 apiece. The new money order form meets American Bankers Association standards for rapid handling, and the processing of all money orders has been centralized at the Postal Data Center in St. Louis, which uses optical character recognition and computer techniques in administering the money order program.

**Registered Mail.**   All classes of mail, particularly those of unusually high value, can be given additional protection, together with evidence of having been delivered, if registered. Registering mail also helps trace delivery. When sending a registered letter it is necessary to go to the post office and fill in the necessary forms. All articles to be registered must be thoroughly sealed (do not use cellophane tape) and postage paid at first class or air mail rates. Upon receipt of the item, the recipient is required to sign a form, acknowledging receipt of delivery. A registered letter may be released to the person to whom it is sent or to his agent. For an additional fee, a personal receipt may be requested. This assures that the letter will be released only to the individual to whom it is addressed. Such pieces bear the label "To Addressee Only." Registered mail is accounted for by number from time of mailing until delivery and is transported separately from other mail under a special lock. In case of loss or damage the customer may be reimbursed up to $10,000, providing the value of the registered articles has been declared at the time of mailing and the appropriate fee has been paid. Minimum registry fee is 95 cents, in addition to postage, and is based upon declared value.

**Special Delivery.**　Any class mail that has been so marked will be charged the special delivery rate. Such pieces may be regular first or second class mail, air mail, registered, insured, or C.O.D. (Collect on Delivery) pieces. Special delivery instruction generally does not speed up the normal travel time between two cities but does assure immediate delivery of the item when it arrives at the designated post office. Air mail special delivery is the speediest mailing method. Special delivery stamps may be purchased at the post office or the equivalent value in regular stamps may be placed upon the envelope, which should always be clearly marked "Special Delivery." Consult the post office for current rates. Use Special Delivery when you need delivery the same day the item is received at the addressee's post office, including weekend delivery not available with regular mail. Do not use for mail addressed to a Post Office box or military installation.

**Special Handling.**　Applied only to third and fourth class mail. For a small additional fee, these two classes will receive the fastest handling and ground transportation practicable, about the same as first class mail. This does not include insurance or special delivery at the destination, but special delivery, if desired, is available at an added fee. If a parcel is sent air mail, special handling is of no additional advantage because it is already traveling at the greatest possible speed. Fees are determined according to weight: up to 2 pounds, 25 cents; from 2 to 10 pounds, 35 cents; over 10 pounds, 50 cents. These fees are in addition to regular postage.

## Handling Special Problems

**Forwarding Mail.**　First class mail only may be forwarded from one city to another without paying additional postage. It may also be reforwarded. First class surface mail may be forwarded by air if additional postage amounting to the difference between surface and air rates is attached.

**Obtaining Change of Address.**　If the mailer wants to know an addressee's new address, he can get this service from the post office by placing the words

"Address Correction Requested" beneath the return address on the envelope. This can be handwritten, stamped, typewritten or printed. The post office will charge ten cents for this service. For first class mail, the post office will forward the piece of ma.l and return only the notification to the sender.

**Recalling Mail.**   If you have dropped a letter in the mailbox and want it back, do not ask the mail collector to give it to you; he is not permitted to do this. Mail can be recalled, however, by making written application at the post office, together with an envelope addressed identically to the one being recalled. If your letter has already left the local post office, the postmaster, at the sender's expense, can telephone or telegraph the postmaster at the addressee's post office to return the letter.

**Returned Mail.**   If a letter is returned to the sender after an attempt has been made to deliver it, it cannot be remailed without new postage. It is best simply to prepare a new envelope with the correct address, affix the proper postage and remail.

**Tracing Lost Mail.**   Receipts issued by the post office, whether for money orders, registered mail, or insured mail, should be retained until receipt of the item has been acknowledged. If after a period of time elapses no acknowledgment of receipt for such mailing arrives, notify the post office to trace the letter or package. Regular first class mail is not easily traced, but the post office will make every attempt to find it for you. In tracing a lost letter or package, the post office requires that a special form be filled out, on which data from any original receipt should be written, along with any other identifying information.

## Preparing the Outgoing Mail

**Sealing and Stamping Hints.**   Here's a suggestion for speeding up the sealing of a number of envelopes. At statement time, for example, many envelopes will be going into the mail at once. Fan out unsealed envelopes, address side down, in groups of six to ten. Then draw a damp sponge over the flaps and, starting with the lower piece, turn down the flaps and seal each one. Do not use too much moisture as this will cause the glue to spread and several letters will stick together.

A similar process simplifies stamping several letters at a time. If possible, purchase your stamps by the roll. Tear off about ten stamps. Fanfold them on the perforations so that they will separate easily. Again fan the envelopes, this time address side up. Wet a strip of stamps with the sponge and, starting at one end of the fanned envelopes, attach the stamp at the end of the strip, tear it off, and proceed to the next envelope. No secretary should be too busy to put a stamp on straight.

**Sorting and Banding.**   Local letters should be separated from out-of-town letters and foreign letters which require special postage. Keep a supply of mail banding tapes on hand. The post office will supply these free of charge upon request — blue bands for local mail, red for out-of-town mail. The tapes are self-sealing and require no glue or rubber bands. Sort the mail according to destination and put a tape around each bundle before dropping it in a pickup box or taking it to the post office. This presorting greatly assists the postal clerks in the rapid routing of your mail.

## Getting Faster Mail Service

Post offices which handle a large volume of mail will appreciate your mailing early in the day whenever possible. Letters or packages that are to be rushed on their way should be taken directly to the post office for mailing. Never leave packages on top of public mail boxes; it is too easy for them to be stolen. Do not trust patients leaving the office or others to mail your letters or packages—do it yourself. If you place a letter tray on your desk, you can keep all outgoing mail together until you are able to send it on its way yourself.

**Postage Meters.**  The postage meter machine is the most efficient way of stamping the mail in a business office. A postage meter prints its own postage, from one cent to $99.99. You set the lever to the amount of postage you need, push a button, and out comes the postage. It's moistened, dated, and post-marked. Some postage meters also seal the envelopes. The meter registers the amount of postage used, and the amount remaining in the meter.

In order to use a postage meter, the mailer applies to the post office for a license, on which he indicates the make and model of the meter he plans to use. He purchases the machine and leases the meter mechanism from the manu-facturer. The meter must be taken to the post office, where it is set for the amount of postage purchased. When the postage is used up, the meter locks until it is again taken to the post office and more postage is purchased. Metered mail does not have to be canceled or postmarked after it reaches the post office. This means it can move on to its destination faster.

In-town letters that are dropped into a mailbox no later than the last mail pickup of the day is fairly sure to be delivered the next day.

**One-Star Mailboxes.**  Have you noticed the mailboxes with the one big white star on the side located along busy streets and in many shopping centers and business areas? These boxes have a pickup at 5 p.m. or later.

**Two-Star Mailboxes.**  The two-star mailboxes have the latest pickups—no earlier than 6:30 and as close to 8 p.m. as possible. These boxes are located in bigger towns—in business areas, and in front of post offices.

**Air-Mail-Only Boxes.**  If you are mailing beyond 150 miles, you should use air mail. It is kept separate from other mail all along the way. Air mail letters and packages are also handled first—before all regular mail in the post office. For next-day delivery to most major cities, you should use an air mail envelope and mail before 4 p.m. in a special air-mail-only box, or by 5 p.m. at your main post office. The air-mail-only box has an all-white top with AIR MAIL in large letters on the side. They are found in front of post offices and in major business sections of large cities.

## VACATION MAIL

When the doctor is away from the office, it is generally the responsibility of his secretary or assistant to handle all mail. In this event, all pieces should be studied carefully. The assistant must then make her decision in regard to handling each piece on the basis of these questions:

1. Is this important enough so that I should call or wire the doctor?
2. Shall I forward this to him for his immediate attention?
3. Shall I answer this myself or send a brief note explaining that there will be a slight delay because the doctor is out of his office?
4. Can this wait for attention until the doctor returns without appearing negligent?

If you are unable to contact your employer or forward important mail to him, always answer the sender immediately, explaining the delay and asking his cooperat.on. Most modern offices have some kind of copy machine as part of the office equipment. Instead of forwarding the original of important pieces of mail to your employer when he is away, and risking possible loss, make a copy for forwarding. Then if he wishes you to answer the letter he can make notations on the copy and return it to you without defacing the original letter.

If your employer is traveling from place to place, each envelope you send him should be numbered consecutively. By doing this he can easily determine whether any mail has been lost or gone astray. By keeping your own record of each piece of mail sent out, with its corresponding number, anything that does not reach him can be identified and remailed if necessary.

Correspondence which does not require immediate action, but which the secretary is unable to answer until the doctor returns, should be placed in a special folder on the doctor's desk, marked "Requires Attention." Mail which the assistant can answer, but which requires the doctor's approval before mailing, should be put into another special folder, marked "For Approval." When the doctor returns, he can then rapidly check and sign these letters for mailing.

Letters marked "Personal" which you hesitate to open and are unable to forward should be acknowledged to the return address on the envelope. The brief acknowledgment should state that the doctor is out of town for a certain period of time and will give the letter his attention upon his return. Your acknowledgment should also offer your help in any way possible in the meantime.

Discard any mail which it is unnecessary for the doctor to see, if at all possible. Some promotional literature will fall into this class. (Make sure, however, that mailings from his professional organizations, whether they are first, second, third, or fourth class, reach his desk.)

Although it is rare, there may be occasions when the entire office is closed. In such cases, the local post office should be notified to forward all first class mail to an address supplied by the doctor, if possible. If forwarding is out of the question, place a request with the post office to hold the mail until your return. Never leave mail unattended to gather outside a mailbox or clutter up a doorway in a hall. Even mail slots may become filled or magazines become stuck in them, causing important mail to pile up outside the slot. There is far too much money sent to doctors' offices to take chances on mail theft. In addition, other important pieces of mail for the doctor may become lost under such circumstances.

If you set up a system for handling all incoming and outgoing mail, what might be a dreaded daily task becomes merely an efficient, routine procedure.

## REFERENCE

*The Postal Manual,* Superintendent of Documents, U.S. Government Printing Office, Washington, D.C.

# Chapter 11

## BEHAVIORAL OBJECTIVES

*The medical office assistant should be able to:*

Produce good typewritten copy of dictated correspondence.
Compose original letters.
Demonstrate knowledge of correct letter form.

Address envelopes in accordance with United States Postal Service recommendations.

# Letter Writing

Letter writing is an important part of the armamentarium of the administrative medical office assistant. The assistant should be able to compose a letter that is professional in looks and language, courteous to the reader, correct in content, concise without being curt—a letter that will create a favorable impression of the writer on anyone reading it.

Although the letter writing responsibilities of the medical office assistant may not be as voluminous as those of a secretary in a business office, there are many other written communications for which she is responsible, such as consultation reports, surgical reports, requests for insurance information, and so forth.

## Prerequisites

Good written communications begin with good equipment and stationery supplies. The typewriter used should be one that will produce good copy; the typewriter ribbon should be dark enough that the letters will be easily read but not so heavily inked as to result in smudged copy. The keys to the typewriter must be kept clean. This is easily accomplished by the regular use of a commercial cushion sheet made especially for this purpose that cleans the keys as you type on it. There is absolutely no excuse for typewriter keys such as the *a, e, o, b,* and *p* being filled with ink from the typewriter ribbon. Good quality watermark bond paper should be used for the professional letterhead. Plain bond paper of matching quality is used for continuation pages of a letter. Letterhead paper is *never* used for the second page of a letter.

## Transcription Skills

The medical office assistant should have received basic instruction in English composition, and have a knowledge of sentence structure, spelling, and punctuation. Much of the doctor's correspondence is dictated either to a machine for transcription by the assistant, or directly to the assistant who writes shorthand. In transcribing such dictation, the assistant must be able to check for errors in composition, punctuate sentences correctly, and spell every word. In many instances, it is the "simple" everyday word that gives trouble—not the technical terms. The assistant is much more inclined to consult a dictionary for the spelling of a technical word because she recognizes the likelihood of misspelling. Too often she does not question her spelling of the common word.

## Composing Responsibilities

Every person who writes letters develops his own personal style. Most physicians conform to a highly professional, dignified style in their dictation. The assistant who is given the responsibility of composing some of the correspondence for the medical office should try to use about the same degree of formality as does her employer. It would be inappropriate for the assistant to write in a breezy, informal style when she is acting as the representative of an employer who is strictly formal in approach.

## Using Form Letters

Many situations that require a letter, such as collections of outstanding accounts, are repetitive; therefore, a few good form letters may be a great timesaver for the busy office assistant. Suggestions for some collection letters will be found in Chapter 16.

## Letter Placement

Standard letter forms have the following components: date line, inside address, salutation, body, complimentary close, signature, and reference initials. Many physicians' letters will also have a subject line; some may have an attention line. These components of the business letter all have a designated place in the standard letter form.

The two letter forms most commonly used in the physician's office are the *block* (Fig. 11–1) and *modified block* (Fig. 11–2). The block form is considered the most efficient because all lines start flush with the left margin. The modified block is more balanced on the page and, consequently, is more pleasing to the eye.

Unless your employer is just starting in practice, he probably has already shown a preference in letter form. You can easily discover his preference by looking over carbon copies of previous correspondence in the files. It is usually best to follow the established pattern unless you find that it is actually very poor or possibly incorrect. If you do decide to make changes, be certain they are improvements.

**Date Line.** The date line is typed on the second line below the last line of the printed letterhead, or it may be typed on the fourth line above the first line of the inside address if a "floating dateline placement" is preferred. The name of the month is written in full, followed by the date and year. The date should not be abbreviated. Ordinal numbers such as 1st, 2nd, and 3rd should not be used following the name of the month.

**Inside Address.** The inside address has two or more lines, starts flush with the left margin, and contains at least the name of the individual or firm to whom

```
                    U. R. GOODE, M.D.
                  1000 SOUTH WEST STREET
                     LONDON, FLORIDA

March 14, 19__




Medical Arts Professional Annex
3578 North Willow Avenue
Anytown, FL    33000

Attention Richard Fluege

Gentlemen:

Please send me full particulars on the professional suites you
expect to offer for sale or rent in about six months.

I definitely plan to re-locate my practice, and am exploring
several possibilities at present.  I shall require approximately
2000 square feet, and prefer a suite at street level rather than
on an upper floor.

After I have had an opportunity to study the information you
send me, I will write or telephone you if I have further questions.

Very truly yours,



U. R. Goode, M.D.

URG:mk
```

**Figure 11–1**

the letter is sent, and the post office address. When the letter is addressed to an individual, the name is preceded by an appropriate title, such as Dr., Mr., Mrs., Miss, or Ms. When addressing a letter to another physician, type the physician's name, followed by his academic degree. Do not use a title and a degree that mean the same thing, such as *Dr.* Herbert H. Long, *M.D.*

**Attention Line.**   If the letter is addressed to a corporation or business firm for the attention of a given individual, an attention line is used. The attention line is placed on the second line below the inside address (Fig. 11–1).

**Salutation.**   The salutation is typed on the second line below the last line of the inside address, flush with the left margin, and is followed by a colon unless open punctuation is used.

**Subject Line.**   If there is a subject line, type it on the second line below the salutation. It may start (1) flush with the left margin, (2) at the point of indenta-

**U. R. GOODE, M.D.**
1000 SOUTH WEST STREET
LONDON, FLORIDA

March 14, 19__

I. M. Wright, M.D.
123 Main Street
Anytown, FL    33000

Dear Doctor Wright:

Mrs. Elaine Norris

Thank you for referring your patient, Mrs. Elaine Norris, for consultation and care.  She was examined in the office today.

FINDINGS:  The patient complained of pain in the left lower quadrant, and some abdominal tenderness.  She had a temperature of 100.2°.

RECOMMENDATIONS:  The patient was placed on a soft, low-residue bland diet, antibiotics, and bed rest for a few days. Upper and lower gastrointestinal X rays will be performed next week.

TENTATIVE DIAGNOSIS:  Diverticulitis of large bowel.

Mrs. Norris has been asked to return here for re-evaluation in about ten days.

Sincerely yours,

U. R. Goode, M.D.

URG:mk

**Figure 11–2**

tion of indented paragraphs, or (3) centered. The word *Subject,* followed by a colon, may be used, or may be omitted entirely (Fig. 11–2).

**Body of Letter.**   Begin typing the body of the letter on the second line below the subject line, or the second line below the salutation if there is no subject line. The first line of each paragraph may be indented 5 or 10 spaces, or may start flush with the left margin.

The tone of the letter is usually determined by the first sentence. The writer should, therefore, try to make certain that this first sentence is worded to elicit a positive reaction from the reader. It is generally wise to put only one idea in each sentence, avoid overly long sentences or paragraphs, and, if possible, limit the business letter to one page. Medical reports often require several pages.

**Complimentary Close.**   Type the complimentary close on the second line below the last line of the body of the letter. Begin flush with the left margin in the *block* form; begin at the center in the *modified block* letter.

The complimentary close is the writer's way of saying goodbye. The words used are determined by the degree of formality in the salutation. For instance, if the salutation is "Dear Herb:" the close might be "Cordially" or "Sincerely." If the letter is addressed to a business firm, the salutation is "Gentlemen:" and the complimentary close most generally used is "Very truly yours." The complimentary close is followed with a comma, and only the first word is capitalized.

**Typewritten Signature.**   Typewriting the name of the signer of the letter is a courtesy to the reader, especially if the name does not appear on the printed letterhead. Type the signature on the fourth line directly below the complimentary close.

**Reference Initials.**   The reference initials identify the dictator and the transcriber, and are typed flush with the left margin on the second line below the typed signature. If the secretary composes the letter, she uses only her own initials. There is no set form, but the one most generally used has the dictator's initials in caps followed by a colon and the transcriber's initials in lower case (PF:mk).

**Enclosure.**   If the letter indicates an enclosure, type the word *Enclosure* or *Enc.* on the second line below the reference initials. If there is more than one enclosure specify the number (Enclosure 3).

**Second Page Heading.**   If the letter requires one or more continuation pages, the heading of the second and subsequent pages must contain three bits of information: the name of the addressee, the page number, and the date. Two accepted forms for the heading are

*I. M. Wright, M.D.*                         -2-                         *March 14, 19___*

                              or

I. M. Wright, M.D.
Page 2
March 14, 19___

The heading is typed on line 7 and the continuation of the body of the letter begins on line 10.

## Personal Signatures

Some letters are signed by the secretary or office assistant. Although not all authorities agree on the form to be followed, most recommend that a woman's typewritten signature include a title, *Miss* or *Mrs.*, and that the title *not* be enclosed in parentheses. It is not necessary to include the title in the handwritten signature.

## Addressing the Envelope

Most offices prefer to use the large envelope that requires only two folds in a letter. With this size envelope (known as a No. 10) begin typing the address on the 14th line from the top of the envelope, just to the left of center, about 4 inches from the left edge of the envelope. Single space the address. Do not indent the second and third lines of the address. Type the city, state and Zip code on one line.

**Zip Code.** The ZIP (Zonal Improvement Plan) code has become an essential part of every mailing address. The Zip code is a five-digit number which identifies a delivery unit, and associates that unit with a major post office through which mail is routed for delivery. The nation is divided into ten large areas, and the first digit of the Zip code identifies one of these areas, starting with "0" on the East Coast and ending with "9" on the West Coast and Hawaii. The first three digits identify a major city or distribution point, and all five digits identify an individual post office, zone of a city, or other delivery unit. Adding the Zip code to the addresses of your correspondents greatly facilitates the fast handling of your mail, and no address is complete without it. The Zip code should follow two pica spaces or three elite spaces after the state, with no punctuation between. The United States Postal Service recommends that the two-letter state abbreviations be used with the Zip code (Fig. 11–3). Some cities have multiple Zip codes. You may obtain a directory for any of these cities free of charge by addressing a request to the postmaster of the city in question.

## Professional Image

In addition to its intended message, every piece of writing creates an image of the originator. The office assistant who takes pride in her work will see that all letters or reports going out of the physician's office are neat, well-spaced, and professional looking. All words will be spelled correctly. Trite phrases and redundant expressions will be avoided. Typewriting must be impeccable and numerous corrections avoided.

No correspondence should be folded and inserted into its envelope until it has been checked for errors in spelling, punctuation, or subject matter, and the signature verified. Take care that you are placing the right letter in the right envelope if you are mailing several pieces at one time.

Do not file carbons of letters until the original has been signed. Many assistants place the carbon copy on the doctor's desk along with the original. If he accepts and signs the originals, he may then initial the carbon copy. This shows on later reference that the letter was not sent out without his knowledge and that it was personally approved by the doctor.

TWO-LETTER ABBREVIATIONS

UNITED STATES AND TERRITORIES

| | | | |
|---|---|---|---|
| Alabama | AL | Montana | MT |
| Alaska | AK | Nebraska | NE |
| Arizona | AZ | Nevada | NV |
| Arkansas | AR | New Hampshire | NH |
| California | CA | New Jersey | NJ |
| Canal Zone | CZ | New Mexico | NM |
| Colorado | CO | New York | NY |
| Connecticut | CT | North Carolina | NC |
| Delaware | DE | North Dakota | ND |
| District of Columbia | DC | Ohio | OH |
| Florida | FL | Oklahoma | OK |
| Georgia | GA | Oregon | OR |
| Guam | GU | Pennsylvania | PA |
| Hawaii | HI | Puerto Rico | PR |
| Idaho | ID | Rhode Island | RI |
| Illinois | IL | South Carolina | SC |
| Indiana | IN | South Dakota | SD |
| Iowa | IA | Tennessee | TN |
| Kansas | KS | Texas | TX |
| Kentucky | KY | Utah | UT |
| Louisiana | LA | Vermont | VT |
| Maine | ME | Virgin Islands | VI |
| Maryland | MD | Virginia | VA |
| Massachusetts | MA | Washington | WA |
| Michigan | MI | West Virginia | WV |
| Minnesota | MN | Wisconsin | WI |
| Mississippi | MS | Wyoming | WY |
| Missouri | MO | | |

CANADIAN PROVINCES AND TERRITORIES

| | | | |
|---|---|---|---|
| Alberta | AB | Nova Scotia | NS |
| British Columbia | BC | Ontario | ON |
| Manitoba | MB | Prince Edward Island | PE |
| New Brunswick | NB | Quebec | PQ |
| Newfoundland | NF | Saskatchewan | SK |
| Northwest Territories | NT | Yukon Territory | YT |

**Figure 11–3**

# REFERENCES

Hanna, J. M., Popham, E. L., and R. S. Tilton, *Secretarial Procedures and Administration*, 6th Ed., Cincinnati, Ohio, South-Western Publishing Company, 1973

House, C. R. and A. M. Koebele, *Reference Manual for Office Personnel*, 5th Ed., Cincinnati, Ohio, South-Western Publishing Company, 1970

# Chapter 12

**CHAPTER OUTLINE**

**BEHAVIORAL OBJECTIVES**

*The medical office assistant should be able to:*

Assist the physician in maintaining a personal library.

Assist in the preparation of abstracts.

Help gather information for lectures and manuscripts.

Typewrite and proofread manuscripts suitable for publication.

# Library and Editorial Duties

Medicine differs from other fields in two important aspects. First, the doctor never can stop studying. Medical progress is so rapid that each doctor must struggle constantly to keep abreast of what's new. Second, the doctor shares the discoveries, information, and observations he gains in his practice, in research, and in study with others in his field by writing and speaking.

The assistant often is called upon to assist the doctor with the preparation of his articles and speeches. She generally helps him maintain his library of books and periodicals. And sometimes, if she is particularly interested in editorial duties, the doctor may request her aid in the actual researching of a subject.

## THE PHYSICIAN'S LIBRARY

Every physician builds up his own personal medical library which forms the basis for his graduate education and is an important source of information. His own library usually consists of the books he acquires in school, books he obtains because of special interest in later years, files of the *Journal of the American Medical Association*, his state medical society journal, certain specialty journals in his field, trade journals, and some informative material provided by pharmaceutical companies. The individual practitioner's library may not be large, since he can neither afford to build up a huge collection of volumes nor store the materials he acquires. However, the materials he does keep must be systematically organized so that the contents are quickly accessible.

Libraries must have some plan of organization. In setting up or rearranging a small library, books should be classified by subject groupings reflecting medical specialties. Those dealing with related topics should be placed together. Arrange journals and periodicals alphabetically.

Periodicals should be bound at regular intervals, generally by volume, in order to preserve the individual copies. The doctor's assistant should see to it that copies are bound in a consistent manner, as several different types of bindings present an untidy appearance. Most journals in the medical field publish indexes, either yearly, twice yearly, or quarterly. Make sure that the index for the copies is bound with them. In most cities the binding of periodicals is a service which is performed locally.

**Card Catalog of Books.** The books in the doctor's library should be indexed in a card catalog or book. A 3 by 5 card file is useful for this purpose. Generally, three or more cards should be typed for each book: a subject card, an author card, and a title card. Here's how to index a book in this manner, using *Introduction to Medicine and Medical Terminology* by Louise Espey Bollo as an example.

Since the volume is a textbook on medicine and medical terminology, two subject cards should be prepared. "Medicine" should be typed at the head of one and "Medical Terminology" at the head of the other, with the following information appearing on the card: Introduction to Medicine and Medical Terminology, Louise Espey Bollo. Philadelphia: W. B. Saunders Company, 1961. A title card on which the book title appears as the top entry and an author card on which the author's surname and initials appear at the top of the card should also be prepared; the additional information about the book which appears on the subject card should also appear on these cards. Then the four cards should be filed in a lexicographic file (all entries alphabetized together), or in a file broken down into sections for author, subject, or title. With such a file and cross reference system, books can be located very quickly.

**Periodical File.** One of the doctor's commonest complaints is the difficulty in keeping up with medical literature. His problem becomes clear when it is pointed out that hundreds of medical and scientific journals are published in English in this country alone each year. The system which a physician uses for examining periodical literature will determine the method of filing periodicals.

It is unlikely that the individual doctor will want to maintain a complete index of all articles appearing in the periodicals he receives. This is a task for a skilled medical librarian. Most doctors do want to keep track of those articles which are of particular interest to them. Abstracts are of great value to professional men and help them in the continuing task of keeping abreast of scientific developments.

## PREPARATION OF AN ABSTRACT

An abstract is a kind of summary or epitome of a book, paper, or case history. It is brief, indicating the nature of the article and summarizing the most important points and conclusions. The value of abstracts to busy doctors is indicated in this statement by Dr. Lewis J. Moorman:

"It is obvious that both the general practitioner and the specialist need the help of those who read for the express purpose of sifting, culling, choosing, and epitomizing the pertinent facts for publication. Placing the kernel of medical knowledge stripped of all superfluous verbiage before the busy physician represents a great service."

Many doctors prepare abstracts of the articles which they find of particular value, and in some offices the secretary-assistant is trained to do abstracting for the doctor. A girl who can prepare a good abstract of an article can save the doctor from reading ten to twenty pages of the original article and can help focus his attention upon information in the article of particular interest to him.

A number of medical and scientific publications contain abstracts of articles. The *Journal of the American Medical Association* contains a section entitled "Selected Abstracts" in which medical literature is reviewed and summarized. Here is an example of an abstract taken from the April 3, 1972, issue of the *Journal.*

**Acute Renal Failure and Open Heart Surgery**—E. D. Yeboah et al (Hammersmith
  Hosp, London) *Br Med J* **1**:415–417 (Feb 12) 1972
  Retrospective studies of 428 open heart operations showed a 26% incidence of mild
renal failure and a 4.7% incidence of severe renal failure. The mortality was 38% in mild,
and 70% in severe cases of renal failure. Autopsy showed significant renal pathology in
half the patients who developed renal failure. When perfusion exceeded 60 minutes,
mean perfusion pressures were less than 80 mm Hg, preoperative blood urea values exceeded 40 mg/100 cc; there was an increased incidence of renal failure when multiple
valve replacement operations were done. Peritoneal dialysis was effective in 15 patients
with severe renal failure and hemodialysis was required in 7.

Abstracts, as you can see, must clearly indicate the nature of the information
contained in the article. Each should note any new procedures or revealed facts,
as well as results of studies and experiments and conclusions noted. Naturally,
the length and character of the article itself will determine the type and length of
the abstract. In most scientific articles, the writer himself will summarize his
conclusions at the end of the piece. This summary is of great help in preparing
an abstract. There is a uniform style for abstracts which is shown in the abstract
taken from J.A.M.A. The title, surname, and initials of the author, publication,
volume, pages, month, and year precede the text for the abstract.

In addition to the abstracts which appear in the *Journal of the American Medical Association,* abstracts are published in certain other journals, and regular volumes of abstracts in special fields are published, such as *Physiological Reviews, Nutrition Abstracts and Reviews, Chemical Abstracts, Biological Abstracts,* and *Excerpta
Medica.* These are available in medical libraries.

**Abstract File for Periodical Literature.**  A system for keeping track of significant literature by use of abstracts is suggested by a number of physicians. The
doctor examines the abstracts section of the journals he receives and checks
those of particular interest. The assistant then makes up a list of the articles
checked and secures the original articles, either by borrowing the periodicals in
which they appear from a medical library, writing to the journal for a single
copy, or writing to the author for a reprint. The doctor then reads the original
articles and prepares brief abstracts based on the facts in the article; later the
assistant types the abstracts and files them in the office. One physician states
that merely by following this procedure with the "Selected Abstracts" section in
the *Journal of the American Medical Association,* he is able to see the articles in
which he has a particular interest in about 300 different journals covering some
13,000 articles per year.

Many doctors prepare abstracts or ask their assistants to prepare abstracts
only of those articles they find particularly valuable in their practices. Today
many professional men dictate abstracts using a sound-writing system at their
leisure and their secretaries transcribe them later. Short summaries of these articles are typed on cards on which the exact references to the periodical, author,
title, volume, date of publication, and so forth are also indicated. These cards are
then filed. If abstract cards are kept, it is not necessary to clip and file the actual
articles separately. The journals in which they appear can be kept in the usual alphabetical order.

Since the early 1970s several medical journals have regularly published, for
their subscribers, abstracts of all their articles on sheets of perforated cards

which can be separated and indexed in a 3 by 5-inch file box. Some of these are the *New England Journal of Medicine, American Journal of Medicine, Postgraduate Medicine,* and *American Journal of Medical Sciences.* Another popular source of information for physicians is *Current Contents,* published biweekly by the Institute for Scientific Information. It contains abstracts and title pages from most of the leading medical journals.

**Reprints.**  When doctors write articles or present papers before scientific meetings, their work is often published in a periodical and reprints of it made available to their colleagues. A portion of each doctor's library is usually composed of a collection of such reprints. In some cases the reprints come into the office unsolicited, owing to the doctor's interest in a particular man's writing in the past; in other cases, the doctor may request his secretary to write for a particular reprint. Sometimes the doctor may have a special postcard form made up for ordering reprints:

Please send me (no.) copies of your article,_____ (title) _____ ,

_____which appeared in_____ (publication) ____ , ____ (date ___ .

_____

(Doctor's signature)

Other doctors prefer to write personal letters in which they compliment the author upon the excellence of his article and request copies of it for their files. Reprints often present a storage problem in the office, since they are not of uniform size. However, references to these reprints can be placed in the library card file and the reprints themselves placed in a separate drawer.

**Other Reference Files.**  Doctors must have at their finger tips a variety of miscellaneous medical information. For this reason some doctors build up, in addition to periodical and book collections and indexes, a separate reference file of valuable information. The system proposed by Dr. Lyon Steine in *GP* magazine (1950) has considerable merit.

To keep track of dosages, certain medical techniques, and other useful information, Dr. Steine uses a 4 by 6 card file. As he reads medical periodicals, he marks in the margin material of interest and then marks those pages to be clipped on the cover of the magazines. One of his staff later clips this marked material and pastes the entries on subject cards headed appropriately. The title of the article, its author, the periodical in which it appeared, the page number, volume, and date of publication also are placed upon the card. The periodicals are then discarded. The clipped material is filed by subject alphabetically in the card file.

For example, if Dr. Steine has a patient with angina who wants to know if it is safe to travel, he checks his card file under "angina" for information and comes up with a clipping of an article pointing out that travel is safe for such patients if the maximum altitude is 5000 feet and oxygen is available. This article also states that air travel would be inadvisable unless the plane were pressurized to 5000 feet. A variety of information, ranging from the name and address of the local Alcoholics Anonymous contact, information on immunizations necessary for travel in foreign countries, and so forth, is thus easily accessible. The information about medications provided in card form by various drug companies also can be placed in such a file.

Neither the doctor nor his assistant should try to index material without first becoming familiar with the content. As personalized a method as possible should be used—that is, material should be indexed in terms of how it might later be used.

**Diagnostic Files.**  Physicians often draw material for their writing and speaking from the case histories of their own patients. For this reason, many doctors like to set up diagnostic files so that they can quickly pull out information on the incidence of certain side effects among patients treated with a particular medication, for example. The assistant familiar with basic nomenclature will have no difficulty in maintaining such a file. The system used will vary from office to office, but subject cards generally will carry the name of the disease or surgical procedure, with subheadings for various aspects with the patient's name, diagnosis, and type of treatment listed below. For example, one subject entry might be "blood diseases" with subheadings for anemia, leukemia, toxemia, and so forth. Personal or patient cards will be headed with the patient's name with diagnosis, treatment, prognosis, and miscellaneous information below. By keeping such a file a doctor can readily obtain the charts from his case history file of all patients with a particular condition. This is particularly valuable to those men who do a great deal of teaching, writing, or research.

**Patients' Library.**  Many doctors today keep a small library of educational information for patients. This library generally contains some books written in language that the average patient can understand and a number of pamphlets and reprints that the patient can take home for his own file. Dr. George Schmitt, a Miami, Florida, internist, for example, has built up a good-sized library of information on such subjects as diabetes, heart disease, first aid, and other subjects, which he provides to patients. This personalized library service saves the doctor considerable time in repeating simple educational information and is generally welcomed by patients.

The Department of Health Education of the American Medical Association has developed a whole series of pamphlets called the "MD-Patient Information Service," which provides specific information in various health areas. Many physicians use these to complement the information that they personally give their patients. A special rack for displaying the pamphlets may be purchased from the A.M.A., and the pamphlets are available at a very low cost to the physician.

# HELPING GATHER INFORMATION

An intelligent secretary-assistant employed by a doctor who teaches, writes, or speaks frequently can increase her value as an employee by actually assisting him with the preparation of the paper. She may make up a list of references for a particular paper or talk or may even do actual research and preparation of abstracts. Any assistant who is called upon to assume such responsibility must know how to make the best use of the available library and reference facilities.

**Library Facilities.**  Almost every doctor, even though he may be practicing in a rural area, has access to medical libraries. The doctor who practices in a metropolitan area or is located near a medical center such as a university is particularly fortunate, since these areas offer good library facilities. All general hospitals also maintain medical libraries comprising a basic collection of carefully selected, authoritative medical textbooks and reference works of the latest edition and files of current journals. The Medical Library Association sets standards for member libraries. A physician usually has access to a county society library or can utilize the package library services of his state society. In addition, extension library facilities can be used to obtain information from special supplemental collections. The American Medical Association, for example, and some other specialty societies, offer periodical lending services and package library services to their members. The facilities of the National Library of Medicine can also be used by doctors. The National Library of Medicine has established a system whereby doctors may get materials from a Regional Medical Library Program when information is not available locally. In those instances when the Regional Program cannot satisfy the need, the request is channeled to the National Library of Medicine.

HOW TO USE A LIBRARY.  All libraries systematically organize the books, periodicals, and other materials in a fairly uniform manner in order that the information be easily located and accessible. The doctor's assistant who finds it necessary to go to a library to do special work should introduce herself to the librarian or her assistant and get an idea of what the library has to offer in the way of materials. At this time she can also learn about the arrangement of materials, privileges, rules, and regulations for use of the library. The trained medical librarian, after a brief discussion, usually can suggest short cuts that are of great help in locating references or doing research.

CARD CATALOG OF BOOKS.  All books, monographs, treatises, handbooks, dictionaries, and encyclopedias contained in a library are indexed by author and subject and sometimes by title in the card catalog. This catalog is really an index of the book contents of the library. Cards are arranged alphabetically, with subject, author, and title cards alphabetized in one series, or are alphabetized within separate sections for subject, author, or title.

There are a number of schemes for classifying library books. In library procedure, classification means putting together materials on a given subject with related materials placed nearby.

Medical libraries use various classification systems. The Dewey decimal system, used not only in medical but all types of libraries, is sometimes used for arranging medical library collections. This system utilizes decimal numbers to indicate particular subjects and arranges the book collection in numerical sequence for easy location. For example, 616 indicates Pathology, Diseases, Treatment. Here's an example of how the Dewey decimal system works:

616.1     Diseases of the cardiovascular system
616.9     Communicable and other diseases
616.96    Parasitic diseases
616.99    Other general diseases
616.992   Neoplasms and neoplastic diseases

The Library of Congress classification system is also used. This consists of a number of separate, mutually exclusive classifications based upon combination of letters of the alphabet and numerals:

QR: Bacteriology
RD: Surgery
RC 321–431: Diseases of the nervous system

The National Library of Medicine classification system is replacing the Library of Congress system in many medical libraries.

There are some other systems, such as the Boston Medical Library Classification, the Cunningham Classification and the Barnard Classification, which are used by some medical libraries. However, a brief discussion with the librarian and a quick look at the card catalog will generally help acquaint you with the system used.

How the Card Catalog Can Help You Locate Books. No matter what system of classification is used, the main purpose is to help those who use the library to locate volumes quickly. The symbol for the particular book, whether it be a numeral, a letter, or a combination of numerals and letters, appears on the card for the book in the card file. This symbol is called a "classification mark." It also appears on the spine of the volume. To locate a volume, check the (classification) mark on the card and if an open shelf system is used, find that shelf in the library where corresponding symbols appear. If a closed shelf system is used in the library, give the number of the book and its title to the librarian and she will locate it for you.

Using Periodical Reference Books. The bulk of current medical literature appears in medical periodicals and journals. It is estimated that approximately 50,000 scientific journals are published in the world each year carrying some 1,850,000 scientific articles. Consequently, some reference system for these hundreds of articles is required. In medical libraries at least three indexes are available to help researchers and others locate various periodical references: the *Cumulative Index Medicus*, the *Current List of Medical Literature*, and the *Cumulative Index to Hospital Literature*.

The *Cumulative Index Medicus*, a kind of reader's guide to medical literature, was published until 1960 twice each year by the American Medical Association. This index covered both books and periodicals and their contents published during the preceding six-month interval. In January 1960 the National Library of Medicine began publication of a monthly *Index Medicus*. Annual cumulated volumes of this index were published by the American Medical Association. Both the monthly and the annual volumes are now published by the National Library of Medicine. An author and subject index to periodicals in many languages is contained in the volume, along with a list of new medical books published recently.

Let's say a doctor is interested in background information on barbiturates used in anesthesia. Turning to anesthesia in the *C. I. M.* the following reference might appear:

Anesthesia, barbital and barbital derivatives—choice of anesthesia in endoscopic procedures (with special reference to thiopental with curare), (A. C. Jones, Jr.) Tr. Pacific Coast Oto-Ophth. Soc. 32:103–107, '51.

Or, let's say that A. C. Jones' work in anesthesia is known to the doctor. He is interested in locating all his recent articles in the field. Turning to the author's name section in *C. I. M.*, this reference might appear:

Jones, A. C., Jr. Choice of anesthesia in endoscopic procedures, Tr. Pacific Coast Oto-Ophth. Soc. 32:103–107, '51.

The National Library of Medicine has developed two bibliographic retrieval systems, MEDLARS and AIM-TWX. According to Wilhelm Moll, Director, Medical Center Library, University of Virginia, Charlottesville, in a letter appearing in *Library Journal*, March 1, 1972:

... MEDLARS (or Medical Literature Analysis and Retrieval System) has been operating for eight years. It is a computer-based system in operation at the National Library of Medicine designed to achieve rapid bibliographical access to the library's store of information. Becoming operational in January 1964 with the publication of the first computer-produced issue of *Index Medicus*, the system has been turning out the monthly and annually cumulated indexes to the world's (approximately 2500) biomedical journals. It also makes possible retrospective demand bibliographical searches, recurring bibliographies on specialized subjects, and a host of other important bibliographical publications. These publications are used in practically every country of the world today.

AIM-TWX, on the other hand, is an on-line, remote-access retrieval service used by some 65 hospital and medical libraries presently. It allows a librarian with access to a TWX (teletype) machine to search a five-year file of the 122 most commonly used clinical medical and nursing journals, including the 100 titles in *Abridged Index Medicus.*

In 1960 the *Index Medicus* was contained in three volumes; in 1970 it required eight volumes. The development of MEDLARS and AIM-TWX has provided an invaluable service to the profession by making possible easy access to references on an unlimited number of medical subjects. A library with a small staff could never provide this service to physicians without such electronic assistance.

Bibliographies for reference work can be prepared by referring to such volumes as the *Cumulative Index Medicus*. The *Current List of Medical Literature*, a former publication of the National Library of Medicine, is a similar volume listing by subject the contents of current medical journals. Each volume contains an author and subject index and an alphabetical listing of journals. A numerical system is used to locate various references. For example, in the author index the following entry might be found:

English O S 13935

In the Register of Articles under the publication *Geriatrics* (Minneapolis) the number 13935 would indicate the following reference:

English O S (Climacteric neuroses and their management, pp. 139–45).

The *Cumulative Index To Hospital Literature* contains an author and subject index to more than 300 journals in the hospital and related fields, including references to hospital literature in medical, nursing, public health, business, architectural, and other periodicals. It is published quarterly with five-year cumulative indexes by the American Hospital Association in Chicago.

Also valuable in some instances is the index to the *Journal of the American Medical Association*, published three times a year.

OTHER REFERENCE SOURCES. There are a number of other specialized reference volumes which a medical librarian may use to locate particular literature. The *Monthly Catalog of U S. Government Publications*, for example, contains certain medical listings, and is sometimes valuable in research work. Or, in securing biographical information about physicians or professional men, it is often necessary to turn to such books as the *Directory of Medical Specialists, American Men of Science*, the *American Medical Directory*, or *Who's Who Among Physicians and Surgeons*. Encyclopedias such as *Encyclopedia Britannica* and the *Practical Medicine* series also are sometimes helpful in obtaining basic information.

**Preparing a Bibliography.** Utilizing the various reference sources of the medical library, a bibliography or list of references on a specific topic can be made up with comparatively little difficulty. It does take time, since the list of references must be accurate. Many researchers recommend listing each reference separately on a 3 by 5 card or in a small loose-leaf notebook. This simplifies the actual preparation of the formal bibliography which always accompanies any published medical paper. Take down all this information: subject, author, title of book or article, publisher or periodical, volume, date of publication, and pages. Sometimes card catalogs and other periodical references will list brief summaries of the specific reference cited; this information is also helpful in research and should be taken down.

Some libraries will prepare medical bibliographies free of charge or for a small fee. Some also will abstract or review literature, translate articles, and collect case reports. The American College of Surgeons library, for example, offers this service at a modest fee to its members. It is best to remember, however, that most medical librarians do not have the time to perform such complete services, although they are ready and willing to help the doctor or his assistant make up individual bibliographies.

## MANUSCRIPT PREPARATION

In most cases the secretary's tasks in connection with the preparation of a talk or a manuscript for publication are mainly mechanical; the doctor himself is responsible for the actual writing. However, since many professional men ask their assistants to serve in the capacity of editorial secretaries, smoothing out and actually editing their copy before submitting it for publication, a basic understanding of the style, format, and characteristics of medical papers is necessary.

A good medical paper must present established new facts, modes or practices, or principles of value, results of suitable original research, or a review of facts on a subject from which the reader can draw a legitimate conclusion. The subject should be limited to a definite area or problem before writing is begun and the purpose determined in advance.

The writing style for a scientific paper should be simple and straightforward. Excess words should be ruthlessly pared from the article. Grammatical construction should be correct in order to facilitate direct, clear expression. Slang, colloquialisms, personal allusions, and reminiscences should generally be avoided in papers for publication; they are often acceptable and add a friendly tone to a paper to be delivered in person before a medical meeting. The paper should be well organized and proceed smoothly from beginning to end in a direct fashion.

Dr. Morris Fishbein, former editor of the *Journal of the American Medical Association*, states in his book, *Medical Writing:* "A florid, roseate style, full of polysyllabic, metaphorical phraseology, distracts the reader's attention. Seldom is it necessary in scientific writing to employ other than simple English terms to express an idea or to state a fact."

Summing it up very simply, Selma DeBakey says, "Clarity, unity and coherence, with emphasis in the right direction, combine to make pleasing style."

There are a number of excellent books which aid the medical writer in preparing this copy. Dr. Fishbein's book, *Medical Writing*, 3rd ed., New York, McGraw-Hill Book Company, 1957, has long been considered a top-notch text in this field. The University of Chicago has also published a guide for writers entitled *A Manual of Style*, 12th ed., Chicago, University of Chicago Press, 1969. Other good reference sources include *The Manuscript: A Guide for the Author*, by W. Jaggi, White Plains, New York, Karger-Phiebig, 1966; *The Preparation of Medical Literature*, by Louise M. Cross, Philadelphia, J. B. Lippincott Company, 1959; and *How to Write Scientific and Technical Papers*, 3rd ed., by Sam F. Trelease, Baltimore, Williams and Wilkins Company, 1958.

Each medical periodical usually has its own style for publishing papers. It is a good idea to check the journal in advance and prepare the manuscript accordingly in order to minimize editorial changes. There are certain fairly uniform procedures, however, in mechanical preparation of a manuscript to be submitted for publication.

**Rough Drafts.**   Triple-space rough or first drafts of the article to provide plenty of space for corrections and revisions. In some offices different colors of paper are used to distinguish between first, second, and final drafts of the article.

**Final Drafts.**   Double-space the finished paper on 8½ by 11 inch standard size paper. It is unwise to single-space a manuscript, since this makes it difficult for the editor who receives it to make corrections or insert instructions for the printer. Type on one side of the paper only and make at least one, preferably two, carbons. The original article is submitted to the editor; the author retains at least one carbon for later checking of proofs. Allow at least an inch margin at each side and clearly indicate all paragraphs. Gauge bottom margins carefully.

In the center of page one the title of the article should appear. If there is a subtitle, this appears under the shorter main title. Then the author's name and identification is listed. If the paper was presented at a particular scientific meeting, this information should appear either below the author's name or at the bottom of page one with an asterisk.

Skip at least three spaces before beginning the text of the article. No title page is necessary for manuscripts submitted for publication. Subsequent pages should be numbered, either in the center of the top or bottom margin or in the upper right- or upper left-hand corner. Generally, the author's name should also appear with the page number on each sheet for identification purposes.

## PREVALENCE AND SIGNIFICANCE OF ANEMIA AS SEEN IN A RURAL GENERAL PRACTICE
### J. J. Kirschenfeld, M.D.
### and
### H. H. Tew, M.S., Fort Deposit, Ala.

The typical medical article leads off with an introductory section outlining the nature of the material or problem to be covered, follows with actual discussion of the subject, and concludes with a summary in which conclusions are usually noted in numerical form. The format for case reports is somewhat similar. Case reports based on clinical information should be written clearly in smooth narrative style and should not read like a collection of telegraphic notes. There should be a clear presentation of sequence of events. A brief abstract may appear at the beginning or end of any article. This summary should be rigidly condensed and should contain the deductions as well as clearly reflect the author's viewpoint. Only the actual conclusions reached should be numbered.

**Footnotes.**   When a paper is based upon a study of the writing of others, it is necessary to acknowledge the sources used. In medical and scientific papers, footnotes usually provide exact references to sources of material. Forms of footnotes differ slightly, depending upon the style of the particular periodical, but in general a footnote contains the author's name, the title of the work cited, the facts of publication, and the exact page from which the citation was taken. Footnotes may be typed in the copy directly below the statement referred to and separated by two solid lines, or placed at the bottom of the page. Or, some editors prefer that footnotes be numbered in the paper and typed on a separate sheet of paper at the end of the article. Here is how a footnote would appear if the first system were used:

> A suitable title, informative subheads, a clear summary and cogent conclusions represent the frame work of a well constructed paper. [1]

1. Fishbein, M. D., Morris: *Medical Writing*, New York, The Blakiston Division, McGraw-Hill Book Company, Inc., 1957, p. 34.

The first time a book or article is mentioned in a footnote, all the information about publication should appear in the footnote; after that, references to the same source can be shortened to the author's last name and the page number cited. When a periodical is concerned, a later reference need contain only the author's name, the magazine, and the page number.

The abbreviation "ibid.," which means "in the same place," can be used with a page number to indicate subsequent reference to the same book or article already cited if it directly follows the first reference. For example, second reference to the Fishbein book coming right after the first one in the paper described would read:

2. Ibid., p. 33.

Detailed information about footnote preparation can be obtained from the University of Chicago's *Manual of Style* or a similar reference book.

**Final Bibliography.** All scientific papers carry a complete bibliography of source materials. Great care should be exercised in making up the final bibliography to make certain all references are correct. List only those sources which directly pertain to the paper and were used in its preparation. The form of bibliographies is fairly uniform. A periodical listing includes the author's name and initials, title of article, name of periodical (either in a commonly used abbreviated form or written in full), volume number, pages cited, and date of publication. A book reference includes the author's name and initials, title, edition, place of publication, name of publisher, year of publication, and volume number.

> Book: Miller, B. F., and J. Burt, *Good Health: Personal and Community*, 2nd ed., Philadelphia, W. B. Saunders Co., 1966.
> Periodical: Dunning, Gordon M., Protecting the Public During Weapons Testing at the Nevada Test Site, J.A.M.A., *158*:900–904, July 16, 1955.

Punctuation in bibliographies varies, depending upon the style of the particular publication. The main parts of the entry can be separated either by periods or by commas. The period at the end of the line is sometimes omitted.

Certain types of references present problems, since they do not fall into either the book or periodical categories. Government bulletins, for example, should be listed in this manner: author's name, title of article, number of the bulletin, name of the department, name of the bureau, and date of publication. Monographs and reports should be treated as books.

Bibliographies may be arranged alphabetically according to author's names or numerically as the references appear in the text. The main point to remember is that whatever punctuation and form is used, it should be consistent throughout the entire listing.

**Illustrations.** All drawings, photographs, and other illustrative material submitted with a manuscript should be pasted or attached to separate sheets. Never include such materials in the body of the manuscript. Illustrations add value to a paper but are expensive and should be used with restraint and judgment. The explanation of the drawing or illustration should appear in a legend. Glossy photographs reproduce best. Captions for photos should be typed on separate sheets or may be pasted with rubber cement below the photo. On the back of the photograph or drawing the author's name and the number of the illustration should be penciled lightly. Do not use pins or paper clips on photos. Credit lines should be given for copyrighted or commercial photos or illustrations. If x-ray films are submitted, make sure the prints are shiny; indicate on the back where they may be cropped, but leave localizing landmarks.

Charts and line drawings must be carefully prepared in order to get good reproduction. Such drawings preferably should be done with India or black ink on heavy white bond paper. The charts should be condensed and simplified as much as possible. Letters and identifying numerals can be placed on the face of the chart with the explanation in the legend below.

Tables should be typewritten on separate sheets in a uniform style, each numbered consecutively and with a descriptive heading.

All illustrative material should be keyed to the manuscript. In other words, illustrations should be numbered and indications placed in the manuscript as to where each illustration should be placed. The editor may not be able to place the illustration at exactly the spot indicated, but he must have this information in order to group the pictures and charts correctly.

**Revision.** An important step in the preparation of any manuscript is a careful revision of copy. This is a duty often assigned to the secretary. Revisions should be made with these specific objectives in mind: (1) organization, (2) accuracy, (3) content, (4) conciseness, (5) correct sentence and grammatical construction, (6) clarity and smoothness. The secretary should check for correct spelling, using a medical dictionary as well as a regular dictionary to aid her in this task.

**Mailing the Manuscript.** Generally, manuscripts should not be folded but should be mailed flat in a large envelope. However, sometimes a paper of less than four pages can be folded twice and mailed in a regular business envelope. Or a manuscript running from four to eight pages is sometimes folded once and mailed in a 6 by 9 envelope. A letter stating that the manuscript is being submitted for publication should be enclosed. Photos and illustrations should be mailed flat with protective cardboards.

**Proofreading.** A paper accepted for publication will be set in type, and proofs of the article will usually be returned by the editor to the doctor's office for checking. Since changes in a manuscript once it is set in type are costly, revisions should be limited to correction of errors and minor changes. It is best to work in a team with someone when checking galley proofs, with one person holding the proofs and the other person reading from the original copy. Check for typographical errors, omitted lines and words, and so forth. Use a different-colored pencil for corrections on the proofs than the one used by the proof-reader on the publication. Corrections should be entered in the margins of the proof, on a line with the error to be corrected.

The assistant whose employer does a great deal of writing for publication should become familiar with the proofreader's marks commonly used. A list of these appears in *A Manual of Style*, published by the University of Chicago Press, and in other books on writing for publication. A few common proofreader's marks are shown on the next page.

One corrected galley should be returned to the editor and one set of proofs should be retained in the office. If a second set of proofs is sent later, check the first corrected set against the second set to make sure all corrections have been made.

**Indexing.** Often it is necessary to provide an index for a long paper or a book. An author and subject index can be made from page proofs. One system for indexing is to use slips of paper or 3 by 5 cards. Each index entry is listed on a separate card or slip; this simplifies alphabetizing under major headings later. The whole index can then be typed from the alphabetized cards.

**Reprints.** At the time the article is set in type the doctor should order the quantity of reprints he feels he will need. Most doctors send copies of their articles to colleagues, to professional men who have evidenced an interest in their work, and to hospitals and teaching institutions with which they have had contact. The secretary will generally handle the ordering of the reprints; the doctor may request from one to 500 or more. Order enough to cover future needs, since type is often destroyed after the original press run. When the reprints arrive, it is best to count them to make sure the order is complete.

## PROOFREADER'S MARKS

| | | | | |
|---|---|---|---|---|
| ⋏ | Insert comma | ⌄² | Superscript (number specified) | |
| ⌄ | Insert apostrophe | | | |
| ⌄⌄ | Insert quotation marks | ⌃₂ | Subscript (number specified) | |
| ⊙ | Insert period | | | |
| ⊙ | Insert colon | # | Insert space | |
| ;/ | Insert semicolon | *hr* # | Hair space between letters | |
| ?/ | Insert question mark | ⨃ | Push down space | |
| =/ | Insert hyphen | ⊏ | Move to left | |
| ₁⁄ₘ | One-em dash | ⊐ | Move to right | |
| ²⁄ₘ | Two-em dash | ⊔ | Lower | |
| *en* | En dash | ⊓ | Elevate | |
| ⎮·⎮·⎮·⎮ | Ellipsis (If preceded by a period there will be 4 dots.) | X | Broken letter | |
| | | ⌢ | Ligature (A͡Esop) | |
| ⤴ | Delete | ⓢⓟ | Spell out ((U.S.)) | |
| ⌒ | Close up | *stet* | Let it stand (some-day) | |
| ⤴ | Delete and close up | *wf* | Wrong font | |
| Ɔ | Reverse; upside-down | *bf* | Set in boldface type | |
| ⋀ | Insert (caret) | *rom* | Set in (roman) type | |
| ¶ | Paragraph | *ital* | Set in italic type | |
| *no* ¶ | No paragraph; run in | *sc* | Small capitals | |
| *tr* | Transpose (their, only is) | *caps* | Capitals | |
| = | Align | *lc* | Set in lower case | |
| | | *ld* > | Insert lead between lines | |

A list of those to whom reprints are to be sent should be made up. Some doctors maintain a separate card file in which the names and addresses of those to whom they want to send reprints are kept. Addresses should be checked from time to time in the *American Medical Directory* or by scanning membership and request lists. Some record of reprints should be kept and acknowledgments checked. A man who does not acknowledge two or three reprints should be taken from the mailing list.

An enclosure card, printed up in advance, is sent by some professional men with a copy of the reprint. Others prefer to enclose a short letter stating that the reprint is a complimentary copy. Reprints usually are mailed as third class printed matter; postal regulations permit handwritten phrases such as "With the author's compliments."

**Speeches.**   Not all papers are prepared for publication. Some are prepared for presentation before medical and scientific meetings. Speeches should be double spaced; in some offices a jumbo or magnatype machine is used so that the speech is easy to read. At the bottom of each page, in the lower right-hand corner, type the first two or three words that appear at the beginning of the next page. The final draft of the paper should be carefully checked for typographical errors. At large meetings a professional man is usually allotted from 10 to 20 minutes to present his paper; at county society and small meetings he may have from 30 minutes to an hour for his presentation. Check in advance to find out exactly how much time will be allowed. The doctor or his assistant should time the speech. It takes about two minutes to read a page of copy on which there are about 200 to 250 words. If slides or other illustrations are planned, arrangements for showing this material must be made in advance.

## OTHER DUTIES

**Meeting Calendars.**   A calendar of all meetings which the physician plans to attend should be kept by the assistant. A carbon copy of this schedule should always be prepared. The calendar can be merely a sheet of paper listing name of meeting, date, place, and time. It must be accurate. Any changes or additions to the calendar should be made as notices are received. A reminder a few days in advance of each meeting is usually appreciated. It is extremely annoying to a busy doctor to find himself in the wrong place at the wrong time for a meeting.

**Transportation Arrangements.**   To the secretary also falls the task of making transportation arrangements for the doctor and sometimes for his family, too. She often must set up a complete itinerary for him, even making hotel reservations. For this reason she should keep a list of the phone numbers of railroads, airlines, and buses in a separate file at the office. A file folder containing a list of hotels is also valuable. The doctor who is a member of a motor club can use his membership privileges to obtain names of good hotels, road maps, and other vital travel information. Although the doctor who is located in a metropolitan area will probably use a travel agent for many of his arrangements, the secretary-assistant will be charged with the responsibility of working with the agent and preparing the detailed itinerary. Most doctors want to leave at the last minute and return quickly, so transportation is usually booked accordingly. Even though reservations are made in advance, recheck a day or two before the doctor is scheduled to leave, since slip-ups sometimes occur. When all arrangements are final, typewrite the itinerary. Keep one copy in the office file and give the doctor the original and several copies for distribution to members of his family or other individuals. Since it is sometimes necessary to reach the doctor during his absence, it is important that his itinerary be carefully prepared so that he can be reached at any point in his trip.

## REFERENCES

Fishbein, M.D., M. *Medical Writing,* New York, The Blakiston Division, McGraw-Hill Book Company, Inc., 1957
*Library Journal,* October 1, 1971
*Library Journal,* March 1, 1972
Strunk, Jr., W. and E. B. White, *The Elements of Style,* 2nd Ed., New York, The Macmillan Company, 1972

# Chapter 13

**BEHAVIORAL OBJECTIVES**

*The medical office assistant should be able to:*

State the reasons for keeping patient
    records.
Request essential subjective
    information for the record from
    the patient.
Correctly make necessary additions
    or corrections to the patient record.

Keep the record orderly, in correct
    form, and current.
Understand the concept of the
    problem-oriented medical record.

# The Patient Record

Complete and accurate records are essential to a well-managed medical practice. They provide a continuous story of a patient's progress from the date of his first visit to his last. The treatment and therapy prescribed are noted, along with regular reports on the patient's condition; when a patient is discharged, the degree of improvement is placed upon the record.

## REASONS FOR MEDICAL RECORDS

There are three important reasons for carefully recording medical information:

1. **To Provide the Best Medical Care.** The doctor examines the patient and reports his findings on the medical record. These are the clues to diagnosis. Sometimes the doctor orders many types of tests to confirm or augment his clinical findings. As the reports of these tests come in, the findings fall into place like the pieces of a jigsaw puzzle. The physician, on the basis of his diagnosis and the confirmation data, now can prescribe treatment and form his opinion about the patient's chances of recovery, assured that he has utilized every technique to arrive at a correct judgment.

Keeping good medical records helps a physician provide continuity in his patients' medical care. Earlier illnesses and difficulties which appear on the patient's record may supply the key to current medical problems. For example, the information on a patient's record that he was treated for rheumatic fever when he was a child can be extremely important in determining the course of treatment the doctor prescribes when he develops an illness a number of years later.

2. **To Supply Statistical Information.** Medical records may be used to evaluate the effectiveness of certain kinds of treatment, or to determine the incidence of a given disease. Correlations of such statistical information may result in a new outlook on some phases of medicine and can lead to revised techniques and treatments. The statistical data from medical records also are valuable in the preparation of scientific papers, books, and lectures.

3. **To Avoid Legal Difficulties.** Sometimes a physician must produce case histories and medical records in court. For example, a patient may wish to substantiate his claims to an insurance company for damages resulting from an accident in which he was injured and required medical treatment. A patient may involve a physician in litigation. The physician's records can be a help or a hindrance, depending on the care with which they were kept. In an article appear-

ing in the October, 1969 *Physician's Management* (Would Your Records Survive Cross Examination?), the author states:

> A proper patient record to furnish adequate legal protection should include the patient's medical history, results of examinations, records of treatment, copies of laboratory reports, notations of all instructions given, copies of all prescriptions, and any other pertinent data.

> When a patient fails to follow instruction or refuses to undergo a recommended treatment, a letter should be sent containing a "warning" and a carbon copy retained in your files. A similar type of letter should be sent if the patient leaves your care or if you feel it necessary to withdraw your services.

> Sometimes a record introduced in court may be of more significance because of an omission than for what was included. If information which should have been included in a record is not, a jury may form the opinion that the omission was deliberate and intended to conceal the truth.

## TYPES OF CASE HISTORIES

The style and form which a physician will select to record his case histories will depend partly upon the nature of his practice. General practitioners and some specialists keep very detailed records. The specialist who sees patients only on a consultant basis, or the specialist who is likely to see a patient only once, such as the dermatologist, the radiologist, or the anesthesiologist, need not keep complex records. The nature of the patient's complaint is also a factor determining just how detailed a record should be. If a patient comes into a physician's office to have a foreign body removed from his eye or to have some minor injury treated, a detailed report on his past medical history or that of his family is unnecessary. However, the cardiac, hypertensive, or diabetic patient seeking medical attention should provide a complete hisotry.

In some medical offices where detailed histories are not required, a simple patient registration slip (see Fig. 13–1) can be used to record personal data and a plain card or sheet of paper used to record the complaint and treatment given. In the great majority of offices, however, the 8 ½ by 11 letter-size form, with an individual folder for each patient, is preferable.

Some physicians use just a plain sheet of paper for the patient record. The physician generally develops an outline which serves as a guide to taking down the information he requires for a history. He then dictates the history and the secretary types it according to the established format and places it in the patient's folder.

There are many different types of forms available from printing companies: forms for general practice, obstetrics, surgery, pediatrics, internal medicine, or any other of the established specialties. Some physicians design their own forms which they feel are best suited to their particular practice and have them printed to order. Companies that specialize in medical forms will sometimes provide a planning kit for the physician to use. Local printers, too, often can be very helpful in form design. Regardless of the form it takes, the case history will contain certain basic information.

PATIENT REGISTRATION RECORD

Date _4-20-73_

Patient _SAM A. MORRIS_ _____ Age _43_

☒ MARRIED   ☐ SINGLE   ☐ WIDOWED   ☐ DIVORCED   ☐ SEPARATED

Home Address _3810 COMMONWEALTH AVE._

City _LOS ANGELES 90056_ Zone _____ Home Phone _862-9917_

Patient Employed by _SELF-MORRIS APPLIANCES_ Occupation _MERCHANT_

Business Address _5400 HOLLYWOOD BLVD._ City _L.A. 90034_

Name of Spouse _LOUISE M._

Spouse Employed by _____ Occupation _____

Business Address _____ City _____

Patient referred to doctor by _DR. GENTRY_

If patient is minor, name of responsible parent _____

Is this visit payable by health insurance?  ☐ Yes;  ☒ No.   Policy Number _____

Name of Insurer or Group _OCCIDENTAL (HOSP. + SURGERY)_

Signed _Sam Morris_

Figure 13–1

# CONTENT OF THE COMPLETE CASE HISTORY

Recordkeeping in the hospital medical records department is deemed important enough that it is entrusted only to specially trained individuals. The job of medical record librarian requires a Master's degree; a medical record technician requires an associate degree with specialization in the specifics of cataloging and recordkeeping in the hospital medical records department. Although it is not necessary for the medical assistant to be a trained medical record librarian or technician, she must be familiar with some of the basic essentials of the work.

The medical case history is the most important record in a doctor's office. For completeness each patient's record should contain:

Subjective Information Provided by the Patient
(1) Routine personal data about the patient
(2) Patient's personal and medical history
(3) Patient's family history
(4) Patient's complaint (in the patient's own words) and date of onset

Objective Information Provided by the Doctor
(5) Physical examination and findings, laboratory and x-ray reports
(6) Diagnosis and prognosis
(7) Treatment prescribed and progress notes
(8) Condition at time of termination of treatment

If these entries are completed, the case history will stand the test of time. No field of medicine is exempt from the necessity of keeping records. Records aid the physician in the practice of medicine, as well as provide for his legal protection.

## SUBJECTIVE INFORMATION

1. **Routine Personal Data About the Patient.** The patient's case history begins with routine personal data which the patient usually supplies on his first visit. The basic facts needed are: (a) patient's full name, spelled correctly; (b) if patient is child, names of parents; (c) date of birth, marital status, name of spouse, number of children; (d) home address and telephone number; (e) occupation; (f) business address and telephone number; (g) source of referral; (h) health insurance information. When a new patient comes into the doctor's office, certain additional information should be secured for the financial record. This is described more completely in Chapter 15, Medical Fees; Credit Arrangements.

2. **Patient's Personal and Medical History.** This portion of the medical record, which is often obtained by having the patient complete a questionnaire, provides information about any past illnesses or surgical operations which the patient may have had, and includes data about injuries or physical defects, congenital or acquired. It also furnishes information about the patient's daily health habits.

3. **Patient's Family History.** The physical condition of the various members of the patient's family, any past illnesses or diseases which individual members may have suffered, and a record of the causes of death comprise the patient's family history. This information is important, since a definite hereditary pattern is often present in the case of certain diseases.

4. **Patient's Complaint.** This is a concise account of the patient's symptoms, explained in his own words. It should include nature and duration of pain, if any, the time when patient first noticed his symptoms, his opinion as to the possible causes for his difficulties, any remedies he may have applied, or other medical treatment he has already had for the same condition.

## OBJECTIVE INFORMATION

5. **Physical Examination and Findings; Laboratory and X-ray Reports.** This section of the case history varies greatly with the specialty of the physician and the complaint of the patient. After the physician has completed his examination of the patient, his findings are recorded on the history. Results of other tests or requests for these tests are then recorded, or, if they appear on separate sheets, attached to the history.

6. **Diagnosis.** The physician, on the basis of all evidence provided by the patient's past history, the physician's examination, and any supplementary tests, places his diagnosis of the patient's condition upon the medical record. If there is some doubt, it may be termed "Provisional Diagnosis."

7. **Treatment Prescribed and Progress Notes.** The physician's suggested treatment is listed following the diagnosis. Generally, instructions to the patient to return for follow-up treatment in a specific period of time are noted here too.

On each subsequent visit, the date must be entered on the chart, and information about the patient's condition and the results of treatment added to the history, on the basis of the physician's observations. Notations of all medications prescribed or instructions given, as well as the patient's own report about his condition and progress, should be placed upon the record. Any home visits are noted. If the patient is hospitalized, record the name of the hospital, the reason for admission, the dates of admission and discharge. Much of this information may be obtained from the hospital discharge summary.

8. **Condition at Time of Termination of Treatment.** When the treatment is terminated, the physician will record that information. For example,

"August 18, 1974. Wound completely healed. Patient discharged."

## OBTAINING THE HISTORY

It has been pointed out that four kinds of subjective information must be secured from the patient in order to prepare the initial history: (1) routine personal data; (2) patient's personal and medical history; (3) patient's family history; and (4) patient's complaint. The assistant usually secures the routine personal data. The personal and medical history, and the patient's family history, may be secured by asking the patient to complete a questionnaire, with the physician augmenting this during his interview with the patient.

If the doctor delegates the taking of patients' histories to his assistant, care must be exercised to assure that the patient's answers are not heard by others in the reception room. If privacy is not possible, it is better to give the patient a form which he can fill out himself and then transfer this information to permanent records later. If convenient, it is timesaving to ask the patient questions and at the same time type the answers directly on the record. This method offers you an opportunity to become better acquainted with the patient as you complete the necessary records.

The patient may have indicated his chief complaint to the assistant, but the physician will question the patient in more detail on this. The majority of doctors write their own entries on the chart in longhand. Others may dictate the material, either to the assistant or to a recording device. If the material is dictated and typed, each entry should be checked by the physician for accuracy and then initialed by him.

## MAKING ADDITIONS AND CORRECTIONS

As long as the patient is under the physician's care, his medical history will be building. Each laboratory report, x-ray report, and progress note is added to the record, in chronological order, with the latest information always on top. Although each item is important, it is usually the most recent which is of greatest significance to the patient's care.

**Laboratory Reports.** Different colors are often used for different procedures. For example, urinalysis report forms may be yellow, blood count forms pink, and so forth. Laboratory slips are usually smaller than the history form and should be placed on a standard size sheet of colored paper. Type the patient's name in the upper righthand corner, then, with transparent tape, fasten the first report even with the bottom of the page. The second laboratory report will be taped or glued in place on top of and about ½ inch above the first slip, allowing the date to show on the first report. By this method, called "shingling," the latest report always appears on top. When checking previous reports, it is only necessary to run your finger down the slips until you find the desired date; then flip up the slips above. Fifteen to twenty slips may be kept on one sheet by using this method, which is illustrated in Figure 13–2.

**X-ray Reports.**   X-ray reports are usually typed on standard letter-size stationery. Some offices prefer to retype these reports onto the patient's case history, but this requires extra time and sometimes errors slip in when copying. X-ray reports are placed in the patient's history folder with the most recent report on top. All x-ray reports may be stapled together.

**Progress notes.**   Reports on the patient's progress are continually being added to the case history. Each visit of the patient should be entered on his record, with the date preceding any notations about his call. The assistant can type or stamp the date on the chart when she pulls the folder. Every instruction, prescription, or telephone call for advice should be entered with the correct date. If there are several persons handling and making entries on a patient's record, it is advisable to initial each entry. This aids in tracing entries about which there may be some question.

**Corrections.**   Sometimes it is necessary to make corrections on medical records. Erasing and obliteration must be avoided. If an error is made in a handwritten entry, it should be struck out by drawing a line through it and the correction written above or immediately following. The word "correction" or "Corr." is then written in the margin and the initials of the person making the correction are placed on the record, along with the date. Errors made while typing are corrected in the usual way. An error discovered in a typed entry at a later date, however, is corrected in the same manner as described above for a handwritten entry.

**General Instructions.**   The appearance of the case history is important. Keep all information orderly and in correct form. Type reports and entries whenever possible with a typewriter that is kept clean and has a fresh ribbon. Although completeness is important in medical records, the information should be concise.

Coding of information on records is sometimes a helpful shortcut, but any coding system used should be a standard one — not some system that you as a secretary may invent. It must be understood by anyone who needs to consult the chart. If the coding in an office does vary somewhat from the standard methods, a key should be prepared and placed in the front of the files for immediate reference.

Every doctor has certain technical terms that he uses frequently. When in doubt about the spelling, be sure to check with your dictionary. Because of close similarity in some medical words, it is wise to also check the definition to be sure the word fits the context in which it is used. You may find it helpful to get a small, alphabetized address book and write the words in it that give you trouble most frequently. There are many excellent books on medical terminology that include lists of standard abbreviations. A list of the more common abbreviations will be found in the appendix on Medical Terminology.

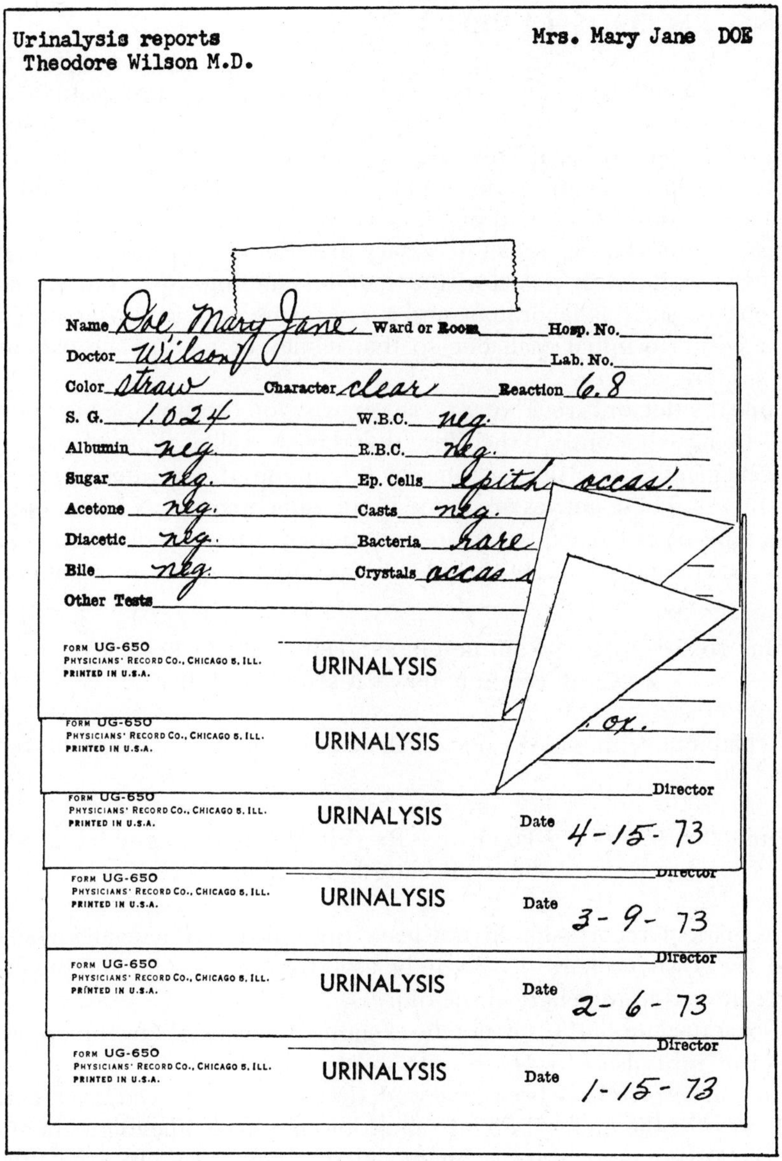

Urinalysis reports                                    Mrs. Mary Jane   DOE
Theodore Wilson M.D.

Name *Doe, Mary Jane*  Ward or Room_____  Hosp. No._____
Doctor *Wilson*  Lab. No._____
Color *straw*  Character *clear*  Reaction *6.8*
S. G. *1.024*  W.B.C. *neg.*
Albumin *neg.*  R.B.C. *neg.*
Sugar *neg.*  Ep. Cells *Epith occas.*
Acetone *neg.*  Casts *neg.*
Diacetic *neg.*  Bacteria *rare*
Bile *neg.*  Crystals *occas*
Other Tests_____

FORM **UG-650**
PHYSICIANS' RECORD CO., CHICAGO 5, ILL.   **URINALYSIS**
PRINTED IN U.S.A.

FORM **UG-650**
PHYSICIANS' RECORD CO., CHICAGO 5, ILL.   **URINALYSIS**
PRINTED IN U.S.A.

FORM **UG-650**
PHYSICIANS' RECORD CO., CHICAGO 5, ILL.   **URINALYSIS**   Director
PRINTED IN U.S.A.   Date *4-15-73*

FORM **UG-650**
PHYSICIANS' RECORD CO., CHICAGO 5, ILL.   **URINALYSIS**   Director
PRINTED IN U.S.A.   Date *3-9-73*

FORM **UG-650**
PHYSICIANS' RECORD CO., CHICAGO 5, ILL.   **URINALYSIS**   Director
PRINTED IN U.S.A.   Date *2-6-73*

FORM **UG-650**
PHYSICIANS' RECORD CO., CHICAGO 5, ILL.   **URINALYSIS**   Director
PRINTED IN U.S.A.   Date *1-15-73*

Figure 13-2

Correspondence relating to the patient's medical history may be stapled together in chronologic order and placed in a pocket in the patient's folder or kept in the back of the folder.

## KEEPING RECORDS CURRENT

One of the greatest dangers to good record keeping is procrastination. The record must be kept current methodically. Many physicians are predisposed to putting off paper work, and the assistant must be relentless in her reminders.

The case histories and reports will probably accumulate on the doctor's or the secretary's desk at the end of the day. After the last patient has left, check each history to make certain all necessary material has been recorded and that each entry is sufficiently clear for future understanding. Give your employer all extra reports, such as laboratory and x-ray forms, to read. After he has read them, ask him to initial each one so that it may be filed in the patient's case history folder.

While the doctor is reviewing these reports, you can pull the histories of the patients he has seen outside the office that day, as well as those of patients who have been given special instructions by telephone or for whom prescriptions were sent out. These entries are made in the same manner as for an office visit, but the type of call is explained in parentheses after the date. For example, here's what the history might include about a home visit to see a patient:

"May 16, 1975 (Res.) Routine ph. ex. Temp. 98.6. Chest clear.
Cont. Rx. May now eat semi-bland diet."

When a patient telephones the doctor, the entry should be made on his record as follows:

"June 26, 1975 (Tel.) To change Rx (Vit. B Comp) to one b.i.d.
Force fluids. Feeling much better."

The patient record should not leave the office. A Physician's Pocket Call Record, as shown in Figure 13–3, can be used for outside calls, and the information transferred to the chart in the office.

Also, at the end of the day notations should be made of any unkept appointments or of refusals to cooperate with instructions.

After all records have been reviewed, they should be placed in a file tray and locked away for the night, if the assistant does not have time to file them before she leaves. Do not leave histories out in view at night, especially if the office has a night cleaning service.

When the office assistant arrives the next morning she can index the histories for filing. Attach extra reports and information sheets; don't just drop them into the folders. It is best to attach them to the case histories with tape or rubber cement. When this is done, the records are ready for filing.

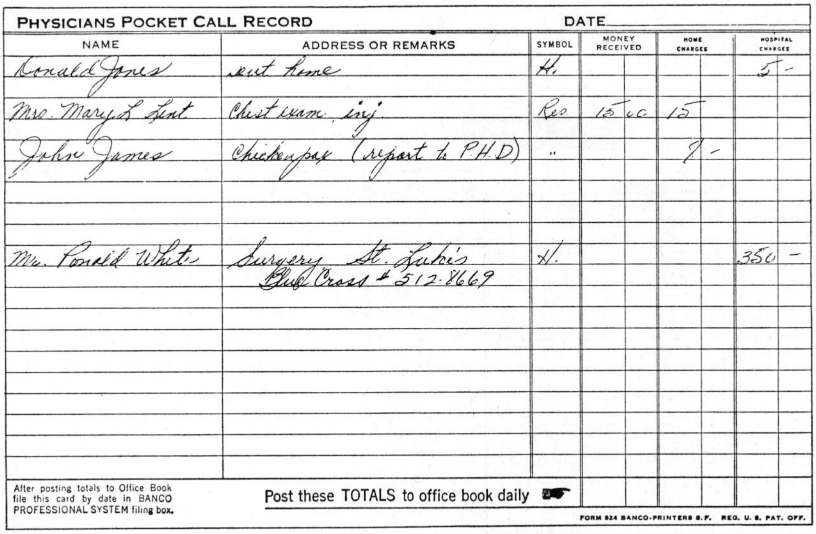

| PHYSICIANS POCKET CALL RECORD | | DATE | | | | |
|---|---|---|---|---|---|---|
| NAME | ADDRESS OR REMARKS | SYMBOL | MONEY RECEIVED | HOME CHARGES | | HOSPITAL CHARGES |
| Donald Jones | out home | H. | | | | 5 - |
| Mrs. Mary L. Lint | Chest exam inj | Rev | 15.00 | 15 | | |
| John James | Chickenpox (report to P.H.D) | " | | 7 - | | |
| | | | | | | |
| | | | | | | |
| Mr. Ronald White | Surgery St. Luke's Blue Cross # 512-8669 | H. | | | | 350 - |

After posting totals to Office Book file this card by date in BANCO PROFESSIONAL SYSTEM filing box.

Post these TOTALS to office book daily ☛

FORM 824 BANCO-PRINTERS S.F.   REG. U. S. PAT. OFF.

**Figure 13–3**   Physicians Pocket Call Record. (Courtesy Banco-Printers, San Francisco, Calif.)

## THE PROBLEM-ORIENTED MEDICAL RECORD

A chapter on the patient record would be incomplete without some discussion of the problem-oriented medical record (POMR), sometimes referred to as the "Weed System." The POMR, originated by Lawrence L. Weed, M.D., a professor of medicine at the University of Vermont's College of Medicine, is a major innovation and a radical departure from the traditional system of keeping patient records. The traditional record is "source-oriented;" that is, observations and data are catalogued according to their source — physician, laboratory, x-ray, nurse, technician — with no recording of a logical relationship between them. In an article appearing in the February, 1973 issue of *Medical Opinion* (Who is Dr. Weed — and Why is He Saying All Those Nasty Things About My Charts?), the editors describe the POMR:

> This is a record of clinical practice that divides medical action up into four bases. First you put down information for a carefully defined, standardized data base. That includes chief complaint, present illness, patient profile; and also a review of systems, physical examination, and lab reports. Next you write out a numbered and titled list of every problem the patient has had that requires management or work-up. We believe this should include social and demographic troubles as well as strictly medical or surgical ones.
>
> Then you write a treatment plan for each problem. That is, "What am I going to do to make this patient well?" This includes management, additional workups needed, and therapy. Each plan is titled and numbered with respect to the problem. Finally, you write progress notes, each also labelled according to these problems. This is the universe of information.

*(Text continued on page 170.)*

**ROCOM** PATIENT RECORD

NAME _Robert Billings_
Number _4270_ | Blood Type: O

ALLERGIES/SENSITIVITIES _Sulfa_

| TESTS | Dates and Results | | | | |
|---|---|---|---|---|---|
| CBC | 10/6/66 | 12/3/68 | | | |
| Hcrit | 42 | 41 | | | |
| Hgb | 14.2 | 14.4 | | | |
| RBC | 4.1 | 4.3 | | | |
| WBC | 7900 | 8000 | | | |
| Differential | | | | | |
| ESR | 14 mm | 14 mm | | | |
| Pro Time | | | 10/5/69 12 sec. | | |
| Chemical Screen | | | | | |
| Cholesterol | 250 | (330) | | | |
| Glucose | 93 | 92 | | | |
| Uric Acid | 4 | 4 | | | |
| BUN | 18 | 20 | | | |
| | | | | | |
| | | | | | |
| PBI | | 4.6 | | | |
| T₃ or T₄ | | | | | |
| Urinalysis | — | — | | | |
| Pap | | | | | |
| Tuberculin | — | | | | |
| | | | | | |
| | | | | | |
| ECG | — | — | | | |
| Pulmonary function | | | | | |
| Vision | 20/30 | 20/30 | | | |
| Tonometry | — | — | | | |
| Audiometry | –– | — | | | |
| | | | | | |
| | | | | | |
| Chest x-ray | neg. | neg. | | | |
| Ht | 5'7" | | | | |
| Wt | 182 | 183 | 2-6-70 | | |
| BP | 140/85 | 170/95 | 148/80 | | |
| PR | 68 | (95) | 71 | | |
| Periodic Health Examinations | Dates | 10/6/66 | 12/3/68 | | |

| Problem No. | Date | PROBLEM DESCRIPTION | Index |
|---|---|---|---|
| 1 | 1/5/67 | Rheumatoid Arthritis | X |
| 2 | 12/3/68 | Essential Hypertension | X |
| 3 | 8/20/69 | Myocardial Infarction | X |

### CONTINUING MEDICATIONS

| Medication | Start | Stop | Medication | Start | Stop |
|---|---|---|---|---|---|
| aspirin 10 gr. qid | 1/5/67 | 1/27/67 | exercise program | 10/5/68 | |
| Phenylbutazone | | | | | |
| 100 mg. qid | 1/5/67 | 1/12/67 | | | |
| 100 mg. bid | 1/13/67 | 1/27/67 | | | |
| aspirin 10 gr. PRN | 2/12/67 | | | | |
| low salt diet | 12/3/68 | | | | |
| 1200 c diet | 12/3/68 | | | | |
| diazepam 5mg tid | 12/3/68 | 8/20/69 | | | |
| low cholesterol diet | 12/6/68 | | | | |
| diazepam 5mg tid | 10/5/69 | | | | |
| flurazepam 30mg HS | 10/5/69 | 11/5/69 | | | |

### CONSULTATIONS

| Date | Name | + or - | Date | Name | + or - |
|---|---|---|---|---|---|
| 9/21/69 | Dr. Ray Robbins | + | | | |

**A**

**Figure 13–4**

IDENTIFICATION DATA

NAME  Billings  Robert          STATUS  M   CHART #  4270
    Last     First       (SMDW)        (571)
ADDRESS 723 Central Ave.  Larron, Mich.  71261  TELEPHONE 644-5377
    Street     City     Zip
BIRTH DATE  9-17-15        SEX  M

NEXT OF KIN
                              (571)
  NAME  Sally      RELATIONSHIP  Wife      TELEPHONE 644-5377
  ADDRESS  723 Central ave

BILLING NAME (if other than patient)
  NAME  Patient        RELATIONSHIP        TELEPHONE
  ADDRESS
EMPLOYER  General Products   ADDRESS  Detroit  Mich
OCCUPATION  Salesman          TELEPHONE  (571) 687-5261
SOCIAL SECURITY #  317-29-4023
INSURANCES
  Blue Shield #  Blue Cross - FMC 317-29-4023
  Medicare #
  Others

| IMMUNIZATIONS | Dates | | | | |
|---|---|---|---|---|---|
| Smallpox | 1950 | | | | |
| Sabin | | | | | |
| Salk | 1963 | | | | |
| DTP | | | | | |
| DT | | | | | |
| Tet Tox | | | | | |
| Measles | | | | | |
| Rubella | | | | | |
| Mumps | | | | | |
| TPT | | | | | |
| Flu | | | | | |
| Hong Kong | 10/6/66 series | | | | |
| Tetanus | 1960 | | | | |

| EDUCATION: | Children's Names | Children's Birthdates |
|---|---|---|
| 8 Years Elementary | Stanley | 6-9-43 |
| 4 Years High School | William | 5-12-45 |
| 4 Years College | | |
| Technical, Business, etc. | | |

| Dates | HOSPITALIZATION DESCRIPTION |
|---|---|
| 1940 | Hernia Chicago General - Non compl. |
| 8/20/69 | Post Wall Myocardial Infarction |

| Date | SPECIAL NOTES |
|---|---|
| 10-6-66 | Referred by John Spartes - Patient |

**B**

**Figure 13-4** *Continued.*

Patient Name _Robert Billings_       Number __4270__    Page _1_

| Date Problems (No. and Description) | FINDINGS (Subjective and Objective) | PLANS |
|---|---|---|
| 10-6-66 CPE ✓ | Subj: Pt. is easily fatigued anxiety about job, home situations · insomnia last two weeks · Drinking each day for about the last month. Compl. that fingers hurt and are stiff at times. | CBC, urine, x-ray, cholesterol Glucose, uric acid, BUN |
| | Obj: Wt. - 182 Ht. - 5'7" BP - 140/85 PR - 68 Heart & lungs normal x-ray neg Vision 20/30 Joints not swollen, normal movement of fingers | B complex 1m diet aid flu shot Hong Kong FU with positive results |
| 1-5-67 | Subj: stiff finger joints. Pt. says more severe after sleeping or non use. General fatigue stopped, occurred again in last 2 weeks. Stopped drinking some weight loss. | Aspirin 10 gr. qid. phenylebutazole 100mg qid #21 1 wk. " 100 mg bid #24 2 wk. |
| #1 Rheumatoid Arthritis | Obj: swelling + pain around joints of fingers. Symmetrical involvement. x-ray - narrowed joint space osteoporosis at joint BP - 144/85 PR-67 Wt - 178 | Pt. call 2 weeks Uric acid - 4.2 FU visit 1 month x-ray |

Record your findings in the unshaded column, writing through the shaded area if you wish. Record Plans in the shaded column only.

18-28-1800-005-042

16 03 008 00

●⃝ ROCOM Progress Notes

    (OVER)

**A**

**Figure 13–5**

Page ___2___

| Date<br>Problems<br>(No. and Description) | FINDINGS<br>(Subjective and Objective) | PLANS |
|---|---|---|
| 2-12-67 | Subj: Mood improved<br>pain reduced in mornings | |
| #1 | | |
| Rheumatoid<br>arthritis | Obj: swelling reduced<br>pain reduced, movement<br>normal Uric acid<br>level O.K., No change<br>in x-ray finding. | ✓aspirin 10 gr PRN<br>CBC<br>CBC - normal<br>FU - next CPE |
| 12-3-68<br>CPE | Subj: Job-related tension. No<br>fatigue, generally feels<br>well arthritis continue | |
| #2<br>Essential ✓<br>Hypertension | w/aspirin no react, Weight<br>loss substant. but has<br>regained. | ✓CBC, ✓urine, ✓x-ray<br>✓cholesterol, ✓Glucose<br>✓uric acid, ✓BUN, ✓PBI |
| | Obj: Wt. 183✓ BP - ✓170/95 PR-95<br>Heart + lungs normal.<br>Chest x-ray-neg. Vision ✓20/30<br>joints not swollen, movement<br>normal. | ✓low salt diet<br>✓1200 c diet<br>✓diazepam 5 mg tid<br><br>FU - w/test results if posit.<br>✓low cholesterol diet<br>FU - 2 months |
| 2-20-69 | Obj: Wt 175 BP - 150/90<br>PR - 80 | ✓Stop diazepam<br>✓Continue low salt,<br>cholesterol + 1200 c diet |
| 10-5-69<br>#3<br>Myocardial ✓<br>Infarction<br>post Hospital | ✓Hosp. for MI (8-26-69)<br>hospital summary w/ECG<br>included. | Care - Dr Roy Robbins - Cardiologist<br>St. Mary's Hosp.<br>✓Protime |

**B**

**Figure 13-5** *Continued.*

One designer* of forms for use in recording the POMR recommends that the progress notes follow a structured plan referred to as SOAP:

Number and name of
problem for reference:

S–the patient's *symptoms* or complaints
O–*objective* findings related to the
    problem
A–the *assessment of the patient's status*
P–the *plan* (diagnostic, therapeutic
    and/or educative)

Figure 13–4 illustrates the inside of the patient folder in the ROCOM system and Figure 13–5 shows the progress notes for the same patient. This same structured plan can be applied to hospital admission and discharge summary, reports of consultations and referrals, as well as to the office record.

A prime requisite of the POMR is the patient data base. The data base can be obtained by having the patient complete a general health history and physical examination questionna.re. A specialist might also use a questionaire designed for screening problems related to his specialty (cardiovascular screen, respiratory screen, and so forth). From these questionnaires the physician isolates the patient's problems. ROCOM, in the first of its series of booklets on practical applications of the problem-oriented medical record, states:

> As the trend toward problem-oriented medical records gains momentum, more and more doctors agree that it *is* possible to impose some order and organization on the information added to a patient's medical record. The practitioner who embraces the problem-oriented concept finds that his records are more easily reviewed, his intellectual stimulation increased, his approach to patient care is more considered and more rational, and he is, therefore, less likely to mismanage patients with difficult problems.

> Of course, problem-oriented records in themselves are not a panacea; they will not directly improve the quality of medical care. Their value is in disciplining the physician to rely less on his memory, and to avoid "impressions," "clinical judgment," or "provisional diagnoses"—the guesswork of medicine. This record system is best regarded as a tool of medical management, assisting in:

> > · definition of patient's problems
> > · honest appraisal of their status
> > · formulation of logical and orderly plans of care

The POMR was practically unheard of before 1970. By 1973 a majority of the medical schools in the United States were either teaching or preparing to teach the problem-oriented system, and problem-oriented medical practices existed in at least 22 states, according to the American Medical Association (American Medical News, February 19, 1973.). While the long-established physician

---

*Patient Care Systems, Inc., ROCOM Division of Hoffman-La Roche Inc.

may continue to use the source-oriented record, clearly the assistant working with the recent medical school graduate will need to be acquainted with the POMR.

## REFERENCES

*American Medical News*, published by American Medical Association, 535 North Dearborn Street, Chicago, Illinois 60610

*Medical Opinion*, published by Weston Communications, Inc., 575 Madison Avenue, New York, New York 10022

ROCOM division of Hoffmann-LaRoche Inc., Nutley, New Jersey 07110

# Chapter 14

## BEHAVIORAL OBJECTIVES

*The medical office assistant should be able to:*

Select suitable equipment and
    supplies for records management.
Organize the files in a
    physician's office.
Utilize the advantages of color coding.
Apply the rules of indexing to
    records management.

File and retrieve correspondence
    and records.
Establish a retention and destruction
    schedule for office records.

# Records Management

Unless the medical office assistant has had formal secretarial training or extensive experience in secretarial procedures, she may find filing to be her Waterloo. Assembling the medical record is important, as was stressed in the previous chapter. But this record must be filed so that it can be easily and quickly found when needed. A filing system is only as good as the "findability" of everything in the files.

The point of view of the person in charge of the files often makes the difference between efficiency and chaos. Some persons equate "filing" with "storing"; the term "records management" is more appropriate to the medical assistant's filing responsibility.

Management of the records will include (1) filing, (2) finding, (3) transferring, (4) protection, and (5) retention, storage, and destruction. The *Records Management Handbook* published in 1964 by the U.S. Government Printing Office (Files Operations, Federal Stock No. 7610-985-6973) comments on estimating finding and filing costs:

> The cost on a national average for initially filing a single page letter is from 3 to 6 cents. On a national average, the annual cost of files operations is about $340 for an uninsulated five-drawer letter-size cabinet. This figure is computed by adding together the following annual costs:
> Rent and maintenance per square foot of cabinet space including working area
> Equipment depreciation
> Filing supplies
> Labor
> Labor cost, which is the largest factor in determining the overall cost, is the proportionate share of the worker's salary representing the time spent in filing.

These figures would be considerably higher today. You can readily understand, then, that this is a responsibility which warrants more than a casual approach.

## EQUIPMENT AND SUPPLIES

### Equipment

Most records in the solo practitioner's office will be stored in four-drawer steel cabinets. In offices where space is limited the trend is toward shelf filing. The rotary circular file is also increasing in popularity. Some kinds of records

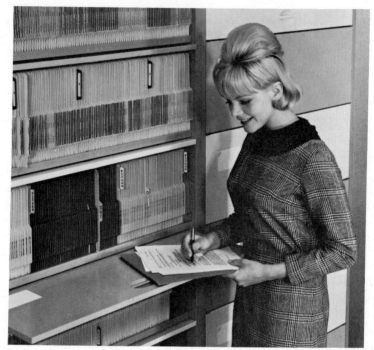

**Figure 14–1**

will be kept in card or tray files. Regardless of the type or style of equipment, the best quality is always an economy.

Drawer files should be full-suspension; they should roll easily, close securely, and be equipped with a locking device. The best cabinets will have a center trough at the bottom of each drawer with a rod for holding divider guides. Floor space of twice the depth of the drawer must be allowed so that the drawer can be pulled out to its full extent.

Shelf files should have doors to protect the contents. A popular type of shelf file has doors which slide back into the cabinet; the door from a lower shelf may be pulled out and used for work space (Fig. 14–1). About 50 per cent more material per square foot of floor space may be filed in shelf files as compared with the usual drawer file. Shelf files are available in many attractive colors and can add a decorative note to the business office. Special storage or shelf space should be provided for x-rays if many films are stored.

Rotary circular files can hold a large volume of records. They save space and clerical motion. The files revolve easily; some come with pushbutton controls. Several persons can work at one rotary file and use records at the same time. They afford less privacy and protection than files which can be closed and locked.

Almost every office will have some occasion to use a card file. This may be for patient ledgers, a patient index, library index, index of surgical tray set-ups, telephone numbers, or numerous other records. A good quality steel box or tray is a sound investment.

**Special Items.**   Metal framework is available which will convert a regular drawer file into suspension-folder equipment. The assistant with a great deal of filing may wish to purchase a portable filing shelf which fits on the side of an opened drawer and can be moved from place to place as needed. A sorting file can be a great timesaver. One general purpose sorter has six means of classification: alphabetic sections, numbers 1 to 31, days of the week, months of the year, numbers in groups of 5, and space on the tabs for special captions to be taped where desired.

## Supplies

Filing supplies include guides, OUTguides or OUTfolders, folders, vertical pockets, and labels.

**Divider Guides.**   Each file drawer or shelf should be equipped with plenty of dividers or guides. Some authorities recommend one guide for approximately each inch and a half of material, or every 8 to 10 folders. Guides should be of good quality pressboard. "Economy" guides will soon become bent and frayed and have to be replaced. Divider guides have a protruding tab, which may be either an integral part of the card or may be made of metal or plastic. The guides reduce the area of search and serve as supports for the folders. They are available in single, third, or fifth cut (one, three, or five different positions). The guide may have a projection at the bottom edge with a ring or hole through which a rod may go. This type of guide card is used in drawers that have a trough for the projection and a rod to hold the guides in place.

**OUTguides.**   An OUTguide is a heavy guide that is used to replace a folder which has been temporarily removed. It may be of a distinctive color for quick detection. This makes refiling simpler and alerts the file clerk that a file is missing. The OUTguide may have lines for recording information, or it may have a plastic pocket for inserting an information card.

**Folders.**   Most records to be filed are placed in tabbed folders. The most commonly used is a general-purpose third-cut kraft folder which may be expanded to ¾ inch. These are available with a double thickness reinforced tab that will greatly lengthen the life of the folder. Folders kept in drawers will have tabs at the top; those kept on shelves will have tabs at the side. There are many variations of folder styles obtainable for special purposes. One example is the classification folder, which will separate the papers in one file into six categories yet keep them all together. The OUTfolder is used like the OUTguide but provides space for temporary filing of materials. Another example is the vertical pocket, which is heavier weight than the general purpose folder, has a front which folds down for easy access to contents and is available with up to 3½ inch expansion. These are used for bulky histories or correspondence. Hanging or suspension folders are made of heavy stock and hang on metal rods at the side of a drawer. They can be used only with files equipped with suspension drawers. Binder folders have fasteners with which to bind papers within them. These offer some security for the papers but are time-consuming in filing the materials.

**Labels.**   Each shelf, drawer, divider guide, and folder will have a label. The label is a necessary "filing and finding" device. Labels may be prepared with a mechanical tapewriter or the typewriter. Paper labels may be purchased in rolls of gummed tape; or they may have adhesive backs which are peeled from a protective sheet after typing. Labels are available in almost any size, shape, or color to meet the individual needs of any office. Visit your stationer and study the catalogs to find the best product for you.

The label on the drawer or shelf identifies the nature of its contents. It should also indicate the range (alphabetic, numeric, or chronologic) of the material filed in that space. For example:

A. PATIENT HISTORIES (Active)
A–F
B. GENERAL CORRESPONDENCE
1973–1976

The label should be easy to read. The tapewriter is probably preferable to the typewriter for these labels.

The final step in locating a record in the file is identification of the individual folder. Every reasonable filing aid should be used to ensure reaching this as speedily as possible. The folder label must be descriptive and legible.

## MECHANICS OF FILING

A little time invested in learning the principles of filing will save a great deal of time in the practice of filing and finding procedures.

**Filing Methods.**   There are four basic methods of filing: (1) alphabetic by name; (2) numeric; (3) geographic; and (4) subject. A fifth method, chronologic, is sometimes used.

In the doctor's office, the patients' records will usually be filed alphabetically by name. The office with a large volume, or the office where an unusual degree of privacy is desired, may use a numeric system. In this case, each new patient is assigned a sequential number, and a cross-index alphabetic card is prepared to identify the name. Because of the need for a cross-index, the numeric method is referred to as an *indirect* method of filing. General correspondence will, in most cases, be filed by subject or by the name of the correspondent.

**Steps in Filing.**   All materials to be filed will involve several steps. In the language of filing, these steps are called *conditioning, releasing, indexing,* and *coding.*

Papers to be filed are *conditioned* by removing all pins, brads, and paper clips; related papers are stapled together; clippings or items smaller than page size are attached to a regular sheet of paper with rubber cement or tape; damaged records are mended or reinforced with tape.

The term *releasing* simply means that some mark has been placed on the paper indicating that it is now ready for filing. This will usually be either the secretary's initials or a FILE stamp placed in the upper left corner.

*Indexing* means deciding where to file the letter or paper, and *coding* means placing some indication of this decision on the paper. This may be done by underlining the name or subject, if it appears on the paper, or writing, in some conspicuous place, the indexing subject or name. If the material could logically be filed in more than one place, it may be necessary to prepare a cross-reference sheet.

## COLOR CODING

If the files are extensive, a system of color coding is recommended for the folder labels. In the patient history files, for instance, the *second* letter of each name would determine the color of the label to be used on the folder. Any selection of colors may be used, and the division of the alphabet determined by your own needs. However, studies have shown that there is wide variation in the frequency with which different letters occur. The following division is one which has been successfully used:

| Color of Label | Letters of Alphabet | Example |
|---|---|---|
| Red | A B C D | Canfield<br>Eberhart<br>O'Connor<br>Adams |
| Yellow | E F G H | Decker<br>Effron<br>Igawa<br>Thill |
| Purple | I J K L M N | Histed<br>Bjork<br>Akron<br>Ullman<br>Imhoff<br>Anderson |
| Green | O P Q R S T | Gordon<br>Epperley<br>Aquino<br>Greiner<br>Osterberg<br>Atherton |
| Blue | U V W X Y Z | Auer<br>Uvena<br>Owsley<br>Oxford<br>Nye<br>Azzaro |

When a color coding system is used, both filing and finding are expedited. Misfiled folders are kept to a minimum. Instead of using colored labels, colored folders in the same array of colors may be used.

There are many ways to make color work for you. Small self-adhesive tabs in a variety of colors may be used to identify certain types of insured patients. For example, a patient on Medicaid may have a red tab over the edge of his folder; a Champus patient may be identified by a blue tab; a workmen's compensation patient by a green tab, and so on. Matching tabs may be attached to the ledger cards. Research cases may be identified by a special color tab. In a partnership practice, it may be desirable to use a different color folder or label for each doctor's patients. Self-adhesive tabs are easily removed, less bulky than metal or plast.c tabs, and not so likely to be inadvertently pulled from the record.

The business records files may also utilize color coding. Main divider guide headings may be of one color, subheadings in a second color, and subdivisions in a third color. For example:

| Main Heading | DISBURSEMENTS | | Red label |
| Subheading | Equipment | | Blue label |
| Subdivisions | | Typewriter | Yellow label |
| | | Copier | Yellow label |
| | | Calculator | Yellow label |

A fourth color might be used for personal items. The use of color in the files is limited only by the imagination. One word of caution, though. Every person in the office who uses the files should know the key to the coding, and the key should also be written in your procedures manual.

## SYSTEMATIC ORGANIZATION OF FILES

**Patient Records.** It is very difficult for a physician to study a disorganized history. Some systematic method must be followed in placing the material in the patient folder. Details of the patient record were discussed in the preceding chapter. From the filing standpoint, it should be stressed that when a patient record is not in actual use, there is only one place it should be—in the filing cabinet. Many precious hours can be lost in searching for misplaced or lost records that were carelessly left unfiled. The patient's full name, in indexing order, should be typed on a label and attached to the folder tab. The patient's full name should also be typed on each sheet within the folder. A strip of transparent tape can be placed over the label to prevent smudging if this is a problem.

**Medical Correspondence.** Correspondence pertaining to patients' medical records should be filed with the case history. Other medical correspondence will probably be filed in a *subject* file.

**General Correspondence.** The physician's office must be operated as a business, as well as a professional service. There will be correspondence of a general nature pertaining to the operation of the office. In all likelihood a special drawer or shelf will be set aside for the general correspondence. The correspondence will be indexed according to subject matter or names of correspondents. The *guides* in a subject file may appear in one, two or three positions, depending upon the number of headings, subheadings, and subdivisions. Examples were shown in the section on color coding above.

**Miscellaneous Folder.**    Papers which do not warrant an individual folder are placed in a *miscellaneous* folder. Within the folder, all papers relating to one subject, or with one correspondent, are kept together in chronologic order, the most recent on top, and then filed alphabetically with other miscellaneous material. Related materials may be stapled together. *Never* use paper clips for this purpose. When as many as five papers accumulate with one correspondent or subject, a separate folder should be prepared.

**Business and Financial Records.**    The most active financial record is, of course, the ledger. In most offices this will be a card or vertical tray file and the ledgers will be arranged alphabetically by name. There will be at least two divisions: *active* and *paid* accounts. Special categories may be set up, for example:(1) government-sponsored insurance; (2) workmen's compensation; (3) delinquent accounts; (4) collection accounts, and so forth.

Other business files include records of income and expense, financial statements, income and payroll tax records, canceled checks, and insurance policies. These papers may be filed chronologically.

**Follow-Up File.**    The most frequently used follow-up method is that of a *tickler* file. It "tickles" the memory that something needs to be done or followed up on a particular date. The tickler file is always a chronologic arrangement. In its simplest form it consists of notations on the daily calendar. If information concerning a patient who has an appointment to come in is expected, such as an x-ray report or laboratory report, the medical assistant might make a note on her calendar or tickler file a day ahead to check on whether the report has arrived. The tickler file is often a card file with 12 guides for the names of the months, and 31 guides printed with numbers 1 through 31 for the days of the month. The guide for the current month, followed by the 31 day guides, is placed at the front of the file. Notations of actions to be taken are placed behind the guides for specific days of the current month. Notations for future months are placed behind the guide for that month. In order to be effective, the tickler file must be checked the first thing each day. It is a useful reminder for recurring events, such as payments, meetings, and so forth. On the last day in each month, all the notations from behind the next month's guide are distributed behind the daily numbered guides and the guide for the completed month is placed at the back of the file.

**Transitory or Temporary File.**    Many papers are kept longer than necessary because no provision is made for segregating those that have a limited usefulness. For instance, if the secretary writes a letter requesting a reprint, the carbon may be placed in the transitory folder. When the reprint is received, the request letter is destroyed. This file is used for materials having no permanent value. The paper may be marked with a "T" and destroyed when the action involved is completed.

## FILING PROCEDURES

Filing should be done daily. Try to establish a definite time for this. You may think you don't have time, but searching for records which have not been filed is even more time-consuming and costly.

**Sorting.**    Sorting is arranging the papers in order for filing. Sort papers before going to the file cabinet. Do any necessary stapling of papers at your desk or filing table. If possible, invest in a desk sorter with a series of dividers between which papers are placed in filing sequence.

You can make your own desk sorter by stapling together a series of four or five folders, leaving about one inch of each folder visible for labeling. The folders may be labeled A–E, F–K, L–R, S–Z, and SPECIAL. In the preliminary sorting you will place the papers in the appropriate folder in the sorter. Then it is comparatively simple to arrange these groups into the proper sequence for filing.

**Placing in Folders.**   Items should be placed face up, top edge to the left, with the most recent date to the front of the folder. Lift the folder an inch or two out of the drawer before inserting material so that the sheets can drop down completely into the folder.

**Indexing.**   Arrange all folders to be filed in indexing order before going to the file cabinet.

**Preventing Accidents.**   File drawers are heavy and can tip over, causing serious damage, unless reasonable care is observed. Open only one file drawer at a time and close it when the filing has been completed. A drawer left even slightly open can cause injury to a passerby.

**Locating Misplaced Files.**   Unless files are promptly replaced after use, they may become lost. Papers may be misfiled, requiring a thorough search to find them. After you have made a methodical and complete search through the proper folder, there are several places you may look for a misplaced paper: in the folder in front of and behind the correct folder; between the folders; on the bottom of the file under all the folders; in a folder of a patient with a similar name; in the sorter.

## RULES FOR INDEXING

Approximately 90 per cent of all indexing and filing is based on the alphabetic arrangement of words or names. It is impossible to file or find successfully until one has mastered all the rules for alphabetic filing. If you can find a word in the dictionary or a name in the telephone directory, you already know some of the rules.

Here are a dozen basic rules for the operation of a simple, efficient filing system in a physician's office:

1. Last names of persons are considered *first* in filing; given name (first name), *second*; and middle name or initial, *third*.

2. Compare the names from the first letter to the last. The first letter that is different in two names is the letter that determines the order of filing. Example: abe, abi, abx, acl, acm, ada, ade, adi, and so on.

3. Initials precede a name beginning with the same letter. Example:

> Smith, J.
> Smith, Jason

This illustrates the librarian's rule, "Nothing comes before something."

4. Hyphenated names: Authorities are about evenly divided on indexing

hyphenated names as one unit or two units. Whichever rule you adopt should be followed consistently.

5. Unusual names of individuals, such as Ah Hop Akee, should be filed under the last name and cross-indexed.

Akee, Ah Hop
Ah Hop Akee (see Akee, Ah Hop)

6. Names with prefixes are filed in the usual alphabetic order. DeLong is filed as Delong; LaFrance as Lafrance; von Schmidt as Vonschmidt.

7. Abbreviated names are indexed as if spelled in full: St. John as Saintjohn; Wm. as William; Edw. as Edward; Jas. as James.

8. Mac and Mc are filed in their regular place in the alphabet:

Maag
Mabry
MacDonald
Machado
MacHale
Maville
McAulay
McWilliams
Meacham

If your files contain a great many names beginning with Mac or Mc you may, for convenience, wish to file them as a separate letter of the alphabet.

9. The name of a married woman is indexed by her legal name (her husband's surname, her given name, her middle name or maiden surname). For example:

Doe, Mary Jones (Mrs. John L.)
NOT
Doe, Mrs. John L.

10. Titles, when followed by a complete name, are disregarded in indexing:

Breckenridge, John J. (Prof.)

Titles without complete names are considered the first indexing unit:

Madame Sylvia
Sister Mary Catherine

Degrees are disregarded in filing but placed after the name, in parentheses:

Wilson, Theodore (M.D.)

11. Articles such as "The" or "A" are disregarded in indexing:

Moore Clinic (The)

12. Terms of seniority, such as "Jr." or "2d" are not indexing units but are included as identifying elements to distinguish between two otherwise identical names: In filing, "Junior comes before "Senior," but place "2d" before "3d" or "4th" (in numerical order):

> Woods, Robert (Jr.)
> Woods, Robert (2d)
> Woods, Robert (Sr.)
> Woods, Robert (3d)

## TRANSFER OF FILES

Some system should be established for regular transfer of files. In most medical offices, records are filed according to three classifications: active, inactive, or closed. Active files are those of patients currently receiving treatment. Inactive files generally are histories of patients whom the doctor has not seen for six months or more. When such individuals return for care, their folders are replaced in the active file. Closed files are records of patients who have terminated their relationship with the physician, died, or moved away.

Charts for patients who are currently hospitalized may be kept in a special section for quick reference, then placed in the regular active file when the patient is discharged from the hospital.

In a surgical practice, there is frequently a specific date on which the patient is discharged from the doctor's care and the notation made on the chart, "Return prn." This record may safely be placed in the inactive file.

In a general practice office, the outside of the folder may be stamped with the date of the patient's visit each time he is seen. It will then be a simple matter to determine when the chart should be transferred to the inactive status. In the parlance of filing, this is called the perpetual transfer method.

## RECORDS PROTECTION

Occasions may arise when records are temporarily out of the office. Some physicians release case histories to their colleagues, or a record may be subpoenaed by the courts. In such instances, an OUTfolder should be placed in the drawer in place of the regular folder, and a notation made of the name, date, and to whom the record was released. Interim papers may be placed in the OUTfolder until the original is returned.

The sending out of actual case histories should be avoided if possible. Instead, prepare a resume, or photocopy the materials needed for reference, and retain the original in the physician's office. Drawers and cabinets should be kept closed at all times when the office is unattended, for further protection of the records.

# RETENTION AND DESTRUCTION

There is no simple rule to follow in establishing a records-retention schedule. Each office must develop its own method, but government and legal requirements will have some influence.

**Case Histories.**    Space permitting, these will probably be kept permanently, or at least as long as the doctor is in practice. Then, if the patient is still living, his records may be made available to another doctor of his own choosing. The record would not be given to the patient himself because of the possibility of misinterpretation.

**Tax Records.**    Income tax returns are kept indefinitely; the last three returns are retained in a fireproof filing cabinet or safe; older returns are filed in dead storage.

**Insurance Policies.**    Keep current policies in a fireproof cabinet or safe, When superseded by a new policy, throw away the old one UNLESS a claim is pending. *Professional liability policies are kept permanently.*

**Cancelled Checks.**    Keep in a fireproof file three years, then indefinitely in dead storage.

**Receipts for Business Equipment.**    Keep until item is fully depreciated.

**General Correspondence and Business Records.**    These should be reviewed periodically, as time permits, and any papers which are no longer of value destroyed. If the slightest doubt exists as to whether a paper should be destroyed, be sure to check with the doctor or retain the paper in the file.

**Miscellaneous.**    Many papers that are filed should instead be destroyed. Examples of these are letters of acknowledgment, announcements of meetings, duplicate copies, and letters of transmittal. Any document that is superseded by another in the file should be removed. For instance, when a new catalog is filed, destroy the old one; when a new fee schedule is received, destroy the old one. Blue Cross and Blue Shield representatives say that retaining old copies of fee schedules and claim forms causes countless problems. The Army has developed the technique of discarding papers to the highest level, and every document receives a date of destruction notation before it goes into the file.

# STORAGE

Large clinics and offices may find it advisable to microfilm records for storage. This permits storage of a considerable number of histories in a small space, saves time in searching, offers protection, and eliminates loss and misfiling. However, the cost is high, microfilm is hard to read for prolonged study, it is difficult to produce film in court, and if a patient returns, it is too small for refiling.

Some papers which should be kept but which need not be readily accessible may be placed in storage. Sturdy storage file boxes may be obtained from your stationery supply house. These boxes should be labeled to identify their contents in case it should be necessary to reclaim a file or refer to a record. The boxes are uniform in size and are available with a lift-off lid or in a drawer model. These can be kept in some out-of-the-way place. If no room is available in the office, they can be placed with a storage company for a low monthly rental. In this case, a record of the contents of each box should be kept in the office. A telephone call to the storage company will produce the record within a very short time.

### Can't Find Things?*

Usually, it's because you've permitted your desk—or closet— to become a catch-all for outdated papers. Mountains of old correspondence, cartoons yellowing with age, magazines never referred to, advertisements, half-finished crossword puzzles, old receipts, outdated manuals, 1958 Christmas cards, wedding announcements—are just some of the papers that add confusion to our lives.

Except for canceled checks and old receipts (which belong in an expanding envelope against the day you figure out your income tax), these space wasters are time-killers, for they force you to spend hours every month searching for the papers you do need.

It has been estimated that 90 per cent of the collection of papers of both a business and an individual is worthless. The word: get rid of them.

Sound ruthless? So's a clock!

## PERSONAL RECORDS

Many times the medical office assistant is required to file or otherwise dispose of documents, receipts, and other records of her employer's personal affairs. An article appearing in *Medical Economics* (November 29, 1965) gives some valuable guidelines for retention of personal records (see below).

### The right place for your personal papers

The accompanying article tells why and how you should keep such personal papers as income tax returns, canceled checks, records of gifts and bequests received, inventory lists and appraisals, contracts and insurance policies. The list below covers other personal records and tells where to store them and how long to keep them.

*Keep in safe or safe-deposit box*

| WHAT | HOW LONG |
|---|---|
| Birth certificates, marriage and divorce records, passports, professional certificates, licenses | Permanently |
| Real-estate deeds, leases, registration receipts, title abstracts, surveyors' reports, auto titles, original of burial plot deed | Until sale of property or settlement of estate; then to dead storage |

*Reprinted by permission of *Physician's Management* (Vol. 2, No. 9) Sept., 1962, p. 26.

| | |
|---|---|
| Stocks, bonds, promissory notes, mortgages | Until sold, paid or collected |
| Originals of wills, powers of attorney or appointment | Until revised, probated or exercised |

*Keep in desk or filing cabinet*

| WHAT | HOW LONG |
|---|---|
| Current bank statements | Three years; then to dead storage |
| Bank deposit slips | Three years; then to dead storage |
| Receipts for paid bills | Three years if needed for tax purposes; otherwise two months to cover crediting errors; then to dead storage or (if trivial amounts are involved) discard |

*Keep in dead storage*

| WHAT | HOW LONG |
|---|---|
| Old bank statements | Permanently |
| Old family health records | Permanently |
| Old partnership and other business agreements | Permanently |
| Old real-estate deeds, major property records | Permanently |
| Old receipts for major paid bills | Until purchased item has been sold or discarded |

*Medical Economics,* November 29, 1965.

## REFERENCES

*Files Operations,* General Services Administration, National Archives and Records Service, Office of Records Management, Washington, D.C., 1964.

Hanna, J. M., *Secretarial Procedures and Administration,* 5th Ed., Cincinnati, Ohio, South-Western Publishing Company, 1968.

Johnson, M. M., and N. F. Kallous, *Records Management,* Cincinnati, Ohio, South-Western Publishing Company, 1967.

Kahn, G., Yerian, I., and J. R. Stewart, *Filing Systems and Records Management,* 2nd Ed., New York, Gregg Division, McGraw-Hill, 1971.

# Chapter 15

**BEHAVIORAL OBJECTIVES**

*The medical office assistant should be able to:*

Explain how medical fees may be
    determined.
Avoid the pitfalls of fee adjustments.
State the advantages of advance
    discussion of fees.

Obtain necessary information from
    patient before extending credit.
Assist patient in planning financing of
    medical care.

# Professional Fees and Credit Arrangements

## PROFESSIONAL FEES

The doctor is trained to view his profession from the standpoint of *service*. Little attention is given to the business side of medicine. But the doctor must charge and collect for his services in order to continue providing medical care to all his patients.

The assistant, too, has some inhibitions to overcome in relation to professional fees. She probably has not given much thought to finances from the viewpoint of the physician; her experience has been from the viewpoint of the patient.

The tasks of charging fees and collecting money from patients in exchange for medical services are often viewed by both the doctor and his assistant as unpleasant and difficult. These duties must be placed in their proper perspective, and a positive attitude toward the financial side of medical practice cultivated in the minds of the doctor, the assistant, and the patient.

## How Fees are Determined

It is not easy to set a "fair fee". A doctor sells his time, his judgment, and his services—yet the value of these commodities is never exactly the same to two different individuals. Medical care has little value except to the patient himself, and the value to that patient may not be consistent with his ability to pay. In every case, the doctor himself must place an estimate upon the value of his services. This value may then be modified by other considerations.

**Prevailing Rate in the Community.** One of the bases for determining medical fees is the nature of the community itself. In some communities the entire cost of living scale is much higher than in other communities. This situation is reflected in medical fees, too. Consequently, the prevailing rate in the community—the average composite fee—must be taken into consideration by each individual doctor. Strangely enough, fees that are too low drive patients away just as quickly as do fees that are too high.

**Usual and Customary Fee.** Some insurance plans do not publish a fee schedule but agree to pay all or a percentage of the *usual and customary fee* for any given procedure. The physician's *usual fee* is the charge he makes to his private patients. The *customary fee* is a range of the usual fees charged by the majority of physicians with similar training and experience practicing in the same geographic and socioeconomic area.

For example, let us suppose Dr. Wallace charges his private patients $15 for a first office visit. This is his *usual* fee for this service. The usual fees charged for a first office visit by other doctors with similar training and experience in the same community range from $8 to $16. The insurance company that pays a usual and customary fee would then allow payment of $15 to Dr. Wallace. If, on the other hand, the range of usual fees in the community is from $8 to $12, the insurance company would allow only the maximum within the range, or $12, to Dr. Wallace.

**Doctor's Fee Profile.**   The fiscal agents for certain government-sponsored insurance programs keep a continuous record of the usual charges submitted for specific services by each individual doctor. By compiling these fees over a given period the doctor's *fee profile* is established. This fee profile is then used by the fiscal agent in determining the amount of third party liability for services under the program.

**Insurance Allowance.**   In some individual cases, the physician may feel that he does not wish to charge the patient in addition to what will be allowed by his insurance coverage. The full fee should be quoted to the patient and charged to his account, with the understanding that after the insurance allowance has been received, the balance will be discounted. If a smaller fee is quoted and charged several problems may arise: (1) the lower fee will disturb the doctor's fee profile; (2) if it should become necessary to bring suit for payment of the fee, only the reduced fee can be recovered; and (3) the insurance allowance may be paid on the basis of a certain percentage of the doctor's fee. If a lower fee is charged, the insurance allowance will be correspondingly lower.

**Relative Value Studies.**   Many doctors do not know just how to determine fees for certain procedures. This is particularly true in situations where the procedure is either rare or one performed infrequently by the physician. Some physicians may wonder whether their fees are in line with others in their community. The relative value study provides a guideline.

What is a relative value study? It is a published index of hundreds of the most commonly performed procedures in medicine, surgery, anesthesia, radiology, and pathology. Listed alongside each procedure is its *relative value* expressed in numbers of units. These units represent the value of this service in relation to other procedures commonly performed. No dollar values are given. Each doctor determines his own value per unit, and then uses this as the conversion factor in arriving at a monetary fee.

When the California Medical Association pioneered this approach with the publication of its 1956 Relative Value Study, all procedures were assigned a four-digit number and the unit values were based upon a single conversion factor for all procedures listed. The California Relative Value Study (CRVS) was adopted in its original form or in some modified version by many other medical societies and specialty groups. After several minor modifications, the CRVS underwent a major revision with the publication of the 1969 CRVS. In this later version, five-digit procedure codes emerged, as well as the use of modifiers to signify special circumstances that warrant increasing or decreasing a normal fee, *i.e.*, night calls, holidays or Sundays, new patient or established patient, and so forth. Additionally, a different unit value is used in determining the fee for procedures in each of the five major categories. The use of relative value studies has spread nationally, and the majority of medical office assistants will need to have some acquaintance with them.

## Adjusting or Canceling Fees

**Care for Those Who Cannot Pay.** The medical profession has traditionally accepted the responsibility of providing medical care for those individuals who are unable to pay for these services. In spite of the increased scope of government-sponsored care for the medically indigent, doctors still donate thousands of dollars' worth of such medical services each year.

In many instances, medical care for the indigent is available, but those who need it may be unaware that such assistance is available. The doctor's assistant should acquaint herself with the various local organizations and agencies that can aid the patient in obtaining the necessary assistance. The doctor himself can furnish only his services—other agencies must provide hospitalization, for example, or arrange for paying costs of special therapy, rehabilitation, or drugs.

If a doctor accepts a case for which he will not be paid, complete records must still be kept on the patient. The only deviation in procedure is that the financial record will indicate "n/c" (no charge) in the debit column.

**Adjusting or Canceling Fees.** Sometimes a doctor is faced with the problem of deciding whether to reduce or cancel a fee in a hardship case or in a case accompanied by special circumstances. Proper financial investigation prior to the setting of a fee eliminates considerable discounting later. In most cases it is far better to adjust the fee at the beginning of treatment than to reduce it later. A fee should never be reduced on the basis of a poor result, or as a means of obtaining payment to avoid the use of a collection agency. A reduction for these reasons will degrade the doctor and his practice.

Before adjusting or canceling a fee, the doctor or his assistant should encourage a frank discussion of the patient's financial problem. Next, an investigation should be made to determine whether or not this person is eligible for local and state public assistance programs. If so, direct the patient to the proper agency. Find out whether the patient is entitled to insurance settlement. Check locally to find out whether the person is a bona fide needy case or not.

The doctor must decide whether it is better to reduce a fee or cancel it entirely. Many feel that the patient who pays at least a part of the fee retains his personal pride and has more appreciation for the care he receives. Other physicians feel that a doctor should not bargain with his patients, and the entire fee should be canceled in needy cases.

**Pitfalls of Fee Adjustments.** Great care should be taken in reducing the fee for care of a patient who dies. The doctor's sympathy may be with the family in such instances, but the doctor's generosity in reducing a fee could be misinterpreted and result in a suit for malpractice.

If the doctor agrees to settle for a reduced fee in a situation where the patient is disputing the fee, he should make certain the negotiations are "without prejudice." By taking this precaution the doctor protects his right to collect the original sum should the patient refuse to pay the lowered fee. The offer of a discount, therefore, should be made in writing, with the insertion of the words "without prejudice," and a definite time limit in which payment is to be made should be stated. Make two copies of the agreement, one for the doctor and one for the patient, and have the signatures witnessed.

Sometimes after a doctor and his patient have agreed upon a fee, special circumstances arise that constitute a hardship case. If the doctor agrees then to reduce the fee, the patient should be advised that the reduction will be effective only after the adjusted amount is paid in full. For instance, if a fee of $300 is reduced to $200, the full amount of the $300 charge should appear on the ledger and when $200 has been received, the remainder can be written off as an adjustment.

**Professional Courtesy.** Traditionally, doctors do not charge one another or their immediate dependents for medical care. In some areas, and especially in the case of specialists, giving of professional courtesy represents the loss of a large amount of potential income. If there is a substantial outlay in the cost of materials, the professional colleague will probably wish to reimburse the physician for the materials used. Many doctors subscribe to a health insurance plan. If the care they receive is covered by insurance, it is entirely ethical for the attending physician to accept the insurance benefits in payment for his services.

If the care involved is frequent enough to involve a significant proportion of the doctor's professional time, or in cases of long-term treatment, the doctor may wish to charge on an adjusted basis.

If professional courtesy is offered, but the recipient insists upon paying, the physician need not hesitate on ethical grounds to accept a fee for his services.

Professional courtesy is often extended beyond fellow physicians and their dependents. Most physicians treat their own assistants without charge, and grant discounts of 20 to 50 per cent to nurses and assistants not in their direct employ. In still other instances, professional courtesy is extended to others in the health care field, for instance, to pharmacists, dentists, and clergymen.

**Charges to Avoid.** It is generally considered inadvisable to charge for *telephone calls*. Some physicians, especially pediatricians, find they must give considerable medical advice over the telephone. Many of these calls, however, are fairly routine to the office (although not to the worried mother or patient) and an able assistant can be trained to answer many of the questions, or a special time can be set aside for telephone calls.

Levying *late charges* on fees for professional services not paid within a prescribed time is not in the best interest of the public or the profession, according to the A.M.A. Judicial Council.

Most physicians feel that charging for a *missed appointment* or for one not canceled 24 hours in advance, although not unethical if the patient is fully advised, is nevertheless not in the best interest of their patients or their practices.

If a patient has multiple insurance forms to be completed, the physician is justified in making a charge but may antagonize if he charges for the *first insurance form*.

October 28, 19___

Mr. John Jones
1234 East Street
Cincinnati, Ohio   45202

Dear Mr. Jones:

Your account in the amount of $135 is long past due.
Understanding the financial circumstances that make it
difficult for you to make any payment on these past
services, Dr. Johnson has instructed me to consider the
debt canceled.  We will see that you are no longer billed
for it.

The doctor wants you to feel free, however, to call on
him for any future services you may require.

Sincerely yours,

CLAYTON L. SCROGGINS

Auditor for Dr. Johnson

**Figure 15-1**  Example of Letter Canceling Fee

The end of the year will find at least some of the patients requesting a *summary of their charges and payments for the year* just completed. There is a temptation to make an additional charge for this service. In most cases, it is probably unwise to do so.

## Advance Discussion of Fees

It is natural for the patient, once he has seen the doctor, to wonder, "How much is this going to cost?" He may be reluctant, however, to voice this concern. The patient who seems least concerned about the fee may very likely be the patient who creates the biggest collection problem.

It is the responsibility of the doctor or his assistant to raise the discussion of fees if the patient does not do so. In this preliminary discussion of fees, the doctor must not sidestep the issue by saying "Don't worry about the bill, let's just get you well first." He must also avoid an attempt to calm a worried patient about to undergo surgery by saying, "There's really nothing to it." He may find that the patient later complains loudly about the bill since the doctor himself said it was a simple procedure. Even in those cases where the doctor quotes a fee, the assistant is often charged with the responsibility of explaining the doctor's fees to the patient. She must know how fees are determined and why charges vary. She must have special knowledge of her own employer's practice and policies in order to handle perplexing situations involving fees.

The neophyte assistant is in the position of having to educate her viewpoint to that of the doctor. She can be something of a "saleswoman" for the doctor's services by gently convincing patients that money spent for medical care is an excellent investment in the future. Sometimes it is impossible for a patient to see or understand the intricate procedures involved in diagnosis and treatment. He rarely is aware of the long years of training and study and the heavy expenses that a doctor incurs in securing his education. Furthermore, he does not always realize that running a modern professional office is a costly process relying upon day-to-day income in return for services. These are factors which the assistant can point out to patients and thus convince them that money paid for care is well spent.

When a doctor frankly discusses fees in advance with his patients, even to the point of describing how he arrives at a fee, misconceptions about overcharging and fee frictions are usually eliminated. One doctor wrote the American Medical Association that, with 95 per cent of his patients, three minutes at the end of the visit spent in explaining the medical bill ensures financial success.

Advance fee discussions help the patient to plan ahead for his medical expenditures. Most patients want to pay their financial obligations but rightly insist upon an accurate estimate of those obligations before they contract for purchase of goods or services. Because many physicians and patients are reluctant to broach the subject of fees, the American Medical Association sells, for a very modest price, an attractive office plaque which encourages fee discussions, with this message:

> TO ALL MY PATIENTS—I INVITE YOU TO DISCUSS
> FRANKLY WITH ME ANY QUESTIONS REGARDING MY
> SERVICES OR MY FEES. THE BEST MEDICAL
> SERVICE IS BASED ON A FRIENDLY, MUTUAL
> UNDERSTANDING BETWEEN DOCTOR AND PATIENT.

This plaque should be placed in the physician's office, not in the reception room.

Explanations of medical costs should extend beyond the doctor's own charges. For example, if a patient is to undergo surgery, the doctor should explain the costs of the operation, the anesthetist's and radiologist's charges, the laboratory fees, and the approximate hospital bill, as well as his own charges. The importance of calling in another physician for consultation should be explained to patients when consultation becomes necessary. It should be made clear, in advance, that there will be a separate bill submitted by the consulting physician.

The public is inclined to blame doctors for all medical costs — even hospital charges. (In 1970, doctors' fees accounted for only one-fifth of medical costs.) The doctor and his assistant can avoid misunderstanding by giving the patient an idea of what the entire medical procedure will cost. Some physicians give patients an estimate of medical expenses before hospitalization. A few medical societies cooperatively develop such estimate sheets with local hospitals. Individual doctors occasionally work up their own estimate forms when a patient is embarking upon long-term treatment. The doctor should, however, always point out that he is providing an estimate only and that the total cost may vary somewhat.

Estimate slips should be written in duplicate so that the patient may have a copy and the other can be retained in the office files. This eliminates the danger of misquoting the fee later or forgetting the charge originally discussed. Advance estimation and explanation of medical fees simplifies collection, since it eliminates later misunderstanding and confusion over bills.

## CREDIT ARRANGEMENTS

### Extending Credit

The word "credit" has numerous definitions and shades of meaning. A student receives educational *credit* for successful completion of a unit of study. To the accountant, *credit* means the righthand side of an account. Credit may mean belief in the genuineness or truth of something. When the doctor "extends credit" to a patient, *credit* implies a given time limit during which payment will be made, and sometimes includes an oral or written promise to pay. When the patient makes a payment, the assistant *credits* the patient's account with the amount paid.

Every collection for a doctor's services is preceded by an extension of credit. Credit arrangements are best made during the patient's initial visit; successful collection of an account may depend upon the skill and tact with which the first interview is conducted.

**Information from the Patient.** Good records are essential to follow-up of collections. It is extremely important that the assistant get adequate information about the patient's ability to pay — on his first visit to the office, if possible. It is neither unprofessional nor time consuming to get full credit information from patients. The public is conditioned to supply such information, and will respect a businesslike approach if it is done tactfully and without apology. Although a patient needing medical care will rarely be turned away because of his credit risk, the information provided on the initial visit may alert the assistant to be cautious about allowing an account to fall in arrears.

Many doctors inform a patient, when he telephones for his primary appointment, that new patients are expected to pay cash for their first visit, at which time credit arrangements can be established if further care is needed. This

# PATIENT REGISTRATION

Age_____ Date of birth_____ Miss
Mrs.

Patients Name _____
Last                    First                    Maiden

Address _____
Street & No.            City & State          Zip Code

Home Telephone_____ Social Security No._____

Employed by _____

Employers Address _____
Street & No.            City & State          Zip Code

Business Telephone_____

Name of Spouse_____
Last                    First                    Initial

Spouses Employer _____

Employers Address _____
Street & No.            City & State          Zip Code

Business Telephone_____

Referred by _____

## MEDICAL INSURANCE

Type:  Group_____    Private_____

Group No. _____ Policy No. _____

Nearest relative other than husband _____

Address _____

Telephone_____

**Figure 15–2**  Application for Credit

(*Illustration continued on opposite page.*)

CARBON COPY

31669

**INFORMATION FOR CASE HISTORY FILE** — PLEASE FILL IN COMPLETELY   DATE   /   /

| | DATE OF BIRTH | AGE | RELIGION |
| | / / | | |

PATIENT
(MR.-MRS.-MISS-MASTER)        FIRST        MIDDLE        LAST

RESPONSIBLE PARTY                                   RELATIONSHIP
(IF MINOR - GIVE FULL NAME AND RELATIONSHIP OF PERSON LEGALLY RESPONSIBLE)

HOME ADDRESS                                   PHONE
            STREET        CITY AND STATE

EMPLOYED BY                                   S.S.N.
            NAME OF FIRM OR CO.    STREET    CITY AND STATE

OCCUPATION                    PHONE

NAME OF SPOUSE                                   OFFICE USE ONLY
                                              /   /

SPOUSE
EMPLOYED BY                                   PHONE
            NAME OF FIRM OR CO.    STREET    CITY AND STATE

RELATIVE
OR FRIEND (IN AREA)                           PHONE
                          STREET    CITY AND STATE

REFERRED BY
            NAME            STREET        CITY AND STATE

MEDICAL OR SURGICAL INSURANCE?    YES    NO    INSURANCE CO.

---

# PATIENT HISTORY INFORMATION

Date_____

Patient _____ Age _____

☐ MARRIED        ☐ SINGLE        ☐ WIDOWED        ☐ DIVORCED        ☐ SEPARATED

Home address_____

City_____ Zone_____ Home phone_____

Patient employed by _____

Business address _____ City_____

Occupation _____ Business phone _____

Name of Spouse _____

Spouse employed by _____

Business Address _____ City _____ Zone ____

Occupation _____ Business phone _____

Patient referred to doctor by _____

If patient is minor, name of responsible parent _____

Is this visit payable by health insurance?   ☐ Yes;   ☐ No. If yes, give details to secretary now.

THE D.B.B. SYSTEMS - MADISON 7-1252 - HEMLOCK 5-6317

**Figure 15–2**   *Continued.*

approach informs the patient in advance that he will be expected to complete a credit application. Although the registration form the patient completes in the doctor's office is usually not as detailed as an application for credit in, for example, a department store, it must establish an information base, should future collection steps become necessary. The forms illustrated in Figure 15–2 are typical.

Sometimes the assistant will ask questions of the patient, and type his answers on the form; in other offices, the patient will be handed a form to complete himself. This affords him more privacy if there are others present, and tends to eliminate the impression that the assistant is overly inquisitive. The medical assistant should check the form carefully to make certain that nothing was overlooked. The new patient will view these questions as reasonable, but the established patient may resent such an inquiry. Consequently, *it is important that the form be completed on the first visit.*

Irrespective of the form or techniques used, the following information should be obtained:

1. *Patient's Full Name,* correctly spelled. J. A. Brown is not sufficient if later collection follow-up is necessary. John Allen Brown would be more helpful.

2. *Date of Birth.* May be useful as identification if there are two patients with similar names. Also, you will be able to determine the patient's exact age at any future time.

3. *Social Security Number,* if any. Many insurance policies use the patient's social security number as his certificate number.

4. *Marital Status and Number of Dependents.* May be useful in determining ability to pay. When couples are divorced or separated, credit and collections sometimes become complicated.

5. *Current Address and Past Addresses for at Least Two Years.* From this information you can judge the person's stability. Multiple residences in a short time may indicate financial instability; the class of neighborhood may give indication of a patient's financial status.

6. *Telephone Numbers for both Residence and Work.* If patient has no home telephone, get number of nearest telephone. It may be necessary to call the patient or contact his employer.

7. *Name and Relationship of Person Legally Responsible for Payment.* See paragraph on third party liability, page 197.

8. *Patient's and Spouse's Occupation, Name and Address of Employer.* If a man lists his employer as Gord's Department Store, find out his employment title and the name of his immediate superior. He may be a shipping clerk, salesman, or he may be the vice president.

9. *Name, Address, and Telephone Number of Person* to be notified in case of emergency.

10. *Name of Neighbor or Friend in Area.* If a patient moves after receiving medical care, a friend or neighbor may be able to provide information on his whereabouts.

11. *Who Referred Patient to Doctor.* If patient is referred by another physician, you will want to send a report to the physician. If referred by another patient, the doctor may wish to thank the referring patient on his next visit to the office.

12. *Health Insurance Information.* See paragraph on page 197.

**Third Party Liability.**   If financial responsibility is attributed to an individual other than the patient, spouse, or parent, be sure to obtain full name, address, employment data, and other credit information about that person. Also, contact the named individual for verification of the obligation. If a third party's agreement to pay is contingent upon the patient's failure to pay, such an agreement must be in writing to be enforceable and must be made prior to treatment. Any agreement made after completion of treatment could be considered as a moral obligation only. The guaranty of a person to pay the account of another may be very simple. It may be typewritten or in longhand, and stating:

I, the undersigned, do promise to pay for the medical services rendered by Theodore Wilson, M. D., to my nephew, Robert L. Smith.
> Date:
> Signed:

or

I, the undersigned, promise to pay the medical bill of Robert L. Smith, if his mother, Mrs. Lydia Smith, does not pay by the 15th of July, 19— —.
> Date:
> Signed:

Accounts rendered to a wife or child should always carry full data about the party responsible, in most cases the husband or father. Generally, a husband or father pays the account for which he is obligated without any necessary follow-up collection procedures.

If you foresee legal difficulties in collecting on an account in a situation in which divorce, legal guardianships, or emancipated minors complicate the matter, it is best to contact your doctor's attorney for advice. The laws governing such matters vary according to each state. One reminder, however, is that you must always have the signature of the third party responsible for the debt if he is not obligated by law. An oral agreement is not binding.

**Health Insurance Information.**   The initial interview is the best time to get full information on the patient's insurance coverage. The patient registration form usually provides a place for the name of the insurance company. Ask to see the patient's identification card; if he has one, make a photocopy for your records. The card will usually show the name of the subscriber, the group and member number, and often will include a service code indicating the patient's coverage. Also obtain information on any supplementary coverage, for instance, a plan in which the spouse is the subscriber and the patient is covered as a dependent. There may also be major medical or supplementary benefits to the patient's policy.

**Assignments.**   Many doctors' offices ask the patient to execute an assignment of insurance benefits at this time. The assignment, authorizing the insurance company to pay benefits directly to the doctor, may be stamped on the insurance form, or may be subsequently attached to a completed insurance form.

**Consent for Release of Information.**   If a standard claim form is used or if the patient has brought along his own form, this is an appropriate time to have the patient sign the consent for release of information which is necessary on most claims, so that the insurance form can be processed without delay as services are performed.

## Installment Buying of Medical Services

Because installment buying is so much a part of our economic system today, the physician's office must be prepared to help patients budget for their medical care. Patients expect to use their credit resources, and will appreciate business-like assistance in establishing a payment plan. The medical profession has too long suffered a poor collection record because of its fear of appearing "too commercial." The doctor should be ready to arrange credit when medical bills will be high or when a patient for some reason is financially unable to pay his bills. Fees for routine office calls and small medical bills should be kept on a pay-as-you-go basis.

**Credit Cards.** The acceptance of credit cards in the doctor's office is becoming more commonplace every day. A few years ago this would have been shocking to most physicians.

The A.M.A. Code of Ethics discourages the use of a bank card in connection with the payment of large fees which might normally be paid to the physician in installments. However, it does set forth certain guidelines for physician participation in bank card programs:

(1) the county medical society should be satisfied as to the financial and professional integrity of the plan . . .

(2) the individual physician may not, because of his participation, increase his fee for medical service rendered the patient. He may not use the plan to solicit patients. He may not encourage patients to use the plan. His position must be that he accepts the plan as a convenience to patients who desire to use it. Plaques or other devices indicating participation in the plan within the physician's office shall be kept to a discreet and dignified minimum. Plaques, signs, or other devices indicating such participation visible outside the physician's office are unacceptable.

**Bank Financing.** Some banks have set up plans to do the financing job for patients in a manner consistent with professional ethics. The dental profession has pioneered in this field, and many dental societies have worked out arrangements with banks to help patients meet dental expenses.

Here is how bank financing of bills works: the bank checks the patient's credit and, if it appears acceptable, agrees to take the patient's promise to pay. The bank then forwards the doctor the total sum which the patient owes him, less a small discount. This provides the doctor with the full amount due him immediately. The bank really is lending the money to patients at a small rate of interest; doctors often deduct the interest charges from their fees as a further encouragement to patients to take advantage of these budget plans. Literature and introductory cards to the bank or a similar professional budget bureau can be provided to patients who are interested in exploring these special budget and financing plans.

Before seeking outside financing help on behalf of patients, it is important that the doctor carefully investigate available plans and determine whether or not their use is justified. There are some unscrupulous organizations that press patients for payment in an unethical manner and create considerable ill will for the profession.

**Special Budget Plans.**   If a patient appears upset at the prospect of meeting his obligations, the doctor or his assistant can suggest in a tactful way: "Mr. Elwood, if you think you will have difficulty paying for your treatments at one time, we can work out some special arrangements." This allows the patient to ask what sort of plan you have in mind, and the discussion progresses very easily into various payment plans. It is well to ask the patient what arrangements will be best for him rather than to suggest a plan. If he is still reluctant, the assistant then can say, "Mr. Elwood, would you be able to pay $50 each month until the account is paid in full?" or "Usually an account of this size can be settled in three to four months. Would you be able to pay $100 down, then $50 a month until the account is paid in full?" When the amount of each installment has been agreed upon, it is then wise to establish definite dates on which the payments will be expected.

**Truth in Lending Act.**   Regulation Z of the Truth in Lending Act, which is enforced by the Federal Trade Commission, requires that when there is a bilateral agreement between doctor and patient to accept payment in more than four installments, the doctor is required to provide disclosure of information regarding finance charges. Even if there are no finance charges involved the form must be completed stating that this is so. One copy of the form is retained by the doctor and one must be given to the patient. Specific wording is required in the disclosure. The form in Figure 15–3 meets the requirements.

It is recognized that physicians generally permit their patients to pay in installments, and as long as there is no specific agreement on the part of the physician for payment to be made in more than four installments, and he does not make a finance charge, he is not subject to the regulation. If the patient chooses to pay installments instead of the full amount for which he is billed, this is considered a unilateral action and the physician, in accepting such payments, probably would not subject himself to the provisions of the regulation.

Helping patients budget their medical expenses is a rather new aspect of the business side of practice. However, it is a real service to patients and demonstrates that the doctor and his office staff are sincerely anxious to help patients pay their own way. From the assistant's standpoint, use of such plans solves many of her collection problems, thus making her work easier.

# Credit is Confidential

Always remember that credit information is confidential. It should be guarded as carefully as a confidential medical history, and should not be disclosed to anyone. When you ask for credit information from patients in the office, make sure that you do so in a place where others cannot overhear the conversation. Credit information is personal—it should be kept that way.

# TRUTH IN LENDING FORM FOR PHYSICIANS

Doctor's Name_____

Doctor's Address_____

_____

Patient's Name_____

Patient's Address_____

_____

| | |
|---|---|
| Cash price (total fee) | *500.00* |
| Less cash down payment | *200.00* |
| Unpaid balance of cash price | *300.00* |
| Amount financed | *300.00* |
| FINANCE CHARGE | *none* |
| ANNUAL PERCENTAGE RATE | *none* |
| Total of payments | *6* |
| Deferred payment price | *500.00* |

Patient hereby agrees to pay to_____at
(physician's name)
his office, the address of which is given above, the total of payments

shown above in___*6*___monthly installments of $___*50*_____, first

installment being payable_____, 19__, and all such install-

ments on the same day of each consecutive month until paid in full.

_____          _____
(date)                              (signature of patient)
**Figure 15–3**

**Credit Bureau.**  Some doctors, particularly in large cities where it is more difficult to gauge informally the patients' ability to pay, join a credit bureau. Credit bureaus round up credit information from many sources, pool it, and make it available to local businessmen who become bureau members by paying dues. Before joining such a credit organization, it is a good idea for the doctor or his staff to check to make sure it is an ethical bureau with no unscrupulous practices.

**Bureaus of Medical Economics.**  In a number of localities, the medical societies maintain bureaus of medical economics which either have their own credit information service or have access to a reputable credit bureau. Such a society-operated bureau can be of great help in determining a patient's medical credit rating and also in helping develop good collection procedures. If there is a bureau of medical economics in your area, this will probably be your best source for determining a patient's medical credit. The county society-owned bureau maintains a master file on all accounts assigned and will advise you if an individual has a poor medical credit record.

**Medical-Dental-Hospital Bureaus.**  The Medical-Dental-Hospital Bureaus of America, with headquarters in Chicago, is a national organization of agencies serving physicians, dentists, and hospitals. It seeks to maintain the highest standards among its members and is committed to following the collection methods most acceptable to physicians. Doctors who use their collection services have access to credit information on accounts assigned by other clients. Member bureaus of the M.D.H.B.A. frequently assist the medical office assistant by sponsoring collection seminars, as well as by providing speakers for medical assistant society meetings.

Even though your office uses the services of a credit bureau or collection agency, do not rely upon such organizations completely to supply you with credit information. Sometimes the information you obtain from patients in the office will be more up-to-date than that on the bureau records. Unfortunately, many people with an A.A.A. rating on auto, bank, and charge accounts still do not like to pay medical bills.

# Chapter 16

---

## BEHAVIORAL OBJECTIVES

*The medical office assistant should be able to:*

Assist in choosing appropriate
    statement forms.

Prepare statements for medical care.

Establish and follow an efficient billing
    schedule.

Explain the reasons for pursuing
    collections.

Prepare an age analysis of patient
    accounts.

Compose effective collection letters.

Apply general rules for telephone
    requests for payment.

Handle special collection problems.

# Billing and Collecting Procedures

Management consultants for the medical profession say that the accounts receivable on a doctor's books should ideally equal no more than two to three months' gross charges. They also agree that a collection ratio of less than 90 per cent indicates that something is wrong with the collection procedure. Keeping accounts receivable down and collections up is neither impossible nor difficult if proper procedures are developed and consistently followed. With all financial records (including patients' account cards) kept up-to-date, and a well-developed collection procedure, collections can be a very satisfying challenge. Without such a basis, however, end-of-the-month billing day can be the most psychologically difficult day of the month for the medical assistant.

The major portion of the doctor's fees will be paid without question upon presentation of a bill, provided correct procedures are being followed. Collection of professional accounts can be divided into three distinct stages:

1. Informing the patient of what his charges will be and what professional services these cover.

2. Providing an opportunity for the patient to pay at the time of service for smaller amounts and sending bills out promptly for larger fees.

3. Conscientiously following up on uncollected accounts. In many instances, particularly if surgery or long-term treatment is involved, the first stage of collection will be done by the physician himself. The medical assistant is customarily charged with the responsibility of stages two and three, the subject of this chapter.

## BILLING PROCEDURES

### Statement Forms

Statements should carry the doctor's letterhead and should be of good quality paper. Statement heads are usually smaller than letter stationery, but they should be large enough to allow itemization of bills.

Many doctors' offices use self-addressed return envelopes to mail statements. This procedure is mainly for the convenience of patients who do not always have stationery available for sending a return payment or are less likely to

203

send a return payment immediately if they must search for an envelope. Occasionally there is the complaint that when statements are sent on self-addressed return envelopes, the patient has no record of the bill once he sends in his payment. A statement form is now available that allows the patient to tear the bill into two parts along a perforated line. The top half, which carries the patient's name, address, and amount owed, is returned to the doctor's office along with the payment; the bottom half, on which the bill is itemized, can then be retained by the patient in his files. The return envelope can be sent in a window envelope, thus avoiding duplicate typing of the patient's name and address (see Fig. 16–2). Because of income tax laws, patients like to keep complete records of expendi-

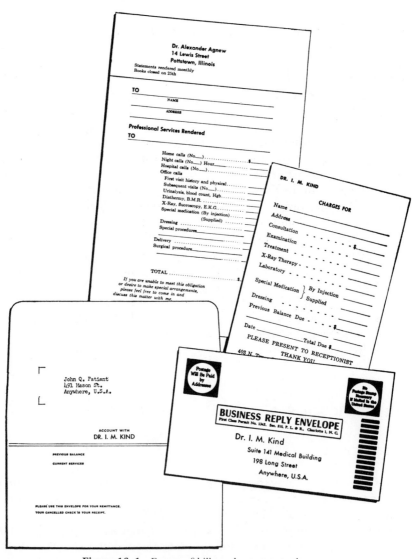

**Figure 16–1** Forms of bills and return envelopes.

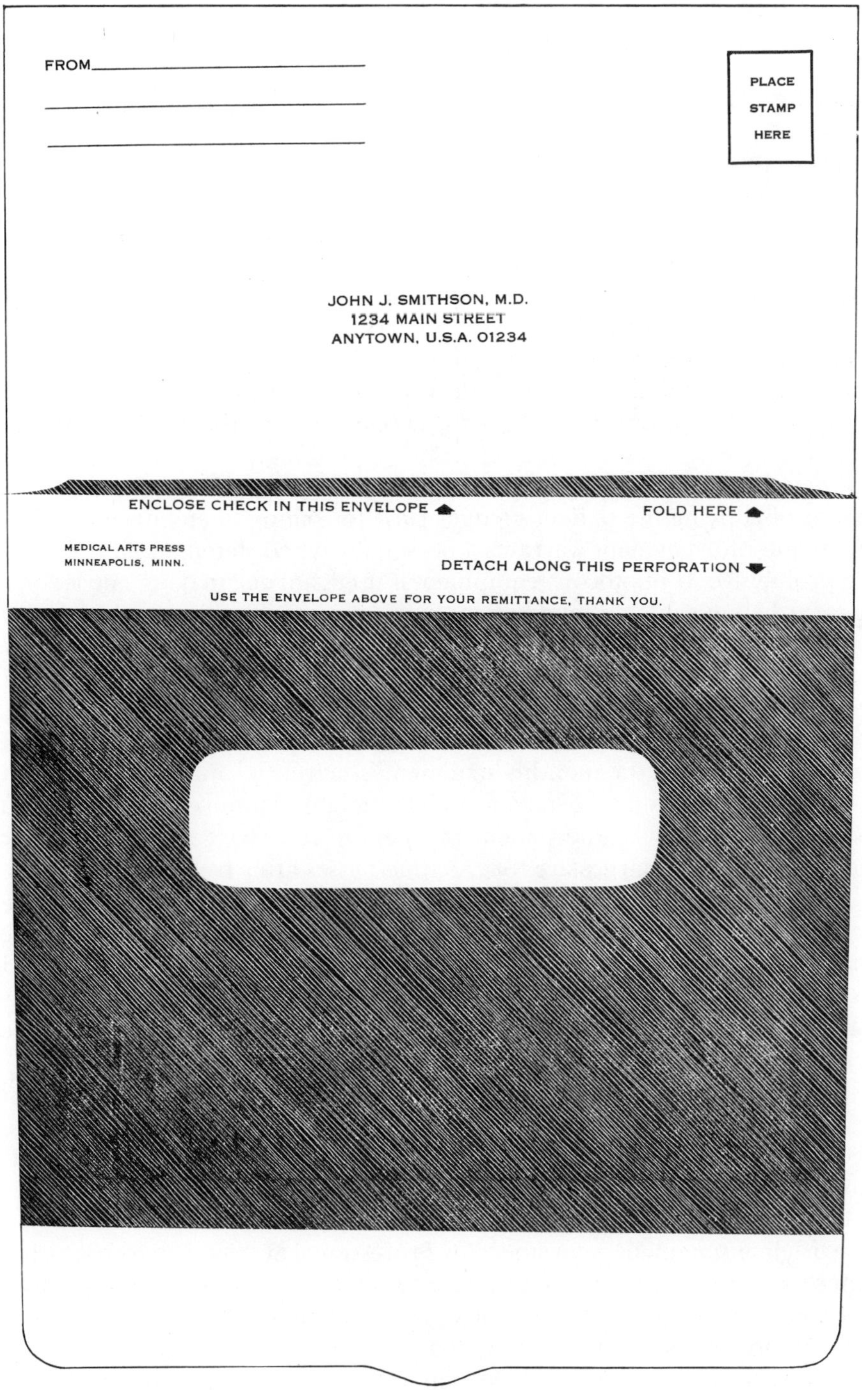

FROM_____

_____

_____

PLACE
STAMP
HERE

JOHN J. SMITHSON, M.D.
1234 MAIN STREET
ANYTOWN, U.S.A. 01234

ENCLOSE CHECK IN THIS ENVELOPE ▲              FOLD HERE ▲

MEDICAL ARTS PRESS
MINNEAPOLIS, MINN.                    DETACH ALONG THIS PERFORATION ▼

USE THE ENVELOPE ABOVE FOR YOUR REMITTANCE, THANK YOU.

Figure 16–2

tures for medical care. Use of such statements saves your time, too, for it eliminates that last-minute pre-income-tax itemization of accounts for patients who want complete records of their yearly payments to you.

## Preparing Statements

Three things should be remembered in preparing statements: bills must be (1) correct, (2) itemized, and (3) mailed promptly.

**Send Correct Bills.**  Take care in preparing statements to assure that all items are correct, including the patient's name and address as well as the amount owed. If your financial records have been carefully maintained each day, there is little likelihood of accounting errors occurring in your statements. Not only should statements be correct; their appearance is every bit as important as the professional correspondence from a doctor's office. A carelessly typed statement has the psychological effect of suggesting carelessness in other activities in the office.

Though the current trend is toward the use of photocopy and other methods of copying the patient's ledger card for billing, many doctors still feel that a request for payment warrants a personally typed statement, if the volume is not prohibitive. If photocopy equipment is used, anyone making entries on the ledger card should be cautioned about making personal notes on these records in pencil or in an ink that will be picked up by the photo equipment. Inasmuch as the patient receives an exact copy of his statement card, he might obtain information that should remain in the office.

**Itemize Bills.**  If the medical fee has been explained in advance, as discussed in Chapter 15, the monthly statement is merely a confirmation of what is owed, and there should be no misunderstanding. However, it is good business—and a courtesy to the patient—to itemize the charges. Patients are entitled to know what charges are for. As time passes after treatment, the patient may forget that he was treated at your office four times, not three. On receiving an unitemized bill, it may appear to the patient that he has been overcharged. Also, remember that he may not have been told, or he may have forgotten under the stress of seeking aid, just exactly what was done to help his condition. Tests unfamiliar to the patient are sometimes ordered at his expense, without an explanation. Even though professional men are making a concerted effort to provide more careful, understandable explanations to patients regarding their care, patients often must be "sold" on the necessity for the various services rendered them. The careful itemization of the bill contributes to greater understanding.

Itemizing bills is not difficult. The simplest method is merely to allow space on the original statement below the "For Professional Services" line on which the doctor's secretary can list the separate charges for office, house, or hospital calls, or for treatments or tests. A typical itemized statement is shown in Figure 16–3.

Many doctors, some of them specialists, have devised their own itemized charge slips, which are given to the patient if he wishes to pay before leaving the office or are mailed in a combination statement-reply envelope later. Use of such charge slips simplifies the itemization procedure, since filling out the slips is

LEDGER CARD

Mr. Paul Allan
123 Main Street
Anytown, CA   90000

| NUMBER | DATE | PROFESSIONAL SERVICE | CHARGE | | PAID | | BALANCE | |
|--------|------|----------------------|--------|---|------|---|---------|---|
| 90050 | 5/29/75 | Office call | 12 | 00 | | | | |
| 85010 | | CBC | 10 | 00 | | | 22 | 00 |
| 90050 | 6/5/75 | Office call | 12 | 00 | | | 34 | 00 |
| | | | | | | | | |
| | | | | | | | | |
| | | | | | | | | |
| | | | | | | | | |
| | | | | | | | | |
| | | | | | | | | |
| | | | | | | | | |
| | | | | | | | | |
| | | | | | | | | |
| | | | | | | | | |
| | | | | | | | | |
| | | | | | | | | |
| | | | | | | | | |
| | | | | | | | | |
| | | | | | | | | |

FORM 5110 COLWELL CO., CHAMPAIGN, ILLINOIS

®
THIS IS A "THERMO-FAX" BRAND SYSTEMS PAPER MASTER

**Figure 16–3**   Itemized statement.

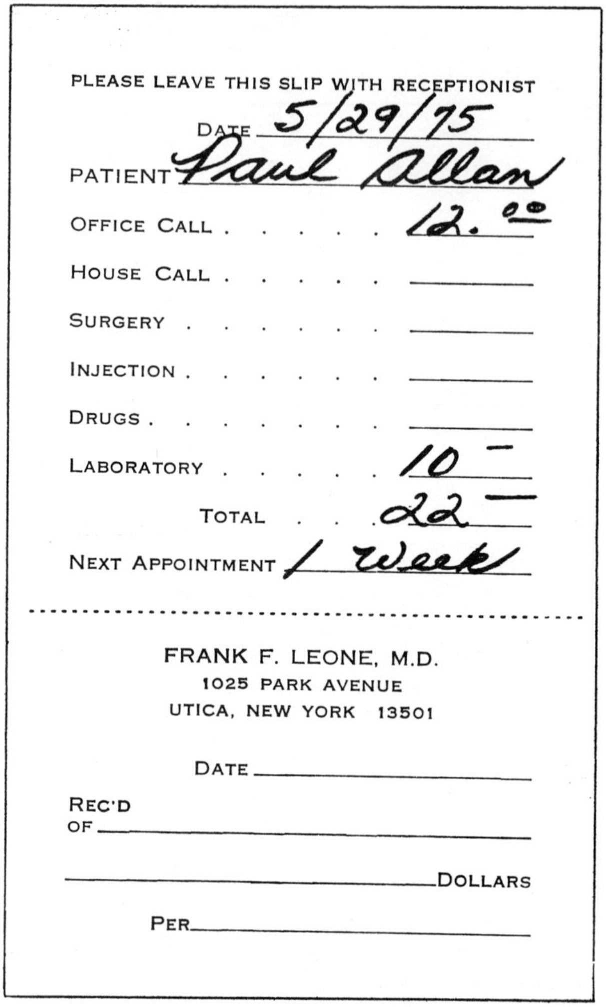

PLEASE LEAVE THIS SLIP WITH RECEPTIONIST

DATE *5/29/75*

PATIENT *Paul Allan*

OFFICE CALL . . . . . *12.00*

HOUSE CALL . . . . . _____

SURGERY . . . . . . _____

INJECTION . . . . . . _____

DRUGS . . . . . . . _____

LABORATORY . . . . . *10*

TOTAL . . *22*

NEXT APPOINTMENT *1 Week*

- - - - - - - - - - - - - - - - - - - - - - - - - - - - - - - - -

FRANK F. LEONE, M.D.
1025 PARK AVENUE
UTICA, NEW YORK 13501

DATE _____

REC'D
OF _____

_____DOLLARS

PER_____

**Figure 16–4**   Charge slip.

usually just a matter of checking procedures lists. An itemized charge slip is shown in Figure 16–4.

First statements, and statements going to a third party responsible for the bill, should always be itemized. If there are any legal involvements—for instance, if a legal guardian is paying a bill for a minor—the statement should be sent in duplicate so that the administrator may retain a copy for his file. Statements to insurance companies also should be itemized.

While the itemization of bills may seem an unnecessary waste of time, in the long run you will spend less time explaining services provided, clearing up misunderstandings with patients over bills, and following up on delinquent accounts if you routinely itemize all bills. The itemization of bills is a plus for public relations, also.

**Mail Bills Promptly.** Most people expect to receive statements from their creditors, and they plan their budgets around first-of-the-month bills received. The bill that arrives late remains unpaid. Punctuality in billing encourages prompt payment.

**Time and Frequency of Billing.** A regular system of rendering statements should be put into operation. Patients are entitled to know the date on which payment of their medical bill is expected. Statements should be sent at least once each month. Some doctors send bills immediately after treatment has been given; others bill at the first of each month. In other offices statements are mailed twice a month, on the first and the fifteenth.

ONCE-A-MONTH BILLING. If a monthly pattern is followed, bills should leave your office no later than the last day of each month. Planning ahead for the typing of statements can lighten the burden of once-a-month billing. The statement can be typed at the time of service or during slack periods, postdated, and mailed at the end of the month.

CYCLE BILLING. Many physicians prefer to use the cycle billing system, which calls for the billing of certain portions of the accounts receivable at various times during the month instead of preparing all statements at the end of each month. Cycle billing has been used for some time in large businesses such as department stores and other companies extending credit. There are certain advantages to this method, and the system is becoming increasingly popular in the physician's office.

Under this plan your accounts are divided into fairly equal sections, usually on the basis of alphabetical breakdowns. The number of sections varies from approximately 15 to 20, depending upon the number of accounts receivable in the office. Regardless of constant changes in the accounts themselves, the mailing dates for accounts in each section remain constant. A schedule for processing and mailing of accounts is thus established, apportioning the load of work throughout the entire month.

This is how the cycle billing system works: patients whose names begin with A, for example, are billed on the first of the month, patients with names beginning with B are billed on the second day of the month, and so on. Small alphabetical groups can be doubled up to keep your accounts-receivable divisions by date fairly equal in size.

The use of cycle billing can enable a secretary to continue all her routine duties each day, handling the statements on a day-to-day schedule rather than in one intensive period at the end of the month. This means that she need never sacrifice whole days from her assisting duties in order to get statements into the mail. By spacing the billing throughout the month, she can give more time and consideration to each statement. The itemization of bills will be less burdensome, and the likelihood of error will be decreased.

Patients generally accept the cycle billing system quickly, often with enthusiasm. However, if your office decides to change from a once-a-month billing to a cycle billing system, patients should be notified in advance and the new plan explained to them.

A reasonable length of time should elapse between the new patient's first visit to the doctor's office and the mailing of a bill. It would be poor policy, for example, to see a new patient on the ninth of the month and then send him a statement on the tenth. Many would feel that the doctor is being overanxious to collect his fee. When the statement is sent, a notice explaining his future payment date should accompany it. To explain the new system to established patients, enclose a notice in each statement the month prior to the transfer, describing the plan and indicating the future dates on which each patient will receive his bill.

Before adopting the cycle system a doctor should take several factors into consideration. First, what is the income of the community, and how and when does the average patient receive his pay? Do local companies pay employees at various times during the month or are most pay checks handed out at the beginning of the month? Would cycle billing benefit patients, as well as the overall operation of the office?

Regular billing and itemizing of statements not only is a service to patients but it is valuable to the doctor, since prompt payments are usually forthcoming if these practices are followed.

## COLLECTION PROCEDURES

### Reasons to Pursue Collections

Collecting for professional services is a very necessary aspect of medical practice. The reasons for pursuing collections go beyond the obvious one that a physician must be paid for his services in order to meet his own expenses. Human nature operates in strange ways. A doctor often loses the good will of patients by not collecting from them. A man who owes the doctor money and is not prodded gently into payment may stay away from the doctor's office in embarrassment or he may even change doctors. Noncollection of medical bills may also imply guilt. A patient may infer that the doctor felt he gave inadequate or improper care, and a malpractice suit may result. Nor is it fair to honest patients to make no attempt to collect from nonpaying patients. Abandoning accounts with no collection follow-up encourages deadbeats and, as a result, honest patients indirectly subsidize the cost of medical care for those who can pay but do not.

According to the American Medical Association (*The Business Side of Medical Practice*), the three most common reasons for patients' failure to pay are *negligence, inability to pay,* and *unwillingness to pay.* Most patients are honest; it is estimated that probably less than 4 per cent are financial deadbeats who never intend to pay. There may be a larger percentage who may be financially "shipwrecked" and temporarily unable to pay. Also, you may encounter a certain percentage of patients who are living beyond their incomes. The man living beyond his means can be identified by his desire to "spare no expense." When faced with questions about nonpayment, this patient says, "I'll pay it all in the future," whereas the average honest patient says, "I'll pay you a certain amount each month."

Though it is important to pursue collections, mercenary business methods have no place in the professional world. As a result, collections must be handled in a special way and must be approached with a humanitarian but businesslike attitude. The underlying elements to success in collections are a good collection system and a good attitude on the part of the assistant.

## The Assistant's Attitude

There are certain attitudes that will help the medical assistant meet with greater success in dealing with collection problems. She should give individual attention and personal consideration to each case. She must at all times be courteous and show a sincere desire to help the patient with his financial problems by working out special payment arrangements. She should always try to find out the patient's reasons for nonpayment. Even though she must be courteous and considerate in such instances, she must still balance her humanitarianism with firmness. After all, a patient has received medical services, and in exchange the doctor has justly earned his fee. However, the medical assistant must not be overeager in her desire to boost her collection percentage. This results in ill will toward the doctor, as well as toward the assistant.

## Using Credit Symbols

It is a good idea to place a credit symbol on the account card of a patient who does not pay promptly. You can place such a symbol on the card discreetly, using an inconspicuous code. Sometimes it becomes necessary to show this card to a patient to explain or clarify a statement, and if he should ask about "that small number in the corner," you can noncommittally reply that it is used for filing purposes.

Most credit ratings will be in one of the numbered classes listed below. This scale is widely used in professional offices:

> Rate 1 – good pay
> Rate 2 – good pay but slow
> Rate 3 – slow to pay because cannot afford to pay
> Rate 4 – slow to pay but can afford to pay
> Rate 5 – poor pay because cannot afford to pay
> Rate 6 – poor pay but can afford to pay
> Rate 7 – does not pay; very poor risk

## Aging Accounts    *Statute of limitations.*

All accounts receivable should be "aged." This is a term for keeping a close monthly record of the status of each account, showing to what stage collections have been pursued. Aging of accounts helps collection follow-up, since it enables the assistant to tell at a glance what the next step should be.

Use a coding system for aging accounts. It is a collection blunder to repeat a collection letter or to backtrack in your follow-up procedures by, for instance, sending a polite reminder notice to a patient who has already received sterner collection letters. Such an error can easily occur unless a specific collection pattern is followed. To the patient such mistakes indicate that you do not really mean what you say in your collection letters, and therefore there is no reason to worry about payment.

Many offices use colored metal clip-on tabs to show the age of the account under collection. For example, after two statements have been sent, a green tab is placed on the record, indicating that a courteous reminder was sent with the last statement. The following month the green tab is replaced with a yellow tab, showing that second payment request was sent in the form of a polite letter. An orange tab is substituted the next month, indicating that the patient received a letter requesting prompt attention to his account. Red tabs may be reserved for accounts that, as a last resort, have been notified of a specific time limit in which payment must be made or sterner measures will be taken. If you reach this stage in pursuing a particular account, make certain you record the date of the time limit on the patient's card so that he does not think you are merely calling "wolf."

Another code system, based on letters, can be used. For example, "N 1" on a patient's card indicates that one notice has been sent; "N 2," that a second notice has been sent. "L 1" can be used to indicate that one letter has gone out, and so on. For an illustration of an analysis of accounts according to their age, see Figure 16–5.

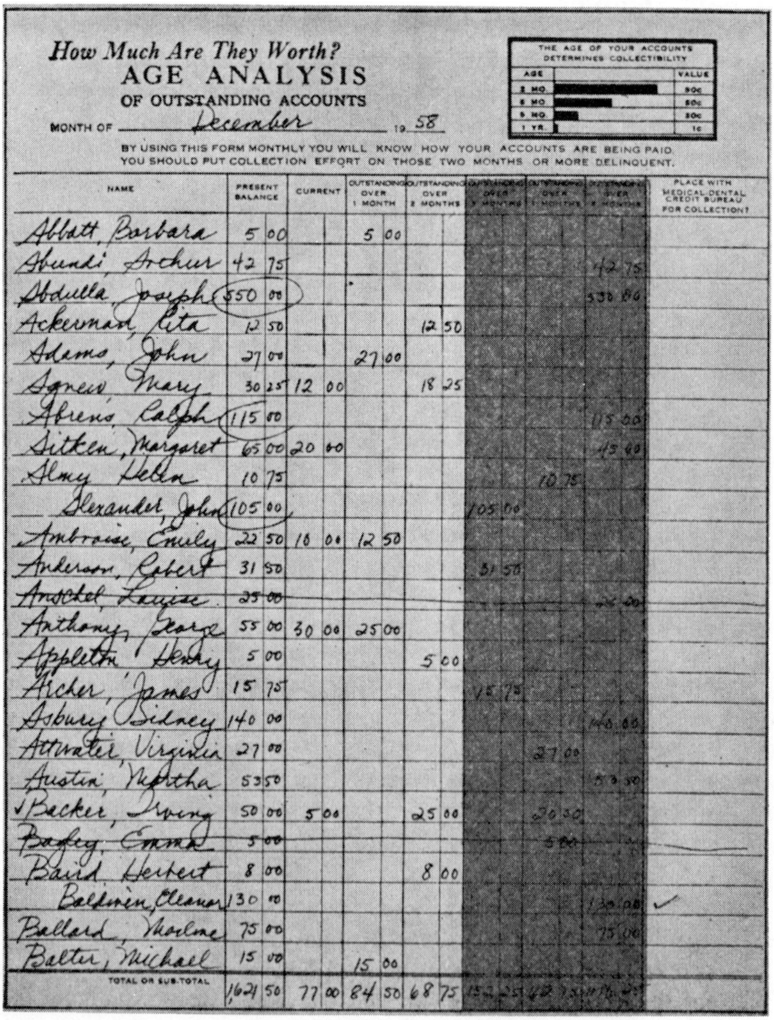

**Figure 16–5** Age analysis of outstanding accounts. (Reprinted with permission. From *Medical Economics*.)

## Collection System

In the introduction to this chapter, it was pointed out that the collection of professional accounts can be divided into three distinct stages, the second of which was "providing an opportunity for the patient to pay at the time of service for smaller amounts and sending bills out promptly for larger fees."

**Immediate Payments.**    If patients get into the habit of paying their bills before they leave the office, monthly billing is lightened and bookkeeping costs are lowered. Set up a system in your office to make it easier for patients to follow this pay-as-you-go system. For example, when the patient stops at your desk to make another appointment, you can reach for your receipt book and say, "Would you like to pay for your visit today?" Most patients are hesitant to ask about charges and are unsure whether to offer to pay or to wait until a statement is received. You will make it easier for them by offering to accept their payments, since most people are prepared to meet small bills on a cash basis. Avoid saying to the departing patient, "I do not know what the charge is today. I will have to send you a bill," or, "I do not know how much it will be, but why don't you pay me ten dollars and if it is more I will bill you." In both cases, the patient leaves the office with an uneasy feeling about the unknown bill. Care should be taken to place positive reactions toward payments in the patient's mind. Compare these two questions:

(a) "The charge today will be five dollars, Mrs. Jones. Do you want me to send you a bill?"

(b) "The charge today will be five dollars, Mrs. Jones. You may pay me now if you wish."

It is obvious which of the two statements will lead to immediate payment.

**Charge Slip System.**    One of the advantages of a charge slip system in the office is that it prefaces immediate payments nicely. The doctor checks what has been done for the patient on a particular visit and gives the slip to the patient. The patient takes it to the assistant, who can tell at a glance exactly what the charges will be. The patient is then psychologically prepared to pay immediately.

If the patient seems reluctant, the assistant can say, "It is so much easier if you pay for each visit. Then it will not accumulate into a sizeable account." A pleasant smile and a ready receipt book are two excellent devices for encouraging on-the-spot payments.

**Why Medical Bills are Paid Last.**    It is well known that people pay their medical bills last. Occasionally, you hear a gracious patient say, in all good faith, "Thank goodness, we have all our bills paid off now, except the doctor. We will start paying him as soon as we catch our breath." Strangely enough, many people do not look upon the doctor's bill as a "debt" in the usual sense of the word. They must be motivated to pay.

People will pay their rent because of the danger of eviction and sometimes because the landlord is frequently encountered in their daily lives. They will pay their utility bills because the service can be terminated. They will make regular payments on their automobile and furniture because these goods can be repossessed. Banks and small loan companies have a reputation for strict enforcement of contracts, and they follow up on accounts which are only a few days late. A patient's commercial credit may be very good and his medical credit poor.

What then causes people to delay payment to the doctor? Oftentimes there is no specific arrangement made for payment. Follow-up is delayed, and in many offices the account is not even considered delinquent until at least three months have elapsed from the date of service. Even people who are educated to the necessity of paying their bills are frequently not concerned about paying them on time unless this is brought to their attention. Failure of the doctor's assistant to consistently and quickly follow up on overdue accounts may contribute to the patients' lack of concern.

Since the fee for medical services is far more intangible than any commercial account, collection efforts must not be delayed too long. Any responsible, sincere patient will call or write the doctor's office within four months of receiving a bill and explain why he cannot pay or ask for a payment plan. If it becomes necessary to refer the account to a collector, a good agency should have a 50 to 60 per cent recovery rate with an account that is assigned within four or five months. This may drop to 25 per cent if the account is held only a few more months.

It must be remembered that the value of medical accounts diminishes in direct proportion to the length of time that has elapsed since service was rendered. The following figures, based on a report from the United States Department of Commerce, show that the chances for recovering the full amount on a bill diminish rapidly as time passes:

> After 2 months one dollar is worth 90 cents
> After 6 months one dollar is worth 67 cents
> After 1 year one dollar is worth 45 cents
> After 2 years one dollar is worth 23 cents
> After 3 years one dollar is worth 15 cents
> After 5 years one dollar is worth 1 cent only

Do not fight the "law of diminishing returns." All collection activity is costly. Each notice you mail costs your doctor at least 60 to 70 cents, for stationery supplies, postage, and typing time. In 1973 it cost $3.31 to prepare and mail one ordinary business letter.

Continued efforts on the old accounts also will allow the current accounts to become delinquent. Know when to stop. At this time call on the services of a professional agency.

## Collection Letters

The ideal method of pursuing collections, in the opinion of many doctors and professional management officials, is the personal letter approach. A letter which is recognized as being a form letter by the recipient is of dubious value. Letters should be friendly requests for an explanation of why payment has not been made. These letters should indicate that the doctor is sincerely interested in the patient's story and wants to help him straighten out his financial obligations. The patient should be invited to visit the doctor's office to explain his reasons for nonpayment so that, if possible, special arrangements can be worked out. To give the patient an opportunity to save face, these letters can suggest that the patient may have overlooked previous statements.

Upon receipt of such a letter, most patients will make some effort to explain their delinquency. If a patient really is in financial straits, the doctor may be able to get public assistance for him. Or, if it is a temporary financial difficulty, the doctor and the patient may together be able to work out a satisfactory installment plan type of payment program as described in Chapter 15.

The doctor's assistant often is given a free hand in the designing of collection patterns and the composition of collection letters. Many secretaries work up a group of such letters which they have found to be effective. Such a series usually includes at least five letters, of varying degrees of forcefulness. One would never use the same type of collection letter for a patient with a good rating as for one who is known to neglect his financial obligations. The assistant can code the range of letters as to severity and credit rating. For example, "Rate 1, Letter 1" might indicate a first collection reminder letter sent to a patient in the top credit rating bracket, that is, good pay. These code symbols should be written on the patients' records so that a record can be kept of what letter was sent and the proper sequence of mailings can be continued if payment is not forthcoming.

Even though the assistant adopts a specific series of letters, each one should sound like a personal message, not a form letter. Use care and thought in designing your collection letters and avoid the ordinary.

**Some Steps to Avoid.**    Never use a mimeographed letter on which the patient's name and the amount due are inserted in blank spaces. Use as few "I's" and "me's" and "my's" as possible, and avoid the use of trite or flippant phrases.

AVOID THESE:

"Unless we receive your check within seven days . . ."

Use instead, "Please send us your check or an explanation within one week."

"I feel sure you must have overlooked the last statement . . ."

Try, "Your cooperation is needed."

"I am disappointed that you have not paid this account."

"In glancing over the accounts, I find that you have not made a payment for several months."

The patient is not apt to believe that you were just casually looking over the accounts and to your great surprise you found that the patient owed money.

"In order to meet our bills, it is necessary for you to pay your account."

The patient is well aware the payment or nonpayment of his particular account will not make or break the doctor financially.

"When you needed the doctor, he came to your aid. Now won't you please return this courtesy?"

This is "biological blackmail"; your doctor's reputation should not be jeopardized in this manner.

"Can you recommend a good collection agency? We may need one to collect your account."

"Enclosed is a stamp—maybe this will help you send in your payment."

Amusing, perhaps, but such flippant phrases are unprofessional and discourteous.

### General Guide for Composing Collection Letters

1. The letter should be brief; three to four sentences is usually sufficient.
2. Use simple language and short sentences and avoid stereotyped phrases.
3. Motivate through one specific appeal, such as *cooperation, pride,* or *preservation of credit rating.*
4. State the amount you expect the patient to pay and suggest specific action he should take, for example, telephone your office, arrange a time-payment schedule, pay within 15 days, or a similar plan.

**Who Signs Collection Letters?**   The question sometimes arises as to who should sign collection letters. In many medical offices the secretary signs them with the identification "Secretary to Dr. _____" below her name. Other physicians feel that they should personally sign these communications. Generally, however, since financial procedures are handled by the secretary-assistant, she also signs the collection letters.

**Sample Letters.**   On the following pages are suggested reminder and personalized collection letters. These can serve as a guide for composing your own letters to suit the circumstances involved.

---

Your account has always been paid promptly in the past, so this must be an oversight. Please accept this note as a friendly reminder of your account due for $_____.

---

Since your care in this office last (March) we have had no word from you in regard to how you are feeling or your account due.

If it is impossible for you to pay the full amount of $_____ at this time, please call this office within the next ten days so that satisfactory arrangements can be worked out.

---

We've sent you three statements for the care you received last (March). Medical bills are payable at the time of service unless special credit arrangements are made.

Please send your check in full or call this office before (June 30).

---

For the patient who has started on a payment program, and then discontinued:

---

We've had no word from you since (April) about your balance of $_____ which has been on our books since (October, 19___).

If you have some question about your statement, we'll be happy to answer it for you. If not, may we have a payment from you before the end of this month?

Enclosed is your statement as of (September 1) showing balance still due in the amount of $180. This account has been reduced by only $30 in the last eight months.

While we are quite willing to go along with you on a monthly payment basis, we do ask that *regular* payments of at least $10 be made each month.

May we have your payment by the 25th of each month?

---

Unless some definite arrangement is made to reduce your balance of $_____, we can no longer carry your account on our books.

Delinquent accounts are turned over to a collection agency on the 25th of the month.

---

When a payment plan has been established, it can be re-enforced by recognizing the first installment with a letter of acknowledgment.

Thank you for the recent payment of $_____ on your account. We are glad to cooperate with you in this arrangement for clearing your account on a regular monthly basis.

We will look for your next check at about the same time next month.

When a payment schedule has been arranged by a telephone call, it can be confirmed by letter:

As agreed upon in our telephone conversation today, we will expect you to mail a payment of ten dollars on Friday the 10th, and ten dollars on each successive Friday until the balance of one hundred dollars is paid in full.

If some emergency should prevent your making one of these payments on time, please notify us immediately by telephone.

The "thank you" letter also has a place in your collection program and is a valuable public relations tool.

Thank you for your $300 check in full payment for your recent surgery. It is much appreciated. Best wishes from the entire office staff for your continued good health.

---

Thank you for your check for $25. This is the final payment on your account of $200, and a receipt for payment in full is enclosed.

We appreciate the promptness with which your payments have always been made.

My very best wishes for your continued good health.

The collection letters in this chapter will provide the medical assistant with a limited variety of styles with which to work in composing her own communications. It is important to remember that letters should sound as though each one were written personally to the individual concerned. Do not send letters with a firmer tone until you have sent one or two friendly reminders. Always imply that the patient has good intentions to pay until lack of reply over a period of time proves otherwise. Your early letters should be merely reminders of debt. Sometimes even a deadbeat will pay his bill if he is treated with respect and consideration.

No medical assistant should ever go beyond the authority given her by her employer in pursuing collections. If she has questions about special collection problems, she should always check with the doctor before proceeding. This is particularly important when she is hesitant about initiating collection procedures with patients whom she does not know personally — for example, patients the doctor has seen in the hospital or at home — and others for whom she is unable to obtain a credit rating. The best rule to follow is this: when in doubt about a collection problem, always check with the doctor before proceeding. It is difficult to say whether pressing collections too hard loses more good will of patients than not pursuing collections diligently enough. The doctor and the secretary together should agree upon general collection policies to be applied in the office.

**Collection by Personal Interview.** Direct collection methods sometimes can be used in eliciting payments. Often, by talking to a patient face to face, you can come to an understanding of his problems more quickly and reach an agreement about future payment plans. Personal interviews with patients are usually more effective than a whole series of collection letters.

Occasionally, a patient may undergo a long course of treatment and yet show no sign of willingness to pay anything on his account. Perhaps he is only waiting for the doctor or the assistant to suggest that a payment be made. When there is advance knowledge that the patient will require extensive treatment, the matter of payment should be discussed early in the course of treatment, and some agreement reached as to a payment plan.

If for some reason the doctor feels that it would be unwise to press the matter at the time the patient completes his treatments, you can make an appointment for him to come back in a month. If the patient does not keep his appointment, or does not offer to make payment, then you have good reason to call or write him about the amount he owes.

**Telephone Collection Techniques.** Sometimes you can use the telephone to follow up on overdue accounts, especially in cases in which a patient has been requested by letter to contact the office and has failed to do so. It is also a nice gesture to call a patient to remind him about his bill when you are genuinely concerned about him and do not wish to press him with collection letters. It is sometimes possible to work out payment arrangements by telephone, and it is certainly easier to do so than by letter. One word of caution, however: the assistant who is uncomfortable with making collection calls will probably be unsuccessful and should not use this approach.

GENERAL RULES TO FOLLOW IN TELEPHONE COLLECTIONS

1. Determine the identity of the person with whom you are speaking. If you ask, "Is this Mrs. Noble?" and she answers "Yes," it may be the patient's mother-in-law who is also "Mrs. Noble."

2. Be dignified and respectful in your attitude. You can be friendly and formal at the same time.

3. Ask the patient if it is a convenient time to talk with you. Unless you have the attention of the called party, there is little to be gained by continuing. If you are told that you have called at an inopportune time, ask for a specific time when you may call back, or get a promise for the patient to call you at a specified time.

4. Assume a positive attitude. For example, convey the impression that you know the patient intends to pay, and it is only a matter of working out some suitable arrangements.

5. After a brief greeting, state the purpose of your call. You expect payment and are interested in helping him meet his obligation.

6. Try to get a definite commitment—payment of a certain amount on a certain date.

7. Keep the conversation brief, to the point, and avoid threats of any kind.

8. Follow up on promises. This is best accomplished by a tickler file or a note on your calendar. If the payment does not arrive on the promised date, remind the patient with another call. If you fail to do this, your whole effort has been wasted.

9. Do not call patients about their accounts when there are others within hearing distance in the reception room.

10. Make no apology for calling but state your reason in a friendly, business-like way. Identify yourself as "Dr. _____'s secretary" as soon as you have made a friendly introductory statement. A well-placed pause at this point in the call sometimes elicits an immediate response from the patient in regard to his non-payment. Use this method cautiously, however, since you do not wish to embarrass the patient unduly.

There are no hard and fast rules for pursuing collections by use of the telephone. You must "play by ear" each individual case on the basis of your own acquaintance with the person concerned.

It is poor policy to call an individual at work. If this is the only phone contact you have and you feel he must be reached, place the call without disclosing the nature of the call to others in his place of employment. You can tell the patient the reason for your call and request that he return your call at a specific time if it is not convenient for him to discuss his account now. If you do call him at work and he cannot come to the telephone, you can leave a message asking him to "call Mrs. Black at 727-5938," not "Dr. Jones's office" or "the secretary to Dr. Jones." In the professional world it would be a rare instance in which the assistant would resort to calling a patient's employer to press for payment of a bill. This is far too commercial; furthermore, it could cost the patient his job and eliminate the possibility of collection entirely. It should be remembered, too, that most states have a "right of privacy law," and you are risking a lawsuit if you reveal to a third party that John Doe owes money to Dr. Jones. Therefore, be certain you have properly identified the party before talking about the account.

Whether dealing with patients by telephone or in person, do not lose your temper or your dignity. An angry patient is a poor-paying patient. Insulted patients often do not pay at all. Never proceed with telephone collections without the consent of your doctor. Some medical business managers feel that telephone collections are unprofessional, and they advise against the technique.

## Special Collection Problems

**Tracing "Skips."**   When a statement is returned marked "Moved—no forwarding address," you may consider this account as a "skip." This generally is accepted as an indication that the patient is attempting to avoid liability for his debts. Many so-called skips are innocent errors. The person may have been careless in not leaving a forwarding address. Or the mistake may have occurred in your office; the wrong name or address may have been placed on the statement. However, immediate action should be taken in regard to returned statements. Do not wait until the next billing time to attempt to trace the patient. Here are some suggestions for tracing skips:

1. Examine the patient's original office registration card.
2. Call the telephone number listed on the card. Occasionally, a patient may move without leaving a forwarding address but will transfer his old telephone number. Or the new phone number will be given when you call the old number.
3. If you are unable to contact the individual by telephone, make a few discreet calls to the references listed on the registration card to get leads.
4. Check the city directory to secure the name and telephone number of neighbors or the landlord and contact these persons to secure information about the patient's whereabouts.
5. Drop a card to the state motor vehicle department; in the event that the patient owns a car this department may be able to provide information. According to law, this department must be notified of changes of address.
6. Check with your client's bank. Sometimes banks will have information about the new addresses of skips.
7. Check the patient's place of employment for information. If the patient is a specialist in his field of work, the local union or similar organizations may be contacted. Although they may not give you his current address, they will relay a message to him so that he will know you are seeking to contact him. Often, people will be stirred into paying a bill if they think their employer may be notified about their payment failure.

The tracing of skips is a challenge to any secretary. A registered letter can be sent to the patient; this letter requires the returning of a receipt and will give information about the patient's new address. If a registered letter is sent, it should be mailed in a plain envelope so that the patient will not refuse to accept the letter because of the letterhead. However, whenever calls are made in an attempt to locate an individual, discretion should be practiced. There is little reason to tell the persons to whom you speak why you are anxious to locate the individual.

If all other methods fail, then turn the account over to your collection agency. Do not keep a "skip" account too long, since the trail may become so cold as time elapses that even expert collection men will be unable to follow it.

**Claims Against Estates.**   A bill owed by a deceased patient is often a troublesome problem to a secretary. Sympathy for the family tends to cause hesitancy in following proper collection procedures. Do not cut the fee because the case terminated in death. The doctor has served the patient to the best of his ability and is entitled to his fee. Furthermore, as was pointed out earlier, failure to pursue collections may indicate that the doctor did not feel he did all he could for the patient and could be misconstrued as the basis for a malpractice action. Of course, if the death has caused extreme financial difficulties and the patient's estate is unable to provide the necessary funds, or if there is no family that is responsible, the fee may be cut at the doctor's discretion.

The first step for the secretary in such cases is to obtain the name and address of the person responsible for the debts of the deceased. This name may be obtained from the family, but usually one does not like to disturb them. The hospital or mortuary may be able to supply this information; obituary notices in the local newspaper will usually list the names of the nearest relatives that you may call.

If you are unable to obtain the name of the party responsible for the estate, you can write to the county seat in the county in which the estate is being settled. A letter to the Probate Department of the Superior Court, County Recorder's Office, will usually provide you with the name of the individual responsible.

Thirty days may pass before a statement is sent to the family of the deceased if you are hesitant to contact the family immediately. But do not wait too long to submit your bill. There are definite laws governing the collection of bills from a deceased individual, and many an account has been lost because of timidity to send a bill or ignorance of these laws. Often a family will contact the doctor and request the bill so that the estate may be settled as quickly as possible.

## When and where to file estate claims

*When.* The various state laws specify that a doctor must file his claim on an estate within the number of months indicated in the table below, starting:

(A) From the date a court of probate recognizes an executor or administrator.
(B) From the date of the first publication of notice to creditors.
(C) From the date of the second publication.
(D) From the date of death.
(E) From a date that has been or will be determined or approved by the court.

The appearance of a range of months indicates that the time limit on filing a claim depends on the amount of the estate, as specified by state law.

*Where.* A doctor must file his claim with the person or place indicated in the table as follows:
S  As selected by the court.
P  With a court of probate.
R  With the executor or administrator or other representative of the estate, as specified by state law.

| State | Time limit (in months) | Where filed | State | Time limit (in months) | Where filed | State | Time limit (in months) | Where filed |
|---|---|---|---|---|---|---|---|---|
| Ala. | 6 (A) | P | Ky. | 9 (D) | R | N.D. | 3 (B) | P |
| Alaska | 6 (B) | R | La. | Indefinite | R | Ohio | 4 (A)–9 (D) | R |
| Ariz. | 4 (B) | R | Me. | 12 (A) | P or R | Okla. | 4 (B) | S |
| Ark. | 6 (B) | P or R | Md. | 6 (B) | P & R | Ore. | 6 (A) | R |
| Calif. | 6 (B) | P or R | Mass. | 6 (B)–12 (A) | R | Pa. | 12 (D) | R |
| Colo. | 6 (A) | P | Mich. | 2–4 (B) | R | R.I. | 6 (B) | P |
| Conn. | 6–12 (A) | R | Minn. | 4–12 (D) | P | S.C. | 5 (B) | P or R |
| Del. | 9 (A) | R | Miss. | 6 (B) | P | S.D. | 4 (B) | P or R |
| D.C. | 6 (A) | R | Mo. | 6 (A)–9 (D) | P & R | Tenn. | 1 (A)–9 (B) | P |
| Fla. | 6 (B) | P | Mont. | 4 (B) | R | Tex. | 12 (A) | R |
| Ga. | 12 (A) | R | Neb. | 3–18 (B) | P | Utah | 3 (B) | R |
| Hawaii | 4 (B) | R | Nev. | 3 (B) | P | Vt. | (E) | S |
| Idaho | 4 (B) | R | N.H. | 3–12 (A) | R | Va. | 6 (A) | R |
| Ill. | 9 (A) | P | N.J. | 6 (A) | R | Wash. | 6 (B) | R |
| Ind. | 6 (B) | P | N.M. | 6 (B) | P | W. Va. | 4–6 (B) | S |
| Iowa | 6 (C) | P | N.Y. | 6 (B)–7 (A) | R | Wis. | 3–12 (A) | P |
| Kan. | 9 (B) | P | N.C. | 6 (B) | R | Wyo. | 6 (B) | R |

After the name of the administrator or executor of the estate has been obtained, you send a duplicate itemized statement of the account to him. This should be sent by certified mail, return receipt requested, so that you'll know who received it. If no answer is received in ten days, you should then contact the executor or the county clerk where the estate is being settled and obtain forms for filing claim against the estate. (Some states do not have special claim forms but will accept simple itemized statements.) This claim against the estate must be made within a certain length of time, varying from one to eighteen months, depending on the state in which it is filed, or the account is lost.

The executor of the estate will either accept or reject the claim. If it is accepted, he will send an acknowledgment of the debt. Payment is often delayed, owing to the legal difficulties in settling an estate, but if the claim has been accepted you will receive your money in due time. If the claim is rejected, and you have full justification for claiming the bill, then you must file claim against the executor within a limited amount of time, according to state laws. The time limit in such cases starts with the date on the letter of rejection which he sends you in response to your original claim.

Because of the various state time limits and statutes in regard to such matters, it is advisable for the secretary to contact her employer's attorney or the local court for the exact procedure to follow in such instances in her area.

**Statutes of Limitations.**    A statute of limitations assigns a certain time after which rights cannot be enforced by action.

*Malpractice.*    In many states there are Statutes of Limitations in regard to malpractice lawsuits, which set a limit to the time during which malpractice actions can be filed. It is usually best to wait until this time has passed before pressing the account of a patient who may feel he is entitled to sue the doctor. However, this should not be made a blanket policy; each case should be judged on its own merit.

*Collections.*    Statutes of Limitations in regard to collections prescribe the time within which a legal collection suit may be rendered against a debtor; the term "outlaw" is sometimes used to refer to debts on which the time limit has passed. This legal time limit varies according to the specific state in which a doctor practices. On page 223 are listed the time limits for collections in various states.

Generally, accounts may be placed in one of three groups: open book accounts, written contracts, or single entry accounts.

*Open book accounts* are accounts on the books that are open to charges made from time to time. The bill for each illness or treatment is computed separately, and the last date of entry, debit or credit, for that particular illness is the time designated by the Statutes of Limitations for starting that specific debt. As you can see, it is almost impossible to have a time limit on an account of a patient with a chronic condition, since there is no actual termination of the illness or treatment unless the patient changes physicians or dies. When legal time limits are set, they usually refer to these "open book accounts."

*Written contracts* are contracts which usually have the same time limit as the open book accounts, but occasionally they vary in different states. The time limit on written contracts starts from the date due.

| 2 years | 4 years | Indiana |
|---|---|---|
| Texas | California | Maine |
| | Georgia | Massachusetts |
| | Idaho | Michigan |
| | Nebraska | Minnesota |
| | Nevada | New Hampshire |
| 3 years | New Mexico | New Jersey |
| Alabama | Utah | New York |
| Arizona | | North Dakota |
| Arkansas | | Ohio |
| Delaware | 5 years | Oregon |
| Dist. of Columbia | Illinois | Pennsylvania |
| Florida | Iowa | Rhode Island |
| Kansas | Kentucky | South Carolina |
| Louisiana | Missouri | South Dakota |
| Maryland | Montana | Tennessee |
| Mississippi | West Virginia | Vermont |
| North Carolina | | Wisconsin |
| Oklahoma | 6 years | |
| Virginia | Colorado | 8 years |
| Washington | Connecticut | Wyoming |

*Single entry accounts* are accounts that have only one entry or charge. These accounts are usually short-lived and are for small amounts. Some states, such as California, place a shorter Statutes of Limitations span on such accounts.

In many states, even though the legal time limit set by the Statutes of Limitations has passed, the account may be reopened and the date extended if you are able to obtain an acknowledgment of the debt due from the patient in writing. Often, a letter from the patient saying "Yes, I know I owe you $150 but I do not intend paying Dr. _____" can be secured. If this letter is signed and dated, keep it and contact your collector; he can then, on the basis of this letter, proceed with collection. Also, a small payment on account may extend the date. Sometimes a belligerent patient will send one dollar on account, thinking it is only a teaser; he is unaware that such a payment keeps his account open.

Sometimes a patient will ignore a bill if he does not feel responsible for the account. He may have neglected to give you the necessary information about the party responsible for the bill, and you may be billing the wrong party.

**Bankruptcy.**  Bankruptcy laws are federal, thus eliminating the confusion of local and state laws. When you are notified that a patient has declared bankruptcy, you should no longer send statements or make any individual attempt to collect the acount.

Bankruptcy laws were passed to secure equal distribution of the assets of an individual among his creditors. There are two types of bankruptcy—a straight petition in bankruptcy and a "wage earner's" bankruptcy. In both, the debtor becomes a ward of the court and has its protection. A creditor can be fined for contempt of court if he continues to proceed against the debtor.

In a wage earner's bankruptcy, the debtor pays a fixed amount, agreed on by the court, to the trustee in bankruptcy. This is then passed on to the creditors.

During this period none of the creditors can attach his wages or bother him.

In a straight petition in bankruptcy you should file a claim on the proper form, which can be obtained from a stationery store or by writing the referee in bankruptcy. Although you may be notified of a creditor's meeting, it is usually a waste of time to attend. A doctor's fee is an unsecured debt and, therefore, one of the last to be paid.

## Suing for Recovery on Overdue Accounts

When you have done everything possible in your office to follow up on an outstanding account and have not secured payment, the question arises as to what step to take next. Should the doctor sue for the amount? Should he turn the account over to a collection agency? Or should he cross it off the books as a bad debt?

Before forcing an account, you must first consider the time element. Has the patient been given a fair chance to pay this bill? Have you sent statements regularly and used a systematic method of following up the account? Ask yourself if there might be a misunderstanding in regard to the fee charged. Did you fully itemize the first statement? A large unexplained bill may frighten a patient into making no payments at all because the whole thing looks too big.

If you have used correct registration forms to secure advance credit information, you should know the financial abilities of the patient in regard to payment. However, his illness may have caused a loss of salary and resulted in temporary inability to pay. A little investigation will reveal such troubles.

Could the patient have been dissatisfied with the care he received? For some unknown reason he may feel that he was not treated correctly. Perhaps he expected a complete cure too soon. Only an explanation of the condition, prognosis, and care can enlighten such patients. This is best explained by the doctor himself. If a bill is pressed too hard and the patient is dissatisfied for some reason, he may file a malpractice suit to "get even."

**Should We Sue?**   Will a doctor lose more good will by suing for a bill than by writing if off as a loss? A management official says that, strangely enough, when a doctor-client sued two patients for large sums, the patients lost the cases, paid up, and were back in his office for treatment very shortly! However, most physicians feel it is unwise to resort to the court to collect medical bills unless there are extenuating circumstances.

An account must be considered a 100 per cent loss to you before legal proceedings are started. Remember that you should never threaten to instigate legal proceedings unless you are prepared to carry out the threat and have the doctor's consent to issue such a warning.

If your employer decides in favor of a legal suit, then investigate thoroughly before taking action. Mr. Leslie S. Kohn, LL.B., former editor of the *New Jersey Law Journal,* says litigation to collect a bill is generally in order in the following instances:

1. When a patient can afford to pay without hardship.
2. When the doctor can produce office records that support the bill.
3. When the doctor can justify the size of the bill by comparison with fee practices in his community.
4. When the patient's general condition after treatment is satisfactory.

5. When the persuasive powers of an ethical collection agency have been exhausted, and the agency advises suing.

6. When the patient can be given ample warning of the doctor's intention of collecting legally.

7. When the patient (or defendant) is not judgment-proof.

8. When the defendant is legally liable for the services rendered to the patient.

9. When the Statute of Limitations has ruled out any possible malpractice action.

10. When the doctor is not bubbling over with indignation or is not in a "he-can't-do-this-to-me" frame of mind.

The experienced practitioner ticks off these ten "whens" before he plunges into costly litigation.

## Selection of Accounts for Collection Agency

The office assistant should try every means possible within the scope of her ability and available time to collect accounts before they become delinquent. It is usually best to set up a definite collection timetable and make few exceptions.

As soon as the account is determined uncollectible through your office—the patient has failed to respond to your final letter, or has failed to fulfill a second promise on payment—send the account to the collector without delay. Skips should be assigned immediately.

Even though collection by an agency will mean sacrificing 40 to 50 per cent of the amount owed, further delay will only reduce the chances of recovery by the professional collector. If the agency finds that the case deserves special consideration, it will probably report this for your consideration.

In an American Medical Association booklet entitled $R$ *Public Relations,* the following paragraph appears in regard to use and abuse of collection agencies:

> Collections cause one of medicine's biggest public relations headaches—an unethical agency which uses unscrupulous tactics such as lumping other accounts owed by the person together for collection purposes or pursuing a threat or scare technique to recover on old bills can ruin a doctor PR-wise. An ethical agency, however, can do a real public relations job for physicians, ferreting out the patients who need special consideration and following through in collecting from people who can pay. Because a different approach is necessary in pursuing medical collections, a physician should thoroughly acquaint himself with the collection methods used by a respective bureau before making use of its services.

There are an increasing number of agencies either owned and operated as an integral part of the county medical society or operated separately from the medical society but supervised by the medical profession. These bureaus provide specialized medical collection services. Agencies or bureaus set up by societies are by far the best. These agencies never lose sight of the delicate professional relationship between doctor and patients. They have an understanding and tolerance of the need for special handling of problems where medical collections are concerned.

Another type of collection agency is a division of the local credit association, recognized by the National Retail Credit Association. If the local credit association does not maintain a collection department, they will be able to recommend a reputable one. A nationally recognized credit association has considerable responsibility and a high standard to maintain. These factors act as monitors to its reliability.

The most common type of collection agency throughout the United States is the privately owned and privately operated agency. Many of these work with the local professional societies and strive to keep their work on a high ethical standard. However, there are a few of these bureaus which are unethical and entirely unscrupulous in their tactics.

If your doctor chooses a collection agency, he should investigate thoroughly to determine whether it is a reliable, ethical one.

1. Investigate the agency by calling the local medical society. Also, write the Medical-Dental-Hospital Bureaus of America, the National Retail Credit Association, and the Associated Credit Bureaus of America for additional information.

2. Check on the ownership of the agency through the Better Business Bureau, Chamber of Commerce, or your own banker.

3. Investigate to find out if the agency has contacts with other services to aid in the collection of out-of-town accounts.

4. Determine whether or not this agency serves other professional men. If so, do they find its services satisfactory?

5. Make sure the agency will not take legal action without the consent of the physician.

6. Find out whether the agency has a "heart." It should be one that is willing to adjust a fee in a sincere hardship case rather than pursuing collections to get every dollar owed to boost its own fee. Will the agency consent to report special cases deserving special consideration to the physician's office? Remember, your collection agency is literally an extension of your office and your policies.

In dealing with collection agencies, do not sign a contract (reputable agencies seldom use them); avoid out-of-town or mail order type agencies; and be sure the agency will take personal instructions about specific cases and make special arrangements on the basis of information about a case.

When your doctor selects a reputable agency and decides to make use of its services, the office must be prepared to provide the agency with all the necessary data to enable it to begin prompt collection procedures on overdue accounts. The agency should receive:

Full name of the debtor
Name of the spouse
Last known address
Full amount of debt
Date of the last entry on the account (debit or credit)
Occupation of the debtor
Business address
Any other pertinent information

Once an account has been turned over to a collection agency, your office makes no further collection attempts. Here are the directions for procedure in the doctor's office, once the collection agency has begun its work:

1. Send no more statements.

2. Mark the patient's card or stamp it so that you know it is now in the hands of the collector.

3. Refer the patient to the agency if he contacts you in regard to the account.

4. Promptly report any payments made direct to your office. (Remember that a percentage of this payment is due to the agency.)

5. Call the agency if you obtain any information that will be of value in tracing or collecting the account.

6. Do not push the agency with frequent calls. The representatives of the bureau will report to you occasionally and keep you posted on collection progress. Continued progress reports are costly to the agency; they cannot report and collect at the same time. After all, you don't want a reporting agency—you really want a collection agency.

## Small Claims Court

Many doctor's offices find the Small Claims Court a satisfactory and inexpensive way to collect delinquent accounts. An action may be filed in the small claims court if you are seeking to recover money in an amount of five hundred dollars or less, provided you have previously demanded payment from the party you intend to sue. A party to a small claims action may not be represented by an attorney at the trial but he may send another person to court in his behalf to produce records supporting the claim. Doctors often send their bookkeepers or office assistants with records of unpaid accounts to show the judge.

In addition to the judgment for the amount owed, the plaintiff in Small Claims Court may also recover the costs of the suit. This rarely exceeds ten dollars. For a very small investment in time and money, the doctor who uses this method has saved the time of a regular court action; he has had no attorney's fees to pay; and he has not sacrificed the 40 to 50 per cent commission charged by most collection agencies.

The forms for filing action and full instructions on the course to follow may be obtained from the clerk of the Small Claims Court. The assistant who has never appeared in the Court would probably be wise to attend once as a spectator only, so that she will understand the procedure followed and feel more at ease when she appears for the doctor.

A collection agency, to whom an account may have been assigned, may not file or handle a small claims action. It must either sue in the regular municipal or justice court, or attempt to collect the debt in some other way.

## Accounts Receivable Protection

The potential income represented by the doctor's accounts receivable ledger is probably considerable and usually the patient ledger is the only record the doctor has of what is owed to him. This potential income deserves insurance protection. The doctor's general insurance representative can obtain insurance protection for these records. Most insurance companies require that the ledgers be kept in a safe place, such as an insulated file cabinet. This is a good practice to follow in any case. They will also require that the accounts receivable balance be reported monthly, for the cost of the insurance is usually based on the average balance during the year. The premium for this type of insurance is nominal. Anyone who has ever lost his records through fire or flood would say it is priceless.

# Chapter 17

---

**BEHAVIORAL OBJECTIVES**

*The medical office assistant should be able to:*

Recognize terms that identify individuals involved in banking exchanges.

Define the various kinds of checks.

Describe the principal kinds of bank accounts.

Apply the rules for writing checks.

Systematize the payment of bills.

Observe basic rules in accepting checks.

Follow proper check endorsement procedures.

Prepare bank deposits.

Reconcile bank balances.

# Banking Services and Procedures

Because practically every financial transaction in the professional office involves the use of checks, it is imperative that the office assistant understand basic banking terminology and procedures. There are many small differences in terminology throughout the various banks. However, the terms as defined in this chapter are fairly common. The medical office assistant must also understand the responsibilities involved in writing checks, in accepting payments, in endorsing and depositing checks, and in maintaining an accurate balance in the checking account. This chapter sets forth basic guidelines involved in these procedures.

## TERMS THAT IDENTIFY INDIVIDUALS INVOLVED IN BANKING EXCHANGES

There are certain legal terms which anyone who deals with banks should understand. Definitions of some of these terms are provided here:

**Agent.**    An agent is a person authorized to represent, or act for, another person, called the principal, in dealing with a third party.

**Endorser.**    This is the person who signs his name on the back of a check for the purpose of transferring his title to the check to another person.

**Guaranty.**    This is an agreement or a contract involving three parties. The first party agrees to see that the performance of the second party is fulfilled. The first party is the *guarantor*, the second party the *guarantee*, and the third party is the *creditor* to whom the amount or service is owed.

**Maker.**    Any individual, corporation, or legal party who signs a check or any type of negotiable instrument is known as a maker.

**Payee.**    The person named on a draft or check as the recipient of the amount shown is a payee. The payee's name is written after the words "Pay to the order of." The payee is the party benefiting from the payment of the instrument.

**Payer.**    The payer is the person who writes the check in favor of the payee. When you write a check to pay a bill at a local store, you become the payer and the store is the payee.

**Teller.**    A teller is an employee of a bank who is assigned the duty of waiting on the bank's customers. He is the contact between the customer and the bank.

Bank tellers are directly concerned with the receiving or paying out of money by the bank.

## CHECKS

The use of checks for the transfer of funds provides a number of advantages. First, when properly used, checks are both safe and convenient, particularly when making payments by mail. Second, one can quickly calculate expenditures or locate specific payments from the check record. Third, a summary of receipts can readily be determined from the deposit record. Fourth, the payer can stop payment on a check, thus protecting himself from lost, stolen, or incorrectly drawn checks. Fifth, checks provide a permanent reliable record of disbursements for tax purposes. Finally, checking accounts protect the money that is deposited.

### What is a Check?

A check is a draft or an order upon a bank for the payment of a certain sum of money to a certain person therein named, or to the bearer, and is payable on demand. It is considered to be a *negotiable instrument.* A negotiable instrument must conform to the following requirements:
1. It must be written and signed by a maker.
2. It must contain a promise or order to pay a sum of money.
3. It must be payable on demand or at a fixed future date.
4. It must be payable to order or bearer.
5. If addressed to drawee, it must be so named.

### Types of Checks

There are many types of checks in use in the business world. Here are descriptions of some:

**Bank Draft.** A check drawn by a bank against funds deposited to its account in another bank.

**Cashier's Check.** A bank's own check, drawn upon itself and signed by the bank cashier or other authorized official. It is also known as an *officer's* or *treasurer's check.* A cashier's check is obtained by paying the bank cashier the amount of the check, in cash or by personal check. Some banks charge a fee for this service. Cashier's checks are usually issued to accommodate the savings account customer who does not maintain a checking account.

**Certified Check.** This is the depositor's own check, upon the face of which the bank has placed the word "CERTIFIED" or "ACCEPTED" with the date and a bank official's signature. The check then becomes an obligation of the bank because the amount of this check is immediately drawn from the depositor's account and held. It is unlawful for a bank to certify a check for an amount which exceeds the sum the depositor has on deposit. In other words, a certified check is a depositor's own check guaranteed by the bank. Because the bank deducts the amount of the check from the depositor's account at the time it certifies the check, the bank can guarantee that the amount is available. A certified check, like a cashier's check, can be used when an ordinary personal check would not be acceptable. If not used, a certified check should be redeposited promptly, so the funds previously set aside will be credited back to the depositor's account.

**Counter Check.** This is a check which a depositor sometimes uses to draw funds from his own account. It is *not negotiable.* Forms for counter checks are available at the bank with the wording "Pay to the Order of MYSELF ONLY" upon it. It is this wording which makes a counter check non-negotiable. The term "counter check" is sometimes applied to the blank checks that are available when a person does not have his own particular bank's checks with him. These are blank checks upon which the bank's name is written by the person writing the check, along with other standard information. The use of these blank checks has declined considerably because of machine bookkeeping and the M.I.C.R. (Magnetic Ink Character Recognition) numbers on checks (Fig. 17-1).

**Limited Check.** This is a check that is limited as to the amount that may be written on it. A statement appears on such checks stating that it is void if written over a certain amount. This type of check is often used for payroll or insurance checks. A limited check may also indicate a definite time limit during which a check may be presented for payment, thus limiting the length of time it is negotiable.

**Money Order.** This is a check purchased for a fee, usually by persons who do not have checking accounts, or in cases when a personal check is not acceptable. The names of both the payee and the payer appear on the face of the in-

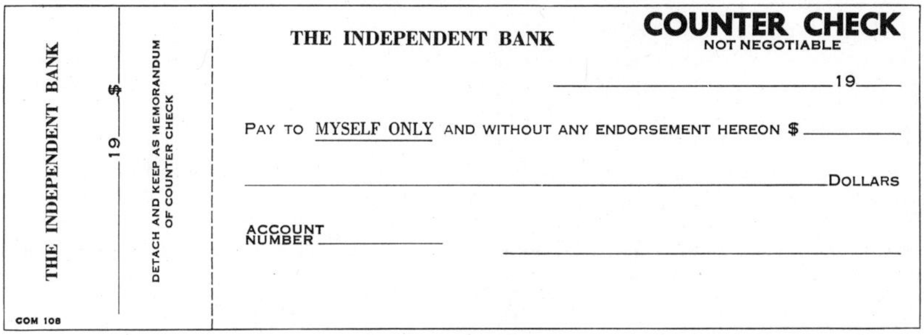
THE INDEPENDENT BANK
19___ $
DETACH AND KEEP AS MEMORANDUM OF COUNTER CHECK
THE INDEPENDENT BANK
COUNTER CHECK
NOT NEGOTIABLE
_______ 19___
PAY TO MYSELF ONLY AND WITHOUT ANY ENDORSEMENT HEREON $ ______
_______ DOLLARS
ACCOUNT NUMBER ______
COM 108

Counter check.

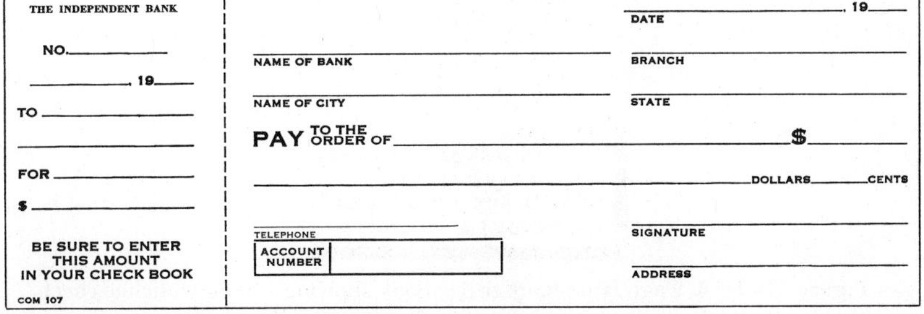
THE INDEPENDENT BANK
NO. ______
______ 19___
TO ______
FOR ______
$ ______
BE SURE TO ENTER THIS AMOUNT IN YOUR CHECK BOOK
COM 107
______ 19___
DATE
NAME OF BANK
BRANCH
NAME OF CITY
STATE
PAY TO THE ORDER OF ______ $ ______
______ DOLLARS ______ CENTS
TELEPHONE
ACCOUNT NUMBER
SIGNATURE
ADDRESS

**Figure 17-1** Blank check.

strument. Postal money orders are drawn on the post office in your city, in amounts up to $300. Express money orders are purchased at the local REA Express office. Bank money orders are drawn on a bank. There are other agencies, large and small, where money orders may be purchased for a fee. All these forms of money orders are considered equally negotiable.

**Traveler's Check.** This check is designed for persons traveling where personal checks may not be accepted or in cases in which it is not advisable to carry large amounts of cash. These checks usually are printed in denominations of $10, $20, $50, and $100. For protection against loss or theft the customer must place his signature on the face of each check, in the presence of a bank witness, at the time of purchase. He later signs his name again on the face of each check when he wishes to cash it. This item is a check and is not to be listed as cash in a deposit.

**Voucher Check.** This is a check with a detachable voucher form. The voucher portion is used to itemize or specify the purpose for which the check is drawn. It is used for the convenience of the payer, showing discounts and various other itemizations. This portion of the check is removed before presenting the check for payment, and provides a record for the payee (Fig. 17-2).

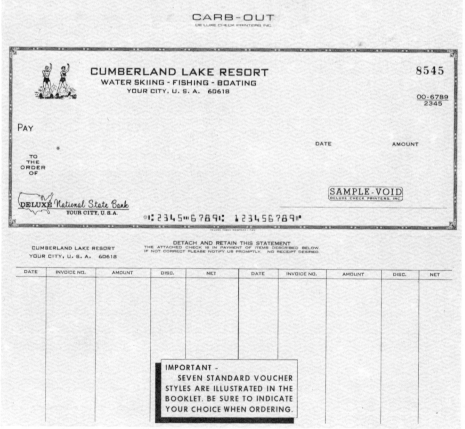

**Figure 17-2** A, Page from bank order book showing sample voucher check.

*(Illustration continued on opposite page.)*

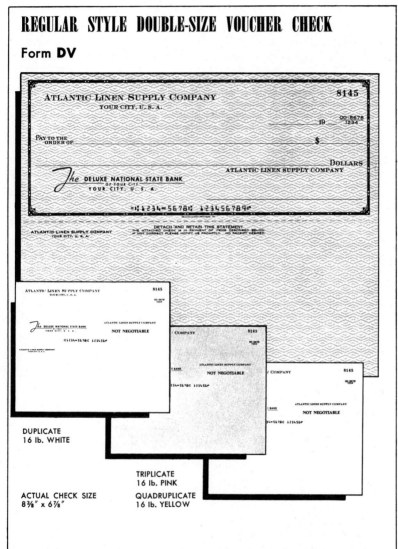

# REGULAR STYLE DOUBLE-SIZE VOUCHER CHECK

## Form **DV**

● This is a regular style double-size voucher check requiring a conventional envelope for mailing. It may be ordered original only or in duplicate, triplicate or quadruplicate in a choice of bindings. Copies are imprinted and numbered same as the original. Seven different voucher styles are also available with the voucher printed at top or bottom as desired. See instructions for ordering various versions at the back of this booklet.

Figure 17–2    **B,**    *Continued.*

**Warrant.** This is a check that is not considered to be negotiable but can be converted into a negotiable instrument or cash. Warrants are evidence of a debt due because of certain services rendered, and the bearer is entitled to certain payment for this service. Government and civic agencies often issue such warrants. A claim draft on an insurance claim is a warrant issued by the insurance adjuster as evidence that the claim is valid. It authorizes the insurance company to pay the claim. Warrants do not have an A.B.A. number (see next paragraph).

## A.B.A. Number

This is a coding system originated by the American Bankers Association, a voluntary association of banks and bank organizations for mutual benefit in the exchange of ideas and information. One division of the American Bankers Association is the American Institute of Banking, whose purpose it is to educate bank employees in banking procedures and banking law.

The A.B.A. number is used on checks as a simple way to identify the area where the bank upon which the check is written is located, and the particular bank within the area. The code number is expressed as a fraction: $\frac{90\text{-}2110}{1222}$ (Fig. 17–3). In the part before the hyphen, the numbers 1 to 49 designate cities in which Federal Reserve banks are located or other key cities. The numbers from 50 to 99 refer to states or territories. As the second part of the number, each bank is issued an A.B.A. number for its own identification purposes. The number in the lower part of the fraction includes the number of the Federal Reserve District in which the bank is located and other identifying information.

## M.I.C.R. (Magnetic Ink Character Recognition)

Characters and numbers printed in magnetic ink are found at the bottom of most checks. They represent a common machine language, readable by machine

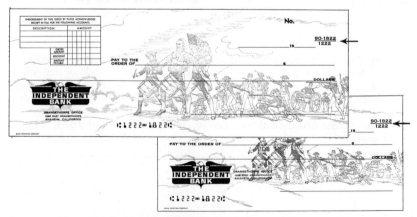

**Figure 17–3**   Sample checks. Arrow indicates A.B.A. number.

and by men. When a check is deposited, the amount of the check can also be printed in magnetic ink below the signature. M.I.C.R. identification facilitates processing through a high-speed machine that reads the characters, sorts the checks, and does the bookkeeping.

## Bank Accounts

**Checking Account.** When an individual places an amount of money on deposit in a bank, he can set up a checking account—that is, he can draw checks upon this amount which are payable on demand. Simply stated, a checking account is a bank account against which checks may be written. Checking accounts usually do not earn interest on the balance deposited.

**Savings Account.** Money can also be deposited at the bank in a savings account (Fig. 17–4). You cannot draw checks upon a savings account. In most cases, savings accounts earn interest upon the amounts deposited; that is, the bank pays the depositor a certain percentage annually for the use of the money in the savings account. When a depositor sets up a savings account, the bank issues a savings passbook in which are entered the dates, amounts deposited, interest earned, and balances on hand each time deposits are made. Withdrawals, which are made by use of special savings account checks, are also shown in the passbook. Savings account checks are not negotiable. Most savings accounts are insured up to $20,000.

**Joint Account.** A joint account is owned by two or more people and is subject to check or withdrawal by the signatures of the persons who share it. It is a common practice for a husband and wife to set up a joint checking account, so that either may draw upon the account. Signatures may be placed on checks singly or jointly, depending upon the stipulations agreed upon when the original account is set up.

**Special Checking Account.** This is a checking account on which a fixed fee is charged for each check written and, in some cases, each deposit made. This differs from a regular checking account, which sometimes requires a minimum balance on hand at all times. The fixed fee may be made on the account before

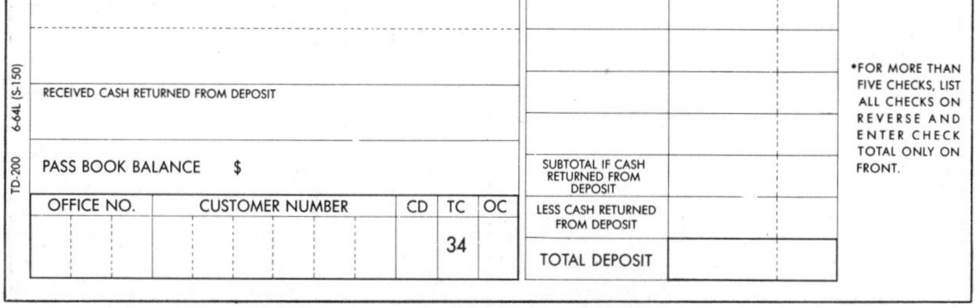
UNITED CALIFORNIA BANK
DATE
CASH
*CHECKS BY BANK NO.
SAVINGS ACCOUNT DEPOSIT
DEPOSITED FOR THE CREDIT OF
RECEIVED CASH RETURNED FROM DEPOSIT
PASS BOOK BALANCE $
*FOR MORE THAN FIVE CHECKS, LIST ALL CHECKS ON REVERSE AND ENTER CHECK TOTAL ONLY ON FRONT.
SUBTOTAL IF CASH RETURNED FROM DEPOSIT
LESS CASH RETURNED FROM DEPOSIT
TOTAL DEPOSIT
OFFICE NO. | CUSTOMER NUMBER | CD | TC | OC
34
TD-200 6-64L (S-150)

**Figure 17–4** Sample of savings account deposit slip.

the checks are written. In this case, the checks are "sold" to the customer for a small fee per check.

**Service Charges.** In all types of accounts, the bank may charge a fee against the account of a depositor for services rendered in bookkeeping. Usually in the case of an individual account, it is a flat fee; in a business account the fee is based on services rendered. If the average or minimum balance is maintained at a specified level, the bank may forego a service charge.

## Rules for Writing Checks

Checks are orders to pay. A check is the most common form of money exchange, with the exception of actual cash. Some of the advantages of making payments by check were outlined earlier in this chapter. However, the handling and writing of checks should be done with extreme care. Here are some basic rules to be remembered when writing checks:

1. Keep all checks numbered and matching with the check stub. Most business concerns have specially printed checks that are pre-numbered with consecutive numbers being used with each successive checkbook.

| CHECK NO. | DATE | CHECK ISSUED TO | AMOUNT OF CHECK | √ | DATE OF DEP. | AMOUNT OF DEPOSIT | BALANCE |
|---|---|---|---|---|---|---|---|
| | | | | | | | |

**Figure 17–5** Sample depositor's record of checks and deposits.

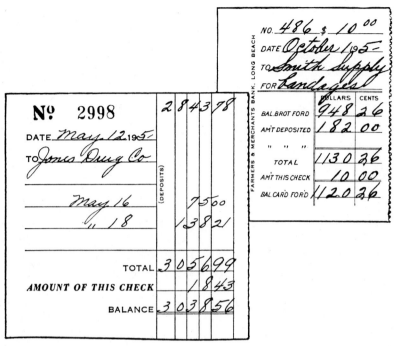

**Figure 17-6**    Methods of filling out check stubs.

2. *Before* you write the check, fill out the stub or the place allotted for recording your expenditures. On the completed stub, there should appear the (a) check number, (b) date, (c) name of person or company to whose order the check is payable, (d) purpose of the payment, and (e) the new balance to be carried forward to the next stub (Fig. 17-6). By following this procedure *every* time you will always know exactly where you stand concerning your balance, and where your money has gone.

3. Checks should be written in ink or typewritten. The typewritten check is preferred by banks and presents a better professional image. A check-writing machine is of value in an office where many checks must be written.

4. Date the check the day it is written (not postdated). If there is an occasion when a postdated check is necessary, you must get the consent of the person accepting the check to hold it until that date.

5. Write the name of the payee after the printed words, "Pay to the order of." Always try to write the name of the payee correctly and as he writes his name (he must endorse the check exactly as his name appears on the face of the check) (Fig. 17-7). When paying bills, you will usually find a notation on the invoice stating "Make check payable to ___" with the necessary information following. Do not use abbreviations unless so instructed or space is limited. Write out in full, if possible. For example, U.S. Dept. of Ed. should be written as United States Department of Education.

6. Leave no space before the name, and follow it with three dashes if there is space remaining.

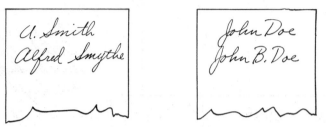

**Figure 17–7** Endorsement of checks. Payee's name incorrect.

7. Omit titles from the names of payees. A check should be made payable to Robert A. Jones rather than Mr. Robert A. Jones. If a married woman is using her husband's name, then it is necessary to put the Mrs. on the check, as, for example, Mrs. John L. Doe. But if the woman is using her own given name, Mary Louise Doe, then the Mrs. is omitted.

If the payee is receiving the check as an officer of an organization, then the title should follow his name, such as John F. Jones, Treasurer, or Paul J. Barnes, Collector. He then accepts the check in his official capacity when he endorses it.

8. Take extreme care in stating the amount of money in both figures and in words. Make certain that the amount stated agrees in these three places: the check stub; the right side of the check close to the dollar sign ($); and the line on which the sum is written in words preceding the word "Dollars." If by chance there is a difference between the two amounts on the check, the bank generally pays the amount in words (or won't pay it at all).

9. Always start writing at the extreme left of each space on the check. Leave no blank spaces. Keep the cents close to the dollars; otherwise, there is room for alteration. If the check is typewritten, use the hyphen or asterisk key to fill in all blank spaces. Draw a line in these spaces if the check is written with pen (Fig. 17–8).

10. The amount of dollars and cents may be expressed in several different ways. Fractions of a dollar are best shown as a numerator of a fraction, i.e., as so many hundredths, when written following the dollar sign, keeping close to the dollars shown. If there are no cents in the amount, write the word "no" as the numerator instead of "00", since the "00" can easily be changed into "66" or "88". A better method is to write "Five dollars only" or "Five dollars and no cents." Double check what you've written and write so that the figures and words can be read correctly by all who need to read them. Capitalize the first word (i.e., Five).

11. If necessary, a check can be written for less than one dollar, but be very careful to emphasize the amount. The figures by the dollar sign ($) may be circled to assure proper attention, as $ 65¢ or enclosed in parentheses, as $–(65¢). The amount of money is written in full with the word "only," as "Only sixty-five cents——" (Fig. 17–10). The word *dollars* should not be crossed out. Figures 17–8 and 17–9 show examples of correct and incorrect check writing.

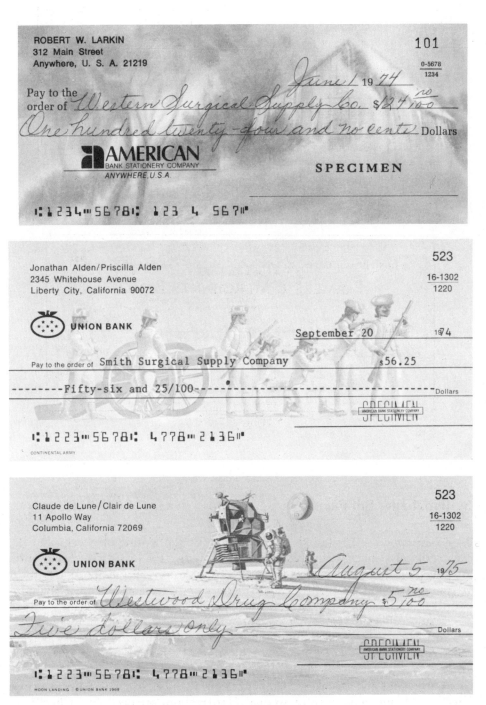

**Figure 17–8**  Correct methods of writing checks.

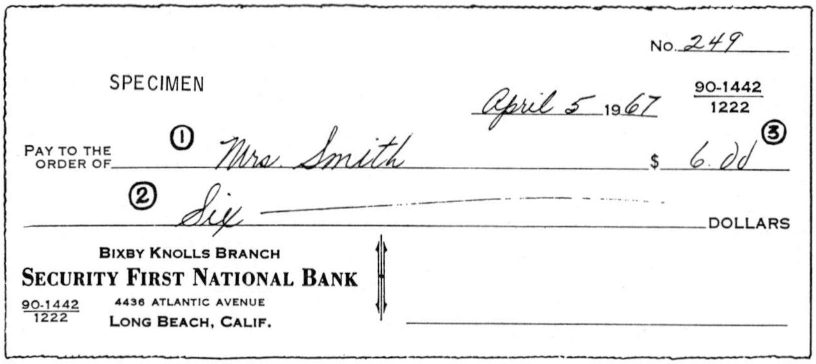

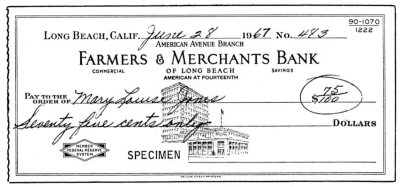

**Figure 17–9**   Incorrect check. 1. Incomplete name; 2. check could be made into $26 very easily; 3. the "00" could be made into 88.

**Figure 17–10**

## Systematizing Bill Paying

A systematic plan should be established for the writing of checks and the paying of bills. Check writing usually is done on the 10th or 15th of each month. An exception sometimes arises when it is possible to realize a good discount if payment of a bill is made within a specified time, for instance ten days. Such discounts usually are indicated at the bottom of invoices or billing forms.

When a check is written in payment of a statement or invoice, it is good practice to write on the invoice the number of the check and the date it was paid. Then if any question arises about whether the bill was paid or when it was paid, you can readily locate the check stub.

**Corrections and Mistakes.**   Do not cross out, erase, or change any part of a check. Take time to be careful, so that no corrections are necessary. Checks are printed on sensitized paper so that erasures are readily noticeable, and the bank has the right to refuse to pay any check that has been altered. If a mistake is made, write the word "VOID" on the stub and the check, but DO NOT destroy the check. It should be filed with the canceled checks so that it is available for auditing purposes. In rare cases, an error is made on a check which cannot be voided. If this situation occurs, it is necessary to strike out the error and write the correct information above. Then initial or sign your name near the correction. The bank will not accept a check in which a correction is made in regard to the name of the payee or the amount of money shown, but it may pass a correction on the date or check number.

**Payment in Full.**   If payment in full is to be recognized in regard to a given check, the statement "Payment in Full to Date" must appear on the back of the check above the endorsement, not on the face of the check. Canceled checks are a receipt for the maker of the check, not for the payee.

**"Cash" Checks.**   A cash check is a check made payable to cash or bearer. Such checks are completely negotiable. Since these checks are easily cashed without positive identification, it is poor policy to write cash checks unless they are to be cashed at the time they are written. Banks may, however, require that the person receiving the cash endorse the check.

**Checkbook Stubs.**   The checkbook stub, the part which remains in the book after the check has been written and removed, is your own record of the checks written, date, amount, payee, and purpose of check. As mentioned earlier in this chapter, it is important that the stub be completed before the check. This prevents the possibility of writing a check and neglecting to complete the stub. If the stub is not completed and the check is sent out, you will have no record of the payee and the amount taken from the account until the canceled check is returned at a later date. Consequently, you will be unable to balance your account or determine the amount on hand until you receive those canceled checks.

If checks are to be typewritten, complete the stub first, then remove the check from the checkbook and type the necessary information on it. After typing the check, compare the amounts appearing on the stub and the check. Differences between amounts listed on check stubs and on the checks themselves are a frequent source of error in banking procedure. Always double check your check stubs against checks to avoid error, and keep checkbook balance up to date. You will be saving yourself time and trouble in the long run.

It is good procedure to keep a separate financial disbursement record with your bookkeeping system as a double check on the status of the bank account.

## Signing Checks

After all checks have been written, place them on the doctor's desk with the invoices or other information so that he can study them and sign the checks. The doctor's secretary or assistant does not sign checks unless power of attorney has been delegated to her for this responsibility (Fig. 17–11).

Never ask your employer to sign a blank check. This places him in a very embarrassing situation, as he is well aware of the dangers involved. Some doctors sign several blank checks before leaving the office on an extended trip to allow the medical assistant to make certain payments during his absence. This is a dangerous procedure even though the assistant is completely trustworthy. Such

Account Number________________

(TO BE FILLED IN BY BANK)

**Union Bank**

Date________________

Robert W. Larker, M.D.

By Joanne Barker

Above is the signature of Joanne Barker, who is hereby authorized as my attorney in fact to sign, cash and draw checks or withdrawal receipts, including checks or withdrawal receipts payable to the order of said attorney in fact, against the above named account only, and to endorse for deposit in such account, or to endorse and cash, checks, notes and drafts and to transact all business with you with respect to such account in my name and as my attorney, until this authorization is revoked by me in writing, delivered to you. I agree to be liable to you and to reimburse you immediately for any and all overdrafts made by my said attorney. I hereby agree to indemnify and save and hold you harmless against any and all loss, expense, damage or claim (including, among other things, court costs and attorney's fees) arising out of, resulting from or incurred in connection with your cashing, paying, honoring or otherwise dealing with any check, withdrawal receipt, note or draft signed or endorsed by said attorney whether during my life or after my death but before you have obtained actual knowledge thereof. This power of attorney includes the power to change the address for delivery of statements and vouchers concerning this account.

Robert W. Larker, M.D.

Cancelled By________________ Date________________

POWER OF ATTORNEY

COM-42 5M 4-61 19906

**Figure 17–11** Application for power of attorney.

checks may be misplaced or they may be stolen and cashed for any amount by anyone completing the check.

Some physicians use two different signatures in conducting the legal aspects of their practices, using one signature on prescriptions, which of course are easily available to forgers, and a second signature for banking purposes. This is an excellent precaution against forged checks on the doctor's bank account.

When checks are sent through the mail, the check should not be visible through the envelope. Either place the check within a letter or fold it into a plain sheet of paper. Checks may be folded at the right end to conceal the amount of money written. Make certain the envelopes are sealed before mailing, and mail all checks yourself as soon as possible after writing. Place these envelopes in a mailbox, not in an outgoing tray, unless you are certain the tray is a safe place in which to leave them prior to mailing.

## Rules for Accepting Checks

The medical assistant is frequently presented with checks by patients or others as payment for the doctor's services. In most cases these will be personal checks. Caution should be used in accepting government checks or payroll checks. Make sure the person presenting the check is known to you. Government and payroll checks sometimes are illegally secured in mailbox robberies.

Acceptance of "third-party" checks is generally unwise. A third-party check is a check made out, for example, to a patient by another person. The patient presents the check for payment on his account. It is necessary to endorse such checks, and the doctor thus becomes responsible in case the check bounces. Do not accept a postal money order for payment if the person paying you has received it from another party; postal money orders cannot be endorsed by more than two persons.

Do not accept a check marked "Payment in full" unless it does pay the account in full up to and including the date on which it is received. If the check received in payment is less than the amount due and it is marked "Payment in full," do not accept it unless you are willing to accept this amount as full payment. You will be unable to collect the balance due on the account once you have accepted and deposited such a check on account. It is illegal for you to scratch out the words "Payment in full."

It is not a good policy to cash checks written for more than the amount due. There are two reasons for avoiding this. First, you will have to return cash for the difference between the amount of the check and the amount owed. If the check is not honored upon presentation at the bank, your office suffers the loss not only of the amount of the check but also of the amount returned in cash. Second, the returned canceled check may indicate the patient paid more on account than he actually did.

The bitter sequel to such a practice was told very well by Dr. W. B. McDonald in *Medical Economics.* Said Dr. McDonald:

> Some years ago I operated on an elderly man and then treated him postoperatively for several months. He had been paying his bill in fifty-dollar installments; but several times, to save himself a trip to the bank, he gave me a check for a larger amount and I gave him the balance in cash. Then he was killed in an auto accident.
>
> Only $200 had by then been paid on his bill of $500. So I sent the estate my statement for the $300 balance. Back came this letter: 'Dear Doctor: We refuse to accept the bill for $300, which you claim is outstanding against the estate of Richard Downes. The canceled checks show that he owed you only $100. We suggest, therefore, that you send us a corrected bill.'
>
> What bothered me even more than the financial loss was to have my integrity questioned. I decided then and there that the penalty for being accommodating in such cases was just too high.*

Such an experience could occur in any doctor's office, as Dr. McDonald points out. It is difficult for the assistant to tell a patient, "We never cash a check for more than the amount due." Dr. McDonald had one suggestion for making this procedure easier. He advised his assistants to explain that it is inadvisable for the office to cash such checks because of tax problems. Most people can appreciate the gravity of an income tax investigation. An alternate "escape" is simply to state that you do not keep extra cash in the office, and suggest that the patient cash the check at a bank or store where he is known and return with the correct amount.

If you do not know the individual and cannot identify his signature, ask for

---

*McDonald, W. B.: Letter to the Editor. Med. Econ., Vol. 31, Nov., 1953.

good identification. An honest person is always willing to show his credentials, such as credit cards or driver's license. Do not hesitate to copy the numbers of these cards on the face of the check; in case the check is returned to you, you will have a means of tracing the person who gave you the bad check. It is wise to have the person make out the check in your presence and then compare the signature with the one on the identification cards.

*Summary of Precautions to Observe in Accepting Checks:*
1. Scan the check carefully for incorrect dates or amounts which do not match.
2. Do not accept a check with corrections on it.
3. An out-of-town check, government check, or payroll check should be accepted *only* if you are well-acquainted with the person presenting it.
4. If you do not know the person presenting a personal check, ask for identification and compare signatures.
5. Do not accept third-party checks unless you are willing to accept responsibility for the value of the check should it prove worthless.
6. Do not accept checks written for more than the amount due.
7. Do not accept checks marked "Payment in full" unless the check does pay the account up to and including the date the check is presented.
8. Remember that money orders cannot be endorsed by more than two persons.

## ENDORSEMENT OF CHECKS

### What is an Endorsement?

An endorsement is a signature plus any other writing on the back of a check by which the endorser transfers his rights in the check to another party. Endorsements are made in ink, either with pen or rubber stamp, on the back of the check across the left or perforated end.

### Necessity for Endorsement

The Uniform Negotiable Instrument Act, applicable in all states, explains the need of an endorsement as follows:

> An instrument is negotiated when it is transferred from one person to another in such a manner as to pass title to another party. If payable to bearer, it is negotiated by delivery. If payable to order, it is negotiated by the endorsement of the holder completed by delivery.

The name of the last endorser of the check shows who last received the money. If a check were cashed for someone who did not endorse it and was returned for some reason, the bank would charge the check to the last endorser, not to the last person receiving the money. For this reason, it is not wise to cash a check made payable to another party without having the endorsement of the person who delivered the check to you for cashing.

## Kinds of Endorsements

If a check is made payable to "Bearer" or "Cash" it is considered to be a negotiable instrument without an endorsement, because no particular party has been named. But a check made payable to a particular party must have an endorsement before it is considered negotiable.

The four principal kinds of endorsements are: (1) blank, (2) restrictive, (3) special, and (4) qualified. Blank and restrictive endorsements are most commonly used.

**Blank Endorsement.**   The payee signs only his name. This makes the check payable to bearer. It is the simplest and most common type of endorsement but should be used only when the check is to be cashed or deposited immediately.

**Restrictive Endorsement.**   This specifies the *purpose* of the endorsement. You will use one kind of restrictive endorsement in preparing the doctor's checks for deposit to his checking account. An example is shown in Figure 17–12.

**Special Endorsement.**   This includes words specifying the person to whom the endorser makes the check payable. For instance, a check naming Helen Barker as payee may be endorsed to the doctor by writing on the back of the check

Pay to the order of
Theodore F. Wilson, M.D.
Helen Barker

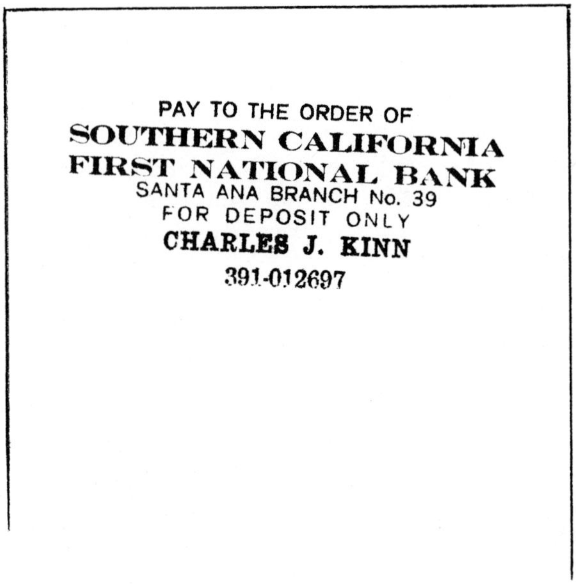

PAY TO THE ORDER OF
**SOUTHERN CALIFORNIA
FIRST NATIONAL BANK**
SANTA ANA BRANCH No. 39
FOR DEPOSIT ONLY
**CHARLES J. KINN**
391-012697

**Figure 17–12**   Example of restrictive endorsement.

The check is still negotiable but requires Dr. Wilson's signature or endorsement.

**Qualified Endorsement.** The *effect* of the endorsement is qualified by disclaiming or destroying any future liability of the endorser. Usually the words "Without Recourse" are written above the payee's signature. This kind of endorsement might be used by an attorney who accepts a check on behalf of a client but who has no personal interest in the transaction.

## Endorsing Procedures

The use of a blank endorsement by the medical assistant will be more or less limited to cashing a petty cash check for the office. If the doctor writes a check to "cash" or "petty cash," the assistant will probably be asked to endorse it when she receives the cash from the bank or any party cashing the check. This endorsement should not be written until the check is actually presented for payment. Although a check made out to "cash" is immediately negotiable, the person who endorses it is verifying that he is the one who received payment.

It is advisable in most medical offices to deposit all receipts in the checking account. For this reason checks may be endorsed for deposit immediately upon receipt, thereby safeguarding them from being negotiable should they be lost or stolen.

Any endorsement should agree exactly with the name on the face of the check. If the name of the payee is misspelled, it is usually necessary for him to endorse the check the way the name is spelled on the face, followed by his name with the correct spelling. The Uniform Commercial Code, Section 3–203, states:

> Where an instrument is made payable to a person under a misspelled name or one other than his own he may indorse in that name or his own or both; but signature in both names may be required by a person paying or giving value for the instrument.

Most banks will accept the routine stamp endorsement that is restricted to "deposit only," if the customer is well known and maintains an established account.

Some insurance checks or drafts require a personal signature endorsement; a stamped endorsement is not accepted. This will be stated on the back of the check. In such cases, ask the payee to endorse with his signature, then stamp immediately below the signature the restrictive endorsement "for deposit only."

## DEPOSITS AND BANK STATEMENTS

It is usually a regular duty of the medical assistant to make deposits of cash and checks received for the doctor's account. She will routinely prepare deposit slips and see that bank statements are reconciled with the checking account.

## Deposit or Cash Checks Promptly

There are several reasons for processing checks promptly:
1. There is possible danger of a "stop-payment order."
2. The check may be lost, misplaced, or stolen.
3. There is the danger that if a delay occurs in presenting the check for payment, the check may be returned because of insufficient funds to cover it.
4. Some checks have a restricted time for cashing.
5. It is common courtesy to cash checks promptly so that the payer does not have checks outstanding when he receives his bank statement.

## Preparing the Deposit Slip

Deposit slips are itemized memoranda of cash or other funds which a customer presents to the bank with the money to be credited to his account. All deposits should be accompanied by a deposit slip. It is good business procedure to make a carbon or photocopy of all deposit slips to keep on file. As in check writing, the bank prefers a typed slip to one handwritten.

There are several different types of deposit slips, sometimes known as deposit tickets. The most common for the average checking account, correctly known as a commercial account, is the commercial slip (Fig. 17–13). There is also the savings slip and the deposit-by-mail slip. These slips may be obtained from your bank and should be kept on hand in your office. Checking account deposit slips are usually printed with the number of the account in Magnetic Ink Characters to correspond with the checks. The slips are frequently bound in the back of the checkbook. Some write-it-once bookkeeping systems include a deposit slip which the bank will accept as the itemization if it is attached to the customer's numbered deposit slip. The deposit slip should be prepared before going to the bank, with the money organized and ready to present to the bank teller.

Each type of money is recorded separately. The coin is first; count it and place in an envelope. If there is a large quantity of a certain coin, then roll it in the rolls provided by the bank. These rolls should be signed by the depositor, as they are not usually counted by the bank.

Currency (paper money) is then counted and organized by placing the larger bills on top, graduating down to the smaller ones. The currency should all face the same direction—that is, the black side up and the portrait right side up.

Checks are recorded by their bank number, each one individually. If the checks are arranged alphabetically by the names of the patient accounts, and these names included on your office copy of the deposit slip, you will have a ready reference of checks deposited should a question arise regarding a patient's payment.

Money orders, either postal, express, or others, are identified by "P.O. Money Order," or "Exp. M.O." Remember that money orders cannot be endorsed by more than two persons.

The deposit slip should be carefully totaled, and the total entered in the checkbook. Clip the currency together, and clip the checks in a separate packet.

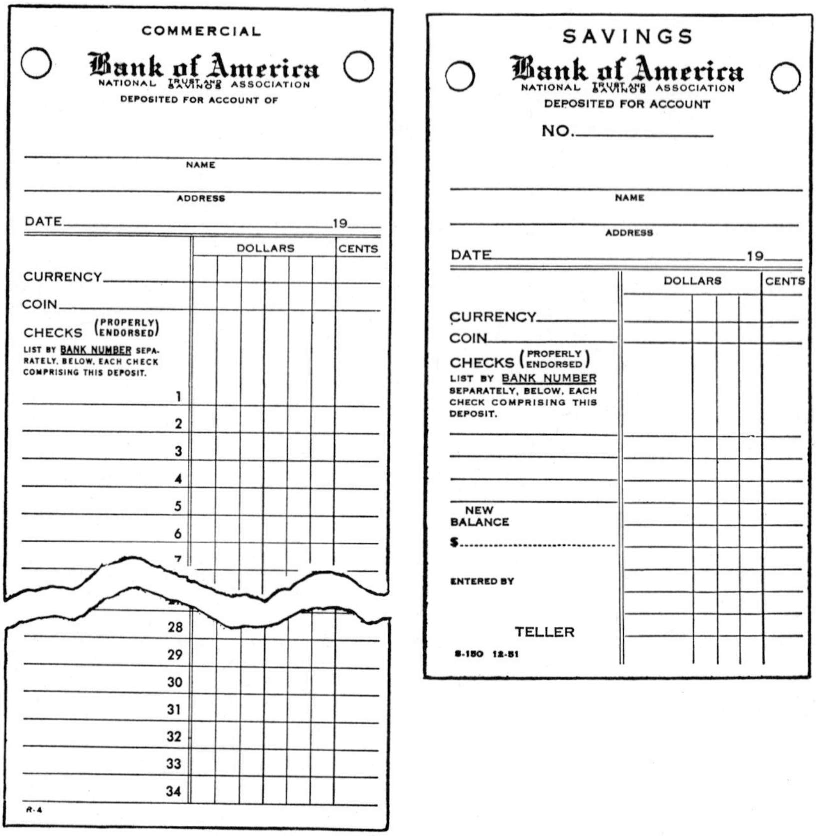

**Figure 17–13** Deposit slips.

Then place the entire amount in a heavy envelope for taking to the bank. Deposit daily if possible. Any torn bills should be mended with transparent tape before taking to the bank.

## Depositing by Mail

Depositing by mail will save you time and is easily accomplished if there are only checks to be deposited. Banks usually supply their customers with special mailing deposit slips and envelopes, upon request (Fig. 17–14). Some mailing deposit slips have an attached portion that the bank will stamp and return as your receipt. Other banks provide the customer with a receipt card which is sent along with the deposit each time for the bank's notation. These deposits are prepared in the same manner as the regular deposits, but certain precautions should be observed:

1. Do not send cash or currency by mail. If this is absolutely necessary, then send it by registered mail.

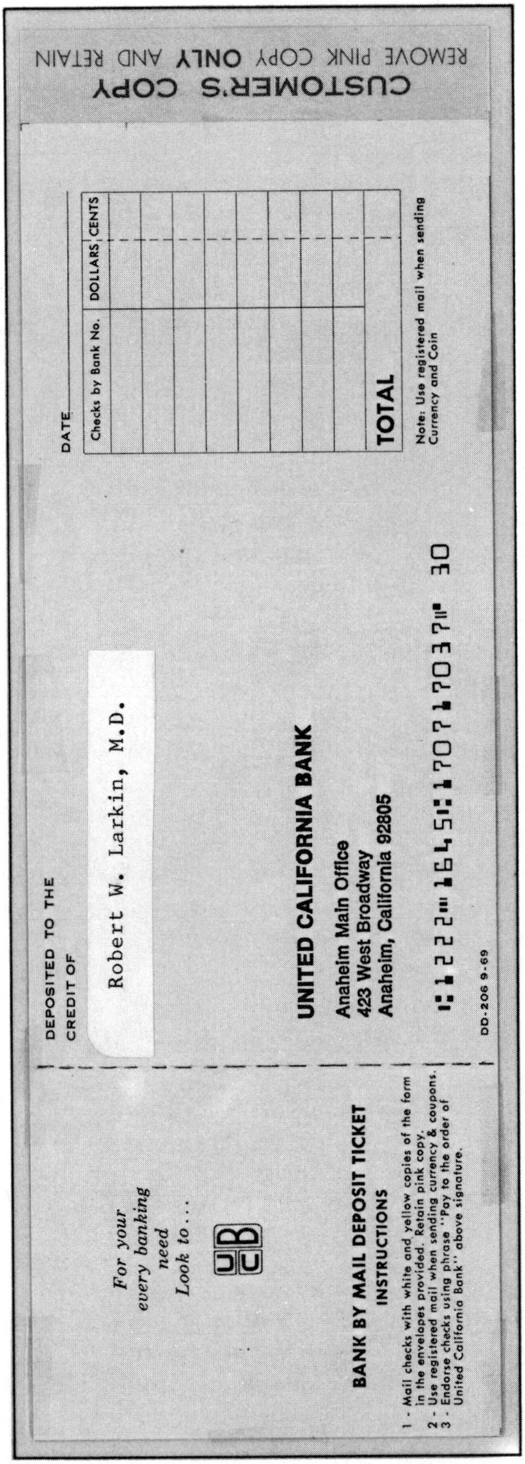

REMOVE PINK COPY **ONLY** AND RETAIN

CUSTOMER'S COPY

DATE

| Checks by Bank No. | DOLLARS | CENTS |
|---|---|---|
| | | |
| | | |
| | | |
| | | |
| | | |
| | | |
| | | |
| | | |
| TOTAL | | |

Note: Use registered mail when sending Currency and Coin

DEPOSITED TO THE CREDIT OF

Robert W. Larkin, M.D.

**UNITED CALIFORNIA BANK**
Anaheim Main Office
423 West Broadway
Anaheim, California 92805

DD-206 9-69

*For your every banking need Look to . . .*

**BANK BY MAIL DEPOSIT TICKET**
**INSTRUCTIONS**

1 - Mail checks with white and yellow copies of the form in the envelopes provided. Retain pink copy.
2 - Use registered mail when sending currency & coupons.
3 - Endorse checks using phrase "Pay to the order of United California Bank" above signature.

**Figure 17–14** Example of Bank By Mail deposit ticket.

2. Do not endorse checks in blank; use a deposit stamp or write the notation "For deposit only to the account of —."

3. If you have not obtained mailing deposit slips or your bank does not provide them, fill out duplicate slips and mail with your deposit. The bank will stamp one copy and return it to you as a receipt.

## Returned Checks

If a check is returned to your office for some reason, usually marked N.S.F. (Not Sufficient Funds), or R.T.M. (Return to Maker), do not delay in contacting the person who gave you the check (Fig. 17–15). Such situations usually arise because of carelessness on the payer's part. Many people just do not attempt to keep close track of their bank balance; they just write checks merrily until one bounces. However, it could be otherwise.

It takes considerable tact to call a patient and inform him that a check has been returned, but it is necessary that such calls be made promptly. The patient may tell you that a deposit was mailed too late to arrive before the check was presented for payment. In that case you may simply re-deposit the check. The patient may ask you to hold the check for a few days and deposit it again. Or he may offer to send another check.

A returned check cannot serve as a receipt for the patient because it has not been "paid" by the bank. Consequently there is no harm in returning it to the maker. However, if you do return it to the maker before receiving a replacement, it is wise to photocopy the N.S.F. check for your records because it does serve as acknowledgment of the debt.

If you are unable to contact the maker of a bad check, waste no time in tracking down all leads, such as referrals, numbers you obtained from credit cards, driver's license, and so forth. There are several places to which bad checks may be reported. Credit associations are often a great help when such a problem arises. If you do not succeed in tracking down and collecting on this account yourself within a short time, turn it over to a qualified collection agency. If a

FM 25M 6-48 F.P. 90-119/1222

**FARMERS & MERCHANTS BANK**
**OF LONG BEACH, CALIF.**

RETURN TO NO.______ REASON______

| | | |
|---|---|---|
| ___NOT ON US AND CHARGED | ___Clearing House Stamp | ___NOT SUFFICIENT FUNDS |
| AMOUNT | ___Restrictive—Official guarantee required | ___Listed to us as $______ |
| ___Altered | ___Pencil—Guarantee | SIGNATURE |
| ___Amounts differ | ___Personal endorsement required | ___Illegible |
| ___Written amount missing | ___Official endorsement required | ___Incomplete |
| ___Written with pencil | ___Voucher missing | ___Irregular |
| DATE | ___Voucher must be receipted | ___Signature required |
| ___Post-dated | | ___Missing |
| ___Altered | ACCOUNT | ___Not authorized |
| ___Missing | ___Closed | ___Not on file |
| ___Stale | ___Unable to locate | ___Not satisfactory |
| ENDORSEMENTS | ___Uncollected funds | ___No authority to pay |
| ___Incomplete | ___Refer to maker | MISCELLANEOUS |
| ___Missing | ___Payment stopped | ___Deceased—Release required |
| ___Irregular | ___Savings account—Not subject to check | ___Payee's name altered |
| ___Unsatisfactory—Guarantee | | ___Payee's name missing |

**Figure 17–15** Returned check slip.

check is returned to your office marked "No account," and it is a check which you had deposited promptly, you have obviously been swindled. This check should be given to the police, the local Better Business Bureau, or your collection agency.

## Reconciling the Bank Statement

The bank customer receives a statement from his bank each month (more often if requested) showing the activity of his account during the month and returning all checks that have cleared the bank during the month (Fig. 17–16). The bank statement balance and the customer's checkbook balance will usually be different, except in a relatively inactive account. The two balances must be "reconciled." The reconciliation will disclose any errors that may exist in the checkbook or, on rare occasions, in the bank statement (Fig. 17–17). Most banks ask to be notified within ten days of any error found in the statement. The bank statement should be reconciled as soon as received each month. You will usually find a form to follow in carrying out this procedure on the back of the bank statement. You may reconcile any bank statement by the following steps:

1. Compare the opening balance on the new statement with the closing balance on the previous statement. They should agree.

2. Compare the entries of the checks on the statement with the returned checks, to see that they are your own checks and that they are listed in the right amount.

3. Now arrange the checks in numerical order.

4. Compare the returned checks with the checkbook stubs. Place a red checkmark on each stub for which a check has been returned (Fig. 17–18).

5. List the outstanding checks (those not returned with the statement).

6. SUBTRACT the total amount of the outstanding checks from the bank balance. *Note*: Do not include any certified checks as outstanding, because the amount has already been deducted from your account.

7. SUBTRACT from the checkbook balance any bank charges (which will be shown as debits on the bank statement). These charges will include service charges, automatic withdrawals or payments, N.S.F. checks, and so on.

8. ADD to the bank statement balance any deposits that appear on your checkbook balance but which have not been included on the bank statement.

9. The balance in your checkbook and the bank statement balance should now agree—they are *reconciled.*

The reconciliation procedure may be put in a formula as follows:

---

| | | |
|---|---|---|
| Bank statement balance | $_____ | |
| Less outstanding checks | _____ | |
| Plus deposits not shown | _____ | |
| CORRECTED BANK STATEMENT BALANCE | | $_____ |
| Checkbook balance | $_____ | |
| Less any bank charges | _____ | |
| CORRECTED CHECKBOOK BALANCE | | $_____ |

---

| PREVIOUS STATEMENT BALANCE | TOTAL AMOUNT OF CHECKS | TOTAL NO. OF CHECKS | TOTAL NO. OF DEPOSITS | TOTAL AMOUNT OF DEPOSITS | SERVICE CHARGE (S/C) | ENDING BALANCE |
|---|---|---|---|---|---|---|
| 1,259.23 | 910.51 | 26 | 3 | 940.03 | .00 | 1,288.75 |

| CHECKS | CHECKS | CHECKS | DEPOSITS | DATE | BALANCE |
|---|---|---|---|---|---|
| | | | BALANCE FORWARD | | 1,259.23 |
| 47.82 | | | | JAN31 | 1,211.41 |
| 5.73 | 28.91 | | | FEB02 | 1,176.77 |
| 35.17 | 71.40 | 106.19 | | FEB03 | 964.01 |
| 7.00 | 57.73 | | | FEB04 | 899.28 |
| 10.00 | 40.00 | 48.41 | | FEB08 | |
| 50.82 | | | | FEB08 | 750.05 |
| 51.54 | | | | FEB11 | 698.51 |
| 14.00 | | | 636.10 | FEB14 | 1,320.61 |
| 7.34 | 8.54 | 37.29 | | FEB15 | 1,266.94 |
| 19.55 | | | | FEB16 | 1,247.39 |
| | | | 38.93 | FEB17 | 1,286.32 |
| 13.00 | | | 265.00 | FEB18 | 1,538.32 |
| 19.13 | 31.24 | | | FEB23 | 1,487.95 |
| 10.24 | | | | FEB24 | 1,477.71 |
| 9.10 | 17.50 | 62.36 | | FEB25 | 1,388.75 |
| 100.00 | | | | FEB28 | 1,288.75 |
| | | | ENDING BALANCE | | 1,288.75 |

AVERAGE DAILY BALANCE      1,169.62

| 1   28 | 910.51 | 26 ( 26) | 940.03 | 3 |
|---|---|---|---|---|
| (EXPLANATION OF CODES) | TOTAL CHECKS THIS PAGE | NO. OF CHECKS | TOTAL DEPOSITS THIS PAGE | NO. OF DEPOSITS |

PLEASE EXAMINE STATEMENT AND CANCELLED CHECKS. REPORT ANY ERASURES, ALTERATIONS OR IRREGULARITIES PROMPTLY. FOR YOUR CONVENIENCE, A RECONCILIATION FORM IS ON THE REVERSE SIDE.

MEMBER FEDERAL RESERVE SYSTEM AND FEDERAL DEPOSIT INSURANCE CORPORATION.

**Figure 17–16**  Example of monthly bank statement.

If these balances agree, you may stop here. If they do not agree, SUBTRACT the lesser from the greater; the difference will usually give you a clue to locating the error.

In searching for a possible error ask yourself these questions:

Did you forget to include one of the outstanding checks?
Is your arithmetic correct?

**UNION BANK**

RECONCILING YOUR CHECKING ACCOUNT

A STEP-BY-STEP PROCESS

1. Sort checks by number or by date.
2. Match each entry with the amount in your register. If you find an error in your register, change its **balance.**
3. Subtract from your register balance any charges deducted by the bank. Enter this **adjusted balance** on line 4 below.

| You Can Figure In This Area | |
|---|---|
| | 5. Enter ending balance of this statement. If ending balance shows OD or ⚬, enter zero and include below as an outstanding check.  $_____ |
| | 6. **Add** any deposits made after last date on the statement.  _____ _____ _____ _____ |
| | NEW BALANCE  $_____ |
| | 7. **Subtract** checks you have written but are not yet paid by the bank. |

OUTSTANDING CHECKS

| Number or Date | AMOUNT |
|---|---|
| | |
| | |
| | |
| | |
| | |
| | |
| | |
| | |
| | |
| | |
| | |
| | |
| | |
| TOTAL | |

4. $_____
Adjusted Register Balance

SHOULD EQUAL

$_____

* SYMBOL REFERENCE

A - ACTIVITY CHARGE
B - RETURNED ITEM CHARGE
D - BANK ORIGINATED CHARGE
I - CASH RESERVE INTEREST CHARGE

L - LIST
OD - OVERDRAFT
P - PAYMENT
R - BANK ORIGINATED DEPOSIT

S - SUB-TOTAL
V - PAYMENT STOPPED
W - CHECK RETURNED
⚬ - CASH RESERVE IN USE

X - CHECK REVERSAL
Y - DEPOSIT REVERSAL
* - FINAL BALANCE

**Figure 17–17** Reverse side of bank statement. Use for reconciling your checking account.

Did you fail to record a deposit or did you record it twice?

Do all stubs and checks agree?

Have you carried your figures forward correctly?

Have you transposed a figure? (if the amount of your error is divisible by nine you probably did)

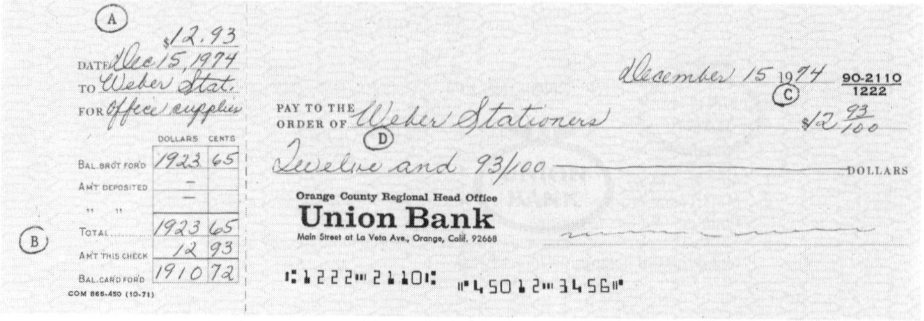

**Figure 17–18** Amounts must correspond in A, B, C, and D.

Did your boss write a check without your knowledge?

Did you fail to correct your checkbook balance at the time of the previous statement?

Once you become familiar with banking procedures, you will find that, by following prescribed procedures, you will simplify the task of "keeping books" in the doctor's office.

## SAFE DEPOSIT BOX

Most commercial banks and many savings institutions have safe deposit boxes which may be rented by their customers. One need not always be a depositor in order to rent a safe deposit box.

Safe deposit boxes provide protection for valuable papers and personal property for a moderate fee. They are obtainable in various sizes to suit the need of the customer; the annual cost will range from five to thirty dollars and is tax deductible. Chapter 14, Records Management, lists certain items which might be placed in a safe deposit box.

The box provides protection in several ways. The box itself is a metal container which is locked with two keys into a compartment in the bank's vault. One key is in possession of the customer; the second key in possession of the bank. The bank is very strict about giving access to the safe deposit boxes. The customer must register on a special form when requesting access to the box. After comparing signatures he is admitted to the vault, accompanied by a bank guard. The guard opens one lock with the bank key and opens the other lock with the customer's key. The box may then be removed and the customer can take it to a private room, or if he merely wishes to place something in the box he can do so and the box can be immediately replaced and locked.

The customer is given two identical keys when he rents the box. These must be guarded carefully because they cannot be duplicated, and he must return both keys to the bank when he relinquishes the box. If a key is lost the bank will charge a fee; if both keys are lost, the fee is considerably higher.

The medical office assistant may be asked to keep a perpetual inventory of the contents of the doctor's safe deposit box. An inventory faithfully kept up to date will save making useless trips to the bank only to discover that the item wanted is not there.

## BANKING TERMINOLOGY

There are certain other banking terms with which the medical office assistant should be familiar, in order that she understand her duties in the handling of a physician's business affairs.

**Bankbook (or Passbook).** This is a book record prepared by the bank for the depositor, listing the amount of deposits and the dates upon which they are made. Because many businesses mail their deposits to the bank, passbooks are not used extensively. Duplicate deposit slips or mail deposit record cards are used instead. Deposit slips with M.I.C.R. numbers are provided with checking accounts. In the case of a savings account, the bankbook lists deposits, withdrawals, interest paid by the bank, dates of all transactions, and the balance on hand. It must be presented with each withdrawal or deposit.

**Bank Statement.** This is a statement sent by the bank to the customer, showing the status of the customer's account on a given date. This statement indicates the beginning balance, deposits received, checks paid, bank charges, and the ending balance at the time the statement is prepared. The bank statement is accompanied by the customer's canceled checks. Such statements are prepared at regular intervals, usually each month. The bank statement is also known as a *bank reconciliation.*

**Countersign.** To countersign is to have another person sign a paper that has already been signed, in order to verify the authenticity of an instrument. The person countersigning is guarantying for the first party and is assuming responsibility.

**Currency.** Paper money issued by the government through an act of law is currency. This paper money has free circulation in trade and is guaranteed to be legal tender by the government.

**Deposit.** An amount of money, either as cash, check, or draft, that is given to a bank for the purpose of establishing and maintaining a credit balance with the bank and is credited to the account of the depositor.

**Deposit Record.** Machine-made receipt for a deposit, presented to customer by bank. This receipt eliminates the necessity for a pen-and-ink entry into a depositor's bankbook.

**Deposit Slip.** An itemized memorandum of cash or other funds that a depositor presents to the bank with the money to be credited to his account. This deposit slip also serves as a record of deposits made.

**Draft.** A drawing on money from a fund or stock, such as an account. Specifically, a draft is an order from one party to another, directing the payment of money. Draft in its broadest sense includes bills of exchange and checks, but the term is more commonly used to indicate a domestic money order. The principal difference between a draft and a check is that, in the case of a draft, the drawer is a bank; in the case of an ordinary check, the drawer is an individual.

**Endorsement.** The act of writing one's signature on the back of an instrument, a legal act of transferring the title of an instrument to another party. When you endorse a check with your signature, you transfer the title of the check to the bank in exchange for the sum written on the face of the check.

**Float.**   A term used to describe the amount of funds in the process of collection represented by checks in the possession of one bank but drawn on the other banks, either local or out-of-town.

**Insufficient Funds.**   A term used to express the fact that the depositor's account is inadequate to cover the amount of a check drawn against his account. The abbreviation "N.S.F." indicates "Not Sufficient Funds" (Fig. 17–15).

**Kite.**   A term used in banking circles to describe the malpractice of individuals in taking advantage of the time element of check collections by the bank. The individual either has a cohort in a distant city, or another account in another city himself. He deposits a check drawn on a bank in a distant city, and then draws from this uncollected balance while the check is in the process of collection. The same individual also sends a check drawn upon this bank, and deposits it in the other bank, where he also draws against uncollected funds by issuing checks against this out-of-town bank. In this manner he uses both bank accounts to his advantage to draw against "non-existent" true balances.

**Note.**   This is a recognized legal evidence of debt, backed only by the promise of an individual giving the note to pay the debt; thus the term, "promissory note." It is a written promise by the maker (or borrower) to pay a given sum of money on a specific date, and it is signed by the maker (or borrower). A "collateral note" requires the pledging of marketable securities, which may be sold by the creditor if the maker of the note fails to pay within the time limit promised.

**Overdrawn or Overdraft.**   When a depositor draws a check for more than the amount he has in his bank account, his account becomes overdrawn. In most states it is illegal to issue a check for more than the amount on deposit in the bank. Should this happen through error or oversight the bank may refuse to honor the check and will return it to the bank that presented it for payment. Such a check is said to "bounce." If the check is written by an established depositor, the bank may honor the check and notify the depositor that he has overdrawn his account. If the bank thus pays or "covers" the check, it issues an overdraft on the depositor's account.

**Postdated Check.**   This is a check on which a future date of payment appears. Postdated checks cannot be presented for payment until the date specified has been reached.

**Power of Attorney.**   This is a legal statement in which a person authorizes another person to act as his attorney or agent. A power of attorney authorization may be limited to the handling of certain procedures or assets listed in the power of attorney statement, or it may give full power over all assets. The person authorized to act as agent is known as an *attorney in fact.*

**Reconciliation.**   (See Bank Statement.)

**Stale Date or Stale Check.**   This term refers to an instrument which is more than six months old or for which a "reasonable time" for presentation and payment has passed. Some payers specify that a check must be presented within 90 days. Stale checks usually are returned to the bank which presented the check for payment and are not honored. This is done to protect the depositor.

**Stop Payment.**   When a depositor or maker of a check wishes to rescind or stop payment of a check he has written, he has the right to request the bank to

**Union Bank**

**STOP PAYMENT ORDER**

OFFICE ____Main_____

| ACCOUNT NUMBER | CHECK PAYABLE TO | | AMOUNT OF CHECK | DATE OF CHECK |
|---|---|---|---|---|
| 45012 3456 | W. B. Saunders Company | | $36.44 | 05/22/74 |

| CHECK NUMBER | CODE | STOP NUMBER | TODAY'S DATE | TIME | EXPIRATION DATE |
|---|---|---|---|---|---|
| 823 | | | 06/18/74 | 11 a.m. | 12/18/74 |

REASON FOR STOP PAYMENT

Check lost in mail

THE UNDERSIGNED AGREES:
1. THAT A CHECK GUARANTEE CARD WAS NOT USED WITH THE CHECK ON WHICH THIS STOP PAYMENT ORDER IS AUTHORIZED.
2. TO INDEMNIFY AND HOLD YOU HARMLESS FROM ALL LIABILITY, DAMAGE, AND EXPENSE INCURRED ON ACCOUNT OF REFUSING PAYMENT OF SAID CHECK;
3. THAT THIS ORDER SHALL AUTOMATICALLY TERMINATE IF THE ACCOUNT ON WHICH THIS CHECK IS DRAWN IS CLOSED OR TRANSFERRED TO ANOTHER OFFICE;
4. TO NOTIFY THIS BANK TO RELEASE THIS ORDER IF AND WHEN THE REASON FOR THE STOP PAYMENT CEASES TO EXIST;
5. THAT THIS ORDER SHALL EXPIRE AND BE OF NO FURTHER EFFECT 6 MONTHS FROM DATE OF ITS RECEIPT BY THIS BANK UNLESS EARLIER RELEASED OR RENEWED BY THE UNDERSIGNED IN WRITING.

AUTHORIZED
SIGNATURE ____T. F. Wilson____        PHONE ___321-4567___

ACCOUNT TITLE____Theodore F. Wilson, M.D._____

CAD-51 A (REV. 7-70)

**Figure 17–19**   Stop-Payment Order.

stop payment on this check. The request to stop payment must be made in writing and must be signed by the maker. (Most banks will accept a stop payment order made by telephone or telegram for a limited time, if it is followed with a written order.) It must give all the required information, such as number of the check, date issued, name of payee, amount of check, and the reason for stopping payment. The stop payment order must reach the bank bookkeeper before the check is presented for payment. It then becomes the responsibility of the bank to refuse payment and return the check to the holder or payee. The holder must then seek his payment from the maker, who has for some reason stopped payment. The customer's account is charged a fee of several dollars for each returned check. Most banks ask a service fee for stop payment requests. Stop payment orders are void after six months unless renewed in writing. Stop payment orders should be used only in extreme emergencies. Reasons for stop payment requests are loss of a check, disagreement about a purchase, or disagreement about a payment (Fig. 17–19).

**Withdrawal.**   The term used for taking funds from a depositor's account. Withdrawal from a checking account is accomplished by writing a check. For withdrawal of funds from a savings account, the depositor must submit his passbook to the bank with a signed withdrawal slip before the bank can pay out funds from the account.

## REFERENCES

Anderson, R. A., Kumpf, W., and R. E. Kendrick: *Business Law, Principles and Cases* (5th Ed.), Cincinnati, South-Western Publishing Company, 1971.

Beckner, C. J.: *Using Bank Services*, Washington, D.C., American Bankers Association, 1970

Hutchinson, L.: *Standard Handbook for Secretaries* (8th Ed.), New York, McGraw-Hill, Inc., and Gregg Publishing Co., 1969

# Chapter 18

**BEHAVIORAL OBJECTIVES**

*The medical office assistant should be able to:*

State the kinds of financial records necessary in the average medical office.
Follow the cardinal rules of any system of bookkeeping.
Briefly explain the three most common systems of bookkeeping.
Account for petty cash in a physician's office.
Keep a single entry set of books.
Maintain payroll records for the small professional office.
Prepare and file payroll reports required by the Internal Revenue Service.

# Keeping Financial Records: Payroll Records

*-locked up*
*- up to date*

The modern doctor recognizes the need for sound business practices in his office. Consequently he looks for a medical assistant who will keep accurate financial records, and who will conduct the nonmedical side of the practice in a businesslike fashion. A doctor's records are the key to efficient management of his practice. No one questions the necessity for keeping adequate *medical* records. The *financial* records are equally important.

Public relations problems are created when records are poorly kept or inadequate, when statements are sent irregularly or incorrectly, and when the collection system is not handled properly.

The reporting of income to federal and state agencies, and the calculating and reporting of payroll deductions necessitate extremely careful and detailed recordkeeping.

## What Kind of Financial Records?

The financial records of any business should, at all times, show
1. how much was *earned* in a given period,
2. how much was *collected*, and
3. the *distribution of expenses* incurred.

Monthly and annual summaries should provide a basis for comparing any given period with another like period. Periodic analyses of the financial records can result in improved business practices, better management of time, curtailment or elimination of unprofitable services, and better budgeting of expenses.

## Who Will Keep the Records?

Bookkeeping and accounting are specialized fields, requiring specific training. *Accounting* has been defined as "the art or system of recording, classifying and summarizing commercial transactions." *Bookkeeping* is mainly the *recording* part of the accounting process. This must be done daily and is the responsibility of the office assistant.

**259**

In many offices, the doctor will employ an outside accounting service to audit the books at regular intervals, and prepare payroll reports, income tax reports, and financial statements. The task of the accountant will be much simpler if he has good daily records with which to work. Since most accountants base their fees on the amount of time needed, the assistant can save the doctor many dollars by keeping clear, accurate records.

**How to Begin.** An important part of bookkeeping is the establishment of good habits, routines, and consistent patterns. When you are introduced to a new office or new bookkeeping system, study it step by step until you are sure you understand it completely.

Do not trust to memory or attempt to use shortcuts. Bookkeeping is either ALL RIGHT or it is ALL WRONG. There is no such thing as *almost correct* as far as financial records are concerned. The books balance or they do not balance. Form the habit of reviewing your work frequently as you proceed.

Bookkeeping procedures are not generally difficult but they do require concentration to avoid errors. The office assistant should set aside a certain time each day for bookkeeping tasks. The early morning when she is fresh, and before patients start arriving, is usually a good time for completing this work. Do not attempt to work on financial records while the office is full of patients, the telephone is ringing continually, and there are other distractions.

**Establish Good Habits**

1. Use good penmanship—no fancy letters or figures.
2. Use the same pen style and ink throughout.
3. Keep columns of figures straight.
4. Write well-formed figures. A careless "9" may look like a "7" or an open "0" may resemble a "6."
5. Carry the decimal point correctly.
6. Check arithmetic carefully; addition and subtraction must be accurate.
7. *Do not erase, write over, or blot out figures.* If an error is made, draw a straight line through the incorrect figure and write the correct figure above it.

## Cardinal Rules to Follow in any Bookkeeping System

1. All fees charged and all payments received must be immediately entered on the daily record or journal.
2. Write a receipt in duplicate for any currency received. Writing receipts for checks is optional—but whatever pattern is followed should be consistent.
3. Endorse checks for deposit as soon as received.
4. All money received should be deposited in the bank. Double check to be sure the total of the deposit plus the amount on hand equals the total to be accounted for on the journal page or day sheet.
5. Post from the day sheet to the patient ledger cards every day.
6. Establish a petty cash fund so that it is never necessary to take funds from patient receipts to pay an office expense.
7. Use the petty cash fund for small, unpredictable expenses. Pay all other expenses by check. A canceled check is your best proof of payment.

8. Check all bills for accuracy and make certain they are paid before due dates. Mark paid bills with the date of payment and the number of your check.

## Bases for Accounting

There are two bases for accounting—the *cash* basis and the *accrual* basis.

Most doctors use the cash basis of accounting. Expressed simply, this means that charges for services are not recognized as income until cash is received, and expenses are not recorded until they are paid.

Commercial enterprises, on the other hand, generally use an accrual basis of accounting. On the accrual basis, income is considered earned when services have been performed (or goods have been sold) even though payment may not have been received. Expenses are recognized and recorded when incurred, even though they have not been paid.

## THREE COMMON SYSTEMS OF BOOKKEEPING

There are many variations in bookkeeping systems, from simple to complex. No one system will meet the needs of every doctor. However, the *basic principles* are the same for all—only the system of recording varies.

## Single Entry System

The simplest of bookkeeping systems, called single entry bookkeeping, will include at least three kinds of records:

1. General Journal, which may be called a daily log, a daybook, daysheet, or charge journal.

2. Accounts Receivable Ledger, which is a record of the amounts owed by each patient. The accounts receivable ledger may be a bound book, a looseleaf binder, card file, or loose pages in a file.

3. Checkbook, which serves as a cash payment journal.

In addition, there may be auxiliary records for petty cash and payroll records.

The single entry bookkeeping system is probably the most popular system for doctors' offices. It is inexpensive, simple to use, and requires very little training. It satisfies the requirements for reporting to governmental agencies. From a negative standpoint, it provides only for daily, monthly, and annual summaries of income and expense. Errors are not easily detected, and there are no built-in controls.

## Write-it-Once, Pegboard, or Accounting Board

Generally termed "pegboard," this system accomplishes all the necessary financial records for each patient with one writing:

1. charge and receipt slip

> 2. ledger card
> 3. journal entry

The board is a lightweight aluminum or masonite board with a row of pegs along the left side or along the top. The accounting forms are perforated for alignment on the pegs. At the beginning of each day a *journal page* is first placed on the board; then a shingled bank of *charge and receipt slips* is placed on top of the journal page. As each patient is taken care of during the day his ledger card is aligned between the charge slip and journal page. Through the interleafing of carbon paper, or carbonized or NCR (no carbon required) forms, the information written on the charge and receipt slip is transferred to the ledger card and to the journal page with one writing.

This system is second in popularity with doctors. It provides for accounts receivable control and daily record of bank deposits, in addition to the record of income and expense. The need for separate posting to patient accounts is eliminated and the chance for error is decreased.

The initial cost of materials is greater than for the single entry system, and the forms are more expensive, although still quite reasonable. The system requires slightly more training than single entry, but is easily mastered.

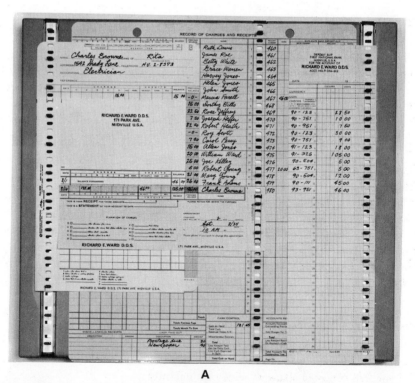

**A**

**Figure 18–1 A,** A Write-It-Once bookkeeping system. (Courtesy of the Todd-Hadley Company, Burroughs Corp., Rochester, N.Y.) **B,** Ledger card used in pegboard bookkeeping.

*(Illustration continued on opposite page.)*

| NAME | JONES, JANE LILLIAN (Mrs.) | | TELEPHONE | 232-7754 |
|---|---|---|---|---|

MALE ☐   FEMALE ☒   AGE 33   S. ☒. W. D.   SPOUSE'S NAME  John W.

REFERRED BY  Dr. Wm. Miller

EMPLOYER  not employed                     OCCUP.  --

ADDRESS  --                                 PHONE  --

SPOUSE'S EMPLOYER  self - City Hardware Company   OCCUP. owner/manager

ADDRESS  306 North Beulah Street, Lakewood  90715   PHONE 432-3924

INSURANCE  Aetna Life & Casualty

| | JAN. | FEB. | MAR. | APRIL | MAY | JUNE | JULY | AUG. | SEPT. | OCT. | NOV. | DEC. |
|---|---|---|---|---|---|---|---|---|---|---|---|---|
| STATEMENT MAILED | | | | | | | | | | | | |

STATEMENT

COMMUNITY HEALTH CARE CENTER
49015 East Cherry Street
Long Beach, California 90808
(213) 444-6789

Mrs. John W. Jones
535 East Woodrow Street
Lakewood, CA  90715

PLEASE PAY
LAST AMOUNT
IN THIS COLUMN

PLEASE DETACH AND RETURN WITH YOUR REMITTANCE

| ✓ | PREVIOUS BALANCE | DATE | O | A | B | C | CODE | MISC. | RVS OR BANK NO. | BY CHECK OR P.M.O. | BY CURRENCY | BALANCE |
|---|---|---|---|---|---|---|---|---|---|---|---|---|
| | new | 4/8/12 | 15 | | | | | | | | | 15 - |
| | 15 - | 2/25/12 | 15 | | | | | | | | | 30 - |
| | 30 - | 3/4/12 | | | | | | | Ins. | 30 | | 0 |
| | 0 | 4/3/13 | 600 | | | | | | | 476 00 | | 600 - |

EXPLANATION OF CHARGES

O—OFFICE CALL
INITIAL VISIT
HISTORY & PHYSICAL
FOR HOSPITAL ADMIT.
HOSPITAL VISIT
HOSP. E.R. TREAT

A—SURGERY
MAJOR GENERAL
MAJOR VASCULAR
B—ANGIOGRAMS
MINOR SURGERY
C—ASSIST. SURGEON

MISCELLANEOUS
D—CONSULT—HOSPITAL
E—CONSULT—OFFICE
F—DETENTION TIME
G—WRITTEN REPORT
H—INSURANCE PAPERS
I—INJECTION

**B**

**Figure 18–1  B,** *Continued.*

## Double Entry Bookkeeping System

In a double entry system there will probably be two general books

1. combined cash journal, and
2. general ledger

plus several auxiliary records:

3. petty cash disbursements record
4. daily service record
5. patients' ledger
6. employees' earnings record, and
7. checkbook

Double entry is the most complete system. It provides a more comprehensive picture of the practice and its effect on the doctor's net worth. Materials are inexpensive. Errors show up more readily than in single entry. The drawbacks are that it requires a specially trained and experienced bookkeeper, and the record-keeping requires more time and skill.

## PETTY CASH

In all systems of bookkeeping a petty cash fund should be established to take care of minor incidental expenses. All major expenses should be paid by check.

## Establishing the Fund

To establish the petty cash fund, a check should be written payable to "Cash" or "Petty cash" and charged to miscellaneous expense or a petty cash account. Twenty-five dollars is sufficient for the petty cash fund in the average medical office. If a larger sum is available, there is a tendency to pay too many bills out of petty cash. When the check is exchanged at the bank for small bills and coin, the money is placed in a cashbox or drawer that can be locked, or kept in the safe at night.

## Responsibility for Fund

One person only should be in charge of the petty cash fund. This person must be able to account for the full amount of the fund at any time. A pad of petty cash vouchers is kept in or near the box. For every disbursement from the fund the petty cashier should either have a receipt or prepare a voucher similar to the one in Figure 18–2.

AMOUNT $ _____     NO. _____

# RECEIVED OF PETTY CASH

_____ 19 _____

FOR _____

CHARGE TO_____

_____

APPROVED BY                    RECEIVED BY

_____        _____

AICO-UTILITY Line Form No. 55-061

**Figure 18–2**  Petty cash receipt.

## Accounting Procedure for Petty Cash

The petty cash fund is a revolving fund. It does not change in amount except to increase or decrease the established fund. The total of the petty cash vouchers and receipts plus the amount of cash in the box must always equal the original amount of the fund.

|  |  |
|---|---|
| Established fund | $25.00 |
| Receipt and voucher total | 15.25 |
|  | ——— |
| Cash on hand | $ 9.75 |

Good bookkeeping procedure includes a formal record of all expenditures from the petty cash fund. Figure 18–3, Petty Cash Disbursements, shows the entries for establishing the fund, recording the expenditures during the month, and replenishing the fund.

When the check is written for $15.25 to replenish the fund, it is accounted for in the monthly distribution of expenditures by posting $5.38 as office expense, $5.00 as donations, $1.50 as auto expense, 62¢ as postage, and $2.75 as miscellaneous expense. In this way the expenditures from petty cash are charged to the actual accounts affected. Only the amount of the original check to establish the fund is charged to petty cash.

Avoid the habit of borrowing from the petty cash fund. This admonition applies to the doctor, as well as to the office assistant. If the doctor requests cash from the fund, ask him to give a personal check or an office check in exchange for cash from the fund. By following this procedure, every cent is still accounted for.

| Date | Description | Vou.No. | Total Amt. | O.E. | Dona-tions | Auto. | Post. | Misc. |
|------|-------------|---------|-----------|------|-----------|-------|-------|-------|
| 4/01 | Rec'd in fund $25 | | | | | | | |
| 4/02 | Postage due | 38 | .17 | | | | .17 | |
| 4/05 | O.R. Nurse benefit | 39 | 2.00 | | 2.- | | | |
| 4/10 | Parking fee | 40 | .50 | | | .50 | | |
| 4/10 | Pen refills | 41 | 1.04 | 1.04 | | | | |
| 4/16 | aerogrammes (3) | 42 | .45 | | | | .45 | |
| 4/17 | scratch pads | 43 | 1.68 | 1.68 | | | | |
| 4/22 | 3 lt. coffee | 44 | 2.75 | | | | | 2.75 |
| 4/24 | Parking fee | 45 | 1.00 | | | 1.- | | |
| 4/28 | Girl Scouts | 46 | 2.00 | | 2.- | | | |
| 4/29 | delivery charges | 47 | 2.66 | 2.66 | | | | |
| | | | 15.25 | 5.39 | 5.- | 1.50 | .62 | 2.75 |
| 4/30 | Bal. $9.75 | | | | | | | |
| | Rec'd in fund 15.25 | | | | | | | |
| | Total $25.00 | | | | | | | |

**Figure 18-3** Petty cash disbursements.

## A TYPICAL BOOKKEEPING SYSTEM

As previously stated, a conventional double entry bookkeeping system requires special skills and training. Therefore, no attempt is made to explain the system here. A simple single entry system can be understood and carried out by using the instructions given here. No special equipment is necessary. Typical forms are shown.

### Kinds of Records in a Typical System

The *daily journal, patient ledger,* and *checkbook* are the general financial records. Auxiliary records for *petty cash* and for *payroll* may also be kept.

### Daily Journal

The daily journal is the chronological record of the practice — the financial diary. All information regarding services rendered, charges, and receipts is first recorded in the daily journal. These entries must be accurate and current. The charges for which payment has not been received are called *receivables*; receivables are amounts owing but not yet received. *Receipts* are cash and checks taken in payment for professional services. In addition, there may be income from other sources, such as rental income, royalties, interest, and so forth. The receipts must be categorized to show the source. Both the office assistant and the doctor must realize the importance of recording *every* transaction. If a patient hands cash to the doctor while he is away from the office, it must be reported to the person responsible for keeping the records as soon as possible.

### Posting to Patient Ledger

Entries made in the daily journal concerning charges to and receipts from patients must be transferred to the individual patient ledger cards. This transfer of information is called *posting*. The ledger is the source of information for answering inquiries from patients about their accounts. Monthly statements are prepared from the ledger cards, as are insurance billings. One can readily appreciate the importance of keeping this information current.

### Checkbook

All receipts are deposited in the checking account, and a record of the deposit is entered on the check stub. A copy of each deposit slip should be kept with the financial records. All bills are paid by check and a record of the payment entered on the check stub and in the disbursements section of the daily journal.

## Accounting for Disbursements

*Disbursements* are funds paid out. *Payables* are amounts owed but not yet paid. All disbursements are recorded in the daily journal. Some systems provide a place for recording disbursements daily at the bottom of each daysheet; others provide a check register page at the end of each month. In either of these plans, the disbursements are distributed among various expense accounts such as

| | |
|---|---|
| auto expense | rent and maintenance |
| dues and meetings | salaries |
| equipment | taxes and licenses |
| insurance | travel and entertainment |
| medical supplies | utilities |
| office expense | miscellaneous |
| printing, postage, stationery | personal withdrawals |

The preparation of income tax reports is simplified if the distribution of expenses in the daily disbursement record is the same as that used for tax reporting.

## Daily Bookkeeping Activities

Figure 18–4 shows one day's entries in a typical *daily journal*.

**Full Name of Patient.**   The patient's full name is written in the left column, last name first. This name may be taken from the appointment book, or a daily sheet similar to this may be used as an appointment record.

**Remarks.**   Next to the patient's name, in the "Remarks" column, is entered a brief explanation of the charge, using a simple code system as suggested on page 270. Some practices use a number system for charge codes instead of abbreviations. If a procedure code number is used for insurance and billing purposes, the same code may be used for recording the services in the daily journal.

**Charges to Patients Today.**   The next section shows a breakdown of various charges to patients today. This section explains the kind of service given: medical, outcall (hospital or residence), surgical, and so forth. These columns show the physician the amount of earnings from each type of service rendered.

**Receipts from Patients.**   All receipts from patients who have been in the office and all receipts by mail are entered in this column. Most receipts will be in the form of checks. If a payment is made by cash, this should be noted on the record. A small (c) above the amount is one way of indicating a cash payment. At the end of each day these columns are totaled. The total of the "Receipts from Patients" plus any cash on hand at the beginning of the day should equal the amount of money in your cashbox. It is good policy to bank the receipts daily. Arrangements can be made to bank all checks by mail, thereby saving frequent trips to the bank.

**Daily Proof of Cash.**   Near the bottom of the page you will find a boxed area for recording a daily proof of cash. On the top line of this section is entered the amount of money (cash and checks) in the cashbox at the beginning of the day.

DAY _Thursday_     DATE _April 16, 1974_

| FULL NAME OF PATIENT | REMARKS | CHARGES TO PATIENT TODAY | | | | | | RECEIPTS FROM PATIENTS | ✓ |
| --- | --- | --- | --- | --- | --- | --- | --- | --- | --- |
| | | MEDICAL | OUT CALLS | SURGERY | OBSTETRICAL | LABORATORY | X RAY | | |
| Brown, John | OC | 5 00 | | | | | | 5 00 | • |
| Sullivan, Mrs B | HC 7/7 | | 10 00 | | | | | 20 00 | • |
| James, Edla | OC + Dim | 8 00 | | | | | | | ✓ |
| Roberts, Mrs E | Inj | 5 00 | | | | | | | ✓ |
| Graves, Ellen | OC | 5 00 | | | | | | | ✓ |
| Johnson, Tom | OC + TIA | 5 00 | | | | 3 00 | | | ✓ |
| Barco, Mrs Edw | OC + BC | 5 00 | | | | 5 00 | | | ✓ |
| Daily, Foster, asst | | | | 35 00 | | | | | ✓ |
| Fredrick, Baby John | Cast | 10 00 | | | | | | 7 00 | ✓ |
| Taylor, Theo | OC | | | | -- | | | 10 00 | ✓ |
| Ahlstrom, Mrs R | Arm | | | | | | 10 00 | | ✓ |
| Bunn, Beatrice | OC | 5 00 | | | | | | | ✓ |
| Zeple, Ticklow | Bandage | 7 00 | | | | | | | ✓ |
| Swanson, Sam | OC | 5 00 | | | | | | 5 00 | ✓ |
| Arnold, Agnes | Math | 3 00 | | | | | | | ✓ |
| Beetson, Edith | OC + Inj | 7 00 | | | | | | | • |
| Camrack, Mrs | OC | 5 00 | | | | | | | ✓ |
| Dietz, Eugene | OC | 5 00 | | | | | | | ✓ |
| Maflow, Eva | HC | | 10 00 | | | | | 15 00 | • |
| Homan, Mrs J | OC | 5 00 | | | | | | | ✓ |
| Saturder, Alice | HC + BXX | | 15 00 | | | 15 00 | | 40 00 | ✓ |
| Burns, Wanda | Hn Phy | 15 00 | N/C | | | | | | • |
| Cogan, Mrs B | OC | | | | | | | | • |
| Bander, Fred | T + A | | | 75 00 | | | | 10 00 | • |
| Boston, Stuart | OC | | | | -- | | | | ✓ |
| Jaro, Ernest | OC | 5 00 | | | | | | | ✓ |
| Ahlers, Mrs L | OC + Inj | 7 00 | | | | | | | ✓ |
| Tasker, Mrs A | PO | | | | -- | | | | ✓ |
| Jinn, Mrs J | Pet Mal | | | | | 175 00 | | | ✓ |
| | | | | | | | | | |
| Thompson, Stan | Mail | | | | | | | 60 00 | 16 -252 |
| Watson, R P | " | | | | | | | 40 00 | 17- 31 |

Sample Record.  (By California Professional Bureau)
Los Angeles 15, California

| DAILY PROOF OF CASH | | RECEIPTS FROM OTHER SOURCES | | MEDICAL | OUT CALLS | SURGERY | OBSTETRICAL | LABORATORY | X RAY | RECEIPTS |
| --- | --- | --- | --- | --- | --- | --- | --- | --- | --- | --- |
| CASH ON HAND BROUGHT FORWARD | 300 00 | Rent - 4 Ave | 80 00 | | | | | | | |
| RECEIVED TODAY | 212 00 | Goodyear | | | | | | | | |
| RECEIVED TODAY | 110 00 | Dividends | 30 00 | | | | | | | |
| RECEIVED TODAY | | | | | | | | | | |
| TOTAL | 632 00 | | | | | | | | | |
| LESS: CONTRA | | | | | | | | | | |
| REMAINDER | 622 00 | TOTALS FOR TODAY | | 116 00 | 112 00 | 35 00 | 116 00 | 175 00 | 23 00 | 10 00 | 212 00 |
| LESS BANK DEPOSIT | 300 00 | TOTALS FROM BOTTOM LINE OF PRECEDING PAGE | | 1561 00 | 74 00 | 1270 00 | 875 00 | 905 00 | 180 00 | 5400 00 |
| BALANCE ON HAND (COUNTED AND PROVED) | 322 00 | GRAND TOTALS FOR THIS MONTH — TO DATE | | 1613 00 | 114 00 | 1400 00 | 1050 00 | 928 00 | 190 00 | 5612 00 |

FORM 300—CALIFORNIA PROFESSIONAL BUREAU—L.A.

**Figure 18–4** Daily record of charges and payments.

The total of the column "*Receipts from Patients*" is entered on the next line. If there are receipts from other sources these are entered next. Then the beginning balance plus receipts from all sources are totaled.

The next item "*Less: Contra*" is seldom used. A contra account is an account which is subtracted from a second account to show the proper net amount for the items recorded in the second account. In this instance it is provided as a means of accounting for money that has been taken out of the cashbox and used for some purpose other than that expended from the bank account or petty cash.

CODES FOR BOOKKEEPING

| | | | |
|---|---|---|---|
| R | residence call | Urn | urinalysis |
| H | hospital call | BMR | basal metabolic rate |
| oc | office call | EKG | electrocardiogram |
| S | surgical | Smr | smear |
| lab | laboratory | inj | injection |
| ph. ex. | physical exam | Del | Delivery OB |
| OB | obstetrical | Wr | Wasserman |
| X | X-ray | Drs | dressing |
| CBC | complete blood count | P. Op. | postoperative |
| def | charge deferred | I/f | In full |
| — | charge already made | M.O. | money order |
| n/c | no charge | Ex. M.O. | express money order |
| ↩ | no balance due | Ins | insurance case |
| c/a | cash on account | Cr | credit |
| ck | check | Dr | debit |

When you have determined the total to be accounted for, subtract the amount of today's bank deposit. The final figure will be the balance on hand at the end of the day. This must agree with the total amount of cash and checks (by actual count) in your cashbox. This final figure is carried forward as the beginning figure for the following day.

**Receipts from Other Sources.**  This is a record of money received from sources other than the practice of medicine, such as dividends, interest, or rent from property owned. There should be a full description of the source of this money, and the balance should be carried forward each day. This money may or may not be shown in the daily proof of cash, depending upon the policy of the office. If the money is kept in a separate bank account, it should not be recorded in the Daily Proof of Cash.

**Totals for Today.**  Review each day carefully before totals are carried down to the line marked "*Totals for Today*" and be very careful to stay in the correct column. Entering a figure in a wrong column is a common cause of bookkeeping errors.

**Totals from Preceding Page.**  Bring the "*Grand Totals*" over from the bottom of the preceding page and enter them on the line marked "*Totals from bottom line of preceding page.*"

**Grand Totals to Date.**  Add the amounts under "*Totals for Today*" and "*Totals from Preceding Page*" to determine "*Grand Totals for this Month—to Date.*" This shows the doctor, at any time during the current month, what he has earned to date and how much has been collected to date.

**Deposits.**  The amount of each bank deposit will be recorded in three places: in the daily proof of cash; in the check register section of the record; and on a stub in the checkbook.

**Daily Posting.**  At the far right of the daily journal page is a narrow column with a checkmark (✔) at the top. When the financial information is posted to the patient's ledger, a small ✔ is placed in this column to confirm that the account has been posted.

**Patient's Ledger or Financial Record.** An individual account record must be kept for each patient whom the doctor treats. While some offices include all members of a family on one financial card, it is generally considered preferable to have separate records for each patient. Several types of ledger cards are shown in Figure 18–5. Note that each card shows the date of service, what service was rendered, the charge and payment if any, and any remaining balance.

The personal information on the card is obtained from the patient at the time of his first visit. When the patient's medical history form is prepared, the financial history form is also readied. Entries on the patient ledger are made from information recorded in the *daily journal.* Under no circumstance is the information recorded directly to the ledger.

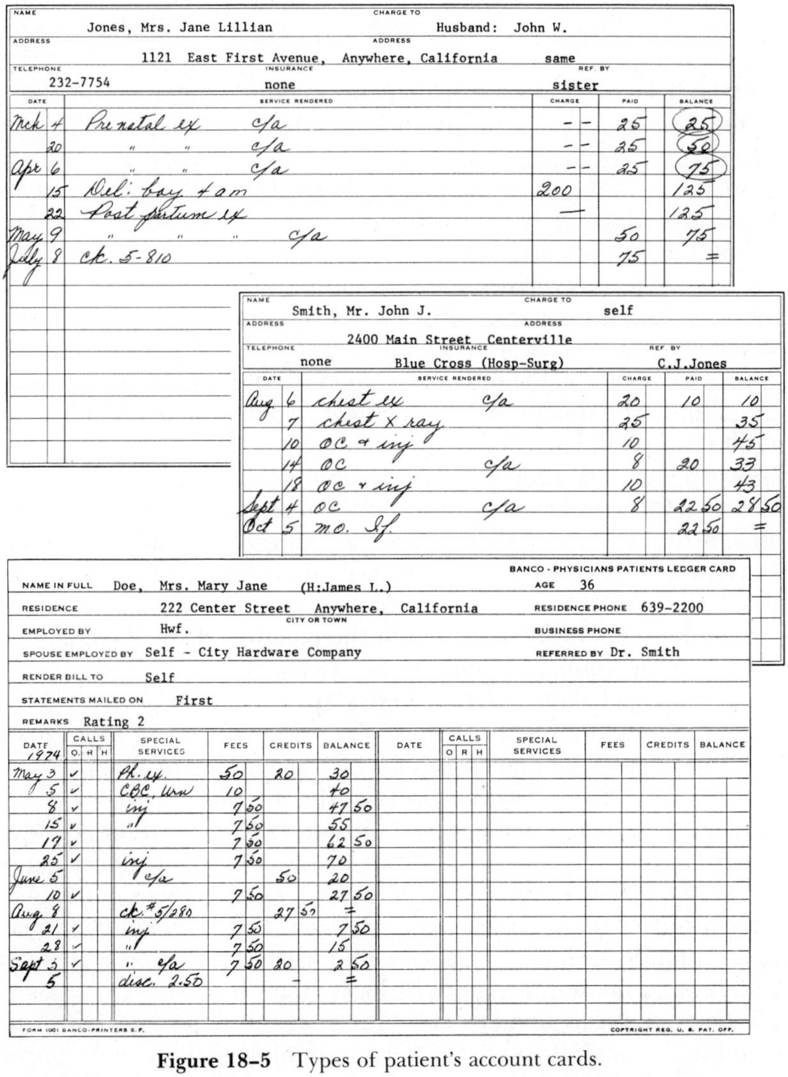

NAME: Jones, Mrs. Jane Lillian — CHARGE TO: Husband: John W.
ADDRESS: 1121 East First Avenue, Anywhere, California — ADDRESS: same
TELEPHONE: 232-7754 — INSURANCE: none — REF. BY: sister

| DATE | | SERVICE RENDERED | CHARGE | PAID | BALANCE |
|---|---|---|---|---|---|
| Mch | 4 | Prenatal ex c/a | -- | 25 | 25 |
| | 20 | " " c/a | -- | 25 | 50 |
| Apr | 6 | " " c/a | -- | 25 | 75 |
| | 15 | Del: boy 4 am | 200 | | 125 |
| | 22 | Post partum ex | — | | 125 |
| May | 9 | " " " c/a | | 50 | 75 |
| July | 8 | ck. 5-810 | | 75 | = |

NAME: Smith, Mr. John J. — CHARGE TO: self
ADDRESS: 2400 Main Street Centerville — ADDRESS:
TELEPHONE: none — INSURANCE: Blue Cross (Hosp-Surg) — REF BY: C.J.Jones

| DATE | | SERVICE RENDERED | CHARGE | PAID | BALANCE |
|---|---|---|---|---|---|
| Aug | 6 | chest ex c/a | 20 | 10 | 10 |
| | 7 | chest X ray | 25 | | 35 |
| | 10 | OC + inj | 10 | | 45 |
| | 14 | OC c/a | 8 | 20 | 33 |
| | 18 | OC + inj | 10 | | 43 |
| Sept | 4 | OC c/a | 8 | 22 50 | 28 50 |
| Oct | 5 | mo. Sf. | | 22 50 | = |

BANCO - PHYSICIANS PATIENTS LEDGER CARD
NAME IN FULL: Doe, Mrs. Mary Jane (H:James L.) — AGE: 36
RESIDENCE: 222 Center Street Anywhere, California (CITY OR TOWN) — RESIDENCE PHONE: 639-2200
EMPLOYED BY: Hwf. — BUSINESS PHONE:
SPOUSE EMPLOYED BY: Self - City Hardware Company — REFERRED BY: Dr. Smith
RENDER BILL TO: Self
STATEMENTS MAILED ON: First
REMARKS: Rating 2

| DATE 1974 | | CALLS O | R | H | SPECIAL SERVICES | FEES | CREDITS | BALANCE | DATE | CALLS O | R | H | SPECIAL SERVICES | FEES | CREDITS | BALANCE |
|---|---|---|---|---|---|---|---|---|---|---|---|---|---|---|---|---|
| May | 3 | ✓ | | | Ph. ex. | 50 | 20 | 30 | | | | | | | | |
| | 5 | ✓ | | | CBC, Urn | 10 | | 40 | | | | | | | | |
| | 8 | ✓ | | | inj | 7 50 | | 47 50 | | | | | | | | |
| | 15 | ✓ | | | " | 7 50 | | 55 | | | | | | | | |
| | 17 | ✓ | | | | 7 50 | | 62 50 | | | | | | | | |
| | 25 | ✓ | | | inj | 7 50 | | 70 | | | | | | | | |
| June | 5 | | | | c/a | | 50 | 20 | | | | | | | | |
| | 10 | ✓ | | | | 7 50 | | 27 50 | | | | | | | | |
| Aug. | 8 | | | | ck. #5/280 | | 27 50 | = | | | | | | | | |
| | 21 | ✓ | | | inj | 7 50 | | 7 50 | | | | | | | | |
| | 28 | ✓ | | | " | 7 50 | | 15 | | | | | | | | |
| Sept | 5 | ✓ | | | " c/a | 7 50 | 20 | 2 50 | | | | | | | | |
| | 5 | | | | disc. 2.50 | | – | = | | | | | | | | |

FORM 1001 BANCO-PRINTERS S.F. — COPYRIGHT REG. U. S. PAT. OFF.

**Figure 18–5** Types of patient's account cards.

There should always be at least three columns for recording figures on the patient ledger. Starting at the left,

> Column 1 is used for entering the fee for service,
> Column 2 is used for entering payments received, and
> Column 3 is used for recording the difference between
>> column 1 and column 2 (account balance).

**Terminology of Accounts.**   You will notice a diversity of terms in the column headings on patient ledger/account cards.

The *left* side of any account is the *debit* side (abbreviation "Dr."). This is column 1 referred to in the explanation above. It is sometimes designated "charge" or "fees."

The right side of any account is the *credit* side (abbreviation "Cr."). This is column 2 described above, and is sometimes headed "paid."

The last column on the right, column 3, is the *balance* of the account.

There may be a fourth column headed "Discounts" or "Adjustments." This would be used to show professional discounts, write-offs, disallowances by insurance carriers, and so forth.

**Account Balance.**   The balance of any account is the difference between the total debits and the total credits to the account. The balance is normally a *debit balance* (charges exceed payments). The account for the patient who pays in advance, for instance in obstetrical care, will have a *credit balance* (payments exceed charges). A debit balance is shown by simply writing the proper figure in the balance column. A credit balance is shown in one of two ways: by writing the credit entry on the card in regular ink and enclosing the figure in parentheses or encircling it; or by writing the credit entry in red ink.

**Discounts.**   Discounts are also credit entries. If there is no adjustment column as described above, the discount is entered with red ink or in parentheses in the *debit* column. By doing this, it is in effect a subtraction from the charges and will not be confused with money received.

**Trial Balance.**   A trial balance should be done at least once a month, preferably before preparing the monthly statements. The trial balance will disclose any discrepancies between the daily journal and the ledger. It does not, however, prove the accuracy of the accounts. For instance, if a charge or payment were posted to the wrong account, or if the wrong amount were entered in the journal and then posted to the patient ledger, the totals would still "balance" but the accounts would not be accurate.

To take a trial balance, follow these steps:

> 1. determine total charges for month
> 2. add the total outstanding at beginning of month
> 3. subtract total receipts for the month

The remainder is the new total of your outstanding accounts, or accounts receivable, and should equal the total of all the balances on the patients' ledger cards. In adding the balances on the patient ledger cards, be sure to *subtract* any numbers in red ink or enclosed in parentheses. If the total of your trial balance equals the total of the ledger balances, your accounts are said to be *in balance*. If the two totals do not agree, you must locate the error.

**Locating and Preventing Errors.**   First find the difference between the two totals, and then search through the ledger accounts and the daily journal for an entry of the identical amount. Check each one you find to see whether it was posted correctly.

If the amount of the error is divisible by 9 you may have transposed a figure. For instance, if the difference is $81, a number divisible by nine, you may find you wrote $209 instead of $290.

If the amount is divisible by 2 you may have posted to the wrong column, that is, posted a debit in the credit column, or posted a credit in the debit column.

Still looking? Did you carry the wrong total forward from one day to the next? Did you *slide* a number? That is, write the initial figure in the wrong column, such as writing 400 for 40, or writing 60 for 600.

Many bookkeepers avoid errors in the cents column by using a line (-) instead of writing 2 zeros when only even dollars are involved. For instance, instead of writing $12.00, the bookkeeper will write $12-. This eliminates the possibility of misreading zeros as other numbers. It also speeds the adding process when columns must be totaled.

**Summary Pages.** In addition to the monthly disbursements pages, most bookkeeping systems include forms for recording payroll deductions and taxes, reconciliation of accounts receivable, and monthly and annual analysis of income and disbursements.

If the accounts are faithfully kept each day and transferred to the monthly summary, then the monthly totals transferred to the annual summary, your financial recordkeeping can be gratifyingly simple.

## Bookkeeping Machines

In larger medical offices and clinics, bookkeeping machines are sometimes used. These automatic accounting machines prepare the patient ledger, the patient statement, and the journal record simultaneously. The medical assistant who must learn to use one of these machines can always secure instructions on how to operate it from the manufacturer.

## Automated Billing Services

In the more metropolitan areas, there is a moderate trend toward using automated billing services, with all accounting for receivables being handled by a service bureau. An automated system can relieve the office staff of the time-consuming repetitive procedures necessary in the recording of charges and in the preparation and mailing of statements, freeing the assistant for more tasks that require her administrative and clinical capabilities.

At the patient's first visit a Patient Master Card is completed and filed with the service bureau. This card provides the basic information that will be needed in future accounting services involving this patient. At the time of each visit a specially coded charge slip is completed for each patient and given to the service bureau. The charge slip includes the date, service rendered, procedure code number, charge, and diagnosis. The service bureau may provide for daily

A-1 Office Equipment

| PATIENT NAME | | PRACTICE NO. **V00101** | VISIT SLIP NO. **151518** | 1 |
|---|---|---|---|---|
| DR. NO. | DATE | ACCOUNT NO. | RECALL M O S / MSG | REMARKS |

| DESCRIPTION | CODE | RVS-MOD | AMT. | DESCRIPTION | CODE | RVS-MOD | AMT. | DESCRIPTION | CODE | RVS-MOD | AMT. |
|---|---|---|---|---|---|---|---|---|---|---|---|
| OFFICE VISIT | 0101 | 90050 | 12\|00 | CHEMOTHERAPY CYT | 0301 | 96030 | | MONITORING | 0133 | 93260 | |
| INITIAL OFFICE VISIT | 0102 | 90010 | 20\|00 | CHEMO-5FU | 0302 | 96030 | | BONE MARROW | 0830 | 85100 | |
| OFFICE VISIT AND PELVIC | 0103 | 90060-22 | 15\|00 | CHEMO-MTX | 0303 | 96030 | | CHEST X-RAY 2 Views | 0701 | 71020 | 20\|00 |
| COMPLETE PHYSICAL NEW PATIENT | 0110 | 90020 | 50\|00 | CHEMO-VCR | 0304 | 96030 | | | | | |
| COMPLETE PHYSICAL EST. PATIENT | 0111 | 90080 | 40\|00 | CHEMO-VLB | 0305 | 96030 | | INFLUENZA IMMUNIZATION | 0170 | 90700 | 3\|00 |
| INSURANCE/SCHOOL PHYSICAL | 0112 | 90022 | 20\|00 | CHEMOTHERAPY | 03_ _ | 96030 | | TETANUS IMMUNIZATION | 0171 | 90700 | 3\|00 |
| | | | | SIGMOIDOSCOPY | 0401 | 45300 | 25\|00 | CHOLERA IMMUNIZATION | 0172 | 90700 | 3\|00 |
| CONSULTATION | 0115 | 90620 | 75\|00 | PAP SMEAR | 0870 | 99000 | 3\|00 | TYPHOID IMMUNIZATION | 0173 | 90700 | 3\|00 |
| CONSULTATION INTER-OFFICE | 0116 | 90610 | 25\|00 | | | | | SMALL POX IMMUNIZATION | 0174 | 90700 | 5\|00 |
| | | | | EKG | 0420 | 93000 | 20\|00 | B12 INJECTION | 0151 | 90705 | 3\|50 |
| EMERGENCY ROOM CARE | 0120 | 90550 10 20 | | PHONO-CARDIOGRAM | 0421 | 93205 | 40\|00 | DEMEROL INJECTION | 0152 | 90705 | 3\|00 |
| INITIAL HOSPITAL ADMIT E.P. | 0121 | 90215 | | VECTOR | 0422 | 93220 | 40\|00 | GOLD INJECTION | 0153 | 90705 | 4\|00 |
| HOSPITAL ADMIT. N.P. | | 90220 | | TREADMILL | 0423 | 93260 | | IMFERON INJECTION | 0154 | 90705 | 4\|00 |
| HOSPITAL CARE | 0122 | 90250 | | | | | | PREMARIN INJECTION | 0155 | 90705 | 5\|00 |
| REST HOME CARE | 0124 | 90350 10 12 | | CARDIOVERSION | 0424 | 96020 | 100\|00 | ARTHROCENTESIS | 0156 | 20610 | |
| DETENTION TIME | 0130 | 99040 | | PULMONARY FUNCTION | 0429 | 94060 | 50\|00 | THERAPEUTIC INJECTION | 0150 | 90705 | |

| DESCRIPTION | CODE | RVS-MOD | EXTENDED DESCRIPTION (25) | LAB | AMOUNT LAB CHARGES | AMOUNT |
|---|---|---|---|---|---|---|
| HOSPITAL VISITS FROM | 0010 | 90250 | | | | |

SKIP 7 | ADM / / DISCH / / | DISABILITY/CONFINEMENT FROM / / TO / / | HOSPITAL NAME OR NUMBER ST. J FCH 01□ 02□

ACTION: P = PERMANENT   T = TEMPORARY        TYPE: 1 = PRIMARY   2 = SECONDARY   P = POSSIBLE   R = RULE OUT

| ACTION | TYPE | DIAGNOSIS | ACTION | TYPE | DIAGNOSIS | ACTION | TYPE | DIAGNOSIS | ACTION | TYPE | DIAGNOSIS |
|---|---|---|---|---|---|---|---|---|---|---|---|
| P T / P R | 1 2 | 4129 A.S.H.D. | P T / P R | 1 2 | 5621 Diverticulosis | P T / P R | 1 2 | 2440 Hypothyroidism | P T / P R | 1 2 | 7123 Rheumatoid Arthritis |
| P T / P R | 1 2 | 6000 Benign Prostatic Hypertrophy | P T / P R | 1 2 | 4920 Emphysema | P T / P R | 1 2 | 2800 Iron Deficiency Anemia | P T / P R | 1 2 | 5030 Sinusitis |
| P T / P R | 1 2 | 4900 Bronchitis | P T / P R | 1 2 | 5350 Gastritis and Duodenitis | P T / P R | 1 2 | 5641 Irritable Colon | P T / P R | 1 2 | 4519 Thrombophlebitis |
| P T / P R | 1 2 | 4279 Cardiac Arrhythmia | P T / P R | 1 2 | 4550 Hemorrhoids | P T / P R | 1 2 | 3840 Labyrinthitis | P T / P R | 1 2 | 4650 Upper Resp. Infection |
| P T / P R | 1 2 | 4370 Cerebrovascular Insufficiency | P T / P R | 1 2 | 5513 Hiatal Hernia | P T / P R | 1 2 | 6270 Menopausal Syndrome | P T / P R | 1 2 | 5990 Urinary Tract Infection |
| P T / P R | 1 2 | 7837 Chest Wall Pain | P T / P R | 1 2 | 2790 Hypercholesterolemia | P T / P R | 1 2 | 7130 Osteoarthritis | P T / P R | 1 2 | 4549 Varicose Veins |
| P T / P R | 1 2 | 6100 Cystic Mastitis | P T / P R | 1 2 | 4010 Hypertension | P T / P R | 1 2 | 5339 Peptic Ulcer | P T / P R | 1 2 | 0088 Viral Enteritis |
| P T / P R | 1 2 | 2509 Diabetes Mellitus | P T / P R | 1 2 | 3052 Hyperventilation | P T / P R | 1 2 | 3919 Rheumatic Heart Disease | | | |

ACTION _____ TYPE _____

SDC COPY

OFFICE

**Figure 18–6**   Charge slip used in automated billing.

pickup, or the information may be mailed or relayed electronically to the service bureau, where it is keypunched for storage in the computer. The service bureau, in addition to regular billing and preparation of insurance forms, can give the doctor almost any type of management report he wants, for instance

> Historical and financial account ledger for each patient
> Accounts receivable and collection report
> Daily transaction journal
> Monthly age analysis printout

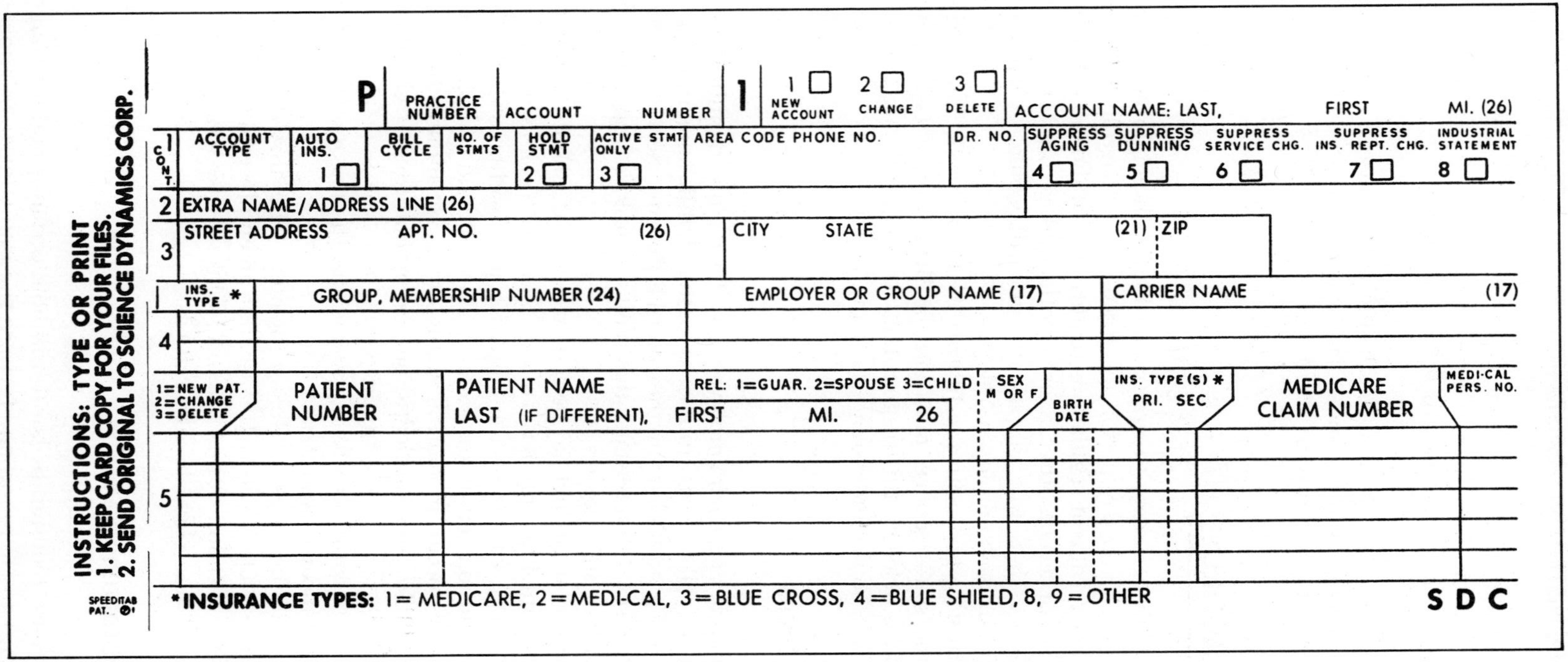
INSTRUCTIONS: TYPE OR PRINT
1. KEEP CARD COPY FOR YOUR FILES.
2. SEND ORIGINAL TO SCIENCE DYNAMICS CORP.

P PRACTICE NUMBER | ACCOUNT NUMBER | 1 | 1 ☐ NEW ACCOUNT | 2 ☐ CHANGE | 3 ☐ DELETE | ACCOUNT NAME: LAST, FIRST MI. (26)

1 CONT. | ACCOUNT TYPE | AUTO INS. 1 ☐ | BILL CYCLE | NO. OF STMTS | HOLD STMT 2 ☐ | ACTIVE STMT ONLY 3 ☐ | AREA CODE PHONE NO. | DR. NO. | SUPPRESS AGING 4 ☐ | SUPPRESS DUNNING 5 ☐ | SUPPRESS SERVICE CHG. 6 ☐ | SUPPRESS INS. REPT. CHG. 7 ☐ | INDUSTRIAL STATEMENT 8 ☐

2 EXTRA NAME/ADDRESS LINE (26)

3 STREET ADDRESS APT. NO. (26) | CITY STATE (21) | ZIP

4 INS. TYPE * | GROUP, MEMBERSHIP NUMBER (24) | EMPLOYER OR GROUP NAME (17) | CARRIER NAME (17)

5 1=NEW PAT. 2=CHANGE 3=DELETE | PATIENT NUMBER | PATIENT NAME LAST (IF DIFFERENT), FIRST MI. 26 | REL: 1=GUAR. 2=SPOUSE 3=CHILD | SEX M OR F | BIRTH DATE | INS. TYPE (S) * PRI. SEC | MEDICARE CLAIM NUMBER | MEDI-CAL PERS. NO.

SPEEDITAB PAT. ©

*INSURANCE TYPES: 1 = MEDICARE, 2 = MEDI-CAL, 3 = BLUE CROSS, 4 = BLUE SHIELD, 8, 9 = OTHER

S D C

**Figure 18–7** Patient master card for automated billing.

Summary of daily transactions
Summary of accounts receivable
Categorized summary of services rendered

The monthly statements can be mailed by the service bureau or returned to the doctor's office for mailing. Insurance forms would be returned to the physician's office for review and signature by the doctor.

## PAYROLL RECORDS

If it were only necessary to write a check to each employee for the agreed upon salary for a given pay period, no discussion of payroll records would be necessary. But government regulations require the withholding of income taxes and the payment of certain other taxes by both employee and employer. A form similar to Figure 18–8 will simplify the recordkeeping. A separate record should be kept for each employee.

Reports must be filed with the Internal Revenue Service quarterly and annually. In some states reports must also be filed with a State agency. Many physicians' offices delegate this responsibility to an outside accountant, but the medical assistant should understand the requirements.

### Preliminary Steps

Each employee and each employer must have a tax identification number. The employee's social security number is his tax identification number. The employer applies for a number from the Internal Revenue Service for federal tax accounting purposes. In those states that require employer reports, he must also apply to the proper state agency.

Before the end of the first pay period the employee should complete an Employee's Withholding Exemption Certificate (Form W-4), showing the number of exemptions claimed. Otherwise the employer must withhold on the basis of a single person with no exemptions. The employee should complete a new form whenever changes occur in marital status or in the number of exemptions claimed. Each employee is entitled to one exemption for herself and one each for other qualified relatives she supports. She may elect to take no exemptions. In this case the tax withheld will be greater and she may qualify for a refund when her annual income tax report is filed.

A supply of all the necessary forms for filing federal returns, preinscribed with the employer's name, will be furnished to an employer if he has applied for an employer identification number. Extra forms may be obtained from the Internal Revenue Office where he files returns.

### Withholding Income Tax

Employers are required by law to withhold certain amounts from their employee's earnings and to report and forward these amounts to be applied toward

(*Text continued on page 280.*)

Name    Dow, Jane      M D W S

Street    456 Main Street

City    East Harbor    Zip 01234

Telephone Number   000-0000

Date Employed   January 1, 1974

Soc. Sec. No.   123-45-6789

No. Exemptions   1

| Pay Period Ending | Gross Wages | DEDUCTIONS Withholding Tax | Employee F.I.C.A. | | | | Net Paid | Employer Taxes F.I.C.A. | F.U.T.A. |
|---|---|---|---|---|---|---|---|---|---|
| 01/31/74 | 500.- | 74.80 | 29.25 | | | | 395.95 | 29.25 | |
| 02/28/74 | 500.- | 74.80 | 29.25 | | | | 395.95 | 29.25 | |

**Figure 18-8**   Payroll register.

☆U.S GOVERNMENT PRINTING OFFICE: 1973 —492 - 951

FOR CLEAR COPY ON ALL PARTS TYPEWRITE OR PRINT WITH BALL-POINT PEN—PRESS FIRMLY
(See Instructions on Reverse)

FORM SS-4 (3-69)

**PART 1**

U.S. TREASURY DEPARTMENT—INTERNAL REVENUE SERVICE
**APPLICATION FOR EMPLOYER IDENTIFICATION NUMBER**

1. NAME *(TRUE name as distinguished from TRADE name.)*

2. TRADE NAME, IF ANY *(Enter name under which business is operated, if different from item 1.)*

3. ADDRESS OF PRINCIPAL PLACE OF BUSINESS *(No. and Street, City, State, Zip Code)*

4. COUNTY OF BUSINESS LOCATION

5. ORGANIZATION Check Type — Individual, Governmental (See Instr. 5), Partnership, Nonprofit Organization (See Instr. 5), Corporation, Other *(specify e.g. estate, trust, etc.)*

6. Ending Month of Accounting year

7. REASON FOR APPLYING *(If "other" specify such as "Corporate structure change," "Acquired by gift or trust," etc.)* Started new business, Purchased going business, Other

8. Date you acquired or started business *(Mo. day, year)*

9. First date you paid or will pay wages *(Mo., day, year)*

10. NATURE OF BUSINESS *(See Instructions)*

11. NUMBER OF EMPLOYEES IF "NONE" ENTER "O" — Non-agricultural, Agricultural

12. If nature of business is MANUFACTURING, list in order of their importance the principal products manufactured and the estimated percentage of the total value of all products which each represents.

A ___ %
B ___ %   C ___ %

PLEASE LEAVE BLANK — R | DO | TA | FR | FRC

13. Do you operate more than one place of business? Yes / No
If "Yes, attach a list showing for each separate establishment:
a. Name and address.   b. Nature of business   c. Number of employees.

14. To whom do you sell most of your products or services? Business establishments, General public, Other *(Specify)*

PLEASE LEAVE BLANK → Geo. | Ind. | Class | Size | Reas. for Appl. | Bus. Bir. Date

FORM SS-4 (3-69)
**PART 2**

DO NOT DETACH ANY PART OF THIS FORM. SEND ALL COPIES TO
**INTERNAL REVENUE SERVICE**

PLEASE LEAVE BLANK

NAME AND COMPLETE ADDRESS

1. Name *(TRUE name as distinguished from TRADE name.)*

2. TRADE NAME, IF ANY *(Enter name under which business is operated, if different from item 1.)*

3. ADDRESS OF PRINCIPAL PLACE OF BUSINESS *(No. and Street)*

*(City, State, Zip Code)*

4. COUNTY OF BUSINESS LOCATION

5. ORGANIZATION Check Type — Individual, Governmental (See Instr. 5), Partnership, Nonprofit Organization (See Instr. 5), Corporation, Other *(specify e.g. estate, trust, etc.)*

6. Ending Month of Accounting year

7. REASON FOR APPLYING *(If "other" specify such as "Corporate structure change," "Acquired by gift or trust," etc.)* Started new business, Purchased going business, Other

8. Date you acquired or started business *(Mo. day, year)*

9. First date you paid or will pay wages *(Mo., day, year)*

10. NATURE OF BUSINESS *(See Instructions)*

11. NUMBER OF EMPLOYEES IF "NONE" ENTER "O" — Non-agricultural, Agricultural

12. Have you ever applied for an identification number for this or any other business? No / Yes
If "Yes," enter name and trade name (if any). Also enter the approximate date, city, and state where you first applied and previous number if known. →

DATE | SIGNATURE | TITLE

**Figure 18–9**  Employer's application for identification number.

# Employee's Withholding Allowance Certificate

The explanatory material below will help you determine your correct number of withholding allowances, and will indicate whether you should complete the new Form W—4 at the bottom of this page.

## How Many Withholding Allowances May You Claim?

Please use the schedule below to determine the number of allowances you may claim for tax withholding purposes. In determining the number, keep in mind these points: If you are single and hold more than one job, you may not claim the same allowances with more than one employer at the same time; If you are married and both you and your wife or husband are employed, you may not claim the same allowances with your employers at the same time. A nonresident alien other than a resident of Canada, Mexico or Puerto Rico may claim only one personal allowance.

## Figure Your Total Withholding Allowances Below

(a) Allowance for yourself—enter 1 . . . . . . . . . . . . . . . . . .    *1*

(b) Allowance for your wife (husband)—enter 1 . . . . . . . . . . . . .    *O*

(c) Allowance for your age—if 65 or over—enter 1 . . . . . . . . . . .    *O*

(d) Allowance for your wife's (husband's) age—if 65 or over—enter 1 . . . . . . . . . .    *O*

(e) Allowance for blindness (yourself)—enter 1 . . . . . . . . . . .    *O*

(f) Allowance for blindness (wife or husband)—enter 1 . . . . . . . . . .    *O*

(g) Allowance(s) for dependent(s)—you are entitled to claim an allowance for each dependent you will be able to claim on your Federal income tax return. Do not include yourself or your wife (husband)* . . . . . .

(h) Special withholding allowance—if you have only one job, and do not have a wife or husband who works— enter 1 . . . . . . . . . . . . . . . . . . . . . .    *O*

(i) Total—add lines (a) through (h) above . . . . . . . . . . . . . .    *1*

*If you do not plan to itemize deductions on your income tax return, enter the number shown on line (i) on line 1, Form W—4 below. Skip lines (j) and (k).*

(j) Allowance(s) for itemized deductions—If you do plan to itemize deductions on your income tax return, enter the number from line 5 of worksheet on back . . . . . . . . . . . . . .    *O*

(k) Total—add lines (i) and (j) above. Enter here and on line 1, Form W—4 below . . . . . . . . . .    *1*

*If you are in doubt as to whom you may claim as a dependent, see the instructions which came with your last Federal income tax return or call your local Internal Revenue Service office.*

## See Table and Worksheet on Back if You Plan to Itemize Your Deductions

### Completing New Form W—4

If you find that you are entitled to one or more allowances in addition to those which you are now claiming, please increase your number of allowances by completing the form below and filing with your employer. If the number of allowances you previously claimed decreases, you must file a new Form W—4 within 10 days. (Should you expect to owe more tax than will be withheld, you may use the same form to increase your withholding by claiming fewer or ''0'' allowances on line 1 or by asking for additional withholding on line 2 or both.)

▼ **Give the bottom part of this form to your employer; keep the upper part for your records and information** ▼

| Form **W-4**<br>(Rev. Aug. 1972)<br>Department of the Treasury<br>Internal Revenue Service | **Employee's Withholding Allowance Certificate**<br>(This certificate is for income tax withholding purposes<br>only; it will remain in effect until you change it.) | |
|---|---|---|
| Type or print your full name<br>ROE, MARY W. | | Your social security number<br>369 12 2468 |
| Home address (Number and street or rural route)<br>123 Main Street | | Marital status<br>☒ Single  ☐ Married |
| City or town, State and ZIP code<br>Anytown, California 90000 | | (If married but legally separated, or wife (husband) is a nonresident alien, check the single block.) |

1 Total number of allowances you are claiming . . . . . . . . . . . .    1

2 Additional amount, if any, you want deducted from each pay (if your employer agrees) . . . . . . . .    $ -

I certify that to the best of my knowledge and belief, the number of withholding allowances claimed on this certificate does not exceed the number to which I am entitled.

Signature ▶ *Mary W. Roe.*           Date ▶ July 1           , 19 73

**Figure 18–10**   Employee's withholding allowance certificate — Form W-4.

payment of income tax. The amount to be withheld is based on: (1) the total earnings of the employee; (2) the number of exemptions claimed; (3) the marital status of the employee; and (4) the length of the pay period involved. Federal Publication 15, Circular E—*Employer's Tax Guide*, includes tables to be used in determining the amount to be withheld. There are two types of tables: one for single persons and unmarried heads of households, and one for married persons. The tables cover monthly, semimonthly, biweekly, weekly, and daily or miscellaneous periods. Circular E also has tables for determining the F.I.C.A. taxes payable.

## F.I.C.A. Taxes

Taxes are imposed on employers and employees for old-age, survivors, and disability insurance benefits (O.A.S.D.I.) and health insurance for the aged (H.I.P.). Both of these taxes are covered under the Federal Insurance Contributions Act (F.I.C.A.). The rate is reviewed frequently and is subject to change by Congress. It is currently (1974) 5.85% on the first $12,000, with employee and employer each paying a like amount. The employee's 5.85% is withheld from salary; the employer's 5.85% is paid by the employer with the monthly federal tax deposit or with the quarterly report. It should be noted that the *total* F.I.C.A. tax on salaries paid is 11.70% of the first $12,000 paid to each employee.

## Deposit Requirements

Generally, the employer must deposit withholding and social security taxes with an authorized commercial bank or a Federal Reserve bank. Federal Tax Deposit Form 501, sometimes called a Depositary Receipt, must accompany each deposit.

The amount of taxes determines the frequency of the deposits. The rules are subject to change and are set forth on the reverse side of the Employer's Quarterly Federal Tax Return. In 1973 the regulations state:

1. If at the end of a *quarter* the total amount of undeposited taxes is less than $200, no deposit is required. The taxes may be paid directly to the Internal Revenue Service along with the quarterly Form 941.

2. If at the end of a *quarter* the total amount of undeposited taxes is $200 or more, the employer must deposit the entire amount on or before the last day of the first month after the end of the quarter. The required dates are April 30, July 31, October 31, January 31.

3. If at the end of any *month* (except the last month of a quarter) the cumulative amount of undeposited taxes for the quarter is $200 or more, the taxes must be deposited within 15 days after the end of the month.

## Quarterly Reports

The Employer's Quarterly Federal Tax Return (Form 941) must be filed by employers on or before the last day of the first month after the end of the

Form **941**
(Rev. Apr. 1973)
Department of the Treasury
Internal Revenue Service

## Employer's Quarterly Federal Tax Return

**SCHEDULE A**—Quarterly Report of Wages Taxable under the Federal Insurance Contributions Act—FOR SOCIAL SECURITY
IF WAGES WERE NOT TAXABLE UNDER THE FICA MAKE NO ENTRIES IN ITEMS 1 THROUGH 9 AND 14 THROUGH 18

| 1. (First quarter only) Number of employees (except household) employed in the pay period including March 12th ▶ | 2. Total pages of this return including this page and any pages of Form 941a ▶  1 | 3. Total number of employees listed ▶  2 |
| --- | --- | --- |

List for each nonagricultural employee the WAGES taxable under the FICA which were paid during the quarter. If you pay an employee more than $10,800 in a calendar year report only the first $10,800 of such wages. In the case of "Tip Income" see instructions on page 4.

Please report each employee's name and number exactly as shown on his Social Security card.

| 4. EMPLOYEE'S SOCIAL SECURITY NUMBER 000 00 0000 ▼ | 5. NAME OF EMPLOYEE (Please type or print) ▼ | 6. TAXABLE FICA WAGES Paid to Employee in Quarter (Before deductions) Dollars / Cents | 7. TAXABLE TIPS REPORTED (See page 4) If amounts in this column are not tips check here □ Dollars / Cents |
| --- | --- | --- | --- |
| 369  12  2468 | Mary W. Roe | 1500  00 | |
| 258  34  1357 | Jane U. Doe | 500  00 | |

If you need more space for listing employees, use Schedule A continuation sheets, Form 941a.
Totals for this page—Wage total in column 6 and tip total in column 7 ▶  | 2000  00 |

**8. TOTAL WAGES** TAXABLE UNDER FICA PAID DURING QUARTER.
(Total of column 6 on this page and continuation sheets.) Enter here and in Item 14 below . . . $ ............  2000  00

**9. TOTAL TAXABLE TIPS** REPORTED UNDER FICA DURING QUARTER.  (If no tips reported, write "None.")
(Total of column 7 on this page and continuation sheets.) Enter here and in Item 15 below . . . . . . . . ▶  $ none

Employer's name, address, employer identification number, and calendar quarter.
(If not correct, please change)

☐ Name (as distinguished from trade name)  Date quarter ended  September 30, 1973

Trade name, if any  ▶ Community Health Care Center   Employer Identification No.  97 0343652

Address and ZIP code  49015 East Cherry St., Long Beach, Ca  90808
........Entries must be made both above and below this line; if address different from previous return check here ☐ ............

Name (as distinguished from trade name)  Date quarter ended  September 30, 1973

Trade name, if any  ▶ Community Health Care Center   Employer Identification No.  97 0343652

Address and ZIP code  49015 East Cherry St., Long Beach, CA  90808

| | T | | FP |
| --- | --- | --- | --- |
| | FF | | I |
| | FD | | TOT |

| | | |
| --- | --- | --- |
| 10. TOTAL WAGES AND TIPS SUBJECT TO WITHHOLDING PLUS OTHER COMPENSATION . . . . . . . . . . . ▶ | 2,000 | 00 |
| 11. AMOUNT OF INCOME TAX WITHHELD FROM WAGES, TIPS, ANNUITIES, etc. (See instructions) . . . . . . . . . . . . . | 317 | 90 |
| 12. ADJUSTMENT FOR PRECEDING QUARTERS OF CALENDAR YEAR . . . . . . . . . . . . . . . . . . . | -0- | |
| 13. ADJUSTED TOTAL OF INCOME TAX WITHHELD . . . . . . . . . . . . . . . . . . . . . . . ▶ | 317 | 90 |
| 14. TAXABLE FICA WAGES PAID (Item 8) . . . . . . . . . $ 2,000 ............ multiplied by 11.7%=TAX | 234 | 00 |
| 15. TAXABLE TIPS REPORTED (Item 9) . . . . . . . . . . $ -0- ............ multiplied by 5.85%=TAX | -0- | |
| 16. TOTAL FICA TAXES (Item 14 plus Item 15) . . . . . . . . . . . . . . . . . . . . . . . . ▶ | 234 | 00 |
| 17. ADJUSTMENT (See Instructions) . . . . . . . . . . . . . . . . . . . . . . . . . . . . | -0- | |
| 18. ADJUSTED TOTAL OF FICA TAXES . . . . . . . . . . . . . . . . . . . . . . . . . . . ▶ | 234 | 00 |
| 19. TOTAL TAXES (Item 13 plus Item 18) . . . . . . . . . . . . . . . . . . . . . . . . . . | 551 | 00 |
| 20. TOTAL DEPOSITS FOR QUARTER (INCLUDING FINAL DEPOSIT MADE FOR QUARTER) AND OVERPAYMENT FROM PREVIOUS QUARTER LIST IN SCHEDULE B (See instructions on page 4) . . . . . . . . . . . . . . . . . . . . . | 368 | 60 |

**Note:** If undeposited taxes at the end of the quarter are $200 or more, the full amount must be deposited with an authorized commercial bank or a Federal Reserve bank. This deposit must be entered in Schedule B and included in Item 20.

| | | |
| --- | --- | --- |
| 21. UNDEPOSITED TAXES DUE (ITEM 19 LESS ITEM 20—THIS SHOULD BE LESS THAN $200 ). PAY TO INTERNAL REVENUE SERVICE AND ENTER HERE . . . . . . . . . . . . . . . . . . . . . . . . . . . . . . ▶ | 183 | 30 |

22. IF ITEM 20 IS MORE THAN ITEM 19, ENTER EXCESS HERE ▶ $ ____  AND CHECK IF YOU WANT IT ☐ APPLIED TO NEXT RETURN, OR ☐ REFUNDED.

23. If not liable for returns in succeeding quarters write "FINAL" here ▶ ____  and enter date of final payment of taxable wages here ▶

Under penalties of perjury, I declare that I have examined this return, including accompanying schedules and statements, and to the best of my knowledge and belief it is true, correct and complete.

Date  October 31, 1973   Signature  R. Williams   Title (Owner, etc.)  Business Manager

**Figure 18–11**

quarter. The return must show the number of employees, the names of all employees with their social security numbers, the total wages paid, the amount of withholding tax, the amount of wages subject to F.I.C.A., the F.I.C.A. taxes paid, the total deposits for the quarter, and any undeposited taxes due.

## Annual Reports

**Form W-2,** Wage and Tax Statement, must be furnished by the end of January to all employees of record at the close of December. If employment is terminated prior to December 31, the statement should be furnished within 30 days after the last payment of wages. The employee gets two copies, the employer keeps one, and the original is sent to the Internal Revenue Service.

**Form W-3,** Transmittal of Wage and Tax Statements, is the transmittal document for the originals of W-2, and must be filed on or before February 28. It may be filed along with the fourth quarter Form 941.

## Federal Unemployment Tax

If an employer paid wages of $1500 or more in any calendar quarter, or had one or more employees for some portion of at least one day during each of 20 different calendar weeks, he is subject to Federal Unemployment Tax.

The Federal Unemployment Tax is imposed on the employer; it must not be collected or deducted from the wages of the employee. The rate is 3.28% on the first $4200 of wages paid to each employee during the calendar year. The employer may receive credit for up to 2.7% of the wages for State Unemployment taxes he paid or for having been granted a favorable experience rate by the state. For this reason the net Federal liability may be as low as 0.58%.

**Federal Unemployment Tax Deposits.** If the liability for undeposited Federal unemployment tax exceeds $100 for any calendar quarter and any preceding quarter, the employer must deposit the tax with an authorized commercial bank or a Federal Reserve bank within one month following the close of the quarter. The deposit must be accompanied by a Federal Unemployment Tax Deposit form (Form 508).

**Annual Return.** An annual return must be filed on Form 940 on or before January 31, following the close of the calendar year for which the tax is due. Any tax still due is payable with the return. Form 940 may be filed on or before February 10, following the close of the year if all required deposits were made timely and full payment of the tax due is deposited on or before January 31.

## State Unemployment Taxes

All of the states and the District of Columbia have unemployment compensation laws. In most states the tax is imposed only on the employer, but a few states require employers to withhold a percentage of wages for unemployment compensation benefits. An employer may be subject to Federal Unemployment tax and not subject to state unemployment tax. In some states, for instance, the

1

| Wage and Tax Statement 1973 | | |

COMMUNITY HEALTH CARE CENTER
49015 East Cherry Street
Long Beach, CA   90808    97 0343652
Type or print EMPLOYER'S Federal identifying number, name, address and ZIP code above.

| Employer's State identifying number | **Copy A** For Internal Revenue Service Center |

| FEDERAL INCOME TAX INFORMATION | | | SOCIAL SECURITY INFORMATION | | | STATE OR LOCAL INCOME TAX INFORMATION | | | | | |
|---|---|---|---|---|---|---|---|---|---|---|---|
| 1 Federal income tax withheld | 2 Wages, tips and other compensation | 3 FICA employee tax withheld | 4 Total FICA wages | | | 6 Tax withheld | 7 Wages paid | 8 Name | | | |
| 897.60 | 6,000.00 | 351.00 | 6,000.00 | | | | | | | | |

EMPLOYEE'S social security number ► 369 12 2468

| 5 Uncollected employee FICA tax on tips | 9 Tax withheld | 10 Wages paid | 11 Name |
|---|---|---|---|
| none | | | |

Mary W. Roe
123 Main Street
Anytown, CA   90000

| STATUS | OTHER INFORMATION (SEE CIRCULAR E) | |
|---|---|---|
| 1. Single 2. Married  1 | Cost of group term life insurance included in box 2 | Excludable sick pay included in box 2 |

If this is a corrected form, put an "X" to the right of the number in the upper left corner.

Type or print EMPLOYEE'S name, address and ZIP code above.

Form **W–2**    ☆ GPO: 1972—458-023 EI-36-2519832-8    Department of the Treasury—Internal Revenue Service

**A**

Form **W-3**
Department of the Treasury
Internal Revenue Service

**Transmittal of Income and Tax Statements**
(Magnetic tape filers: See the applicable Revenue Procedures regarding transmittal of returns on magnetic tape.)

1973

| Enter number of documents | Place an "X" in the proper box to identify type of document being transmitted | | | All documents are: Place an "X" in the proper boxes. (See Instructions.) | | | |
|---|---|---|---|---|---|---|---|
| | Form W–2 | Form W–2P | Form 1099R | Original | Corrected | With taxpayer identifying number | Without taxpayer identifying number |
| 2 | X | | | X | | | |

PAYER'S identifying number ►  97 0343652

Community Health Care Center
49015 East Cherry Street
Long Beach, CA   90808

Type or print PAYER'S name, address and ZIP code above.

Under penalties of perjury, I declare that I have examined this return, including accompanying documents and to the best of my knowledge and belief, it is true, correct, and complete. In the case of documents without recipients' identifying numbers I have complied with the requirements of the law by requesting such numbers from the recipients, but did not receive them; I assume full responsibility for the accuracy of Forms W–2 that reflect excludable sick pay.

Signature _Williams_    Title  Business Manager    Date  1/30/74

**B**

Please remove this strip at perforation before mailing.

**Figure 18–12**   *A*, W-2 Wage and tax statement. *B*, W-3 transmittal of income and tax statements.

employer with fewer than four employees is not subject to the state unemployment tax. The office assistant should check the requirements in her own state in regard to state unemployment taxes.

## State Disability Insurance

Some states require that employees be covered by disability or sick-pay insurance. The employer may be required to withhold a certain amount from the employee's salary to pay for this insurance. In California, for instance, the employee contributes one per cent of his income up to $8500.

## REFERENCES

Carson, A. B., Carlson, A. E., and M. E. Burnet, *Accounting Essentials for Career Secretaries*, 3rd Ed., Cincinnati, Ohio, South-Western Publishing Company, 1972
Publication 334, Tax Guide for Small Business 1973 Edition, Department of the Treasury, Internal Revenue Service

# Chapter 19

**BEHAVIORAL OBJECTIVES**

*The medical office assistant should be able to:*

Describe the general types of private health insurance plans on the market.

Contrast the principles of *group* and *individual* policies.

Compare the methods of payment under *indemnity* plans and *service benefit* plans.

Define common insurance terms.

Describe the benefits and limitations of government sponsored and mandated insurance plans.

Identify and abstract from the patient record the necessary information for completing insurance claim forms.

Expedite the logging and processing of insurance forms.

Minimize the rejection of insurance claims in the doctor's office.

# Accident and Health
# Insurance

Health insurance in the medical office is no longer a threat – it is a reality. It is a reality to be accepted with a positive viewpoint and good management. With few exceptions, the doctor in private practice receives a major share of his income from his patients' insurance benefits.

To suggest that you view the processing of insurance claims with enthusiasm would be unrealistic. You must, however, recognize the importance of medical insurance and be prepared to complete the claims cheerfully, accurately, and promptly, so that the doctor's fees can be collected.

## PRIVATE HEALTH INSURANCE

The Health Insurance Association of America estimated in 1970 that nearly 182 million persons were covered for hospital benefits under private health insurance and about 168 million were covered for surgical benefits. This is compared to 77 million with hospital coverage and 54 million with surgical coverage in 1950; and 130 million and 117 million, respectively, in 1960.

Benefit payments (excluding Blue Cross–Blue Shield, medical society sponsored plans, and all other independent plans) of 755 million dollars were made in 1950; this figure rose to 9.089 billion dollars in 1970. Total hospital, surgical, and medical care costs, including loss of income, paid to insured persons under age 65 in the United States in the year 1969 amounted to 14.267 billion dollars, according to data published by the United States Government.

**Purpose of Health Insurance.**   Voluntary health insurance is designed primarily for those who can take care of the costs of routine illnesses but to whom a major illness may prove a real financial burden. Practicality dictates insuring against only those risks that would result in a considerable financial loss. It would be impractical, for example, to insure against minor bills for preventive injections, periodic health examinations, and treatment of short-duration ailments such as colds. These should be considered a predictable expense in a family budget. Covering such items in an insurance program boosts administrative costs of the insurance plan out of proportion to the small benefits received.

Few insurance companies pay all expenses resulting from accident or illness. A 100 per cent payment would leave little or no inducement to the disabled employee to return to work. Since health and accident benefits are not subject to income tax, it actually would be more profitable for the patient to remain "sick" if full payment were made.

## Kinds of Policies

There are over 1200 voluntary insurance organizations, writing many different types of plans, in the United States. An individual may carry one type or a combination of policies. Health insurance may be purchased under an *individual* policy or a *group* policy. In 1970 about two-thirds of those insured by private insurance companies were enrolled in group policies, and about one-third had individual policies.

**Group Policies.**   Insurance written under a group policy covers a group of people under a master contract, which is generally issued to an employer for the benefit of the employees. Group coverage usually provides better benefits at lower premiums, and there is seldom a physical examination required for the enrollees. Each person in the group has the same coverage.

**Individual Policies.**   Some people who desire health insurance do not have access to a group policy. Most of the companies that write group plans also write individual policies. Although the premium for the individual will be higher, and in most cases the benefits will be less, health insurance is still a good investment for all.

## Types of Plans

There are several hundred private insurance companies offering both group and individual medical and hospital benefit coverage in this country today, as well as numerous local plans, including those sponsored by medical societies, by rural cooperative societies, labor unions, industries, and other organizations.

**Hospital Plan.**   Hospital coverage pays the cost of all or part of the insured's hospital room and board and special hospital services, such as x-ray and the use of special rooms (surgery, cystoscopic, intensive care, recovery, cast application, and so forth). Most plans cover in-hospital drugs. Many cover laboratory services, physical therapy, and blood transfusions. Hospital insurance policies generally set a specific maximum amount payable per day and a maximum number of days of hospital care to which a patient is entitled under the contract. Some insurance companies require that the hospital be an accredited or a licensed hospital. Most hospital plans *exclude* admission for diagnostic studies.

**Surgical Plan.**   Surgical coverage pays all or part of a patient's surgical expenses. Surgical contracts cover any incision or excision, removal of foreign bodies, aspirations, suturing, or reduction of fractures, in the hospital, office, or home. The insurer usually provides the subscriber with a list of benefits for various types of surgery and also sets maximum amounts payable.

**Medical Plan.**   Medical coverage pays the physician's fees that are nonsurgical, including hospital, home, and office visits (dependent upon the type of policy purchased), special laboratory fees, x-ray charges, pathology fees, and consultant fees. Some policies pay medical bills only while the patient is in the hospital (medical-while-hospitalized, M.W.H). They may pay *detention time;* that is, additional time spent treating a patient who is in critical condition. Policies may pay for a physician consultant when one is requested by the attending physician. Very few plans cover a routine physical examination when the patient does not have a specific complaint or illness.

**Major Medical Plan** (formerly called "catastrophic" coverage).   Major medical insurance provides protection against especially heavy medical bills resulting from catastrophic or prolonged illnesses, and is used as a supplement to basic medical care insurance or as a comprehensive, integrated program providing both basic and major medical protection, including charges for private duty nursing, drugs, and medical appliances. This kind of insurance grew out of the realization that it is not necessary to provide protection against small bills; it is the major medical expenses that constitute the real financial drain.

**Special Risk Insurance.**   Some persons also purchase special risk insurance to protect themselves in the event of a certain type of accident, such as automobile or airplane crashes, or for certain diseases, such as tuberculosis or cancer. There is usually a maximum payment.

**Loss of Income Protection.**   This protection provides weekly or monthly cash benefits to employed policyholders who become unable to work owing to an accident or illness. Many policies do not start payment until after a specified number of days or until a certain number of sick leave days are used. Payment is made directly to the patient and is intended to replace loss of income resulting from illness. It is not intended for payment of specific medical bills.

**Personal Accident Insurance.**   Policies can be secured which provide benefits for loss of time, death, loss of sight or limbs, and for costs of medical care needed as a result of accident only. This is a form of special risk insurance.

**Group Insurance — Accidental Death and Dismemberment.**   Many employers provide such insurance as part of their group insurance program for employees. Lump sums are paid in the event of loss of life, sight, or limb by accidental means.

**Liability Insurance.**   There are many types of liability insurance, including automobile, business, and residence liability policies. Such policies often include benefits for medical expenses payable to individuals who are injured in the insured person's home or car, without regard to the insured person's actual legal liability for the accident. (Professional liability insurance is covered in the chapter on Medicine and the Law.)

**Life Insurance.**   Sometimes the proceeds from life insurance are used to meet the expenses of the insured person's last illness. Some policies provide additional monthly cash benefits if the policyholder becomes permanently and totally disabled.

## The "Blue Plans"

**Blue Cross.**   In the early 1930's hospitals introduced Blue Cross plans to provide protection against *hospital* costs. In 1969 there were 80 local Blue Cross plans operating in the western hemisphere, including all states, the District of Columbia, Canada, Puerto Rico, and Jamaica.

**Blue Shield.** In 1939, state medical societies in California and Michigan began sponsoring health plans to provide *medical* and *surgical* services; these became known as Blue Shield plans. Other states soon followed and there are now more than 80 Blue Shield plans in the western hemisphere. These are sometimes called "the doctors' own plan" because each is sponsored or approved by a state or local medical society. The Blue Shield plans are coordinated by the National Association of Blue Shield Plans, which has headquarters in Chicago.

Blue Cross–Blue Shield operated as a combination plan, with Blue Cross providing hospital coverage in participating hospitals, and Blue Shield providing the medical and surgical coverage from member physicians. Through an evolutionary process, each of the Blue Plans began offering broader coverage, so that now many Blue Cross plans write medical and surgical insurance, as well as providing hospital coverage. Many Blue Shield plans now offer hospital insurance, as well as medical and surgical coverage. In other instances, the Blue Plans still complement each other.

Blue Cross benefits are normally paid to the provider of service. In some cases a check issued jointly to the provider and the insured is sent to the insured, who must then endorse and forward it to the provider.

Blue Shield makes direct payment to physician members. For services of a non-member physician the payment is sent to the subscriber.

## Foundations for Medical Care

A Foundation for Medical Care is a management system for community health services. It takes the form of an organization created by local physicians through their medical society and it concerns itself with the quality and cost of medical care. Under the Foundation concept the following procedure occurs:

*Insurance company* sells and negotiates the policy; collects the premiums; assumes all the risks; reimburses the Foundation for cost of the claims office;

*Foundation* sets policy standards; receives, processes, reviews and pays claims to doctors; sets maximum fees based on going fees in the area; elects doctor-members yearly; continually studies local medical-economic problems;

*Member doctors* agree to accept Foundation fees as full payment under Foundation-approved policies;

*Medical society* legally controls the Foundation; selects Foundation trustees;

*Patient* selects doctor of his own choice; patient, union or employer pays premium direct to insurance company; has certainty of coverage.

The Foundation for Medical Care originated in San Joaquin County, California, in 1954. Foundations now exist in more than 40 states. The American Association of Foundations for Medical Care was organized in 1970 with the avowed purpose of helping individual Foundations provide a better health care system for the American people.

## Payment of Benefits

Insurance benefits are paid in two different ways—through *indemnity* plans and through *service benefit* plans.

**Indemnity Plans.**   In indemnity plans the insuring company agrees to pay the patient a specific amount of money for a certain procedure or service. For example, the company agrees to pay up to $200 for an appendectomy, with no consideration for the time or complications of the surgery. Indemnity plans do not agree to pay for the complete services rendered. Many times there is a difference in the amount paid by the insurance company and the amount of the physician's regular fee. This type of plan takes the major expense out of medical bills and helps to keep the premiums down. It also discourages overuse of a policy. Indemnity payments are usually paid to the patient, who, in turn, pays the physician. When the patient purchases the policy he is given a "schedule of indemnities;" that is, specified amounts payable for specified procedures. The amount of the premium often determines the schedule of benefits.

**Service Benefit Plans.**   In service benefit plans the insuring company agrees to pay for certain surgical or medical services without additional cost to the insured. There is no set fee schedule. Service benefit plans are usually sponsored by medical societies or medical groups. In a service plan, an appendectomy with complications would warrant a higher surgical fee than a routine procedure. Premiums are sometimes higher for this type of coverage, but often payments are larger. Frequently the payments are sent directly to the physician and are considered full payment for the services rendered.


# GOVERNMENT SPONSORED PLANS
## Military Medical Benefits

The term *Medicare* first became an important word in the medical assistant's vocabulary in December, 1956, with the passage of Law 569, authorizing dependents of military personnel to receive treatment by civilian physicians at the expense of the government. This program was at first called Medicare but has since been changed to CHAMPUS (Civilian Health and Medical Program of the Uniformed Services).

On September 30, 1966, the Military Medical Benefits Amendment Act of 1966 became law. This act added outpatient care benefits, including prescription drugs, to the in-hospital benefits previously allowed. The patient pays an out-of-pocket deductible (now $50) each fiscal year (July 1 to June 30), plus 20 per cent of the balance.

Military retirees and their dependents, and dependents of deceased members became eligible for the same benefits in January, 1967, except that their co-payment amount is 25 per cent after the deductible.

The patient pays his share of the charges directly to the physician. This includes the deductible and the 20 per cent. The doctor collects the remainder from the government by filing Form 1863-2 (Fig. 19–1) with the fiscal agent. The patient or sponsor must complete Section I of the form. The doctor completes Section II, and must sign the form personally.

Since details of government sponsored programs are changed from time to time and are regulated by law, the medical assistant is urged to keep a copy of the latest official manual on hand and note any changes that occur.

**SERVICES AND/OR SUPPLIES PROVIDED BY CIVILIAN SOURCES (EXCEPT HOSPITALS)**
CIVILIAN HEALTH AND MEDICAL PROGRAM OF THE UNIFORMED SERVICES (CHAMPUS)
For use of this form, see AR 40-121; the proponent agency is the Office of The Surgeon General.

SEE INSTRUCTIONS ON REVERSE

**SECTION I** *(To be completed by patient or other responsible family member. Please print or type)*

PATIENT DATA | SERVICE MEMBER DATA

1. NAME (last, first, middle initial): Carter, Elaine
2. DATE OF BIRTH: 07-16-53
7. NAME OF SPONSOR (last, first, middle initial): Carter, Scott W.

3. ADDRESS (Include Zip Code): 337 Peppertree Drive, Baldwin, NY 11510
8a. SERVICE NUMBER: 123-45-6789
8b. SOCIAL SECURITY ACCOUNT NUMBER: 123-45-6789
9. GRADE: SSG(6)

4. PATIENT IS A: [X](1) SPOUSE (2) DAUGHTER (3) SON (4) RETIREE

10. ORGANIZATION AND DUTY STATION: HHC, 2nd Batt., 24th Infantry APO New York, NY 10026

5. IDENTIFICATION CARD CARD NO.: S12345
EFFECTIVE DATE: 06 01 74
EXPIRATION DATE: 05 31 76

11. SPONSOR'S OR RETIREE'S BRANCH OF SERVICE: [X](1) USA (2) USAF (3) USMC (4) USN (5) USCG (6) USPHS (7) ESSA

6. BASIS FOR CARE — ACTIVE DUTY DEPENDENTS ONLY: [X](1) RESIDING APART FROM SPONSOR (2) RESIDING WITH SPONSOR DD FORM 1251 ATTACHED (3) OUTPATIENT (4) OTHER

12. STATUS: [X](1) ACTIVE DUTY (2) RETIRED (3) DECEASED

13. CERTIFICATION

I certify to the best of my knowledge and belief the above information in Section I is correct. To the extent that I have authority to do so I hereby authorize the release of medical records in this case to both the contractor and the Government. If a RETIRED MEMBER or dependent of a retired or deceased member, I certify that to the best of my knowledge and belief, that *(Check appropriate box) (Delete portion in parenthesis not applicable)*

[X] (I am not) (the patient is not) enrolled (neither is sponsor) in any other insurance, medical service, or health plan provided by law or through employment.

[ ] (I am) (the patient is) enrolled (so is sponsor) in another insurance, medical service, or health plan provided by law or through employment; however the particular benefits claimed on this form are not payable under the other plan.

Carter, Elaine | spouse | 05-31-75
Name (print or type) | (Relationship to Patient) | Date | Signature

**SECTION II** *(To be completed by Source of Care)*

14. NAME AND ADDRESS OF SOURCE OF CARE (Include Zip Code): John E. Adams, M.D., 94 Kenmore Parkway, Garden City, NY 11530
a. SOURCE OF CARE LOCATION CODE
b. PROVIDER OF SERVICES: [X](1) ATTENDING PHYSICIAN (2) OTHER
c. PATIENT STATUS: [X](1) INPATIENT (2) OUTPATIENT

15. NAME AND TITLE OF INDIVIDUAL ORDERING CARE: John E. Adams, M.D.
16. INCLUSIVE DATES OF CARE: FROM 05 28 75 TO 06 21 75
a. INTL STAT CODE

17. DIAGNOSIS (Use standard nomenclature): Acute cholecystitis with cholelithiasis
(Check when applicable) [X] services were necessary for treatment of a bonafide medical emergency
b. 12 BREAK CODE

18. RELATED HOSPITALIZATION (If applicable): FROM 05-28-75 TO 06-02-75

19. ENTER ESTIMATED OR ACTUAL DATE OF DELIVERY IN MATERNITY CASES. LIST BY DATE SURGICAL OPERATIONS AND/OR CARE FURNISHED INCLUDING VISITS FOR WHICH SEPARATE CHARGES ARE CLAIMED (Type or print) (Attach additional sheets if required)

| DATE(S) OF SERVICE | a. ITEM OR DESCRIPTION OF SERVICE | b. CHARGES | c. PROCEDURE CODE |
|---|---|---|---|
| 05-28-75 | cholecystectomy with open exploration of common duct | $ 500 00 | 3517 |
| d. TOTAL CHARGES THIS STATEMENT FOR CARE AUTHORIZED | | $ 500 00 | |
| e. (PAID BY) OR (DUE FROM) PATIENT (Cross out one) | | $ | |
| f. DUE FROM GOVERNMENT TO SOURCE OF CARE | | $ | |
| g. DUE PATIENT OR SPONSOR, REIMBURSEMENT | | $ | |

20. CERTIFICATION BY SOURCE OF CARE

I certify that the services and/or supplies listed hereon were performed or authorized by the attending physician, dentist or other professional personnel in charge, that payment due from the Government has not been received, and that, except for the amount payable by the patient in accordance with the terms of the Civilian Health and Medical Program of the Uniformed Services, the amount paid by the Government will be accepted as payment in full for the authorized services and/or supplies listed hereon.
I further certify that I am not an intern, resident or otherwise in training status for which I am receiving compensation for services listed on this claim.

John E. Adams | M.D. | 06-30-75
Name (print or type) | Title | Date | Signature

*The persons signing this form are advised that the willful making of a false or fraudulent statement herein renders them liable to prosecution under applicable Federal Laws.*

DA FORM 1863-2 1 JUN 67 (Civilian Sources) | REPLACES DA FORM 1863-2, 1 SEP 61, WHICH IS OBSOLETE. | Form Approved Comptroller General, U.S., 22 Sep 67

1

**Figure 19–1** CHAMPUS Claim Form

## Medicare Under the Social Security Administration

Medicare for the over-65 patient went into effect on July 1, 1966. There are two parts (A and B) to the program.

**Part A.** Hospital insurance, Part A, is financed by special contributions paid by people while they work, with matching contributions from employers, and there is no additional premium required from the insured. These sums are collected, along with regular social security contributions, from wages and self-employment income earned during a person's working years.

Any person who is receiving monthly social security or railroad retirement checks is automatically enrolled for hospital insurance benefits. Some federal employees and former federal employees who are not eligible for social security benefits are also not eligible for hospital insurance, but may enroll in the Part B medical insurance program.

**Part B.** Medical insurance, Part B, is voluntary. The insured must apply for coverage within a specified period and pay a monthly premium. This premium was initially three dollars in 1966. By 1972, it had increased to $5.80. Matching payments are contributed by the federal government from general revenues. The law requires that the premium be reviewed every two years.

A new patient who says he is covered by Medicare should always be asked to show his identification card (Fig. 19–2). This will include his name and identification number and will also indicate whether he has both hospital and medical coverage. Keep in mind that the older patient is frequently confused by the complexity of such programs, and the medical assistant can do much to assist him. The patient may be under the impression that he is "fully covered" under Medicare. Part B has a deductible ($60 in 1973). After the deductible is met, Medicare will pay 80 per cent of the covered benefits; the patient must pay the remaining 20 per cent.

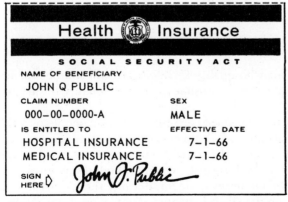

**Figure 19–2** Identification card for the Medicare patient

Some major changes in Medicare were enacted into law in 1972. Beginning July 1, 1973, disabled people under 65 who had been getting social security or railroad retirement checks for two years or more became eligible for Medicare. Persons able to receive disability coverage include disabled workers, persons who became incapacitated before age 22, disabled widows, and disabled dependent widowers.

Also, beginning July 1, 1973, people who had not worked long enough under social security to be eligible for the hospital insurance under Medicare were enabled to buy this protection on a voluntary basis. People who choose to buy hospital insurance protection must also enroll and pay the monthly premium for medical coverage.

**Billing for Medicare Services.**   Billing for Medicare services may be accomplished easily in any one of these three ways:

(1) If the doctor *accepts* assignment (which means that the doctor agrees to accept the charge determination of the Medicare carrier), ask the patient to sign Part I of Form SSA-1490 (Fig. 19–3) on his first visit. Itemize the services on Part II of the claim form, have the physician sign it, and submit it to the Medicare carrier. When the charge determination has been made you then bill the patient for his 20 per cent plus the deductible, if this has not already been met for the current year.

(2) If the doctor *does not accept* assignment, you may bill the patient direct. The patient then must submit Form SSA-1490 to the Medicare carrier. In order to do this he will need from the doctor either an itemized bill which he can attach to the claim form, or an itemization of services on Part II of the form.

(3) Alternatively, if the doctor *does not accept* assignment, he can still submit the claim to Medicare for the patient, and check the box, □ *I do not accept assignment,* in Item 12. A bill for the full amount should then be sent to the patient with the understanding that payment is his responsibility.

Medicare patients are particularly appreciative of your assistance in preparing claim forms. In addition to the public relations value, an advantage of submitting claims directly is that supportive documents, such as operation reports, x-ray reports, and so on, may be attached.

# Medicaid

Some patients who qualify for Medicare will still be unable to pay the portion for which they are responsible. They may qualify for aid from a public welfare agency.

Most states have medical care programs for people of all ages who cannot pay their medical bills and who meet certain income requirements. Title XIX of Public Law 89-97, under the Social Security Amendments of 1965, provides for agreements with states for assistance from the federal government in providing health care for the medically indigent. Because there is great variation from state to state, you should seek information from your local public welfare agency regarding assistance to the needy in your area.

## REQUEST FOR MEDICARE PAYMENT

MEDICAL INSURANCE BENEFITS—SOCIAL SECURITY ACT (See Instructions on Back—Type or Print Information)

Form Approved
Budget Bureau No.
72–R0730

NOTICE—Anyone who misrepresents or falsifies essential information requested by this form may upon conviction be subject to fine and imprisonment under Federal Law.

### PART I—PATIENT TO FILL IN ITEMS 1 THROUGH 6 ONLY

**A** When completed, send this form to:

Occidental Life Insurance Co. of California
Box 54905
Terminal Annex
Los Angeles, California 90054

Copy from your
HEALTH
INSURANCE
CARD
(See example
on back)

**1** Name of patient

Arthur O. Switzer

**2** Health insurance claim number

055   10   6754   Letter
A

☒ Male  ☐ Female

**3** Patient's mailing address
4705 Waring Place

City, State, ZIP code
Los Angeles, CA   90033

Telephone Number
987-6543

**4** Describe the illness or injury for which you received treatment (*Always fill in this item if your doctor does not complete Part II below*)

Was your illness or injury connected with your employment?
☐ Yes  ☐ No

**5** If you have other health insurance or if your State medical assistance agency will pay part of your medical expenses and you want information about this claim released to the insurance company or State agency upon its request, give the following information.

Insuring organization or State agency name and address

Policy No.
Medi-cal Identification No.

**6** I authorize any holder of medical or other information about me to release to the Social Security Administration or its intermediaries or carriers any information needed for this or a related Medicare claim. I permit a copy of this authorization to be used in place of the original, and request payment of medical insurance benefits either to myself or to the party who accepts assignment below.

Signature of patient (See instructions on reverse where patient is unable to sign)

SIGN HERE ▶ *Arthur O. Switzer*

Date signed
11/24/74

### PART II—PHYSICIAN OR SUPPLIER TO FILL IN 7 THROUGH 14

| 7 A. Date of each service | B. Place of service (*See Codes below) | C. Code surgical or medical procedures and other services or supplies furnished for each date given | | D. Nature of illness or injury requiring services or supplies | E. Charges (If related to unusual circumstances explain in 7C) | Leave Blank |
|---|---|---|---|---|---|---|
| | | | Code | | | |
| 07/21/74 | IH | Initial History and Physical | 90220 | Subacute bacterial endocarditis | $   50.00 | |
| 07/22/74 to 08/13/74 | IH | Ext. visits (23) @ $20/visit | 90250 | | 460.00 | |
| 08/14/74 | IH | Complete cardiac re-evaluation | 90270 | | 30.00 | |
| 08/15 to 09/11/74 | IH | Ext. visits (27) @ $20/visit | 90250 | | 540.00 | |
| | | | | | | |

**8** Name and address of physician or supplier (*Number and street, city, State, ZIP code*)

Robert O. Elam, M.D.
300 North Broadway
Los Angeles, CA   90005

Telephone No.
487-0302

Physician or supplier code
A20586-01

| 9 Total charges | $1080.00 |
|---|---|
| 10 Amount paid | $ -0- |
| 11 Any unpaid balance due | $1080.00 |

**12** Assignment of patient's bill (*See reverse*)

☐ I accept assignment   ☒ I do not accept assignment

**13** Show name and address of facility where services were performed (*If other than home or office visits*)

St. Vincent's Hospital
Los Angeles, California

**14** Signature of physician or supplier (*A physician's signature certifies that physician's services were personally rendered by him or under his personal direction*)

▶ *Robert O. Elam, M.D.*

☒ MD  ☐ DO  ☐ DDS
Other degree _____

Date signed
11/15/74

*O—Doctor's Office
IL—Independent Laboratory
H—Patient's Home (If portable X-ray services, identify the supplier)
IH—Inpatient Hospital
ECF—Extended Care Facility
OH—Outpatient Hospital
OL—Other Locations
NH—Nursing Home

FORM SSA-1490D (CA) (10–69)

Department of Health, Education, and Welfare
Social Security Administration

**Figure 19–3**   Medicare Billing Form

CARBON COPY

THE COLWELL COMPANY
CHAMPAIGN, IL

FORM # 6160

ROBERT O. ELAM, M.D.
300 North Broadway
Los Angeles, CA     90005

MEDICARE STATEMENT

Mr. Arthur O. Switzer
4705 Waring Place
Los Angeles, CA     90033

DATE  11/15/74          HEALTH INSURANCE
                         CLAIM NUMBER       055 10 6754 A

| A DATE OF EACH SERVICE | B PLACE OF SERVICE | C FULLY DESCRIBE SURGICAL OR MEDICAL PROCEDURES AND OTHER SERVICES OR SUPPLIES FURNISHED FOR EACH DATE GIVEN | D NATURE OF ILLNESS OR INJURY REQUIRING SERVICES OR SUPPLIES (DIAGNOSIS) | E CHARGES |
|---|---|---|---|---|
| 1974 07/21 | IH | Initial History and Physical RVS 90220 | Subacute bacterial endocarditis | $  50.00 |
| 07/22 to 08/13 | IH | Ext. visits (23) @ $20/visit RVS 90250 | | 460.00 |
| 08/14 | IH | Complete cardiac re-evaluation RVS 90270 | | 30.00 |
| 08/15 to 09/11 | IH | Ext. visits (27) @ $20/visit RVS 90250 | | 540.00 |
| | | | | |

O - DOCTOR'S OFC.          H – PATIENT'S HOME       NH – NURSING HOME
IH – INPATIENT - HOSP.     OL – OTHER LOCATION      ECF – EXTENDED CARE
OH - OUTPATIENT - HOSP.        (SPECIFIED IN C)           FACILITY

TOTAL  $ 1080.00

PATIENT CLAIM COPY

**Figure 19–4** Patient can submit his own claim to Medicare when billed on this form. (Courtesy of the Colwell Co., Ill.)

## Workmen's Compensation

All state legislatures have passed workmen's compensation laws to protect wage earners against the loss of wages and the cost of medical care resulting from occupational accident or disease. This is a form of mandated insurance. The clue to whether an accident or illness is covered by this insurance is this: did the accident or illness occur during the course of or as a result of the patient's employment? If so, the worker's medical expenses are covered in their entirety. The provider of service (doctor, hospital, therapist, and so on) is prohibited from billing the patient. Fees are fixed, and are oftentimes lower than the usual and customary private fees.

Compensation benefits also include weekly cash payments for temporary disability, for permanent disability resulting from industrial injury, and death benefits to dependents of employees fatally injured.

Within 48 hours after the physician has seen the workmen's compensation patient for the first time, he must submit a report of his findings to the (1) insurance carrier, (2) patient's employer, and (3) state workmen's compensation board or commission (Fig. 19–5). This report must be personally signed by the doctor. Since you will need to keep a copy for the doctor's file, the report should be typed in quadruplicate.

The information requested by the insuring company must be completed carefully. The physician's report should set forth:

1. The history of the case as obtained from the patient, noting any pre-existing injuries or diseases.

2. The patient's symptoms and physical complaints.

3. The complete physical findings, including laboratory and x-ray findings.

4. A tentative diagnosis of the condition.

5. An estimate of the type and extent of the disability. Where permanent disability has resulted, there should be a very careful survey, and the extent of disability given in detail.

6. Treatment that is indicated, including type, frequency, and duration. It may be necessary to attach a letter giving more detailed information to assist in making an evaluation of the case.

7. Whenever possible, the date the patient may be able to return to work, if he has been totally disabled.

In severe or prolonged cases supplemental reports should be sent to the insurance carrier at least once per month. At the termination of treatment a final report and bill is sent to the insurance carrier. NEVER SEND A BILL TO THE PATIENT.

**Keep Separate Records.**   The records for workmen's compensation cases, sometimes referred to as industrial cases, preferably should be separated from the doctor's regular patient histories.

If the patient seen for an industrial injury has previously been seen as a private patient, a new chart and ledger should be started to be used only for the treatment rendered under conditions of the workmen's compensation law. The insurance carrier may request, and is entitled to receive, copies of all records pertaining to the industrial injury but not the records of a private patient. There

**DOCTOR'S FIRST REPORT**
**OF**
**WORK INJURY**

STATE OF CALIFORNIA
DEPARTMENT OF INDUSTRIAL RELATIONS
DIVISION OF LABOR STATISTICS AND RESEARCH
P. O. Box 965, San Francisco, Calif. 94101

Immediately after first examination mail one copy **directly** to the Division of Labor Statistics and Research. Failure to file a report with the Division is a misdemeanor. (Labor Code, Sections 6407-6413.) Answer all questions fully.

**A. INSURANCE CARRIER** State Compensation Insurance Fund

| | Do not write in this space |
|---|---|
| 1. **EMPLOYER** Jones Hardware | |
| 2. Address (No., St. & City) 750 Tenth Street, San Francisco, CA 94100 | |
| 3. Business (Manufacturing shoes, building construction, retailing men's clothes, etc.) retail store | |
| 4. **EMPLOYEE** (First name, middle initial, last name) John J. Doe   Soc. Sec. No. 000-00-0000 | |
| 5. Address (No., St. & City) 234 -11th Street, San Francisco, CA 94100 | |
| 6. Occupation clerk   Age 40   Sex M | |
| 7. Date injured 10/13/76   Hour 3 P.M. Date last worked same | |
| 8. Injured at (No., St. & City) 750 Tenth Street, San Francisco   County San Francisco | |
| 9. Date of your first examination 10/13/76   Hour 5 P.M. Who engaged your services? employer | |
| 10. Name other doctors who treated employee for this injury none | |
| 11. **ACCIDENT OR EXPOSURE:** Did employee notify employer of this injury? yes   Employee's statement of cause of injury or illness: | |
| Fell from ladder a distance of four feet to the floor. Twisted right ankle. | |
| 12. **NATURE AND EXTENT OF INJURY OR DISEASE** (Include all objective findings, subjective complaints, and diagnoses. If occupational disease state date of onset, occupational history, and exposures.) | |
| Simple fracture lateral malleolus rt. ankle - undisplaced. | |
| 13. X-rays: By whom taken? (State if none) St. Martha's Hospital | |
| Findings: as above | |
| 14. Treatment:   Short leg cast applied - no anesthesia | |
| 15. Kind of case (Office, home or hospital) office   If hospitalized, date   Estimated stay | |
| Name and address of hospital | |
| 16. Further treatment (Estimated frequency and duration) weekly | |
| 17. Estimated period of disability for: Regular work 3 months   Modified work 6 weeks | |
| 18. Describe any permanent disability or disfigurement expected (State if none) none | |
| 19. If death ensued, give date | |
| 20. **REMARKS** (Note any pre-existing injuries or diseases, need for special examination or laboratory tests, other pertinent information.) | |

Name Friend Hunton   Degree M.D. [ PERSONAL SIGNATURE OF DOCTOR ]   *Friend Hunton, M.D.*
(Type or print)
Date of report 10/14/76   Address (No., St. & City) 450 Sutter Street, San Francisco, CA 94100

FORM 5021   *Use reverse side if more space required*   57939-607 10-65 600M ① Ⓑ OSP

**Figure 19-5**  First Report of Work Injury

**DOCTOR'S FINAL (OR MONTHLY) REPORT AND BILL**

Itemized bills, IN DUPLICATE, are to be submitted at the termination of the case.
Monthly statements are POSITIVELY required on cases under treatment.
Mail to State Compensation Insurance Fund Address 525 Golden Gate Avenue, San Francisco
Services beginning late in month and extending into succeeding month may be itemized on one statement.

EMPLOYER Jones Hardware, 750 Tenth Street, San Francisco, CA 94100
EMPLOYEE John J. Doe                                     Social Security # 000-00-0000
DATE OF INJURY 10/13/76            SERVICES FOR MONTH OF October , 19 76

Patient refused treatment ...........-.-.., 19......       Patient able to return to work ...-.-.., 19......
Patient stopped treatment                                   Patient discharged as cured ...-.-.., 19......
   without orders ...........-.-.., 19......                Condition at time of last visit convalescent
Patient entered hospital ...........-.-.., 19......

Any other charges authorized such as Drugs? ...-.-... Hospital? ...-.-...
                                          (Check)          (Check)

Code: O—Office; V—Home Visit; H—Hospital Visit; N—Night Visit; S—Operation; X—X-Ray.

| Month | 1 | 2 | 3 | 4 | 5 | 6 | 7 | 8 | 9 | 10 | 11 | 12 | 13 | 14 | 15 | 16 | 17 | 18 | 19 | 20 | 21 | 22 | 23 | 24 | 25 | 26 | 27 | 28 | 29 | 30 | 31 |
|-------|---|---|---|---|---|---|---|---|---|----|----|----|----|----|----|----|----|----|----|----|----|----|----|----|----|----|----|----|----|----|----|
| Oct   |   |   |   |   |   |   |   |   |   |    |    |    | S  |    |    |    |    |    |    |    |    |    |    |    |    |    | O  |    |    |    |    |
|       |   |   |   |   |   |   |   |   |   |    |    |    |    |    |    |    |    |    |    |    |    |    |    |    |    |    |    |    |    |    |    |
|       |   |   |   |   |   |   |   |   |   |    |    |    |    |    |    |    |    |    |    |    |    |    |    |    |    |    |    |    |    |    |    |

                                                                    Totals
First aid treatment (describe) ..........................................................  $
Office Visits 10/27/76                    CRVS #90060                            $ 12.00
Home Visits                                                                      $
Hospital Visits                                                                 $
Operations 10/13/76 Short leg walking cast CRVS #29425                          $ 40.00
MATERIAL (Itemized at cost)                                                     $

                                                 TOTAL $ 52.00

Any charges shown above which are in excess of the minimum fee must be explained below regarding nature
of such services, indicating the date rendered.

Make check payable to:

Doctor Friend Hunton                           Signature *Friend Hunton MD*

Address 450 Sutter Street, San Francisco       Date October 31, 1976

Form 5020-B
Crenshaw P. & S., 1326 Wilshire, Los Angeles, Calif. - HUbbard 3-0660

**Figure 19–6**   Monthly Statement: Workmen's Compensation

may be a lawsuit or a hearing before a referee or Appeals Board for which
records are subpoenaed. If separate records are kept, there is no question of
privilege involved.

# LIFE INSURANCE

When an individual makes application for life insurance, the insurance company naturally wants to know the current status of the applicant's health and any

significant previous history. Therefore, there are two kinds of reports for life insurance companies that may concern you:

(1) In the first type, the insurance company authorizes one or more physicians in each community to perform physical examinations of prospective insurers. The examining physician will make a report to the insurance company following the examination. The insurance agent arranges the applicant's appointment for the physical examination — and he will probably want the appointment as soon as possible so that his prospect doesn't get away! The insurance company, or its agent, will supply the necessary forms for completion. The company may require that the forms be completed in the doctor's own handwriting, but the assistant will make sure the forms are on hand at the time of the appointment. She may want to double check the form before mailing it, to be certain no details have been overlooked. The insurance company pays the physician a stipulated fee upon receipt of his report.

(2) For this kind of report, the agent asks the applicant to supply the names and addresses of any physicians consulted in the past. The company, in turn, will request reports from these physicians. Your physician may receive a request for such information concerning a previous patient. Before completing the form, make certain the applicant has signed an authorization for release of information. The request form usually has a voucher check for a minimal fee attached. The doctor may accept the proffered fee or, if he deems it inadequate, may bill the insurance company for "balance of fee." If it is reasonable, it will be paid without question.

## INSURANCE TERMINOLOGY

The medical assistant should be acquainted with the language of the health insurance world. She is not expected to interpret each patient's insurance policy for him, but she must know how to read the instructions from the various companies and know how to complete a form correctly. Many physicians derive a good percentage of their income from insurance payments. Physicians associated with large companies, or those specializing in industrial medicine, may receive as high as 85 per cent of their income from this source.

**Assignment of Insurance Benefits.**   To facilitate prompt payment of bills, a medical assistant should have the patient sign an *assignment of insurance benefits* form. This form is often provided by the insurance company, or a standard form from the printers may be used. Some offices use a rubber stamp. The assignment authorizes the insurance company to make direct payment of benefits to the physician. Most insurance companies honor these assignments.

**Beneficiary.**   The person receiving the benefits of the policy is the beneficiary; the term usually refers to the policyowner, who may sometimes be called the *subscribing member* or the *enrolled member,* rather than to the dependents. (In a life insurance policy the beneficiary is one receiving the proceeds in the event of the death of the policyowner.)

**Claim.**   This is a demand to the insurer by the insured person for the payment of benefits under a policy.

## ASSIGNMENT OF INSURANCE BENEFITS

I, the undersigned represent that I have insurance coverage with and do hereby

authorize_____to pay and assign directly
(NAME OF COMPANY)

to_____all surgical and/or medical benefits, if any, other-
(NAME OF DOCTOR)

wise payable to me for services as described on the attached forms hereof, but not
to exceed the charges for those services. I understand that I am financially responsible
for all charges whether or not paid by said insurance. I hereby authorize said assignee
to release all information necessary to secure the payment of said benefits.

Date_____Signed_____

**Figure 19–7**  Assignment of Benefits Form

**Coinsurance.**   This term means that the insuring company pays a certain percentage of the patient's actual expense, generally 75 to 80 per cent, and the patient pays the remaining 25 to 20 per cent. A policy may or may not have coinsurance over and above a deductible amount. This type of insurance grew out of the realization that it is not as necessary to provide protection against small medical and hospital expenses as it is against major medical bills. *Deductibles* and *coinsurance* help to keep the premium rates at a lower level and, in some instances, have been offered as an alternative to rate increases. The patient who pays for the first two visits on a medical contract also helps hold costs down. This is called *two-visit deductible* (2V.D.).

**Co-ordination of Benefits** (see Non-duplication of Benefits).

**Deductible.**   Many policies, especially "major medical," carry a deductible clause which states that the insuring company will pay the expenses incurred *after* the insured has paid a specified amount. This amount ranges from $25 to $500, depending on how the contract (deductible clause) is written.

**Disability.**   It is said that disability exists when illness or injury makes an individual unable to be employed, either partially or totally. *Total disability* is the inability of the insured to perform any duties of his occupation. *Partial disability* is the inability to perform a part of one's occupation; there may be a partial loss of income. The insured may do limited duties, with shortened hours or lighter work. *Temporary disability* exists when the insured expects to return to work and regain earning power. *Permanent disability* is expected to continue for the person's lifetime.

These disability terms are important when reporting workmen's compensation cases or in the case of cash settlements.

HEALTH INSURANCE CLAIM — GROUP OR INDIVIDUAL                                                   COMB-1 (2-70)

| PART A | TO BE COMPLETED BY PATIENT (INSURED) |
|---|---|
| | *Spaced for Typewriter — Marks for Tabulator Appear on this Line* |

PATIENT'S NAME AND ADDRESS | DATE OF BIRTH

Richard DeWitt, 837 North Harbor Boulevard, Irvine, CA   92705 | 01/23/13

INSURED'S NAME IF PATIENT IS A DEPENDENT

| NAME OF INSURANCE COMPANY | POLICY NUMBER | INSURED'S SOCIAL SECURITY NUMBER |
|---|---|---|
| Pacific Mutual Life Insurance Co. | 32785 | 055-10-6754 |

IF GROUP INSURANCE, NAME OF POLICYHOLDER (*i.e., Employer, Union or Association through whom insured*)

Eckhart Appliance Company

AUTHORIZATION TO PAY BENEFITS TO PHYSICIAN: I hereby authorize payment directly to the undersigned physician of the Surgical and/or Medical Benefits, if any, otherwise payable to me for his services as described below but not to exceed the reasonable and customary charge for those services.

SIGNED (INSURED PERSON)  *Richard DeWitt*   DATE 2/20/75

AUTHORIZATION TO RELEASE INFORMATION: I hereby authorize the undersigned physician to release any information acquired in the course of my examination or treatment.

SIGNED (PATIENT, OR PARENT IF MINOR)  *Richard DeWitt*   DATE 2/20/75

| PART B | ATTENDING PHYSICIAN'S STATEMENT |
|---|---|

1. DIAGNOSIS AND CONCURRENT CONDITIONS
(IF DIAGNOSIS CODE OTHER THAN ICDA* USED, GIVE NAME):    Subacute bacterial endocarditis

2. IS CONDITION DUE TO INJURY OR SICKNESS ARISING OUT OF PATIENT'S EMPLOYMENT?   YES ☐   NO ☒   PREGNANCY? YES ☐  NO ☐   IF YES, APPROXIMATE DATE PREGNANCY COMMENCED. DATE

3. REPORT OF SERVICES (OR ATTACH ITEMIZED BILL) (IF PREVIOUS FORM SUBMITTED TO THIS CARRIER, YOU NEED SHOW ONLY DATES AND SERVICES SINCE LAST REPORT)

| DATE OF SERVICES | PLACE OF SERVICES† | DESCRIPTION OF SURGICAL OR MEDICAL SERVICES RENDERED | PROCEDURE CODE—IF USED (IF CODE OTHER THAN CPT** USED, GIVE NAME) | CHARGES |
|---|---|---|---|---|
| | | | CRVS | |
| 02/20/75 | 0 | Return examination | 90080 | 30.00 |
| | | Multi 033, Diff | 80013 | 21.00 |
| | | Electrocardiogram | 93000 | 18.00 |
| | | | TOTAL CHARGES ▶ $ | 69.00 |
| | | | AMOUNT PAID ▶ $ | —0— |
| | | | BALANCE DUE ▶ $ | 69.00 |

†O—Doctor's Office   IH—Inpatient Hospital   NH—Nursing Home
H—Patient's Home   OH—Outpatient Hospital   OL—Other Locations
*ICDA—International Classification of Diseases
**CPT—Current Procedural Terminology (current edition)

4. DATE SYMPTOMS FIRST APPEARED OR ACCIDENT HAPPENED.
February 1, 1975

5. DATE PATIENT FIRST CONSULTED YOU FOR THIS CONDITION.
February 1, 1975

6. PATIENT EVER HAD SAME OR SIMILAR CONDITION?   YES ☐   NO ☒   IF "YES" WHEN AND DESCRIBE:

7. PATIENT STILL UNDER CARE FOR THIS CONDITION?   YES ☒   NO ☐

8. PATIENT WAS CONTINOUSLY TOTALLY DISABLED (UNABLE TO WORK).
FROM 02/01/75   THRU 02/21/75

9. PATIENT WAS PARTIALLY DISABLED.
FROM n/a   THRU

10. IF STILL DISABLED, DATE PATIENT SHOULD BE ABLE TO RETURN TO WORK.
04/01/75

11. PATIENT WAS HOUSE CONFINED.
FROM n/a   THRU

12. DOES PATIENT HAVE OTHER HEALTH COVERAGE?   YES ☐   NO ☒
IF "YES" PLEASE IDENTIFY

13. I DO NOT ACCEPT ASSIGNMENT. ☐

| DATE | PHYSICIAN'S NAME (PRINT) | DEGREE |
|---|---|---|
| 03/01/75 | Robert O. Elam, M.D. | |

INDIVIDUAL PRACTITIONER'S - SS#

ALL OTHERS - EMPLOYER I.D. #   A20586-01

PHYSICIAN'S SIGNATURE  *Robert O. Elam*   TELEPHONE 987-6543

MUST BE FURNISHED UNDER AUTHORITY OF LAW

| STREET ADDRESS | CITY OR TOWN | STATE OR PROVINCE | ZIP CODE |
|---|---|---|---|
| 300 North Broadway | Los Angeles | CA | 90005 |

MEMORANDUM REGARDING DISPOSITION OF THIS FORM ON REVERSE SIDE

APPROVED BY THE COUNCIL ON MEDICAL SERVICE, A.M.A. 2/70

**Figure 19–8**   H.I.C. Claim Form

**Effective Date.** This is the date the coverage starts to take effect. There may be a *probationary period;* that is, a specific number of days during which no coverage will be available for any sickness commencing during this period. There may be a *waiting period* or a time *limitation,* during which a policyholder is not entitled to benefits for a year for certain pre-existing conditions, such as hemorrhoids, hernia, varicose veins, tonsils, and adenoids.

**Eligible Family Members.** These include the spouse (husband or wife) and any unmarried children under the age of 18 or 21 (or occasionally 23) years of age. There is usually a waiting period of 14 days to one month for a newborn dependent. A *family policy* covers all members of a family, as previously stated.

**Exclusions** (also known as exceptions). Exclusions are usually listed in the insuring clause and are found in all insurance policies. This is a list of the injuries and illnesses, or the conditions under which they are obtained that the insuring company will not pay for. Common exclusions include the following: sickness or accident resulting from warfare; suicide or self-inflicted injury; air travel on nonscheduled flights; any sickness or injury covered by workmen's compensation or cared for in a government hospital, such as a Veterans' Hospital; and the services of a dentist or oral surgeon. Many policies exclude any illness or injury connected with pregnancy, hernia, or plastic surgery for cosmetic purposes; certain major diseases, such as tuberculosis, may also be excluded.

**Fee Schedules.** Most insurance companies have a fee schedule, especially in the case of an indemnifying policy. This is a list of services or procedures and the specific dollars paid for each. A service policy may have a fee shedule, but it is adjustable to the service rendered. Many companies now give a dollar value to a unit, as shown on a relative value scale. These *relative value scales* (R.V.S.) assign a given number of units to each procedure rather than a dollar value. The insurance carrier may have a predetermined conversion factor (specified in cents or dollars), by which it will convert the unit value into monetary value. In this way every procedure has a given relationship to every other procedure. One advantage of using an R.V.S. is that entire fee schedules need not be revised when coverage is increased or decreased. Only the conversion factor need be changed.

**Income Limit.** It is recognized that the income of certain persons determines their ability to pay; therefore, for these income groups the physicians agree to provide the benefits without additional charges. To persons of a lower income group the policy becomes a service policy, while for persons with a higher income, who are charged the additional fee, the policy is an indemnification. The "income" is the gross income as stated for federal income tax purposes for the family (spouse, dependents, and subscribing member).

**Insuring Clause.** This is the insurance company's statement, usually the first paragraph of the policy, stating the benefits and under what circumstances they will be paid. It is a promise to pay if the person insured suffers any of the losses he is insured against.

**Lapse.** This is termination of a policy upon the policyholder's failure to pay the premium within the time required.

**Member Physician.** This term refers to a medical doctor who has joined a group or enrolled with the insurance company and has agreed to accept the contracts. He will meet certain obligations of the contract, such as accepting the insurance benefits as payment in full for care of persons under a certain income.

**Non-duplication of Benefits.** Most group insurance plans have the *non-duplication of benefits* provision, which is also known as a *coordination of benefits* provision (double coverage). Its purposes are to prevent the available benefits from exceeding the covered medical expenses and also to prevent increase in insurance costs. It is important to identify the primary carrier as it will be the first to pay benefits.

**Other Benefits.** These benefits are specified in each instance and often include x-ray, laboratory, anesthesiologist, and assistant surgeon. Some provide benefits for drugs, oxygen, and blood. The contract may read that the insurance company will pay the first $15 to $25 and then one-half of all additional charges. These are usually limited to drugs or other benefits supplied and used while in the hospital.

**Patient Status.** There are frequently stipulations of payment for procedures if a patient is an inpatient or outpatient. An *inpatient* is one who is registered as a bed patient in a hospital; he has been "admitted" to the hospital and is considered a resident of the institution. An *outpatient* is one who is receiving the services of the hospital but is not a registered bed patient; he does not stay overnight and is not considered a resident of the institution.

**Pre-existing Conditions.** Any illness, injury, or physical condition that existed or was incurred prior to the issuance of the policy is a pre-existing condition. Some policies do not pay for pre-existing conditions and therefore attach an elimination rider. This is more common in individual contracts than with group coverage.

**Premium.** This is the rate or the amount charged for the policy. This payment is usually periodic and is determined by many factors, such as occupation, age, and sex of the insured, the amount of the coverage, and the value of the fee schedule.

**Relative Value Scale** (see Fee Schedule).

**Release of Information to Insurance Companies.** The assistant or the physician will, of course, fill out forms for sickness or accident benefits that the patient brings to the office. However, information should not be released to insurance companies without proper authorization from the patient. Sometimes an insurance company will telephone the office and request some medical information. The assistant should indicate that the office will be glad to provide the information if the company will suppy the proper authorization for its release. This same procedure should be followed with an attorney, newspaper reporter, or any third party who calls for information. It may be advisable to have a patient sign a *release of medical information* form. This form authorizes the release of medical information to the insurance company or allows the hospital to release information.

**Termination Conversion.** Most group policies stop coverage when an employee terminates his employment or association with the group. One of the most important benefits given to the person terminating from an insured group is the right to convert from the group plan to an individual plan. In some cases the insuring company agrees, subject to the desire of the individual, to continue coverage of the employee after he retires or is not employed, but usually with a change in benefits; either the premiums are increased or the benefits are

**RECORDS RELEASE**                                    DATE_____

TO_____
                                    DOCTOR

_____
                                    ADDRESS

I HEREBY AUTHORIZE AND REQUEST YOU TO RELEASE

TO_____
                                    DOCTOR

_____
                                    ADDRESS

THE COMPLETE MEDICAL RECORDS IN YOUR POSSESSION, CONCERNING MY ILLNESS

AND/OR TREATMENT DURING THE PERIOD FROM_____TO_____

                                    SIGNED_____
                                            (PATIENT OR NEAREST RELATIVE)

_____      RELATIONSHIP_____
            WITNESS

FORM 122 - EASTMAN, INC.

**Figure 19–9**   Records Release

decreased. The employee does not have the protection of the group any longer and is issued an individual policy.

**Usual and Customary Fee.**   Some insurance plans do not publish a fee schedule but agree to pay all or a percentage of the *usual and customary fee* for any given procedure. The *usual* fee is the charge a physician makes to his private patients. The *customary* fee is one that is within range of the usual fees charged by physicians in the same geographic and socioeconomic area and by physicians with similar training and experience.

## THE PROCESSING OF INSURANCE CLAIMS

The majority of the doctor's patients will carry some type of health insurance, but there is a wide variety of forms to be completed, as well as a great variance in fee schedules. Because few of the policies pay the entire medical bill, many offices bill the patient direct. Exceptions to this, of course, are service-type policies that pay in full, workmen's compensation, and other policies under which the patient is not legally responsible for payment.

Claims are generally paid upon receipt of a doctor's bill, hospital bill, or statement from the policyholder citing the nature and extent of sickness or disability. The benefit application form for medical or surgical insurance almost always includes a statement from the attending physician. Most companies have revised their forms to simplify and standardize the questions as much as possible. They rely heavily on the physician's statement in determining benefits. For this reason it is very important that all insurance forms be carefully and completely filled out. Sometimes the insurance company will also require information from the hospital, such as the date of admission or discharge, and other important details.

The required forms should be completed as soon as possible. Many times payment to the assistant surgeon, anesthesiologist, or consultant is held until the attending physician's statement is received. A patient's loss of income protection payment is also held until the physician's statement is received; this, in turn, could delay payment to the physician.

**Simplified Claim Form.** A great service has been performed for the busy physician—and his busy assistant—by the Health Insurance Council, a federation of eight insurance associations whose member companies account for more than 90 per cent of the health insurance policies written in the United States.

Some years ago, the Health Insurance Council, in cooperation with the American Medical Association's Council on Medical Service, began a program of claim form simplification which won wide support from the nation's insurance companies. The Council first developed two lists of questions designed to elicit the necessary information for handling claims; one list was for individual insurance claims and the other for group claims. Six simplified standard claim forms, covering different situations, were developed and made available to physicians' offices, as well as to cooperating insurance companies.

Refinement of these forms continued, and in 1964 further simplification and standardization was begun. Variations in the group and individual questions were eliminated, one format of questions was adopted, some questions were eliminated and some changed, *authorization to release information* and *authorization to pay physician* clauses were incorporated, and a standard size of 8½ × 11 inches was agreed upon.

This form, generally referred to as the "standard" or "H.I.C. Form," can be used for both group and individual insurance claims and has been found acceptable to almost all insurance companies. Many companies supply the form to the claimant, but in cases where the company has a non-standard form the physician can use the H.I.C. form and attach it to the form supplied by the company. Blank forms can be obtained from most professional printing companies, many of them produced in duplicate with a snap-out carbon (Fig. 19–8).

## SYSTEMATIZING CLAIMS PREPARATION

Whenever you find medical assistants "talking shop" a frequent topic of discussion is the ever-mounting accumulation of insurance forms to be completed. It is not always just the volume of forms that causes the problem. Failure to systematize the work, procrastination, failure to keep informed, and possibly a subconscious resentment contribute to the problem.

So what is so difficult about completing an insurance claim? It is surely easier and less expensive than billing an account for several months, then writing a series of collection letters, and perhaps eventually having to resort to third-party collection procedures. It is also easier to complete five to ten forms per day than it is to find time to complete a stack of forms which have been allowed to accumulate for a week or more. If the volume of insurance is so great that the office assistant, using efficient systematized procedures, cannot keep them up to date, then the wise physician will hire extra help for this purpose. The collection potential in most medical practices is increased in proportion to the proper handling of the patients' insurance. It therefore behooves the medical office assistant and the physician to give proper attention to the processing of the claims.

**Who is Responsible?** The receptionist, the medical assistant, the bookkeeper, the insurance clerk, the nurse, the doctor, anyone who treats the patient, keeps records, or handles the telephone or appointments, plays a role in insurance.

The processing of insurance claim forms begins with the receptionist. When the first appointment is made, she can ask the patient to bring along his insurance information and forms. If the patient has an identification card, first determine that the coverage is current, then photocopy the card for your records. If more than one insurance is involved, get information for ALL companies.

Obtain complete and accurate information on every new patient, including:

1. Full name, address, and telephone number
2. Marital status; name of spouse, if married
3. Occupation, employer, business address and telephone
4. Date of birth
5. Social security number
6. Driver's license number (for skip tracing)
7. Name of insurance subscriber, if patient is a dependent
8. Who referred patient

Insurance information can change. For continuing patients, the receptionist should recheck insurance coverage every six months or so. Date stamp forms as they are received, and keep a log of all insurance forms (Fig. 19–10). A log such as this will immediately enable you to tell an inquiring patient whether or not his claim form has been completed and mailed.

The doctor, office nurse, or medical assistant is responsible for the complete and accurate reporting of diagnosis and services performed. Unless the full information is on the chart, the insurance clerk cannot do her work well.

The person who does the bookkeeping must post the charges promptly and accurately.

## COMPLETING THE FORMS

The importance of systematizing the processing of claims cannot be overemphasized. The work will be much easier if the following items are observed:

1. A definite time is set aside for this task

| PATIENT | INSURANCE CO. | DATE IN | DATE OUT |
|---------|---------------|---------|----------|
| James Bush | Continental Casualty | 3-14 | 3-15 |
| Virginia Ellis | Aetna Life | 3-14 | 3-15 |
| Robert Haskell | Occidental | 3-15 | 3-15 |
| Mary Blodgett | Travelers | " | 3-15 |
| Stan Wilson | Prudential | " | 3-15 |
| " " | State Disability | " | 3-15 |
| Wm. Price | County Employee's Group | 3-16 | 3-18 Returned to pt |
| Earl Jacoby | Fireman's Fund | " | 3-17 |
| Mary Frederick | Aetna Casualty | " | 3-17 |

*(INSURANCE CLAIM FORMS)*

**Figure 19–10**   Insurance Log

2. There is a central location for all insurance forms

3. The necessary manuals, code books, and other references are nearby

4. Standard insurance forms, rubber stamps, and so on are used

5. Forms are completed by category (all Blue Cross, all Medicare, and so forth)

6. Tabulator stops are set for the form being completed (Note these stops so they can be easily found when doing the same kind of form again)

**Reasons for Claims Rejection.** Many complaints made against insurance companies are not the fault of the companies but of the individuals completing the claim forms. The company processors are not mind readers; the claim form must be sufficiently detailed, complete, and accurate. Perhaps recounting some of the reasons for claim rejection will emphasize this point.

1. Diagnosis is missing, or incomplete, or does not correspond with treatment performed
2. Charges are not itemized
3. Patient's group, member, or policy number is missing or incorrect
4. Patient's portion of form is incomplete
5. Birth date is missing
6. Doctor's name or address is missing

## SOME GUIDELINES FOR THE INSURANCE CLERK

When the patient brings in his insurance form, check to see that his portion has been completed.

With your doctor's approval, have the patient sign *Assignment of Benefits* and *Authorization to Release Information* on first visit.

Typewrite all claim forms and keep a copy (either carbon or photocopy).

If insured's statement is on a separate page from the physician's statement, photocopy the insured's completed page. Then use the reverse side of the photocopy for a carbon copy of the physician's statement. You then will have complete information and only one sheet of paper to add to your record.

Use standard nomenclature in diagnosis and procedure. If your state does not have a relative value study, use *Current Medical Terminology* and *Current Procedural Terminology* manuals, published by the American Medical Association, or *International Classification of Diseases, Adapted* (I.C.D.A.) Vol. II (alphabetical list), available from the U.S. Government Printing Office.

List ALL procedures performed; one procedure per line. Be specific. If a laceration is treated, give location, length and depth, number of sutures required, and time of treatment involved. If a sterile surgical tray was used for office surgery, itemize and bill as a separate fee. If treatment injection was given, state injectable material and amount given.

Attach a copy of x-ray report, hospital report, or consultant's report in complicated cases.

State usual and customary fee on all claim forms regardless of what payment is expected.

Never alter a claim as to services performed, date of service, or fees established.

If more than one visit per day is required, state the times of day so that the claims processor will know they were separate procedures.

Fill in ALL blanks. Type D.N.A. (does not apply) or N.A. (not applicable) or simply dash lines (- - - -) rather than leave an item blank. This prevents possible tampering, and is an added assurance that the item was not overlooked.

Note on the copy the date and to whom the form was mailed.

Process all claims promptly and cheerfully.

**Answering Patient's Questions About Insurance.**   Many times patients will ask questions about their policies and the extent of coverage. The assistant should be familiar with basic information about voluntary health insurance but should refrain from attempting to interpret specific contracts, since there are many factors not known to her which will have a bearing on benefits. She should not be expected to be familiar with the details of the countless policies in force. Suggest that the patient take his policy to his local insurance agent or Blue Cross or Blue Shield representative, depending on the type of coverage, for a detailed answer to his questions. If the policy is one held by an employees' group in a large company, the employer or the insurance clerk can probably answer the question.

Blue Cross and Blue Shield representatives may call at the office from time to time. In many areas, representatives hold special meetings for doctors' assistants in order to familiarize them with insurance forms and the types of coverage offered. The medical office assistant should attend such meetings, since the information she obtains will help her complete her own insurance work more rapidly and efficiently.

The medical assistant, since she understands the need for health insurance, should be enthusiastic about its success. When a patient questions her about the purchase of health insurance, there are several bits of advice she can give:

1. The patient should know the company
2. Know the insurance representative
3. Read and understand the policy
4. Do not expect health insurance to cover pre-existing conditions
5. Know whether the company is licensed by the State Insurance Commission. If the company is not licensed, the state has no jurisdiction over it, and the insured has little recourse if the company refuses to pay a claim.
6. Ask what the limitations are, as well as the provisions of the policy. Are there cancellation or renewable clauses? Does it meet the individual's needs and his ability to pay?

Cheap insurance is available, but it is no bargain, since it gives limited coverage. Policies are available for moderate sums that may provide the coverage suitable for the individual's particular need.

**Avoiding Insurance Abuse.**   When patients and physicians abuse voluntary health insurance, premiums for the insurance inevitably rise. No physician should send a patient to the hospital unless it is positively necessary. Few plans cover diagnostic work. Furthermore, there are many procedures which can be done in the office with equal safety and efficiency, and at a considerably lower cost than in the hospital. Procedures which would benefit from the safety of the hospital, but which do not require an overnight stay, may be scheduled in the outpatient department. Inclusion of outpatient services in insurance coverage will help to eliminate over-utilization of hospital services.

It is really no favor to the patient to put him in the hospital overnight for a few tests in order to help him recover on his insurance, since in the long run such practices make his insurance more costly. Many hospitals have a utilization committee which guards against unnecessary admissions. The medical assistant who understands the regulations and the reasons for them can help keep the goodwill of the patient who may not understand these rules.

Continued growth of voluntary health insurance and prepayment plans, and their successfulness as a means of financing costs of illness, depend to a large extent upon proper use of these programs. People must realize that insurance does not create new money, and using, but not abusing insurance actually provides the most value for each health insurance dollar.

# Chapter 20

**BEHAVIORAL OBJECTIVES**

*The medical office assistant should be able to:*

Organize and plan the housekeeping details in a medical office.

Apply proper methods of stain removal.

Observe necessary precautions for office security.

Correctly label and store drug supplies.

Maintain a card system for supply inventory.

Keep the doctor's bag ready for immediate use.

# Housekeeping and Ordering Supplies

A harmonious, orderly office helps create a good working environment and lifts the morale of patients as well as office personnel. Supervision, or actual performance, of certain housekeeping duties in the office often is a responsibility of the medical assistant. Her duties may grow in proportion to the growth of her employer's practice as she becomes an experienced, loyal employee. She should be completely dependable and willing to assume the duties that will help keep the office running smoothly.

The same principles of organization and planning that guide the business management of an office are essential in the assistant's housekeeping duties. To maintain an atmosphere of organization and harmony, she should plan her duties to avoid rushing and confusion. Here's a good housekeeping rule to follow: have a place for everything, keep everything clean, and *ready for use.* This saves time, conserves property, and eliminates incorrect use of materials. Adoption of sound housekeeping procedures also saves the assistant's personal energy. Furthermore, an office managed on a hit-or-miss basis holds potential dangers for patients, doctors, and assistants alike.

Medical equipment and supplies are expensive and sometimes hard to obtain. If properly cared for, they have a longer life and their use is increased. When you receive a piece of equipment in the office, read the instructions carefully. Do not attempt to assemble or use articles you have not first studied. File these instructions in a special folder and save them for future reference or for your successors. If there is a guarantee with the item, copy the code number, fill in the blank, and mail as instructed. Instructions and guarantees are enclosed for a definite purpose; do not misplace them. Keep a service file for equipment that needs regular servicing. This file should contain:

> guarantee dates
> how often item should be serviced
> when and by whom item was last serviced
> cost of servicing

## OFFICE HOUSEKEEPING DETAILS

Patients in a professional office are especially critical of the condition of the office and its contents. Anyone who visits a physician expects cleanliness and order to prevail. He does not want to feel he has been exposed to the diseases of other patients; he should never see any evidence of previous patients in inner office rooms. Here are some suggestions for general office housekeeping.

*Woodwork* should be washed regularly with a mild soap and water solution. It is the assistant's job to see that such work is done and to make arrangements to have someone do it. Many offices have night janitor or custodial service; if not, a patient who is having difficulty paying his account may be glad to perform such services at the regular prevailing wage to help meet his obligations.

*Floors* should be scrubbed and waxed with a nonskid wax. Highly finished floors look beautiful but are very dangerous, especially for those who are ill and inclined to be unsteady on their feet.

*Rugs* should extend wall to wall or should be tacked down to prevent tripping. It is not advisable to use scatter rugs in professional offices; they are too likely to slip and cause falls.

*Radiators or vents* should be dusted with a dampened cloth; use a paint brush to clean the corners. Check the heater and pilot light for leaks. Furnaces should be oiled regularly and the filters cleaned or changed. A professional service may be best.

*Sinks* should be scrubbed daily or more often, if necessary, to prevent pitting and contamination. Frequent polishing with a mild cleanser will keep a smooth, glossy finish on porcelain, preventing acids from collecting. Hot water should be flushed through the tap and a drain cleanser used frequently. A sink is often the source of infection and odors; it needs constant care and disinfection. Any solid material should be removed from the sink, wrapped in paper, and placed in the waste container. Waste containers of the closed variety are lined with disposable plastic bags, especially in the treatment or examining rooms.

*Surfaces* of counters, table tops, and so forth should be covered with clean towels, white paper, or the new plastics, and these coverings should be changed or washed regularly. Stained surfaces are a sign of contamination. If the area is too large for towels, use paper towels directly under any bottles. The newer equipment has a plastic finish counter surface that is highly resistant to acids and medicine stains. These surfaces are heat resistant and do not scratch easily. They are easy to keep clean. They should be scrubbed daily, or after each patient, with a germicidal cleanser. The undersides of towel and tape dispensers are frequently overlooked in the daily cleaning. Tops of cabinets that are exposed should be dusted daily. These last two items are usually noticed by the patient.

*Cabinets* should be kept scrupulously clean and orderly. Many of the modern medical offices are substituting closed cabinets for those which expose contents to view, since displays of instruments are disturbing to many patients. Even though they may not be visible, all instruments should be cleaned and organized for immediate use.

Do not begin cleaning cabinets unless you have time to complete the job. The doctor's afternoon off is a good opportunity for such jobs. Do one shelf at a time, starting at the top.

1. Remove the material from the shelf and place on a table in the same order as on the shelf.

2. Wash the shelf with warm, soapy water and rinse well. Dry.

3. Clean and polish the instruments and check for faults. Examine hinges and blades.

4. Check all labels to make certain of clarity. Retype and reglue labels, if necessary. Cleaning time is a good time to examine supplies for expiration dates, quantity, and deterioration. Make a list of those items that should be reordered.

5. Replace the supplies in their original places on the shelf. Two major dangers in the medical office are the changing of medications from their original locations and the incorrect reading of labels by the doctor or his staff. Even if a bottle has been in the same position for years, its location should never be taken for granted. When using a product, always read the label twice before proceeding and once again after administration.

*Boiler sanitizers* should be cleaned daily, especially if tap water is used in place of distilled or demineralized water. If there is no sediment from the water, the boiler can be cleaned less frequently. At the end of the day the boiler should be left open with the tray clearing the water level. Acquire the habit of turning off the boiler before opening it for the night and you will eliminate the after-hours fear that you left it on. Many an assistant has had to return to the office in the evening to check the boiler for that very reason.

In areas where water forms a heavy scum inside the boiler, it is necessary to boil it out with an 8 per cent hydrochloric acid (muriatic acid) solution each month. Fill the boiler completely with this solution, bring it to a boil, cool, and drain. Rinse the equipment well and it is again ready to use. Vinegar also is a good cleaning agent, but it is not advisable for office use because of its noticeable odor. Some boiler manufacturers advise the use of a 10 per cent solution of hydrochloric acid at room temperature for cleaning. Do not boil this solution; allow it to stand in the boiler until the scale becomes softened and can be scrubbed off with a stiff brush. When using acids for cleaning purposes, be careful not to spill them on the outside of the boiler, as they will remove the chrome finish. Also take care not to spill such substances on cabinet tops.

Sterilizer tablets are excellent for prevention of scale or rust. These tablets often are available from manufacturers of sterilizers and boilers, who distribute them with their own equipment. Sodium bicarbonate also can be used as a rust deterrent, but it does not do as thorough a job as tablets.

*Autoclaves* should be given special care, and instructions for proper use and cleaning should be followed closely. If you are new in an office and cannot find the proper instructions, write the manufacturer of the equipment for another copy. *Use only distilled or demineralized water in the autoclave.* Place instructions in a transparent plastic folder and tack inside a cupboard door near the autoclave.

*Linens,* if owned by the doctor, must be carefully marked with a special linen marker, ink, or linen pen. This ink will not smear or wash out. All laundry should be counted before it is sent and recounted when it is returned. Keep a copy of the laundry list in a special folder, for use in checking the returned laundry. Clean linen should be stored in a clean, dry place free from dust and insects. Provide a definite place for each type of linen. When storing, place folds on the outside toward the front; this gives a neater appearance and makes it easier to pick up one piece at a time.

Never use towels as scrub cloths, even though they are rented from a commercial laundry. Wash your hands immediately after handling dirty laundry and before handling clean linens. Avoid unnecessary waste of linens. If the linens are owned by the doctor, inspect pieces before putting them away and remove damaged pieces for discard or mending. The laundry will perform this checking service if your office uses a laundry rental service. Many offices are now using some disposable towels and examination drapes, *so remember to separate them from the soiled linen going to the laundry. These paper products can cause no end of trouble in the washing processes.*

*Blankets* should never be allowed to touch a patient's body. The blankets should be protected from such contact with a sheet. Blankets should be cleaned regularly. Treatment blankets are usually washable; blanket sheets are also warm and washable.

**Removal of Stains.**   Stains, markings, and discolorations are frequent and inevitable eyesores in the professional office. Such blemishes on linens, furniture, supplies, clothing, or the skin often have a distressing effect on the morale of patients. Immediate action very often results in successful removal of such stains. Various agents for removal of stains should be kept on hand in a convenient place. General directions for stain removals should be memorized.

*Blood stains,* common in the medical office, can be removed by soaking the article in cool, *not hot,* water and then washing it. To remove old blood stains, soak in peroxide or ammonia, then wash. Naphtha or benzene should never be applied to blood; this sets the blood stain, making removal impossible. Peroxide is best for removing blood stains from white materials.

*Acids* should be neutralized immediately with an alkaline substance such as ammonia or sodium bicarbonate, then washed thoroughly. Then test with litmus. *Alkalis* should be treated with a mild acid, such as vinegar or a weak (10 per cent) solution of citric or acetic acid. Wash the article well and test with litmus.

See opposite page for table giving directions for removing stains of various types.

# RECEPTION ROOM

The importance of a neat, attractive reception room was pointed out in Chapter 8, *Your Role as Receptionist.* It is the room from which patients gain their first impression of the office. From a housekeeping standpoint, then, it is particularly vital that the reception room be kept clean, orderly, and in good condition. The assistant must see to it that cleaning duties such as dusting and vacuuming are performed regularly. Even if you have maintenance service in your office, morning dusting is advisable.

Provide plenty of fresh air but guard against drafts, since people who are ill are very susceptible to chills. There should be a constant change of air by means of open windows or air conditioners. If you have air conditioning, do not keep it too cool. The ideal temperature for a reception room is about 74° F. Room thermometers are a great help in maintaining the proper temperature. If your office does not have a thermometer, purchase one and place it in a location where you think the temperature is neither too hot nor too cold in the room.

Lighting should be balanced, and there should be no glare. If it is necessary for chairs to face the windows, keep the blinds drawn slightly to prevent direct reflection into patients' eyes. Lamps are very decorative, but they are useful only if properly placed. Lamps should be at reading height; otherwise, they shine into

| *Substance Causing Stain* | *How to Remove* |
|---|---|
| Aniline dyes | Use lye solution or weak hydrochloric acid solution. Acid alcohol also may be used. Wash. |
| Silver nitrate | Remove fresh stains by soaking in salt water. Treat old stains with a warm solution of sodium thiosulfate, about 10 to 20%. Silver nitrate stains on the skin can be removed by painting the surface with iodine and then applying alcohol. |
| Coffee or cocoa | Wash in concentrated salt water and rinse well. It is sometimes necessary to soften the stain with glycerin before rinsing with cold water and borax. |
| Feces | Soak well in cold water and wash with soap and water. |
| Merthiolate | Remove with Dakin's solution (chlorinated soda). |
| Iron rust | Cover with lemon juice and salt and bleach in sunlight. There are also excellent commercial products for removal of rust. |
| Chlorophyll (grass stains) | Use warm alcohol to remove fresh stains. Kerosene can be used on older stains along with sodium perborate, diluted hydrogen peroxide, or diluted aromatic spirits of ammonia. Some commercial products are excellent. |
| Iodine (on hands or clothes) | Moisten with ammonia or sodium thiosulfate solution. Starch is sometimes a successful removal agent. |
| Mercurochrome | Immerse first in a 20% solution of potassium permanganate and then in a 5% solution of oxalic acid. Rinse well. |
| Petroleum jelly | Use ether, alcohol, or benzol (benzene) and wash with soda and hot water solution. An absorbent material placed under the stain will facilitate absorption while treating the stain. |
| Adhesive plaster | Use ether or benzol. There are special removers on the market that do not sting the tissues and are pleasant-smelling. |
| Ink | Remove ink stains from the skin with glycerin, acetic acid, or citric acid. To remove ink stains from fabric, immerse in tepid water and skimmed milk for a long time. It is sometimes necessary to cover the surface with lemon juice and salt and place in the sun. |

the eyes of others in the waiting room or are so low patients have to slump to read by them.

The supply of accessories such as magazines and ash trays should be constantly checked. Smoking is usually discouraged in a professional office, since some people object to it. If a patient insists on smoking, have an ashtray ready if he asks for it. Then remove it immediately after the patient leaves.

Flower arrangements are a delight to see, but they should be attractively arranged and discarded immediately when they start to wilt. The water should be changed and kept fresh to prevent any odor. Because artificial plants are now so attractive, they are frequently used, but they too take care. Keep the leaves wiped free of dust to give a fresh appearance.

Toys present definite housekeeping problems. They are necessary in offices where children are visitors and have to wait any length of time. Such articles should be chosen for their cleanability and noiselessness. In some offices, the toys are kept in another room and are given to the children as needed, with an explanation to the mother that the article has been washed since the last child used it. Some offices have discontinued having toys and find that large animal pillows and plenty of good picture books satisfy the children and make a quieter waiting area. Television is good but should be mounted high enough to prevent the little patients from adjusting the channel and sound.

Draperies and upholstery should be cleaned regularly. This may be done at vacation time. Today much office furniture is plastic and washable; the dark, gloomy appearance of the reception room furniture of the past is being replaced with lighter colored furniture that is easier to clean.

Step into the reception room several times a day to check on the lighting and temperature and straighten the magazines. In more than one office patients have been left in the dark at the close of the day because the assistant was too busy to attend to her reception room duties properly.

## THE ASSISTANT'S DESK

The office assistant's desk is usually in view of the patients, and consequently it should be neat at all times. Everything should have its place and should be returned to it when you are finished. Provide desk trays for records and business papers requiring attention. Do not leave such items lying around to be lost or to be read by patients. *Keep your personal belongings out of sight.*

In the ideal office, the assistant has a private corner that is separated from the reception room by a glass partition of some sort. She can see entering patients and keep close check on the reception room but can also carry on private conversations with patients out of earshot of those who are waiting.

## THE DOCTOR'S OFFICE AND OTHER ROOMS

The doctor's office should always be kept neat and clean. Give this room a quick once-over after each patient departs, and remove any evidence of the preceding patient. Do not make any changes without first consulting your doctor. Never throw anything away, even a bit of paper with a number on it. It may be important to the doctor. Organize his professional literature in convenient order and to his liking. Check his supplies, such as batteries in the flashlight, tongue depressors, the cuff of his sphygmomanometer and so forth, daily. In offices where the doctor likes to keep some form of appeasement for his little patients, such as candy or pencils, the assistant must also check to see that the supply of these items is adequate.

Inner office housekeeping is a full-time job in many offices. Good system and management are essential here. Consulting, examining, treatment, diagnostic rooms, recovery rooms, and laboratories must be spotless. These rooms should be straightened and cleaned after each patient. All linen must be changed and medications used earlier put out of sight. Often a patient knows who was in the room previously; never leave a telltale bottle of medication in view. Watch the temperature in these rooms, since patients are usually asked to disrobe. These rooms should be kept a little warmer than other parts of the office. Deodorants are often necessary in the examination rooms; these help remove the medicinal odor that many people dislike.

Check supplies and equipment often. Reorder when supplies are low; do not wait until the supply is exhausted. If you are not familiar with the supplies in a new office, ask the doctor; or if you feel he may change brands, check with him on new orders. Expiration dates and deterioration of materials must be watched constantly. Don't jeopardize a life by using outdated or spoiled medication.

The laboratory is often the office catch-all. Even though it is out of sight, it should be kept clean. Accurate work cannot be done in the midst of disorder. All contaminated material must be properly disposed of by wrapping it in paper and placing it in a plastic-lined waste container. Glassware should be immersed in a disinfectant solution and allowed to remain there for several hours. Autoclave any contaminated articles that are not disposable. Sterility must be maintained in the laboratory just as in the examining and treatment rooms.

Laboratory table tops should be scrubbed after contact with any contaminated material. All hose connections should be checked for leaks; electric wires should be protected against moisture. It is a good idea to leave the laboratory window open whenever possible. There are many odors from the laboratory that soon are not noticeable to the office force but are very disagreeable to the patients. Be very careful when using any volatile material, making certain that the burners are shut off.

All solutions and bottles should have definite storage places away from too much light and heat. Most solutions are stored in brown bottles, since light causes deterioration. The laboratory glassware must be spotlessly clean and free from chemicals and contamination. Do not use any glassware that has been cracked or nicked. A cut hand in the laboratory is dangerous.

The recovery room should be comfortable and clean. Provide facilities so that patients can relax and keep warm. Interesting reading material will help the time pass more pleasantly for them. If the patient wishes to sleep, see that no one enters the room. It is a disadvantage in such cases when the recovery room doubles as a storage room.

Decorations are not used in the inner office rooms. These rooms are designed for utility; only necessary equipment and supplies should be found here. They should appear fresh and clean as well as pleasant and comfortable. Stark white examining rooms are almost a thing of the past. Treatment tables and cabinets are now available in colors. Walls are in soft pastels, and the general decor is more attractive. Instruments and much of the equipment are out of sight, but the rooms should be neat and easy to maintain.

Close adherence to good housekeeping principles lightens the assistant's tasks in the long run, since the materials she and the doctor need are always in working condition and always available.

## OFFICE SECURITY

**Protect Your Office Against Theft.** Police say it is the smalltime thief or drug addict who breaks into physicians' offices. Smalltime or not, this kind of occurrence is all toò frequent, and medical offices are far too often making it easy, at times almost seeming to invite the break-in. The drug addict is doubly danger- ous because he is usually desperate and angers easily if he breaks in and cannot find what he wants.

Smalltime or bigtime thieves usually "case" an office before breaking in. The would-be thief is not easy to spot but the office staff can be alert to certain indi- viduals who may be focusing on the office as a possible "easy" target. Be on guard against the extremely nervous person with moist "glassy" eyes and a runny nose, the delivery man or messenger who is unduly interested in the location of your syringe and drug storage, or the person who watches too intently when you make change from the petty cash drawer. Always be suspicious of anyone hang- ing around the parking area or the courtyard of a medical complex. If you notice such an individual, report it to the manager at once.

It is most important to secure all entrances—windows as well as doors. Have good double locks put on by a reliable locksmith. It may be well worth the cost to consult a professional security service and follow their advice. Check with the local police department or the county medical society for the name of such an agency. Making an office "burglar-proof" is impossible, but entry can be made difficult, and this in itself will usually discourage the amateur.

Bright outside lights with unbreakable shields are extremely helpful. Leav- ing a light burning inside the office is another deterrent. Tell the local police which lights will always be left on. If the inside of the office is visible to passersby, all small movable items which might be tempting should be put away out of sight before you leave the office at the end of the day.

Alarms can be helpful if they are reliable and are not easily disconnected by an expert. Loud local alarms are usually sufficient to frighten off a prowler. It is possible, though, to install an alarm that will ring in the local police station or at a special security office.

Police departments are urging that all valuables be protected by etching them with personal identification, such as the owner's name or social security number. This is easily done with an electric engraving tool that cuts into the equipment, and the marking is practically impossible to eradicate. Even if an at- tempt is made to scratch it off, a sufficient mark will be left so that the police, with the aid of a special chemical, can bring the engraved characters up again. Ar- ticles so marked are almost impossible to "fence." Place a sign in the office win- dow (Fig. 20–1) showing that you have identified your valuables.

The most effective step in protecting your office is to remember to check carefully at the end of the day to make certain all doors and windows are doubly locked. Unless you make this an unvarying part of your routine, it is easy to leave a window unlatched. You may as well write an invitation on it or hand the thief the items through the window.

## SUPPLIES

Although the care and ordering of supplies have been mentioned pre- viously, there are some special notations that should be considered.

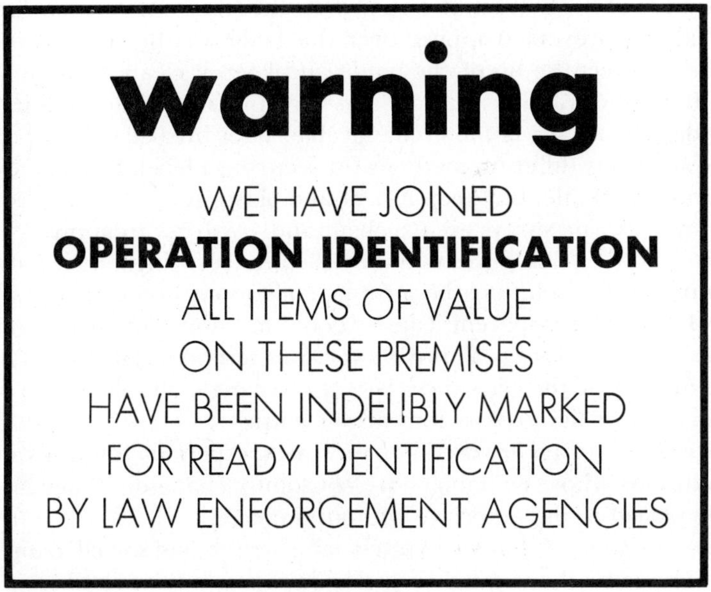

# warning

WE HAVE JOINED
**OPERATION IDENTIFICATION**
ALL ITEMS OF VALUE
ON THESE PREMISES
HAVE BEEN INDELIBLY MARKED
FOR READY IDENTIFICATION
BY LAW ENFORCEMENT AGENCIES

**Figure 20–1**

Follow good housekeeping rules in storing supplies. Supplies should be kept where they are most accessible, yet protected from damage and exposure to moisture, heat, light, and air. Most drugs and solutions should be stored in a cool, dark cupboard because direct light and sunlight cause drug deterioration. Poisons should be stored separately from products used routinely. Have a *distinct label or cap* for these poisons. You might use a bright color, such as red, for their labels or caps. Narcotics must be stored in a secure place, out of sight. Acids and caustics should have special resistant lids; never use metal lids for these substances. Do not store strong acids next to alkalis. Inflammable items must be stored away from heat.

If drugs and solutions are to be stored for some time, the stoppers should be dipped in paraffin to seal them from the air. Do not fill these bottles to the very top; leave a little expansion room.

## Labels

If a bottle is to be used for a long time, the label should be indestructible. The original one is best and should be treated to preserve it when it is first received. If it has not been preserved, however, and shows signs of wear or mutilation, replace it with a neatly typed or printed fresh one.

When you are making new labels (and this cannot be stressed too greatly!), make sure that the new label is an accurate, identical copy of the original. If there are varying strengths or dosages, make certain this information appears correctly. Never change a direction or a name on a label. These labels should be placed on the upper edge of the bottle and on the opposite side from the pouring spout if there is one.

Careful use of the bottles will also protect the labels. Always pour away from the label side to prevent dripping over the label. Plastic screw caps are best because they protect the lip of the bottle and keep it clean. Glass stoppers are necessary for some solutions but are not very practical. They are individually ground and generally are not interchangeable. They break easily and often stick.

There are many different methods for securing a label. Use whatever is best for the particular bottle, but keep it neat and accurate.

1. *Sprays.* Plastic sprays are excellent and very easy to apply.

2. *Scotch Tape.* Although commonly used for securing labels, Scotch tape is not very durable for solutions because it tends to curl on the edges and turn yellow. 3-M Magic Transparent Tape is good and does not curl or yellow.

3. *Glass Ink or Lab-Ink.* This is a superior method of labeling. The ink can be printed directly on the glass and it is very resistant to all solutions. You can obtain inks in dark or light colors for various bottles.

4. *Metal Tags.* Tags are used in many cases, especially for flasks and bottles of stock solutions whose containers are constantly changing. They are durable and can be placed in the autoclave without damage.

5. *Tape Writing.* A hand-operated tape writer has solved many labeling problems. The self-adhering tape is available in many colors and several widths and is quite resistant to damage.

## Ordering of Supplies

Ordering supplies is usually the duty of the medical assistant. Although not an easy task for a new girl, it is an excellent way to learn about supplies and their storage. Never trust your memory to recall amounts, types, or styles to be ordered. Keep an established list or sort of running inventory where you can note dwindling supplies. Record exactly what has been previously used. Do not change brands when ordering unless you consult the doctor and get his consent.

It is advisable to establish good credit with certain reputable supply companies. Very seldom can you save money by purchasing from cut-rate or unknown supply houses. This does not mean that you cannot obtain estimates from competitive houses and purchase wisely. However, do not shift your purchases from company to company without good reason. If you are well known to a supply house, the people there will endeavor to please you and hasten your order. Also, the company will often give you the privilege of trying out a piece of equipment in the office before you actually purchase it. As a result, you will have a better guarantee of the quality of your purchases.

There should be an established method for ordering supplies. Set up a pattern for this task and do not vary it except in emergencies. Many representatives of supply houses will call at regular intervals. This facilitates ordering because you can ask questions and explain to them just what you want.

In some cases, you may save money by purchasing in larger quantities but there are several factors which must be first considered:

1. Will the supply be used in a reasonable length of time?
2. Will it spoil or deteriorate?
3. Is there proper space in the office?
4. Will the doctor continue to use the product?

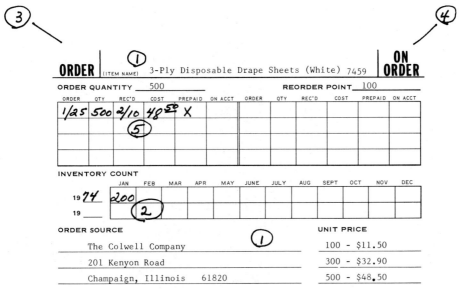

**Figure 20–2**

Before you reorder, be sure you have the correct name of the item and any other identifying information needed. Attention to detail in ordering will be greatly appreciated by the supply houses. It will also speed delivery and assure you of obtaining exactly what you want.

A card system can be used for inventory control of all supplies. Start with 4″ × 6″ Inventory and Order Control Cards (Fig. 20–2).* These can be kept in a file box divided into two indexed sections: one for clinical materials and one for office supplies. Fill in the appropriate data on the cards (1),** using a separate card for each item. Next take inventory and write the amount of stock on hand in the space provided (2). Place a flag, such as the one shown in Figure 20–3, at the point where the supply should be replenished.

When an item needs to be ordered, place a metal tab over the "Order" section of the card (3). When the item is ordered, place the tab over to the right of the card in the "On Order" section (4). Note too the date and quantity ordered at this time.

When the order has been received, note the date and quantity in the correct column (5), remove the tab and refile the card in your file box. If the order is only partially filled, let the tab remain until it is complete. The system is simple, it's accurate, and it can eliminate the problem of running out of needed supplies.

If you have any questions regarding various supplies or if you have a complaint to make, gather the following information before contacting the company: invoice number, date ordered, and name of the person who ordered it. List on paper your questions and the information you desire. If a catalog was used in making the order, open your copy to the correct page and secure additional information.

---

*Available from The Colwell Company, Champaign, Illinois
**Refer to corresponding numbers on Figure 20–2 for location of items on Inventory and Order Control Card.

# RED FLAG
# RE-ORDER TAG

### when this inventory
### point is reached,
### its time to reorder

### Product
### Identification

_____

#### The Colwell Company
#### Champaign, Illinois

Figure 20-3

Even a reputable supply house can make mistakes, so check all the supplies you receive against your original order and the enclosed invoice. Check for correct items, sizes, and styles as well as the number or amount received. Keep all invoices and order forms for at least three years.

Orders for supplies usually should be listed in a set style—that is, the actual title of the supply listed first, then the special name and size. Here are examples: "Scissors, Lister bandage, chrome, $5\frac{1}{2}$ inch" or "pipette, Thoma blood diluting, for white corpuscles."

Your order should state whether payment is to be charged to the doctor's account, paid by check, or C.O.D. Very few physicians use C.O.D. Most doctors have established credit and prefer to pay their accounts by check at given times each month.

It is good business to inventory all equipment and supplies each year. First, list all capital purchases, such as furniture, sterilizers, treatment machines. These items are expensive but are permanent equipment. List date purchased and original price. Next, list the smaller items that are not considered expendable but are less expensive, such as instruments, syringes, and thermometers. Last, estimate the usable supplies and drugs. Keep this inventory to check against the inventory for the coming year. It is also invaluable for income tax purposes.

## Drug Samples

Samples of drugs and medications are continually arriving in the physician's office. These drugs should not be simply discarded. Separate those that are suitable to the doctor's practice and place them in the sample cupboard. The remainder can be saved for charitable agencies. There are many deserving medical missionaries who are very appreciative of medical supplies, but be sure to thoroughly examine the reliability of the drugs and the authenticity of the recipients before releasing the samples. The consent of the physician is, of course, also necessary. Under no circumstances should these samples be sold or given out randomly.

## Storage of Drugs

The sample cupboard should be organized categorically. Place all similar drugs together, preferably in boxes of similar size and shape, with the tops open and plainly labeled on the outside. Clear plastic shoe boxes or sweater boxes are excellent for this type of storage. Color-coded labels are an additional help in identification. Keep all the sedative samples in one box, all the stimulant samples in another, and so forth. It is a good practice to band together drug samples that have the same code number or expiration date. Do not forget to rotate the drugs by placing the most recently received ones in the back of the cupboard. At regular intervals check them for expiration dates, and properly discard those that have expired.

If you frequently receive samples of the same product, you can remove a label and place it on a larger bottle. Then each time this particular sample is received, empty it into the stock bottle. This may provide a good supply of the drug for some patient who is having financial difficulties and is unable to pay for his medicines. A disadvantage of this practice is that the manufacturer's drug batch code number and the expiration date are no longer known.

## THE DOCTOR'S BAG

Minutes mean the difference between life or death in a medical emergency. The doctor's bag must be completely fitted and ready for his use at any hour of the day or night.

The responsibility of caring for the doctor's bag is often delegated to his medical assistant. This responsibility is a serious one and must be given close and continual attention. There is nothing more disconcerting or dangerous than to have the physician arrive at the scene of an emergency only to find that his assistant has not replaced the heart stimulants, the sedatives, or some other equally vital supply. The dangers involved are apparent.

It is a sign of his confidence in your reliability when your doctor turns over to you the care of his bag. So that the bag is always ready, establish a routine for daily examination of its contents. As a guide, keep an inventory of the bag's contents posted inside a cupboard above the place where you check and clean the bag.

If you have no time to check the bag routinely, do not fail to ask the doctor whether or not he made any house calls and find out what medications and equipment he used. You will need this information for your records and case histories.

When checking the bag, remove any specimens and see that they are properly labeled with the patient's full name, the date, and the type of test if the specimen is to be sent out for examination. If the doctor has used any instruments or gloves, remove them and replace with sterile ones. It is a wise idea to have a duplicate set of instruments and extra pairs of gloves handy so that they may be replaced immediately. Even if this equipment has not been used, it should be sterilized weekly. Keep the containers of alcohol, germicides, and other substances filled and check containers often for leaks. Do not fill fluid containers completely full to the stopper, but allow a small space for heat expansion.

If you have not received the information from the physician, you can tell what medications have been used by checking the contents of the bag against your inventory list. Medications should be routinely checked for deterioration and outdated material.

The physician usually carries only a small amount of narcotics in his bag. Whenever narcotics are dispensed from the bag, it is necessary to enter the patient's full name, the date, his address, the amount given, and the doctor's diagnosis in the office narcotic record book. This book will help you in your narcotic inventory.

You will find that the items your employer carries in his bag are determined by his personal preference, professional requirements, and the areas to be covered. When you clean the bag thoroughly each week, be careful to replace everything in its original position. The doctor organizes his bag to fit his individual needs. Often he is in a hurry, and this organization facilitates speed and accuracy. Do not substitute equipment or medications without the doctor's knowledge and consent. The many new disposable supplies make it much easier to care for the doctor's bag.

Here is a list of some items commonly found in a physician's bag:

Blood pressure set
Stethoscope
Thermometers (oral and rectal)
Flashlight and/or pencil light
Sterile gloves and lubricating
  jelly

Sterile syringes and needles
  (preferably disposable)
Sterile swabs
Sterile dressings
Tongue depressors
Scissors

Wooden applicators
Assorted bandages
Adhesive tape (assorted widths)
Safety pins
Towel
Fountain pen
Prescription pads
Sterile suture set
Scalpel
Probe
Tourniquet
Percussion hammer
Illuminated diagnostic set (otoscope and ophthalmoscope)
Tissue forceps
Hemostatic forceps

Dressing forceps
Oral screw and airway
Microscopic slides and fixative
Culture tubes for throat cultures
Medications:
  Morphine
  Codeine
  Sedatives
  Adrenalin
  Digitalis
  Antibiotics (disposable type)
  Alcohol and/or skin disinfectant
  Sterilizing solution
  Spirits of ammonia

Section Three

# *The*
# *Clinical*
# *Assistant*

# Chapter 21

## BEHAVIORAL OBJECTIVES

*The medical assistant should be able to:*

List the Basic Four Food Groups and know the major nutrients contributed by each group.

Identify the Recommended Daily Allowances for a specific nutrient for a given individual using the N.R.C. table.

Evaluate menus using either the Basic Four Food Groups or the N.R.C. table.

Describe the classic deficiency diseases, major food sources, and basic function in the body of the nu-trients required for good health.

Identify the seven basic methods of modifying the normal diet for therapeutic purposes.

Name the general characteristics of a given therapeutic diet and describe its application in terms of the types of conditions for which it can be used.

Describe the function of the medical assistant in teaching and interpreting the therapeutic diet to a patient.

# Nutrition and Diet Therapy

## Lee Weller Callaway, R.D., M.P.H., Ph.D.

## Normal Nutrition

Good health is a state of emotional and physical well-being which is determined to a large extent by a person's diet. We are, quite literally, what we eat, since the food we consume is used to build and repair every part of our bodies. Consequently, it is important that the food choices made are based on sound information and knowledge. A person who is well nourished will probably be more alert in every way and emotionally better balanced. He is also better able to ward off infections than the poorly nourished individual.

The physician, the nurse, and the dietitian are all closely involved in the nutritive care of a patient. The physician prescribes the diet, and, ideally, a dietitian instructs the patient on how to follow it. Frequently, however, such professional aid is not available. In this case, it is often necessary for the assistant to discuss the diet with the patient, answer questions, and explain certain aspects of the modifications involved. Many patients may hesitate to ask the physician details about the diet, or questions may arise after the patients leave the office. Such concerns are usually about preparation methods, information sources, label interpretation, and so forth, and the medical assistant is the one the patient turns to for answers. Consequently, the assistant should be able to answer basic questions on normal nutrition and have a fundamental knowledge of those diets which the doctor prescribes most often.

## Nutrition and Dietetics

The definitions of these terms vary considerably throughout the literature. Basically, the science of nutrition is concerned with studying the nutritive materials taken into the body (food) and the metabolic processes which utilize them. Nutrition, as such, is defined in the *Handbook of Diet Therapy* as the "combination of processes by which the living organism receives and utilizes the materials necessary for the maintenance of its functions and for the growth and renewal of its components." In a slightly different context, nutrition is also used to indicate nutritional status, or the condition of the body due to "the utilization of the essential nutrients available to the body."

Dietetics, on the other hand, is the practical application of nutritional science to individuals. It is "the combined science and art of feeding individuals or groups under different economic or health conditions according to the principles of nutrition and management."

**329**

## Food

There are many materials eaten throughout the world which we in the United States do not consider acceptable food (grasshoppers, sheep's eyes, and so on). Similarly, many substances man can eat are forbidden, some for religious reasons or because of cultural custom. Nevertheless, to be classified as food a substance must perform one or more of three basic functions in the body (Fig. 21–1):

1. Provide a source of fuel or energy.
2. Supply nutrients to build and repair tissues.
3. Supply nutrients to regulate body processes.

Most foods supply both fuel and nutrients; however, no one food supplies all nutrients required for proper metabolism. Consequently, a mixture of different foods is necessary. With a little planning, a well-balanced diet, one that supplies all the elements which the body needs, can be obtained. If one or more of the required nutrients is inadequate, health suffers and the ability to function optimally is lowered. If prolonged deficiencies occur, specific diseases, even death, may follow.

Nutrients are substances from food that the cells of the body utilize. When food is consumed and broken down by the process of digestion, the nutrients derived are absorbed into the system.

Digestion is a series of reactions occurring in the mouth, the stomach, and the small intestine that result in reducing large food molecules into simple absorbable forms. Absorption is the process of assimilation of foods into the body when they are in their simpler form. Most absorption occurs in the small intestines. The blood then carries the digested and absorbed nutrients to all parts of

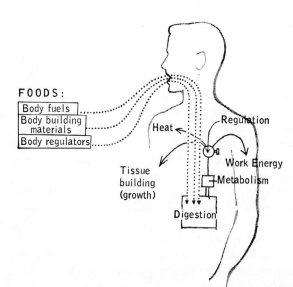

**Figure 21–1** Diagram summarizing the functions of food. To qualify as a food, it must offer substances that act as body fuel to provide energy, serve to build or maintain body tissues, or act as regulators of body processes. Many foods contain substances that serve all three purposes. (From Bogert et al.: *Nutrition and Physical Fitness,* 9th Ed. Philadelphia, W. B. Saunders Co., 1973.)

the body where they are metabolized. The nutrients referred to are divided into seven classes:

1. Carbohydrates
2. Fats
3. Proteins
4. Vitamins
5. Minerals
6. Water
7. Cellulose

All of these must be supplied in sufficient quantities daily for good health.

## Energy

Every bodily action, voluntary and involuntary, requires energy. Even when asleep the body still needs a source of energy for basal metabolism, to keep the heart beating, the lungs breathing, and other vital organs functioning. Voluntary action refers to muscular activities that are consciously carried out. Additionally, the involuntary activities of digestion and respiration also require energy even though not consciously controlled.

There are basically two energy sources available to the body: exogenous and endogenous. If insufficient quantities of food (exogenous) are consumed to furnish the required fuel, the body will begin to break down its own fat reserves (endogenous) in an attempt to supply the necessary energy. Generally, it is desirable for the daily food intake to equal the total energy needs of the body (number of calories needed both for voluntary and for involuntary activities).

Energy, or heat production, is measured in units called calories. In nutrition the "large calorie," or kilocalorie (kcal), is used to differentiate it from the smaller, more widely used calorie. One kilocalorie (or Calorie) is defined as the amount of heat required to raise the temperature of one kilogram of water one degree Centigrade.* Of the seven food constituents, carbohydrates, fats, and proteins are capable of furnishing the body with energy. One gram of either carbohydrate or protein yields 4 kcal/gm, whereas one gram of fat provides 9 kcal/gm. The amount of energy needed by a given individual varies considerably with his activity level and basal requirements; however, most adults require 1800 to 3600 kcal a day.

## Dietary Evaluation

There are two basic methods commonly used for determining the nutritional adequacy of a given diet. The easier is a shorthand method and utilizes the Basic Four Groups. The other, using the recommended allowances, is more time consuming but more accurate.

---

*Although the term calorie is currently being used, nomenclature is expected to change soon. The Joule is a unit of energy that is accepted by all scientists. Conversion: 1 Calorie = 4.184 Joules.

## THE BASIC FOUR FOOD GROUPS

Foods within a group supply similar nutrients, although the foods differ in caloric level and in nutrients supplied. If the Basic Four Food plan is followed and no other foods are included, the average diet will supply 1200 kcal. If the foods from each group are chosen wisely, a person can meet all of his nutrient requirements (with the possible exception of iron for women). Additional calories are easily obtained by either increasing the total quantity of food eaten from the Basic Four, or by adding sugars and fats to these foods (see Table 21–1).

In planning daily menus a person should try to schedule regularly spaced meals. It is not an absolute necessity that three meals be consumed; however, it is extremely difficult to meet all of the nutrient and caloric requirements with fewer meals. Each meal should supply about one-third of the total daily requirements. This means that something from each group should be included at every meal.

## RECOMMENDED DAILY ALLOWANCES

During World War II, the Food and Nutrition Board of the National Academy of Sciences–National Research Council was appointed to examine current research in the field of nutrition and to set up dietary standards. The first edition of the resulting dietary guide was published in 1943, and has been updated approximately every five years since then, as new research data becomes

**TABLE 21–1** BASIC FOUR FOOD GROUPS

| Food Group | Average Amount/Serving | Average Servings/Day | Major Nutrients |
|---|---|---|---|
| Milk and dairy products | 8 oz. fluid milk<br>⅔ cup ice cream<br>1 oz. cheddar cheese | children 4<br>adults 2 | Calcium<br>Phosphorus<br>Protein<br>Riboflavin |
| Meats<br>beef, lamb, poultry, fish, eggs, veal | 3 oz. cooked weight | 2 | Protein<br>Iron<br>Thiamin<br>Niacin |
| Fruits and vegetables | ½ cup | 4<br>(1 citrus daily,<br>1 dark green leafy or<br>deep yellow vegetable<br>every other day) | Vitamin A<br>Vitamin C |
| Breads and cereals | 1 slice bread<br>½ cup cooked cereal<br>¾ cup dry cereal | 4<br>(whole grain or<br>enriched) | Thiamin<br>Iron<br>Protein<br>Niacin<br>Riboflavin |

available. The latest revision (1973) is shown in Table 21–2. The standards are known as the NRC's (National Research Council) or as the Recommended Dietary Allowances (RDA). These are suggested daily nutrient intakes which are "judged to be adequate for the maintenance of good nutrition in essentially all healthy persons in the United States under current conditions of living."* All nutrients, except for calories, allow a safety margin to cover individual physical or environmental variations. The allowances are not, however, meant to be adequate in cases of illness or injury. The allowances are grouped by both age and sex. Activity level is assumed to be moderate.

## Nutrients

### CARBOHYDRATES

Carbohydrates are chemical organic compounds composed of carbon, hydrogen, and oxygen. They are divided into three groups based on the complexity of the molecule: monosaccharides, disaccharides, and polysaccharides.

Monosaccharides and disaccharides are also called simple sugars. That is, they are made of one (mono) or two (di) units (saccharides). They are usually water soluble and sweet if tasted. The most common monosaccharides are glucose and fructose. The best dietary sources of these sugars are fruits and vegetables. Since they are small molecules they are absorbed rapidly into the blood stream from the small intestine. Glucose is an especially important sugar since it is the form of carbohydrate used by the body for energy and the only form of carbohydrate which the brain and nervous system can use for fuel. The most common disaccharides are sucrose and lactose. Sucrose is granulated or table sugar obtained from either sugar cane or beet sugar. Lactose is the major sugar found in milk and is the only common sugar not found in plant sources. It is not as sweet as many sugars and therefore is frequently used to sweeten formulas for tube feedings or to increase the caloric value of juices without appreciably changing the sweetness.

Polysaccharides are complex sugars, composed of many units of simple sugars. They are neither water soluble nor sweet to the taste. Sources of polysaccharides are starches, cellulose, and glycogen. Starches are found in grain products (such as rice and wheat), in vegetables, and in smaller amounts in fruits. Cellulose is the structural component of plants. Digestion of cellulose is very limited in the body so cellulose has little nutritive value. It is, however, important as a source of bulk or roughage which aids in proper elimination. Glycogen in the body is equivalent to starch in plants; it is the storage form of carbohydrate in the body. As such it is stored in liver and muscle tissue. It is used for energy by the body when broken down to glucose in the liver.

---

*Recommended Dietary Allowances, Publication #1694, 8th Ed., Washington, D.C., National Academy of Science – National Research Council, 1973, adapted.

**TABLE 21–2** RECOMMENDED DAILY DIETARY ALLOWANCES,[1] REVISED 1973 FOOD AND NUTRITION BOARD, NATIONAL ACADEMY OF SCIENCES—NATIONAL RESEARCH COUNCIL DESIGNED FOR THE MAINTENANCE OF GOOD NUTRITION OF PRACTICALLY ALL HEALTHY PEOPLE IN THE U.S.A.

| | Age (years) From Up to | Weight (kg) | Weight (lbs) | Height (cm) | Height (in) | Energy (kcal)[2] | Protein (g) | Vitamin A Activity (RE)[3] | Vitamin A Activity (IU) | Vitamin D (IU) | Vitamin E Activity[5] (IU) |
|---|---|---|---|---|---|---|---|---|---|---|---|
| Infants | 0.0–0.5 | 6 | 14 | 60 | 24 | kg × 117 | kg × 2.2 | 420[4] | 1100 | 400 | 4 |
| | 0.5–1.0 | 9 | 20 | 71 | 28 | kg × 108 | kg × 2.0 | 400 | 2000 | 400 | 5 |
| Children | 1–3 | 13 | 28 | 86 | 34 | 1300 | 23 | 400 | 2000 | 400 | 7 |
| | 4–6 | 20 | 44 | | | 1800 | 30 | 500 | 2500 | 400 | 9 |
| | 7–10 | 30 | 66 | | | 2400 | 36 | 700 | 3300 | 400 | 10 |
| Males | 11–14 | 44 | 97 | | | 2800 | 44 | 1000 | 5000 | 400 | 12 |
| | 15–18 | 61 | 134 | | | 3000 | 54 | 1000 | 5000 | 400 | 15 |
| | 19–22 | 67 | 147 | | | 3000 | 52 | 1000 | 5000 | 400 | 15 |
| | 23–50 | 70 | 154 | | | 2700 | 56 | 1000 | 5000 | | 15 |
| | 51+ | 70 | 154 | | | 2400 | 56 | 1000 | 5000 | | 15 |
| Females | 11–14 | 44 | 97 | | | 2400 | 44 | 800 | 4000 | 400 | 10 |
| | 15–18 | 54 | 119 | | | 2100 | 48 | 800 | 4000 | 400 | 11 |
| | 19–22 | 58 | 128 | | | 2100 | 46 | 800 | 4000 | 400 | 12 |
| | 23–50 | 58 | 128 | | | 2000 | 46 | 800 | 4000 | | 12 |
| | 51+ | 58 | 128 | | | 1800 | 46 | 800 | 4000 | | 12 |
| Pregnant | | | | | | +300 | +30 | 1000 | 5000 | 400 | 15 |
| Lactating | | | | | | +500 | +20 | 1200 | 6000 | 400 | 15 |

[1]The allowances are intended to provide for individual variations among most normal persons as they live in the United States under usual environmental stresses. Diets should be based on a variety of common foods in order to provide other nutrients for which human requirements have been less well defined. See text for more detailed discussion of allowances and of nutrients not tabulated.

[2]Kilojoules (KJ) = 4.2 × kcal.

[3]Retinol equivalents.

[4]Assumed to be all as retinol in milk during the first six months of life. All subsequent intakes are assumed to be one-half as retinol and one-half as β-carotene when calculated from international units. As retinol equivalents, three-fourths are as retinol and one-fourth as β-carotene.

The major functions of carbohydrate in the body are to:
    provide a source of energy supplying about 40 per cent of the calories in the American diet;
    aid in metabolism of fat (without a source of carbohydrate, fat metabolism cannot go to completion); and
    spare protein from being used as a source of energy (protein is needed for specific functions in the body which no other nutrient can replace).

**TABLE 21–2**  RECOMMENDED DAILY DIETARY ALLOWANCES,[1]
REVISED 1973 FOOD AND NUTRITION BOARD,
NATIONAL ACADEMY OF SCIENCES—NATIONAL
RESEARCH COUNCIL DESIGNED FOR THE MAINTENANCE
OF GOOD NUTRITION OF PRACTICALLY ALL HEALTHY
PEOPLE IN THE U.S.A. (Continued)

| Water-Soluble Vitamins | | | | | | | Minerals | | | | | |
|---|---|---|---|---|---|---|---|---|---|---|---|---|
| Ascorbic Acid (mg) | Folacin[6] (μg) | Niacin[7] (mg) | Riboflavin (mg) | Thiamin (mg) | Vitamin $B_6$ (mg) | Vitamin $B_{12}$ (μg) | Calcium (mg) | Phosphorus (mg) | Iodine (μg) | Iron (mg) | Magnesium (mg) | Zinc (mg) |
| 35 | 50 | 5 | 0.4 | 0.3 | 0.3 | 0.3 | 360 | 240 | 35 | 10 | 60 | 3 |
| 35 | 50 | 8 | 0.6 | 0.5 | 0.4 | 0.3 | 540 | 400 | 45 | 15 | 70 | 5 |
| 40 | 100 | 9 | 0.8 | 0.7 | 0.6 | 1.0 | 800 | 800 | 60 | 15 | 150 | 10 |
| 40 | 200 | 12 | 1.1 | 0.9 | 0.9 | 1.5 | 800 | 800 | 80 | 10 | 200 | 10 |
| 40 | 300 | 16 | 1.2 | 1.2 | 1.2 | 2.0 | 800 | 800 | 110 | 10 | 250 | 10 |
| 45 | 400 | 18 | 1.5 | 1.4 | 1.6 | 3.0 | 1200 | 1200 | 130 | 18 | 350 | 15 |
| 45 | 400 | 20 | 1.8 | 1.5 | 1.8 | 3.0 | 1200 | 1200 | 150 | 18 | 400 | 15 |
| 45 | 400 | 20 | 1.8 | 1.5 | 2.0 | 3.0 | 800 | 800 | 140 | 10 | 350 | 15 |
| 45 | 400 | 18 | 1.6 | 1.4 | 2.0 | 3.0 | 800 | 800 | 130 | 10 | 350 | 15 |
| 45 | 400 | 16 | 1.5 | 1.2 | 2.0 | 3.0 | 800 | 800 | 110 | 10 | 350 | 15 |
| 45 | 400 | 16 | 1.3 | 1.2 | 1.6 | 3.0 | 1200 | 1200 | 115 | 18 | 300 | 15 |
| 45 | 400 | 14 | 1.4 | 1.1 | 2.0 | 3.0 | 1200 | 1200 | 115 | 18 | 300 | 15 |
| 45 | 400 | 14 | 1.4 | 1.1 | 2.0 | 3.0 | 800 | 800 | 100 | 18 | 300 | 15 |
| 45 | 400 | 13 | 1.2 | 1.0 | 2.0 | 3.0 | 800 | 800 | 100 | 18 | 300 | 15 |
| 45 | 400 | 12 | 1.1 | 1.0 | 2.0 | 3.0 | 800 | 800 | 80 | 10 | 300 | 15 |
| 60 | 800 | +2 | +0.3 | +0.3 | 2.5 | 4.0 | 1200 | 1200 | 125 | 18+[8] | 450 | 20 |
| 60 | 600 | +4 | +0.5 | +0.3 | 2.5 | 4.0 | 1200 | 1200 | 150 | 18 | 450 | 25 |

[5] Total vitamin E activity, estimated to be 80 percent as α-tocopherol and 20 percent other tocopherols.

[6] The folacin allowances refer to dietary sources as determined by *Lactobacillus Casei* assay. Pure forms of folacin may be effective in doses less than one-fourth of the RDA.

[7] Although allowances are expressed as niacin, it is recognized that on the average 1 mg of niacin is derived from each 60 mg of dietary tryptophan.

[8] This increased requirement cannot be met by ordinary diets, therefore the use of supplemental iron is recommended.

## FATS

Also composed of carbon, hydrogen, and oxygen, fats differ from carbohydrates in the proportions of each of these elements. Fats can be classified in several different ways: from their source, by their physical appearance, or by their chemical structure.

### Source: Animal or Vegetable

Animal fats are found in dairy products, meat, fish, and eggs. They are usually solid at room temperature. Vegetable fats are found in plants such as corn, olives, cottonseed, nuts, and beans. They are generally liquid at room temperature.

### Physical Appearance: Visible or Invisible

Visible fats are those which have a fatty appearance, such as butter or the fat around meat. Fats such as those in avocados or eggs are labeled invisible since they are not discernible.

### Chemical Structure: Saturated or Unsaturated

Saturated fats are those fatty acids which contain all the hydrogen possible. They are usually from animal sources and are solid at room temperature. Examples of saturated fats are lard, butter, meat fat, and hydrogenated fats.

Unsaturated fatty acids can take on more hydrogen under the proper conditions. They are found in plants and are usually liquid at room temperature. Examples are oils from corn, cottonseed, peanuts, and safflower.

Fats, such as some of the soft-type margarines, are partially hydrogenated. That is, an unsaturated fat is treated so that it takes up a predetermined quantity of hydrogen and the result is a product which exhibits properties of both a saturated and an unsaturated fat. These fats are usually soft at room temperature.

Cholesterol is a lipid commonly found with saturated fats. It is also made by the body. If abnormally high levels of cholesterol are in the blood (above 250 mg per 100 ml), the risk of deposition in the walls of blood vessels of this compound increases. Such a condition may increase the individual's chances of having a fatal heart attack. For such individuals a low cholesterol diet is usually prescribed. Foods such as egg yolk, organ meats, shellfish, whole dairy products, and meat fat are restricted since they are high in cholesterol and saturated fats.

Fats make up about 40 per cent of the total calories in the American diet. Since they supply 9 kcal/gm, they are the most concentrated source of energy in our diet. The major functions of fat in the body are to:

provide a source of energy;

carry fat soluble vitamins A and D;

supply those fatty acids essential for growth and life; and

slow down emptying time of the stomach, thus increasing the satiety value of the diet.

When fat is stored in the body as adipose tissue, it acts as a reserve energy supply and as insulation and padding for the body and its vital organs.

## PROTEINS

The word protein comes from a Greek word meaning to "take first place," and rightly so, for protein is necessary for all living cells. Chemically, proteins are made of carbon, hydrogen, and oxygen, similar to carbohydrates and fats. However, they also contain nitrogen and several other elements, such as sulphur, phosphorus, and iron. It is the nitrogen that distinguishes proteins from other molecules.

Proteins are very large, complex molecules. They are composed of units known as amino acids, which are the materials that our bodies use to build and repair tissues. They are the form in which proteins are absorbed into the system and metabolized. There are 22 amino acids, of which eight are essential in the adult (possibly ten in children) for normal growth and maintenance of tissues.

Proteins are classified according to whether or not they contain all essential amino acids in good proportions to one another. A complete protein is one which contains a well-balanced mixture of all eight essential amino acids. If it is the only source of protein in the diet it will support life and normal growth. A partially complete protein is one which supplies an imbalanced mixture of essential amino acids. If it is used as the sole protein source, it will maintain life but will not support normal growth. An incomplete protein will neither support life nor normal growth. It must not be the sole protein source, for it is missing or extremely low in one or more of the essential amino acids. Food sources of these proteins are:

  Complete: meat, fish, poultry, eggs, dairy products.
  Partially complete: grain and vegetable proteins.
  Incomplete: corn, gelatin.

Fortunately, most foods have a mixture of proteins that supplement each other. Since there is little, if any, storage of amino acids in the body, it is important that a source of protein be included at each meal. If incomplete or partially complete proteins are used, attempts should be made to balance them. That is, a protein deficient in one amino acid should be eaten with one that is high in the same amino acid. Generally, grain proteins are low in the same amino acids, so they should be balanced with a vegetable protein.

The recommended intake of protein is 0.8 gm per kilogram body weight (see Table 21-2). Of this, at least one-third should be obtained from complete proteins (one-half or more in children) unless the individual is a strict vegetarian, in which case care must be taken to balance the proteins consumed.

Proteins have numerous functions in the body, but the major ones are to:

  build and repair body tissue (cannot be accomplished by any other nutrient);
  provide energy;
  aid in the body's defense mechanisms against disease; and
  regulate body secretions and fluids.

## VITAMINS

Vitamins are defined in the *Handbook of Diet Therapy* as organic substances "occurring in minute quantities in plant and animal tissues; essential for specific metabolic functions or reactions to proceed normally." They do not supply calories to our diet. Rather they function as catalysts and help or allow metabolic reactions to proceed. Originally they were lettered or numbered as they were discovered. However, as they have been identified chemically they have been given more specific names. In many cases their chemical names are as well known as the letter designation.

Vitamins are divided into two groups: fat soluble, A, D, E, and K; or water soluble, C and the B complex. The only vitamins that are stored to any large extent in the body are the fat soluble vitamins A and D, which are held in the liver. In some cases, toxic reactions may result if large quantities are consumed for prolonged periods without consulting a physician.

Deficiencies of a vitamin cause illness. However, vitamins will not cure a disease or illness other than one caused by a lack of that nutrient. For example, vitamin C will not cure bleeding gums unless the condition is specifically caused by a lack of ascorbic acid, an alias for vitamin C.

## Fat-Soluble Vitamins

### VITAMIN A

We can obtain vitamin A by two methods: (1) as vitamin A; or (2) from a compound called carotene which the body converts to vitamin A. Carotene is known as a precursor for vitamin A and is probably a more important source of the vitamin than the preformed compound, since vitamin A, as such, is present in very few foods.

| *Functions of Vitamin A* | *Deficiency Symptoms* |
|---|---|
| 1. Required for healthy skin and mucous membranes in the nose, throat, eyes, gastrointestinal tract, and genitourinary tract. | 1. Tissues become dry, cracked, and unable to resist infection. |
| 2. Necessary for proper vision. | 2. Night blindness—ability to adapt to darkness is impaired. If deficiency progresses the eye dries out, becomes infected, and xerophthalmia occurs, in which the patient goes blind. |
| 3. Required for normal growth and body functions. | 3. Skeletal retardation. |

*Human Requirements.* The recommended daily allowance for the adult male is 5000 I.U. (International Units) per day (see Table 21–2).

*Sources.* The sources of vitamin A are limited to animal products. The best sources are liver, fish liver oils, egg yolk, butter, and cream. Carotene is much more widely distributed in nature and is found in foods that have a deep yellow or dark green color (the green pigment is much stronger and hides the yellow color of the carotene). Foods such as carrots, yellow squash, pumpkin, dark green leafy vegetables, sweet potatoes, apricots, peaches, and cantaloupes are excellent sources.

*Stability.* Vitamin A and carotene are not water soluble and are resistant to heat if not in prolonged contact with it. Consequently, they are not lost through most cooking methods. However, fats will become rancid when in contact with warm air, and once this occurs the major portion of vitamin A and carotene present are destroyed.

*Toxicity.* It is possible to get too much vitamin A. Toxic reactions are characterized by joint and bone pain, loss of appetite, loss of hair, and jaundice. The Council on Foods and Nutrition of the American Medical Association warns that 50,000 I.U. of this vitamin taken for a prolonged period of time can be dangerous.

### VITAMIN D

Vitamin D is also obtained from two sources: (1) foods, and (2) sunshine. The preformed vitamin is not widely distributed. However, through enrichment processes it is added to a number of foods, mainly dairy products.

| *Functions of Vitamin D* | *Deficiency Symptoms* |
|---|---|
| 1. Required for absorption of calcium and facilitates absorption of phosphorus. Necessary for metabolism of calcium and phosphorus in normal nourishment and formation of bones and teeth. | 1. Rickets: bones bend easily and do not form correctly since calcium is not absorbed adequately. Teeth are also malformed. |

*Human Requirements.*   No level is established for adults since exposure to sunlight is considered adequate. The level for children and pregnant or lactating women is 400 I.U. per day (see Table 21–2).

*Sources.*   Enriched milk and milk products, eggs, liver, butter, cream, and fish liver oils. The best source is probably sunlight for most adults.

*Stability.*   Vitamin D is stable to heat and is not affected by most cooking methods.

*Toxicity.*   Excesses of this vitamin can cause toxicity symptomized by nausea, diarrhea, loss of appetite, and calcium deposits in tissues and joints. No exact figure can be given for an overdose since exposure to sunlight varies greatly among individuals.

VITAMIN E

Vitamin E is the vitamin which is still looking for a disease. There have been numerous attempts over the years to link this vitamin with many illnesses in humans, but efforts largely have failed. It does, however, have several very important functions which are linked with its ability to combine with oxygen and thus protect various substances that would otherwise be subject to oxidation (see below). Other functions, such as preventing sterility or curing muscular dystrophy, are at this time only of importance in animals, not in man.

| *Functions of Vitamin E* | *Deficiency Symptoms* |
|---|---|
| 1. Protects red blood cells from breakdown by such substances as hydrogen peroxide. | 1. Anemia, so far seen only in infants. |
| 2. Protects structure and function of muscle tissue. | 2. Some forms of muscle degeneration have been seen in patients with low plasma vitamin E levels. |
| 3. Protects unsaturated fatty acids and vitamin A from oxidative destruction. | |

*Human Requirements.*   Re-evaluated in 1973, the recommended allowance for vitamin E in the adult male was lowered to 15 I.U. per day (see Table 21–2).

*Sources.*   The best sources of this vitamin are vegetable oils and wheat germ. Other sources include milk, eggs, meats, grains, and leafy vegetables.

*Toxicity.*   None identified as yet. This vitamin, unlike other fat soluble vitamins, is stored in adipose tissue.

VITAMIN K

The major function of this vitamin in the body is that it is required for the formation of prothrombin, which is a clotting agent in the blood. Consequently, the vitamin is often used to treat certain types of hemorrhages. Deficiency is rare, usually due to absorption problems rather than inadequate supply of the vitamin.

| *Functions of Vitamin K* | *Deficiency Symptoms* |
|---|---|
| 1. Required for formation of the protein prothrombin by the liver. | 1. Blood will not clot, hemorrhages occur. |

*Human Requirements.* None set.

*Sources.* Good food sources include green leafy vegetables, egg yolk, and organ meats. A form of vitamin K is produced by intestinal bacteria.

*Toxicity.* None known.

## Water-Soluble Vitamins

VITAMIN C

Vitamin C, or ascorbic acid, was first used to treat scurvy in British sailors during the eighteenth century. Of course, at the time the curative factor in the limes each sailor was required to consume daily while at sea was unknown. However, they did know that a lime daily seemed to prevent the dread disease. As a result, the British sailors were nicknamed "limies," a term which is still used today.

| *Functions of Vitamin C* | *Deficiency Symptoms* |
|---|---|
| 1. Required for proper wound healing and helps in the body's resistance to bacterial infection. | 1. Minor illnesses, general listlessness. |
| 2. Necessary for the structure and maintenance of capillary walls. | 2. Gums bleed, small pinpoint hemorrhages appear under the skin. If deficiency continues the disease scurvy develops. Patients with this disease have skeletal malformations which are irreversible. |

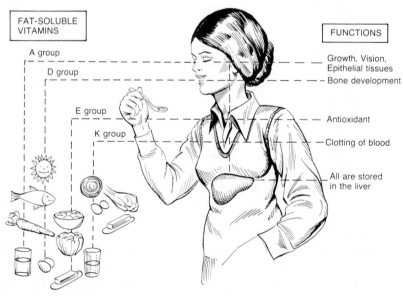

**Figure 21–2** Fat-soluble vitamins and their functions. (From Bogert et al.: *Nutrition and Physical Fitness.* 9th Ed. Philadelphia, W. B. Saunders Co., 1973.)

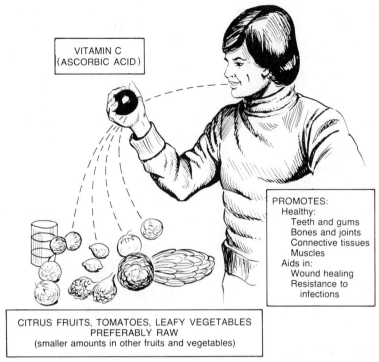

VITAMIN C
(ASCORBIC ACID)

PROMOTES:
Healthy:
    Teeth and gums
    Bones and joints
    Connective tissues
    Muscles
Aids in:
    Wound healing
    Resistance to
        infections

CITRUS FRUITS, TOMATOES, LEAFY VEGETABLES
PREFERABLY RAW
(smaller amounts in other fruits and vegetables)

**Figure 21-3**  (From Bogert et al.: *Nutrition and Physical Fitness*. 9th Ed. Philadelphia, W. B. Saunders Co., 1973.)

*Human Requirements.*  The National Research Council lowered the vitamin C recommendations in 1973 to 45 mg/day for the adult (see Table 21–2).

*Sources.*  Best sources of this nutrient are citrus fruits, cabbage, dark green leafy vegetables, and strawberries. Some sources are relatively low in vitamin C, but are consumed in sufficient quantities so that they can be an important source as, for example, potatoes.

*Stability.*  Vitamin C is very easily destroyed by both heat and exposure to air. Since it is water soluble, care must be used in cooking fruits and vegetables which contain vitamin C. Small amounts of water and short cooking times should be used. An alkaline medium will speed up the loss of vitamin C.

*Toxicity.*  At very large doses, nausea and diarrhea have been reported.

## The B Complex

Vitamin B$_1$, or Thiamin

### Functions of Vitamin B$_1$

1. Necessary for healthy appetite and proper functioning of the digestive tract.

2. Required for the metabolism of carbohydrates in the body and for normal functioning of the nervous system.

### Deficiency Symptoms

1. Loss of appetite, diminished gastric secretions, fatigue, irritability.

2. Edema, foot drop, beri-beri.

*Human Requirements.* Need for the vitamin depends on caloric intake, generally 0.5 mg/1000 calories is adequate. The level set by the National Research Council is 1.0 to 1.4 mg per day depending on sex (see Table 21–2).

*Sources.* Meats are not as good a source of thiamin as they are of most of the other B vitamins, although pork and organ meats, such as liver, can contribute good amounts if consumed in large enough quantities. The best sources are whole grain or enriched breads and cereals, wheat germ, and potatoes.

*Stability.* Thiamin is destroyed by heat and alkaline mediums. Since it is water soluble small amounts of water should be used in cooking in order to preserve this nutrient.

*Toxicity.* None.

Vitamin B₂, or Riboflavin

| *Functions of Vitamin B₂* | *Deficiency Symptoms* |
|---|---|
| 1. Necessary for all tissues, particularly for healthy skin and lips. | 1. Cheilosis, cracking of the corners of the mouth. |
| 2. Required for maintaining healthy eyes. | 2. Itching and burning of eyes, sensitivity to light, headaches. |
| 3. Essential for proper growth. | |
| 4. Composes part of some enzymes. | |

*Human Requirements.* 1.2 to 1.6 mg per day as established by the National Research Council (see Table 21–2).

*Sources.* The major source of this vitamin is milk, since one quart supplies 2 mg. Other sources include meats and enriched grains.

*Stability.* Riboflavin is very unstable in light. Consequently, milk should be stored in either dark glass or plasticized paper containers. Riboflavin from foods other than milk can also be lost in cooking water or drippings since it is water soluble.

*Toxicity.* None.

Niacin

Niacin is available in two forms, either as niacin or the precursor, tryptophan. Tryptophan is an essential amino acid and the body converts it into niacin. About 1 mg of niacin is produced from every 50 to 60 mg of tryptophan.

| *Functions of Niacin* | *Deficiency Symptoms* |
|---|---|
| 1. Composes part of some enzymes and is required for proper growth and metabolism of carbohydrates. | 1. Pellagra: characterized by the three D's (dermatitis, dementia, diarrhea). |
| 2. Necessary for proper function of the gastrointestinal tract and the nervous system. | |

*Human Requirements.* 13 to 18 mg per day is the recommended allowance (see Table 21–2).

*Sources.* Probably one-half of our niacin comes from tryptophan which is obtained from meat and other complete sources of protein. Flour and cereal products are also good sources.

*Stability.*    Niacin is fairly stable to heat and air but it can be lost in the cooking water.

*Toxicity.*    None.

VITAMIN B$_6$, OR PYRIDOXINE

| *Functions of Vitamin B$_6$* | *Deficiency Symptoms* |
|---|---|
| 1. Many generalized functions in relation to muscle and nervous system function. | 1. Convulsions, muscle twitching, irritability seen in infants. In adults, nausea, diarrhea, irritability, and nervous disturbances; no specific disease associated with a deficiency of this vitamin. |

*Human Requirements.*    National Research Council recommends 2 mg per day for adults (see Table 21–2).

*Sources.*    Occurs in many foods, mainly meats and vegetables.

*Toxicity.*    None.

FOLIC ACID OR FOLACIN

| *Functions of Folic Acid* | *Deficiency Symptoms* |
|---|---|
| 1. Essential for all cells, particularly red blood cells. | 1. Smooth, red tongue, diarrhea, anemia. |

*Human Requirements.*    Allowance established at 400 $\mu$g per day for adults (see Table 21–2).

*Sources.*    Best sources are green leafy vegetables, liver and whole grains.

*Stability.*    Folacin is destroyed by heat and frequently lost in cooking water. Storage and cooking losses are usually high irrespective of methods used.

*Toxicity.*    None.

VITAMIN B$_{12}$

Deficiency of this vitamin produces an anemia identical to that produced by a folic acid deficiency. However, if a deficiency of vitamin B$_{12}$ is allowed to continue untreated, mental retardation will result. (For this reason, folic acid cannot legally be added to multi-vitamin capsules except at very low levels so that it will not inadvertently mask the early symptoms of a vitamin B$_{12}$ deficiency.)

*Human Requirements.*    Established for the first time in 1968 at 5 $\mu$g per day, the allowance was reduced in 1973 to 3 $\mu$g per day for adults (see Table 21–2).

*Sources.*    Liver and muscle meats are the best sources.

*Stability.*    Stable under most conditions since it is attached to a protein in foods.

*Toxicity.*    None.

OTHER B VITAMINS

Other vitamins which belong to the B complex, but for which no requirements have as yet been established, are biotin, pantothenic acid, and choline. Biotin is synthesized by bacteria in the gastrointestinal tract and is important in

FOOD SOURCES AND USES IN THE BODY

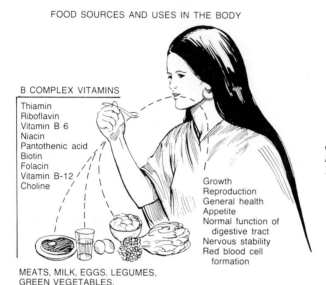

B COMPLEX VITAMINS

Thiamin
Riboflavin
Vitamin B 6
Niacin
Pantothenic acid
Biotin
Folacin
Vitamin B-12
Choline

Growth
Reproduction
General health
Appetite
Normal function of
    digestive tract
Nervous stability
Red blood cell
    formation

MEATS, MILK, EGGS, LEGUMES,
GREEN VEGETABLES,
WHOLE GRAIN BREADS & CEREALS

**Figure 21–4**  (From Bogert et al.: *Nutrition and Physical Fitness.* 9th Ed. Philadelphia, W. B. Saunders Co., 1973.)

several enzyme systems. Raw egg white contains a protein, avidin, which is capable of binding biotin, thus making it unavailable to the body. Avidin is changed by heating, so it will not function in this manner in cooked egg whites. Pantothenic acid is involved in carbohydrate and fatty acid metabolism. It is present in almost all foods and a deficiency should not be seen if a mixed diet is consumed. Choline is mainly important in the body as a constituent of compounds known as phospholipids (primarily lecithin). Among other roles, it is involved in the transportation and metabolism of fats. Choline is found in whole grains, meats, egg yolks, and legumes.

### Minerals

Minerals are inorganic chemical elements that make up about 4 per cent of body weight. Of the many that are used by the body only 13 are felt to be essential, and of those there are allowances established for only six. Most minerals are required in relatively small amounts, but even so they are absolutely essential for life.

Those minerals which are needed in trace amounts only seem either to behave as part of hormone or enzyme systems or to work with vitamins in various metabolic reactions throughout the body. For example, iodine is part of the thyroid hormone, thyroxine, and another hormone, insulin, has zinc as part of its structure. Cobalt, on the other hand, is an essential part of the $B_{12}$ molecule.

Generally, if an individual consumes a well-balanced diet he will receive adequate amounts of most minerals. Those which may require special attention to insure that they are in sufficient quantities are calcium, phosphorus, iron, and, in some cases, iodine. During illness, of course, other minerals may also be of more concern.

CALCIUM

Calcium is the mineral which, in the American diet, is most likely to be deficient. The body requires calcium at all ages, but the highest requirement is during pregnancy, lactation, and childhood.

| *Functions of Calcium* | *Deficiency Symptoms* |
|---|---|
| 1. Forms the body's skeleton and teeth. | 1. Rickets: characterized by retarded growth and malformations of the bones. |
| 2. Aids in forming blood clots. | 2. Delayed blood clotting, hemorrhaging. |
| 3. Required for normal muscle activity, especially the heart muscle. | 3. Tetany, abnormal twitching of the muscles. |

*Human Requirements.* 800 mg per day (see Table 21–2).

*Sources.* Milk of any kind (skim, whole, low fat, buttermilk, chocolate milk, and so forth) or milk products, such as ice cream or cheese. Other sources include dark green leafy vegetables and shellfish, for instance, clams and oysters.

PHOSPHORUS

Phosphorus is a constituent of every living cell and as such has numerous functions in the body. In many cases it works in very much the same manner as calcium. However, in addition it is required for protein, fat, and carbohydrate metabolism, in energy metabolism, and in various buffering systems in the body. It is also involved in a number of vitamin and enzyme reactions. No specific disease is associated with a deficiency of this nutrient.

*Human Requirements.* The same as for calcium, 800 mg per day (see Table 21–2).

*Sources.* Phosphorus is present in most foods, particularly in milk and meat products. Other good sources are cereals and legumes.

IRON

Although required in small amounts in comparison with nutrients like phosphorus and calcium, iron is a vitally important element. It is an essential part of hemoglobin, which is the protein that is responsible for the color of red blood cells and is the oxygen carrying substance in the blood. The body is very conservative with iron, and it reuses it again and again. However, deficiencies do occur, particularly in premenopausal women or during pregnancy or hemorrhagic conditions. A deficiency of iron results in anemia.

*Human Requirements.* The 1973 NRC allowance is 18 mg per day for women. Unless a woman eats liver and other rich sources of iron frequently, the ordinary diet may not supply a sufficient quantity of iron. In this case an iron supplement may be desirable. Ten mg per day is recommended for men (see Table 21–2).

*Sources.* Best sources are liver and other organ meats, egg yolks, whole grain products, and green leafy vegetables. Some other products, such as raisins, dried fruits, and molasses, are good sources of iron if eaten in sufficient quantities.

IODINE

Iodine's only function in the body is as a part of the thyroid gland hormone, thyroxine. Although the requirement for iodine is small, without it the thyroid gland fails to function properly and the condition known as goiter occurs. Iodine deficiency in a pregnant woman can result in cretinism in the infant. This disease is characterized by dwarfing and retarded physical and mental growth.

*Human Requirements.*   Established for adults at 100 to 130 $\mu$g per day (see Table 21–2).

*Sources.*   The iodine content of plants is determined by the amount of iodine in the soil in which they are grown. Generally, vegetables grown in the Atlantic coastal area or regions around the Gulf of Mexico have the highest iodine content. However, the most reliable source of iodine is iodized table salt.

MAGNESIUM

Magnesium is an essential nutrient, most of which is found in combination with calcium and phosphorus in bone tissue. It functions mainly in carbohydrate and amino acid metabolism in the body. A deficiency of this element results in nervous irritability and eventually in convulsions similar to those seen in cases of tetany (hypocalcemia).

*Human Requirements.*   300–350 mg per day for adults depending on sex (see Table 21–2).

*Sources.*   Magnesium occurs in many foods, particularly cereal grains, legumes, and dark green vegetables.

ZINC

Zinc is necessary for growth and gonadal development in man. It has many functions in the body, the major one being that of a coenzyme in several body reactions. A deficiency of this nutrient retards skeletal growth and sexual maturation.

*Human Requirements.*   Established for the first time in 1973 at 15 mg per day for adults (see Table 21–2).

*Sources.*   The best sources of zinc are oysters, herring, whole grains, meats, milk and egg yolk.

SALTS

Sodium, potassium, and chloride are elements which are classified as electrolytes or salts in the diet. Among many other functions they are extremely important in fluid and acid-base balance in the body. A deficiency of sodium usually results in dehydration; however, in severe cases the individual may go into a state of shock. Potassium deficiency is sometimes encountered following excessive vomiting or prolonged diuretic therapy and, if allowed to continue, can lead to improper muscle tone and irregular contractions of the heart.

*Human Requirements.*   None set.

*Sources.*   The major source of both sodium and chloride is table salt. Other sources include meats, milk, and processed foods. Some vegetables are also naturally high in sodium. Potassium is furnished to us mainly by fruits (particularly bananas and oranges), vegetables, and cereal products.

OTHER MINERALS

There are many other minerals which are required by the body. Slowly, as methods improve, deficiencies may be identified and allowances established as, for example, in the following minerals:

Copper:   necessary for red blood cell production.
Sulphur:   used in protein synthesis and in detoxifying reactions in the liver.
Fluorine:   important in preventing dental caries.

It is rare to see deficiencies of these if the diet is adequate in other nutrients.

## THERAPEUTIC NUTRITION

Although the majority of patients a physician sees will be treated medically without using a therapeutic diet, there are some illnesses and diseases which can be cured, or the patient's recovery improved, by the use of a special diet. In such cases, the normal (sometimes referred to as house or regular) diet is used as a basis of planning. This is used for two major reasons:

1. The closer the special diet is to a normal diet, the fewer changes the assistant will be asking the person to accept, and the easier it will be for him to adhere to the diet.
2. It is easier to be certain that the patient's diet supplies adequate amounts of essential nutrients if a regular diet pattern is used as a baseline.

### Modifying a Diet

The normal diet can be modified in the following seven ways (or any combination thereof) to supply a therapeutic diet:

1. Consistency.
2. Caloric level.
3. Levels of one or more nutrients.
4. Bulk.
5. Flavor.
6. Inclusion or exclusion of specific foods.
7. Feeding intervals.

*CONSISTENCY*

Consistency changes are sometimes ordered for individuals who have problems with their mouth, teeth, or esophagus. A texture restriction is also frequently called for in cases of illnesses of the gastrointestinal tract.

**Soft or Light Diet:**   Foods with roughage are eliminated (no raw fruits or vegetables). No strongly flavored or gas-forming vegetables are allowed (onions, beans, broccoli, cauliflower, and so on). In many cases, spices are limited.

**Mechanical Soft:** A regular diet in which the food is either chopped, ground or pureed, depending upon the degree of texture change required. No foods or spices are restricted.

**Liquid:** There are two types of liquid diets. The clear liquid diet includes only broth soups, tea, coffee, and jello. In some cases, apple juice and cranberry juice may be allowed. The full liquid diet includes all foods allowed on a clear liquid diet plus milk, custards, strained cream soups, refined cereals, eggnogs, milkshakes, and all juices.

*Adequacy.* The soft and mechanical soft diets should supply all nutrients required by an individual. The clear liquid diet is not adequate and should be used for very brief periods of time. Full liquid diets can be made adequate, but they are also usually used only for short periods.

## CALORIES

Calories may be either increased or decreased. Increased calories are ordered in cases of chronic underweight, following an illness, for malnutrition and hyperthyroidism, or during times of growth, such as infancy, childhood, pregnancy, or lactation. In such circumstances the total amounts of foods on the regular diet are increased, and the diet is usually higher in fats (since fat supplies more calories per gram than either carbohydrates or proteins). The number of meals eaten may also be increased from three to six or more.

Calories are restricted in cases of obesity and diabetes. Quantities of food consumed should be decreased, but no one food group should be eliminated. For diabetes, foods containing carbohydrates, particularly the simple sugars, are withheld. Lists of foods have been prepared by the American Diabetic Association that enable the diabetic to plan his diet more easily. (The lists are known as Exchange Lists and various modifications of them are frequently used for calorie restricted diets in general.)

*Adequacy.* High calorie diets should be adequate in all nutrients. Low calorie diets can usually be made adequate, unless the calories are restricted to below 1000 calories per day.

## LEVELS OF ONE OR MORE NUTRIENTS

A large number of therapeutic diets fall into this category. This type of diet is used to treat specific deficiency diseases (for example, high iron) or in cases where a patient has had a toxic reaction to a specific vitamin or mineral (for example, low vitamin A). Many inborn errors of metabolism are treated by eliminating or limiting the ingestion of a nutrient (for instance, phenylketonuria is treated by limiting the quantities of the essential amino acid, phenylalanine).

In cases of hypertensive heart disease, sodium is restricted. For patients with atherosclerosis, a low fat or low cholesterol diet may be prescribed. Protein levels are changed for kidney and liver disease therapy. Fat is also restricted for gallbladder or liver disease.

In any case, the normal diet is modified by restricting foods that are sources of the nutrient involved.

*Adequacy.* Except for the nutrient in question, the NRC allowances can usually be met, although if several restrictions are ordered for the same patient a nutrient supplement may be necessary.

## BULK

Bulk or residue is changed when treating problems of the colon or large bowel. In some cases high residue diets are ordered, in others, low residue diets. In either case, foods high in cellulose are considered to be high in residue because the body does not digest this carbohydrate well and a residue is left in the colon. In some instances, a low residue diet is distinguished from a low fiber diet. In this case a low fiber diet eliminates those foods with a high cellulose content, and a low residue diet restricts milk, in addition to fiber content.

*Adequacy.* Either diet should supply all nutrients needed, although if milk is restricted drastically the calcium level must be watched carefully.

## FLAVOR

Flavor restriction generally implies that a bland diet is being used. A bland diet restricts any foods that are chemically (for instance, caffeine, pepper, chili, nutmeg, alcohol, and so on) or mechanically (high fiber) irritating. No fried foods or highly concentrated sweets are included. Gas-forming vegetables belonging to the onion and cabbage family are also eliminated. The diet is usually used for problems occurring in the gastrointestinal tract (such as ulcers).

*Adequacy.* The bland diet should supply sufficient nutrients for the individual to meet the NRC allowances, unless fruits and vegetables are eliminated (in which case, a supplement may be necessary).

## INCLUSION OR EXCLUSION OF SPECIFIC FOODS

Diets that fall into this category are most frequently used to treat allergies of various kinds. In children the most common allergies are to chocolate, wheat, eggs, and milk. A disease known as celiac disease is treated by eliminating those foods which contain a protein called gliadin (found in wheat, oats, and barley products). In any given instance the diet simply eliminates, or restricts, the food or foods containing the allergent.

*Adequacy.* In some cases it may be difficult to meet the NRC allowances for all nutrients. When this situation occurs, supplements should be ordered.

*FEEDING INTERVALS*

Feeding intervals can be changed. Usually more meals are ordered rather than fewer. Generally the increase is from three meals to six or eight meals. Feeding intervals are shortened for treating problems dealing with the gastrointestinal tract, malnutrition, or underweight. An individual who has had part or all of his stomach removed surgically requires more meals. In some cases, the total food consumed per day is the same, but it is fed in smaller quantities at any given time. In other cases more food is added at the extra meals.

*Adequacy.* Unless the number of meals is reduced severely, the NRC allowances should be met.

There are, of course, many other diets which have not been mentioned. If further information is required a text on diet therapy should be consulted (see list at end of this chapter).

## Prescribing a Diet

Since there are so many different types of therapeutic diets, it is frequently impossible for the physician to stay abreast of all of the restrictions and other considerations involved. For this reason he will often rely on either a local dietitian or a nutrition consultant to instruct his patients on the modifications they should follow. If this is not possible, the physician may wish to use a service offered by some firms which develop diets, printed with the physician's name on them, if desired, that can then be handed to the patient. Numerous pharmaceutical or medical suppliers also supply diet lists, which usually are used as additional advertising for the products of that manufacturer. If such diets are used, remember that one list is frequently used for more than one type of diet (for example, several different calorie levels may be listed in chart form), and it is left to the patient to decipher the information. Diets of this nature must be as clear and concise as possible so that the patient is not unduly confused or frightened.

In any event, it is important that the patient return home with something he can read after leaving the office. All questions will not occur to him at the time the diet is first introduced. He must have some method of finding out information, and a written diet list is the easiest method of accomplishing this.

If, as a medical assistant, it is your duty to discuss the diet with the patient, be sure that you understand it well enough to talk with the patient in a convincing manner. There may be some questions you cannot answer. If so, have the patient ask the physician or contact a person more versed in diet therapy. It is important that the patient understand the diet and the rationale behind its use. If he feels uneasy or has a lot of unanswered questions, he will be far less motivated to follow the diet.

You, as the medical assistant, can be a very valuable asset to the physician, the dietitian, and particularly, the patient. A sound understanding of nutrition and especially of diet therapy will enable you to function in your role in the most effective manner possible.

# REFERENCES

Bogert, J. L., Briggs, G. M., and D. H. Calloway, *Nutrition and Physical Fitness,* 9th Ed., Philadelphia, W. B. Saunders Company, 1973.

Krause, M. V., and M. A. Hunscher, *Food, Nutrition and Diet Therapy,* 5th Ed., Philadelphia, W. B. Saunders Company, 1972.

Turner, D., *Handbook of Diet Therapy,* 3rd Ed., Chicago, The University of Chicago Press, 1959.

Williams, S. R., *Nutrition and Diet Therapy,* 2nd Ed., St. Louis, C. V. Mosby Company, 1973.

Wohl, M. G., and R. S. Goodhart, *Modern Nutrition in Health and Disease,* 3rd Ed., Philadelphia, Lea and Febiger, 1964.

# Chapter 22

## BEHAVIORAL OBJECTIVES

*The medical office assistant should be able to:*

Define microorganism and identify the major divisions of microorganisms.

Distinguish which pathogens cause the diseases introduced in this chapter.

Define common, confusing terms allied with the study of microbiology.

Identify the importance of sterilization.

Take a direct smear from a patient's throat, vagina, abscess, or wound.

Prepare culture smears taken from patients.

Stain and prepare smears for microscopic examination.

Define immunity and recognize its importance in defense against disease.

Describe how immunization reinforces natural immunity to infectious agents.

Explain the rejection phenomenon.

Explain allergic reaction in terms of immune mechanisms.

352

# Microbiology

Biology is the science of living things; therefore, *micro-* (small or minute) biology is the science of small or minute living things. Microorganisms (bacteria) were first seen by Antonj van Leeuwenhoek, a Dutch investigator who, about 1664, perfected a magnifying glass strong enough to visualize bacteria which he called "animalcules" (little animals) (Figs. 22–1 to 22–3). He carefully described and drew what he saw, but he did not disclose how he made his lens. Small hand magnifying glasses, reading glasses, and such had been in use for many years, but they did not magnify enough to disclose microorganisms.

It was not until about 1820 that a really useful microscope was perfected. This microscope was similar to those used today in that it used two lenses—one near the object (the objective lens) and one at the other end of the tube (the ocular eyepiece). Present day microscopes have multiple coordination lenses in both objective lens and eyepiece. The modern office microscope will magnify about 900 to 1500 times the size of the original object (Fig. 22–4).

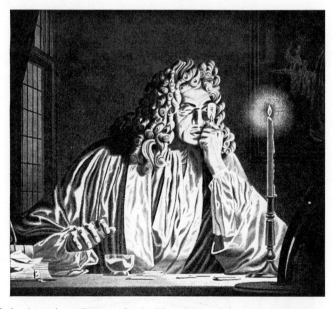

**Figure 22–1** Antonj van Leeuwenhoek. The picture shows accurately the size and shape of the first microscopes, the manner in which they were used, and the simple laboratory apparatus of the "Father of Bacteriology." (Courtesy of Lambert Pharmacal Co.) In Frobisher, M., et al.: *Fundamentals of Microbiology*, 8th Ed., Philadelphia, 1968, W. B. Saunders Co.

**353**

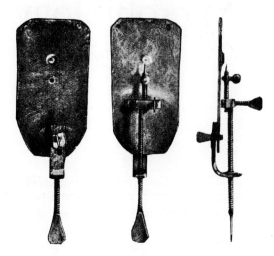

**Figure 22–2** One of Leeuwenhoek's microscopes: front, back, and side views. (From Frobisher, M., et al.: *Fundamentals of Microbiology*, 8th Ed., Philadelphia, 1968, W. B. Saunders Co.)

Microbiology became a science in its own right with the work of such men as Louis Pasteur, Robert Koch, Joseph Lister, and many others. Pasteur was a French chemist. He was asked in about 1837 by the wine makers to try to find out what was making their wine sour. He found out that it was a microorganism. This led him to work in other microbiological areas. He perfected a treatment for the prevention of the development of rabies in persons bitten by rabid animals, a means of controlling anthrax, a disease of sheep, and so on. Koch was

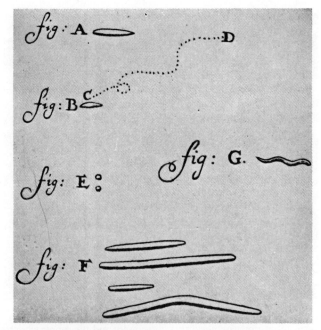

**Figure 22–3** Leeuwenhoek's drawings of bacteria. Here may be seen cocci, bacilli, and (probably) a spirochete. (From Frobisher, M., et al.: *Fundamentals of Microbiology*, 8th Ed., Philadelphia, 1968, W. B. Saunders Co.)

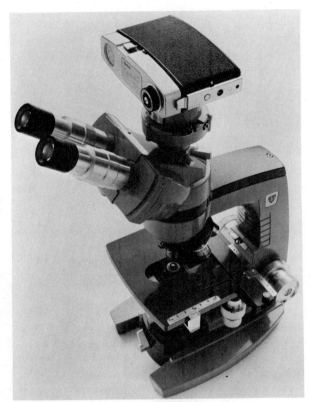

**Figure 22–4**  A modern light microscope. (Courtesy of American Optical Corporation.)

a German physician, and he turned his attention to the causes and transmissions of disease, while Lister was a Scottish surgeon who first tried to "clean" the surgical field of microorganisms by the use of a disinfectant (phenol).

The list of accomplishments of these and a multitude of other scientists since would fill and has filled many books. Actually, the search is still going on, both in the field of microscopes and in the application of the findings to the betterment of mankind.

It was necessary to perfect the electron microscope (which uses a stream of electrons instead of light rays) (Fig. 22–5) before viruses could be seen. Are these the smallest living things? This is a still unanswered question. Actually, viruses are not living in the usual sense of the word but are capable of living under ideal circumstances. More of this later.

## MICROORGANISMS

Before the various types are discussed, it may be advantageous to make a few general statements about these "creatures." First of all, they are omnipresent and multitudinous. They are in you, on you, and all around you. The only place they are *not* is in freshly sterilized materials or in the contents of sealed, sterilized containers.

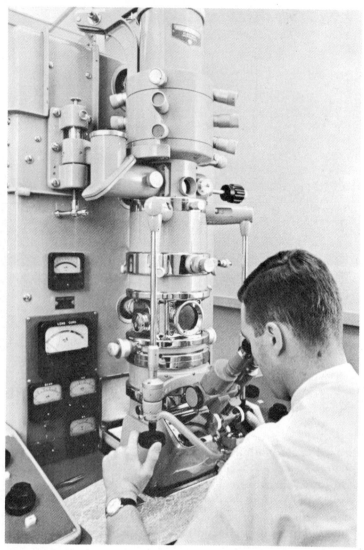

**Figure 22–5** A modern type of electron microscope. (Courtesy of the Perkin-Elmer Corporation.) In Frobisher, M., et al.: *Fundamentals of Microbiology*, 8th Ed., Philadelphia, 1968, W. B. Saunders Co.

In relation to humans, microorganisms are good, bad and indifferent. If it were not for microorganisms, we would not have any bread, wine, cheese, and many other foods. In our intestinal tract, bacteria manufacture vitamins which we need but cannot synthesize ourselves. Some microorganisms produce secretions or excretions which give us our antibiotic drugs; some destroy our waste materials; and some fix nitrogens in the soil which allows our food plants to grow. The list of good bacteria is much longer than the list of those which are bad.

The bad microorganisms (pathogenic—disease producing) are in the minority, but will be discussed in some detail in this chapter.

This brings us to those that are indifferent to us. All that needs to be said is that they are the majority.

Microorganisms are all one-celled organisms, but most are not typical cells, as in the cells of higher animals and plants. Briefly, a typical animal cell has a cell membrane, cytoplasm, and a nucleus or sometimes nuclei (more than one). The membrane is a thin semipermeable membrane which allows full passage of water (osmosis) and the passage of certain dissolved substances (dialysis). The cytoplasm contains numerous and varied structures which are used in cell metabolism. The nucleus (Fig. 22–6) is enclosed within a fine membrane and contains the hereditary (genetic) substances. Plant cells differ mainly in that they have a heavy outer coat called a cell wall. Some microscopic single cell animals have a heavy membrane that approaches the cell wall of the plant, but most do not, nor do any of the multicellular animals.

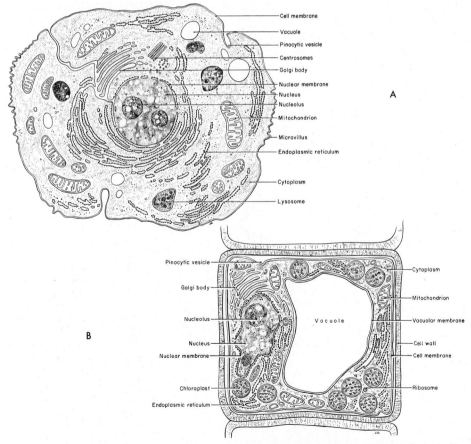

**Figure 22–6**  A. Composite drawing of a "typical" animal cell based on various cytologic studies and use of the electron microscope. B. Diagram of a typical plant cell. (Copyright © 1961 by *Scientific American, Inc.* All rights reserved.) In Villee, C.: *Biology*, Philadelphia, 1972, W. B. Saunders Co.

All true cells contain deoxyribonucleic acid (DNA) in their nuclei. This carries the inherited characteristics of the cell. In the cytoplasm is ribonucleic acid (RNA), which constructs the cell proteins in response to the directions from the DNA.

Bacteria have their RNA scattered through the cell, and they do not have a typical nucleus. Viruses are really different in that they have only RNA or DNA — never both.

## FUNGI

Yeasts (Fig. 22–7), molds (Fig. 22–8), and fungi imperfecti (having some resemblance to both yeasts and molds) are plants that lack chlorophyll. They do not form a major pathogenic group, though some do cause diseases such as athlete's foot, ringworm, and some systemic disorders. Diseases caused by fungi are usually termed mycosis (or mycoses in the plural), since *myco* is used in their scientific terminology. Most fungi replicate (multiply, reproduce) asexually, often by *budding, spores,* or *filaments,* but some reproduce sexually at certain stages. In budding, a "bubble" which gradually increases in size and finally breaks off appears on the cell. However, there may be many bubbles on the "mother" cell, and the daughter cell may start a bubble before it breaks away so that the fungus appears to be a colony. In spore formation a number of spores (usually spherical, hard covered and drought and temperature resistant) may be encased in a capsule or may be scattered singly. With filamentous replication, in place of budding, long thin filaments grow out from the original cell.

Many of the pathogenic fungi infect the skin and scalp; these are especially difficult to eradicate, since a spore or filament may be left hidden under the outer skin cells and under favorable conditions may start multiplying again. Systemic fungal infections are also very difficult to treat. Most anti-infective drugs

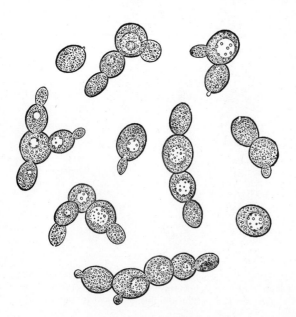

**Figure 22–7**   Yeast cells. Brewers' yeast actively multiplying by budding. This species is called *Saccharomyces cerevisiae.* The single large internal vacuoles and the numerous small fat drops are shown, as are also buds in various stages of development and the cell wall. Nuclei not visible here. (Highly magnified.) (Sedgwick and Wilson.) In Frobisher, M., and Fuerst, R.: *Microbiology in Health and Disease,* 13th Ed., Philadelphia, 1973, W. B. Saunders Co.

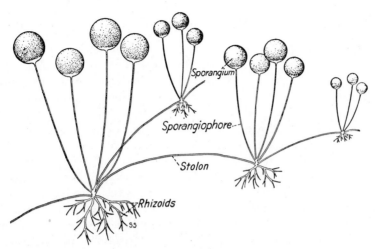

**Figure 22-8** A species of *Rhizopus*, a coenocytic mold. (From Frobisher, M., and Fuerst, R.: *Microbiology in Health and Disease*, 13th Ed., Philadelphia, 1973, W. B. Saunders Co.)

are ineffective against the fungi. Special medications and treatment are needed to cure or arrest the infection. Therapy is usually continued for months to be sure there will be no relapse.

A few of the pathogenic fungi the office assistant may see include ringworm—tinea capitis (head), corpus (body), and others—a relatively common skin condition especially found in the scalp of children, and dermatophytosis (athlete's foot), which can infect the hands as well. These are transmitted by contact. Children playing together, making paper hats, and "swapping" them and so on can readily transmit the tineas. Dermatophytosis is most apt to occur by going barefoot, especially in school shower rooms—hence the common name. All skin fungal infections are treated by local antifungal ointments or drying powders if the area is apt to be damp, as between the toes, in the groin, axilla, or similar areas. If the condition is at all severe, one of the systemic antifungal drugs is given at the same time the local treatment is instituted. Often the drugs are continued even after apparent recovery.

Systemic mycoses are more common in tropical than in temperate areas, but some are not uncommon in the cooler areas. San Joaquin fever, a fungal infection caused by the *Coccidioides immitis* and properly called coccidioidomycosis, and candidiasis, caused by the *Candida albicans* (also called *monilia*), are two such diseases. The former is transmitted by inhalation of infected dust. The *Candida* are opportunist pathogens; that is, they are usually harmless and are often in the nose, throat, gastrointestinal tract, and genital mucosa of apparently healthy individuals. However, debilitating diseases, pregnancy, excessive use of antibiotics (which destroy the *Candida's* normal enemies), and other factors can give the *Candida* a chance to replicate rapidly and to invade areas where they usually do not occur.

All systemic mycoses are treated in two ways: (1) remove the underlying cause, if known and if possible, and (2) give the antifungal systemic drugs. Treatment is always continued for several weeks or months to insure complete eradication of the organisms.

## PROTOZOA

Protozoa, like fungi, are much larger than bacteria, but unlike fungi, protozoa are minute, one-celled animals. Protozoa are true cells with a cell membrane, cytoplasm, and nucleus. Some protozoa have a somewhat thickened cell membrane which gives more support than the membrane of the multicellular organisms. Most protozoa replicate by fission. The nucleus first divides. Then the cell membrane dips in and gradually separates the cytoplasm and the two nuclei. The two cells then separate. Some protozoa reproduce sexually—the two cells meeting, the membrane between them dissolving, and the cells fusing. Then, after the two nuclei have fused, the division described above takes place. Most protozoa are free living and are nonpathogenic. A few form cysts (a rather dormant stage). In the cyst form they are resistant to unfavorable environments as are the spores of certain fungi, but not as completely as bacterial spores. The active stage is called the trophozoite stage (Gr. "tropho" = nutrition, zoon = an animal). In this last stage the protozoan is active, taking in food (even minute solid food such as bacteria which are much smaller) and multiplying. Protozoa are usually classified by their means of locomotion.

1. *Flagellates* move by means of hairlike appendage(s) which moves the organism with a back-and-forth motion (Fig. 22–9).
2. *Ciliates* move by means of numerous hairlike projections called cilia, which are much shorter than flagella. The motion is wavelike (Fig. 22–10).

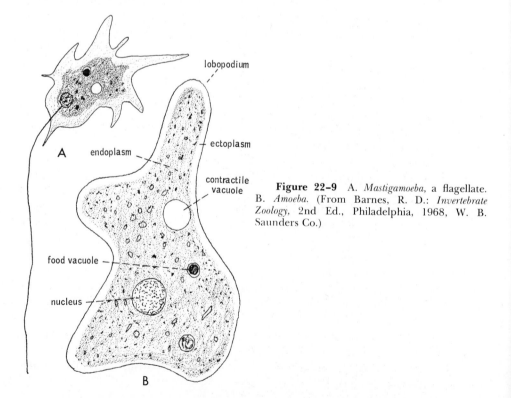

lobopodium

ectoplasm

A   endoplasm

contractile
vacuole

food vacuole

nucleus

**Figure 22–9** A. *Mastigamoeba,* a flagellate. B. *Amoeba.* (From Barnes, R. D.: *Invertebrate Zoology,* 2nd Ed., Philadelphia, 1968, W. B. Saunders Co.)

B

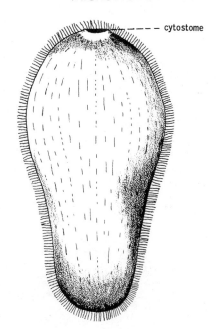

cytostome

**Figure 22–10**   *Prorodon,* a ciliate. (From Barnes, R. D.: *Invertebrate Zoology,* 2nd Ed., Philadelphia, 1968, W. B. Saunders Co.)

3. *Amoebae* move by means of pseudopodia (pseudo — false, podo — feet or foot). The amoeba pushes out a portion of itself and then proceeds to pull itself into the protrusion. It is the slowest form of protozoan movement. The amoeba also uses its pseudopodia to obtain food. By putting out two pseudopodia it surrounds the food particle, pulls it into itself, and there digests it. The protozoa are the only microscopic organisms that can digest solid material. All other forms secure their nourishment by dialysis through the cell membrane.

There are only a few protozoa that are pathogenic to man, and in temperate zones where good sanitary conditions prevail even those few are rarely encountered. However, in some parts of the world, and in the United States in previous years, they caused much illness and many deaths.

Protozoa are usually transmitted by fecal-food contamination or by vectors. The term vector usually refers to an arthropod (insect) which is capable of transmitting the organisms of a communicable disease. The protozoa of interest include the following.

1. The plasmodia which cause malaria. There are four forms: the *Plasmodium vivax* (causing tertian malaria — an episode every 3 days — or really every other day), *Plasmodium malariae* (causing quartan malaria with an episode every fourth day — actually every third day), *Plasmodium falciparum* (causing autumnal malaria — the episodes are irregular; this is the most serious of all the forms and in spite of the name is not limited to the autumn or fall season), and the *Plasmodium ovale* (causing the same episodes as *Plasmodium vivax,* but in a much milder form.) All these are transmitted from a patient with malaria to another person by the female *Anopheles* mosquito. The plasmodia have a very complex life cycle. There is an asexual reproductive stage in the human and a sexual stage in the mosquito. A break in the chain destroys the organism. Various drugs are used to treat malaria when it occurs, but the best treatment is

prevention by the destruction of the mosquito and its breeding ground. This is done by getting rid of standing water and putting a thin oily film over ponds where the mosquitos breed. This prevents the larvae (wiggle tails) from breathing, and they drown.

2. The *Entamoeba histolytica* causes amebic dysentery and can cause severe abscess especially in the liver or gallbladder, but the abscesses may occur in any part of the body. This amoeba forms cysts (Fig. 22–11) which are excreted with the feces, and if anything contaminated with the feces gets on "fingers, food or in drinking water" and is ingested, the cysts will revert to the trophozoite stage. A person who has had amoebic dysentery may become a carrier. A carrier is an apparently healthy individual who harbors pathogenic organisms which,

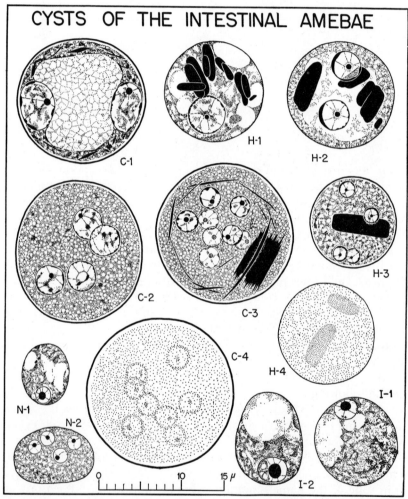

**Figure 22–11** Cysts of intestinal amoebae. C–1, Iron-hematoxylin stained binucleate cyst of *Entamoeba coli.* C–2, Iron-hematoxylin stained quadrinucleate cyst of *E. coli.* C–3, Iron-hematoxylin stained mature cyst of *E. coli.* H–1, Iron-hematoxylin stained uninucleate cyst of *E. histolytica.* H–2, Iron-hematoxylin stained binucleate cyst of *E. histolytica.* H–3, Iron-hematoxylin stained mature cyst of *E. histolytica.* N–1, Iron-hematoxylin stained uninucleate cyst of *Endolimax nana.* N–2, Iron-hematoxylin stained mature cysts of *E. nana.* I–1, I–2, Iron-hematoxylin stained mature cysts of *Iodamoeba bütschlii.* C–4, Unstained mature cyst of *E. coli.* H–4, Unstained cyst of *E. histolytica* showing chromatoid bars. (From Hunter, G. W., et al.: *A Manual of Tropical Medicine,* 4th Ed., Philadelphia, 1966, W. B. Saunders Co.)

under proper circumstances, can infect other people. It is believed that the organisms are usually in the gallbladder in a cystic stage.

3. *Giardia lamblia* is an opportunist pathogen; that is, it is not uncommon in the human intestinal tract, usually in cyst form, and usually harmless. However, under certain circumstances it can cause a serious intestinal infection. It occurs more often in children than in adults. The condition is called giardiasis. The *Giardia* is a flagellate.

4. The *Trichomonas hominis, buccalis,* and *vaginalis* are similar organisms. The first two are relatively harmless inhabitants of the intestines and mouth respectively. The *Trichomonas vaginalis* is a larger protozoan, a flagellate with four tails at its blunt end and an undulating membrane down one side. It is pear shaped. This organism is found in the genital tracts of both male and female. In the male it may cause a whitish urethral discharge but usually causes no symptoms. However, in the female it can cause a severe vulvovaginitis with itching, redness, and a copious whitish or creamy discharge. It is most often transmitted by coitus but may be transferred by other means.

There are many other protozoal diseases, but they are rarely, if ever, seen in North America.

## BACTERIA

Bacteria are minute one-celled organisms which, unlike fungi and protozoa, do not have a typical nucleus; their genetic material is scattered within the cell. Bacteria are usually considered to be minute plants. Like fungi, they do not have chlorophyll, and they are much smaller than most fungi.

Bacteria are classified in many ways. Briefly these are as follows. (Major bacteria in each group will be discussed later.)

1. *By shape.* Spherical—cocci; oblong (ends may be blunt or tapered)—bacilli; curved or spiral—spirilla.

2. *According to divisional grouping.* All bacteria divide by fission, but not all separate into distinct single organisms. Specific prefixes are used thus: diplo—two (diplococci)—appearing in groups of two; strepto—a chain (streptococci)—like a chain of beads; staphylo—grape-like (staphylococci)—like a bunch of grapes.

3. *By their reaction to various stains.* Three are common: gram-positive; gram-negative; and acid-fast. (Staining methods are given later.)

4. *By their reaction to oxygen.* Strict (or obligate) aerobes (these require oxygen to live); strict (or obligate) anaerobes (these cannot live in the presence of oxygen); facultative (these can adapt to an environment with or without oxygen).

5. *By their relation to disease.* Pathogenic—cause disease; nonpathogenic—do not cause disease (in the majority); and opportunists—usually do not cause disease, but may do so under certain circumstances.

There are an almost limitless number of diseases caused by bacteria. Here will be discussed only the more common ones, causative organisms, diseases they cause, and the usual mode of transmission.

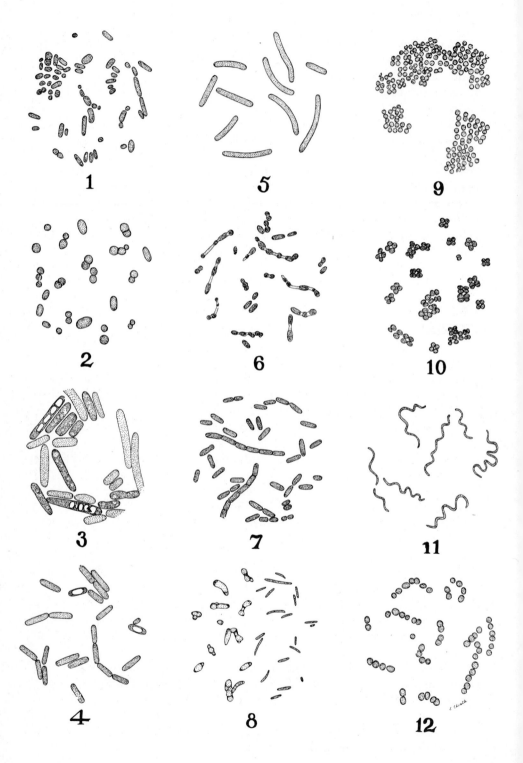

1

5

9

2

6

10

3

7

11

4

8

12

**Figure 22–12** *See opposite page for legend.*

## Diseases Caused by Cocci (Gram-Positive)

Lobar or pneumococcal pneumonia is a common respiratory lung disease that is transmitted by direct contact, droplets, or fomites (inanimate things such as dishes, towels, and the like).

Droplet infection is the most common method of transmission for all infectious respiratory diseases. Coughing, sneezing, and even talking can cause fine droplets of nasal pharyngeal and/or bronchial secretion to be dispersed in the surrounding air. These are then inhaled by anyone nearby, who, if susceptible, will then develop the disease. It has been estimated that talking will force a droplet as far as three feet, a cough, ten feet, and a sneeze, twenty feet. The physician's reception room can be a place of unwittingly spreading diseases. Patients should be taught (if they do not already know) to cover the mouth and nose with facial tissue when coughing or sneezing. The tissue will trap the droplets. The tissue should then be destroyed as soon as possible. Bacteria, of themselves, travel only in a fluid medium (they cannot fly or walk), but they can and do hitchhike on droplets of fluid as above and on minute dust particles.

Pathogenic streptococci cause several diseases, septicemia (septi—septic, poison, and -emia—blood, commonly termed blood poisoning), acute sore throat (it may involve tonsils, pharynx, and larynx), scarlet fever, and erysipelas (a severe skin disease with systemic involvement).

Before the advent of modern drugs such as the sulfonamides and antibiotics, streptococcal infections were always serious and often fatal. The same can be said of many bacterial diseases.

Pathogenic staphylococci may cause a pyogenic (pyo—pus, genic—to produce) infection in almost any part of the body. Actually, the same is true of streptococci. However, staphylococci do not cause any single identifiable disease. Also, staphylococci have become resistant to many drugs which are still effective against streptococci. Most cutaneous abscesses (boils—furuncles, and multiple boils—carbuncles) are caused by staphylococci. Many hospitals and other institutions where a number of patients are gathered together have trouble with staphylococcal infections. Either there are carriers among the personnel, or some inanimate objects harbor the organisms. This can be a serious situation.

## Diseases Caused by Cocci (Gram-Negative)

Of the many gram-negative cocci, only two are of interest to the office assistant, and only one of these will be apt to be seen frequently.

---

**Figure 22–12** Free-living bacteria. (Copyright © 1947, General Biological Supply House, Chicago, Ill.)

1. Aerobacter aerogenes
2. Azotobacter
3. Bacillus megatherium
4. Bacillus subtilis
5. Lactobacillus bulgaricus
6. Mycobacterium smegmatis
7. Pseudomonas fluorescens
8. Rhizobium radicicola
9. Rhodococcus roseus
10. Sarcina aurantica
11. Spirillum rubrum
12. Streptococcus lacticus

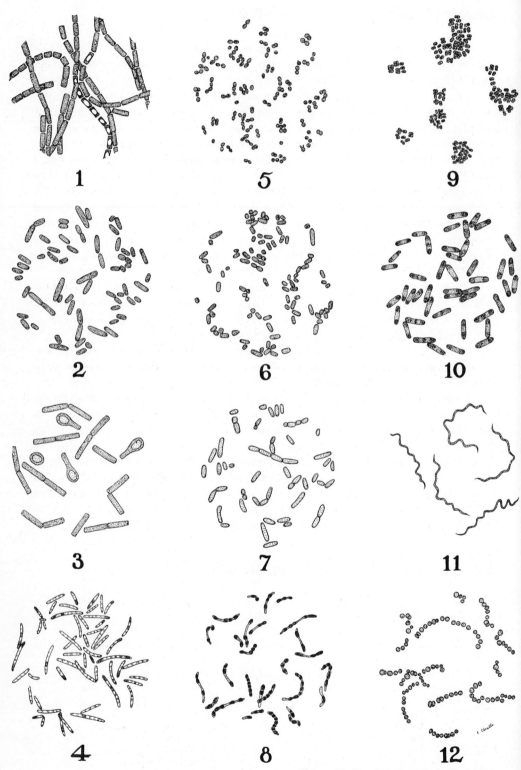

**Figure 22–13** *See opposite page for legend.*

Gonorrhea, caused by the *Neisseria gonorrhoea,* is all too common. Gonorrhea exists in epidemic proportions throughout the country. The disease is transmitted mainly through coitus. However, the handling of contaminated clothing, towels, and the like can be a method of transmission. Individuals, both male and female, may harbor the gonococcus, as the organism is commonly called, and appear to be in good health. In this carrier stage they can inadvertently infect others. It is relatively easy to overcome gonorrhea with modern drug therapy (antibiotics), but many, especially young adults, hesitate to visit the doctor and put off treatment until irreparable tissue damage has been done. In the early stages the disease is localized, but if it goes untreated, it becomes systemic with various symptoms following according to the area involved.

Meningococcic meningitis is caused by the *Neisseria meningitidis.* It is a severe infectious disease affecting the coverings of the brain and spinal cord. It can occur in severe epidemics, but with modern drug therapy, it is not the life-threatening condition it once was. Actually, it has rarely occurred in the United States or Canada in the last ten or fifteen years. The mode of transmission is thought to be contact with the nasopharyngeal secretion which usually harbors the organism.

## Diseases Caused by Bacilli (Gram-Positive)

It is possible to prevent most diseases of the pathogenic gram-positive bacilli by proper immunization. (This subject will be discussed later in this chapter.) Such diseases as diphtheria, pertussis (whooping cough), and tetanus (lockjaw) are rarely encountered now, since they are prevented by routine immunization in childhood. In the face of an imported case or an epidemic, booster immunizations are given.

Tetanus, together with gas gangrene and botulism, is a somewhat specialized case. The organisms causing these diseases are of the genus *Clostridium.* The clostridia are spore bearing, anaerobic, and excrete or secrete very powerful toxins. The spore stage is not a means of reproduction but a reaction to an unfriendly environment. When the environment improves, the vegetative stage is re-established. Spores are very resistant to heat and disinfectants and are killed only by special sterilization methods.

The organisms of tetanus and gas gangrene enter the body through a "dirty" wound. The dirt around animal corrals, feed lots, and such places is very often infected with the spores, especially those of tetanus. In any such cases, the medical assistant should be extremely careful of the soiled clothing or dressings.

**Figure 22–13**    Pathogenic bacteria. (Copyright © 1947, General Biological Supply House, Chicago, Ill.)

1. Bacillus anthracis
2. Eberthella typhi
3. Clostridium tetani
4. Corynebacterium diphtheriae
5. Diplococcus pneumoniae
6. Escherichia coli
7. Hemophilus pertussis
8. Mycobacterium tuberculosis
9. Neisseria gonorrhoeae
10. Yersinia pestis
11. Spirochaeta recurrentis
12. Streptococcus mitior (viridans)

She should inquire whether the patient has been immunized against tetanus. The physician must be notified, and if the patient has had tetanus toxoid, then a booster dose may be ordered. If not, the physician will probably order tetanus antiserum. This immunization is given either by subcutaneous or intramuscular injection. The commercial literature with the medication will indicate the method of injection. This literature should be studied before administering the drug, since it is important to use the correct form (prophylactic, not therapeutic), as they differ in strength.

Before giving any serum, a *skin sensitivity* test should be performed. A minute amount of the antitoxin (0.1 ml) is given intradermally. If the patient is allergic to that serum, a raised reddened wheal will appear in about 20 minutes. Do not give the antitoxin until you ascertain what the physician wishes done. It is customary to give the amount of serum required in a very small dose every 15 to 30 minutes until the total dose is complete. Epinephrine (Adrenalin) and equipment for administering it either I.M. or I.V. should be at hand. If the patient shows signs of allergic reaction, epinephrine will counteract any adverse effects.

Botulism is rarely seen in the physician's office. It is contracted by eating improperly prepared food. The clostridia live best in slightly alkaline media and are anaerobic, living without air, as said previously. If non-acid foods such as beans, meat, and mushrooms are canned and sealed without proper sterilization, the organisms can multiply rapidly. The actual bacteria are harmless but the exotoxin (exo — outside or given off) is so potent there have been cases of one piece of canned string beans' killing a patient. The toxin is destroyed by boiling for at least 15 minutes. In the case noted, the cook tasted the beans before boiling.

One other gram-positive rod of interest is the fusiform bacillus of Vincent's angina (trench mouth and other names). This bacillus is tapered at both ends; hence, its name. This organism alone is nonpathogenic, but in Vincent's angina it lives with a spirochete (a spirillum). Where two or more organisms live together to the apparent benefit of both, the term symbiotic or symbiosis is used. Both organisms are anaerobic. They cause ulceration of the mucous membrane of the mouth and sometimes of the throat. The patient's saliva is highly infectious. Patients with this condition are usually ambulatory and are often treated by the doctor in his office. The doctor usually cleans the ulcers and applies topical medication. Systemic drugs may also be given. The patient should have explained to him the necessity for either sterilizing his dishes and eating utensils or using disposable ones. Disposable disinfectant wash cloths and towels are best. Pillow cases and sheets should be boiled or soaked for several minutes in a suitable disinfectant solution. The physician will designate what solution to use. Since the organisms are anaerobic, the physician will probably order mouth washes of some substance which liberates oxygen, such as hydrogen peroxide.

## Diseases Caused by Bacilli (Gram-Negative)

This is also a large group, and at one time these organisms gave rise to severe plagues. However, modern sanitation has largely eliminated the gram-negative rods as potential killers. Only in disasters (natural or man made) in which the water supply is contaminated with sewage do they pose a threat. Most of these are intestinal parasites. There are three groups — *Salmonella* (including *S. Eberthella*), *Shigella*, and *Escherichia*.

The salmonellae are the cause of typhoid fever and related diseases often classified as paratyphoids A, B, C, and so on. The shigellae cause bacillary dysentery. The *Escherichia coli* is a normal intestinal organism and does not cause trouble unless it gets out of its usual environment. It is a not uncommon cause, especially in females, of cystitis (a bladder infection) which may extend upward causing pyelonephritis (kidney infection). For typhoid there is adequate immunization which has largely eliminated the disease in some areas. However, typhoid carriers are not uncommon and, like amoebic dysentery, it is believed the organisms "reside" in the gallbladder.

There are many other gram-negative rods that cause diseases. However, they are not seen too commonly in North America. Brucellosis (undulant fever) is an animal disease that sometimes causes disease in man. There are three strains, *Brucella melitensis* (Malta fever — a disease of goats which may be transmitted through drinking unpasteurized goat's milk); *Brucella abortus* (a disease of cows transmitted in the same way); *Brucella suis* (a disease of pigs contracted by humans in handling diseased carcasses). The name undulant fever tells the story. It is usually not too serious, but the patient, often a child fed goat's milk, has repeated bouts of fever, and it is often weeks or even months before a diagnosis is made. Once diagnosed, it is not difficult to treat. Any individual who has a series of febrile attacks without apparent cause should be tested for brucellosis.

Tularemia (so named because it was first noticed in Tulare County, California — Tular, -emia — affecting the blood) and plague (bubonic — glandular or pneumonic — pulmonary) are both caused by a small gram-negative rod-like organism. Tularemia (common name rabbit fever, *Francisella tularensis* is found throughout the desert and semi-arid areas of the Southwest. Its common name gives its source. It is almost exclusively contracted by handling jack rabbits afflicted with the disease. If, in preparing the rabbit for cooking, there is a break in the individual's skin, local, and then systemic infection occurs. The cooked meat is not infectious.

Plague caused by the *Yersinia pestis* is more common in the Orient than in the United States. It is transmitted usually by fleas from its normal host, rats, small ground animals such as ground squirrels, chipmunks, and the like. The organism is endemic in these animals in parts of the West, especially the Coast Range of mountains in California. Occasionally, a human case develops, but these are rare.

## Diseases Caused by the Spirilla

(Including vibrio, spirochete, and other curve-shaped organisms. Microbiologists separate these, so the student should realize they are grouped here to conserve space.)

Of this group, by far the most important one in this area is the *Treponema pallidum* — a spirochetal organism that causes syphilis. Like gonorrhea, syphilis is in epidemic proportions throughout the United States. There are many reasons for this, but they are largely sociological. Only one reason is of importance here, and it applies equally to gonorrhea. Many patients hesitate to visit a doctor or go to a clinic for fear of (1) having a venereal disease, (2) being criticized for their "morals," and (3) having their condition made public. The medical assistant can, if she surmises or knows of the situation, assure the patient that the second and third fears will not materialize. Naturally, she cannot tell the person whether or not he has the disease; this is done only by the physician. It is true that venereal diseases, like most communicable diseases, are reportable to the Department of Health authorities, but they are very careful not to disclose the situation though they may contact the individual privately in order to ascertain, if possible, the source of his disease. Syphilis is transmitted mainly by sexual intercourse. In the early stage, the chancre or lesion is highly infectious, though the patient may not even realize he has the lesion. Later, when the disease becomes widespread throughout the body, there may be ulcers of the lips and gums. These are caused by the second most common method of transmission — kissing. After one party of about 30 individuals in which a "kissing" game had been played, nine visited a dermatologist for treatment of sores of the lips (chancres). The organism of syphilis is very fragile and dies quickly when removed from a warm, moist environment.

The only other disease of importance caused by a curved organism is cholera. It is caused by the *Vibrio cholerae* or comma bacteria, so-called since it looks like a comma. It is not seen in North America except as an imported case, because where sanitation is adequate cholera is not a problem. It is an intestinal parasite.

Two other conditions that do not fit easily into any of the preceding categories should be mentioned.

Diphtheria is caused by the *Corynebacterium diphtheriae*. Most commonly a disease of the throat, the organism will grow on any mucous membrane or open wound. Owing to adequate immunization programs, this disease has all but disappeared in the United States and Canada as well as in many other countries. It is a serious disease but can be treated rather easily.

Tuberculosis, caused by the *Mycobacterium tuberculosis,* probably needs little introduction. This is a worldwide disease causing untold suffering and many deaths. Though much less common now than previously, it is still endemic in most areas of the United States and Canada as well as the rest of the world. Tuberculosis can attack any or all parts of the body, but by far the majority of cases are pulmonary. Tuberculosis can be treated and arrested to a point the patient can live a normal life, but treatment is always prolonged.

## RICKETTSIAE AND CHLAMYDIAS

These organisms are specialized types of bacteria. They have some of the characteristics of viruses.

Rickettsiae are larger than the chlamydias but smaller than typical bacteria. Rickettsiae have diffuse genetic material, as do bacteria, and they also contain both DNA and RNA. They are capable of autonomous growth, but unlike typical bacteria they are obligate intracellular parasites. They cannot be cultivated on regular culture media but are grown in chick embryos. Most rickettsial diseases are transmitted by arthropods (insects). One of the most important diseases caused by rickettsiae is Rocky Mountain spotted fever, transmitted by wood ticks from an animal host to the human. Incidentally, the disease is not limited to the Rocky Mountains but is found in the Appalachians as well. The disease can be prevented by vaccines and responds to antibiotic therapy. The other disease is *typhus* (not typhoid). This disease is endemic in Central and Southeastern Europe. It is transmitted by the body louse from one human to another. It is said that typhus killed more German soldiers in their World War I Balkan campaign than were killed by enemy gun fire.

A major distinction between rickettsiae and chlamydias is the fact that the latter are much smaller and cause a different type of disease. Diseases caused by the chlamydias include trachoma, a serious eye disease transmitted by flies, fingers, and so forth; lymphogranuloma venerum, a venereal disease, transmitted usually by coitus or unhygienic personal habits; inclusion conjunctivitis, transmitted to the neonate during its passage through the infected birth canal; and psittacosis and ornithosis, diseases of birds sometimes transmitted to humans who handle the infected animals.

## VIRUSES

Viruses are the smallest living things yet discovered, and in some ways they are only partly living. Viruses, as with rickettsiae and chlamydias, are obligate intracellular organisms. Unlike all other organisms discussed so far, each virus contains only one nucleic acid (DNA or RNA). They do not reproduce themselves but induce the host cell to stop making proteins it needs and produce more viruses. The term *virion* is used to designate individual viral particles. There are many different kinds of viruses, but classification has not been complete. It is common to designate viruses according to the diseases they cause. Viruses infect plants and animals as well as man. Most chemotherapeutic agents are not effective against the viruses. However, for many viral diseases, preventive measures have been perfected. (See Immunity, this chapter.) Some viruses cause destruction of bacteria. They have been termed phages or bacteriophages. Viruses, like the rickettsias or the chlamydias, enter the host by penetrating the cell membrane (and wall in a plant) and then replicate until the cell is ruptured, letting out any number of viruses to find new cells. Viruses cannot live outside a living cell, but they can be dried and later, when given the chance in the presence of moisture and living cells, they will invade the cells and start the cell making new viruses.

There are a number of diseases caused by viruses: influenza, measles, mumps, rubella, yellow fever, small pox, chicken pox, atypical pneumonia or viral pneumonia, hepatitis, and the common cold, to name a few. There is some indication that viruses may be implicated in cancer in ways not yet understood.

## TERMINOLOGY

The following terms are often confusing to medical personnel as well as the layman and need to be briefly defined.
1. *Contagion* or *contagious* is usually used to designate a disease that is rapidly transmitted from one individual to another and affects a large number of people at a time. The term is usually so vague it has been largely replaced by

*communicable.* These diseases are spread by *direct contact*; that is, contact with a body secretion or exudate from a lesion or open sore, and the like, or they are spread by *indirect contact* by inanimate objects such as drinking glasses or bed clothing.

2. *Infection* is a term applied to any disease or condition, such as an abscess or boil, that is caused by a microorganism. It is the invasion of the body by any pathogenic organism. An *infectious disease* is one caused by some parasitic organism and transmitted from one person to another. This term is interchangeable with *communicable.*

3. *Endemic* is a condition in which a certain disease (or diseases) is found in a given area more or less at all times. Endemic diseases are present in a community continuously but occur in small numbers of cases. Some usual childhood diseases are said to be endemic. Smallpox is endemic in countries where vaccination is not routinely performed.

4. *Epidemic* refers to a condition in which a large number of people are afflicted with the same adverse condition. As now used it can even be applied to non-disease phenomena. "There is an epidemic of suicides" or "there is almost an epidemic of accidents," and the like are examples of such applications. Whether this usage is correct or not depends upon the point of view of each individual regarding language. *Epidemic* still refers mainly to disease.

5. *Pandemic* refers to a disease that is widespread, an epidemic that has increased to cover a much larger territory. The "Flu of 1918" was considered a pandemic, "pan" meaning all and "demos" meaning people.

## LABORATORY PROCEDURES RELATIVE TO MICROBIOLOGY FREQUENTLY PERFORMED IN THE PHYSICIAN'S OFFICE

It is hoped by this time, the student will have some specific ideas as to:
1. How diseases are transmitted.
2. How body secretions or excretions are apt to be infective in certain types of diseases.
3. How the physician is helped in making a differential diagnosis of various communicable diseases.
4. The importance of the proper disposal of contaminated materials.
5. Why sterilization is stressed.

Some physicians prefer to do basic identification of the microbial cause of a disease in their office rather than send the specimen to a laboratory for analysis. Of course, this excludes those microbial tests that require extensive laboratory equipment and training. If some procedures are done in the medical office certain items of equipment are essential. These include a microscope, incubator, Bunsen burner, bacteriological loop or point, glass microscopic slides, culture media, various stains, stain rack, and items needed for taking smears.

**Techniques for Smears.** A bacteriological smear is a preparation for microscopic study. The material is spread thinly across the slide with a swab or loop. It is then stained and examined under the microscope.

The medical assistant may be expected to take direct smears from the patient's throat, vagina, abscesses or an infected wound. Indirect smears are taken from a bacterial culture and will be discussed later.

The basic principle is the same for all smears and may vary a little according to the area it is taken from. You will need a sterile swab and two clear microscopic slides. The slides must be absolutely fat free and should be held by the sides only. *Never* put the fingers on the flat surface of the slide, because the fingerprints will make smearing and staining difficult as well as interfere with identification.

THROAT SMEAR AND CULTURE. Aided by a good light, look into the throat and carefully locate the infected area. It is of no value to just "dab in the dark." You may accidentally get to the right spot, but more likely you will not. When the area is located it is touched with the sterile applicator enough to obtain some exudate. For a smear, the applicator is lightly brushed or rolled over the surface of the slide. If the offending material is to be cultured, then sterile technique must be carefully observed. The swab is gently streaked over the surface of the culture medium.

A vaginal culture and smear are done in the same way but are usually obtained by the physician with the medical assistant's holding the culture tube or Petri plate and the microscopic slides.

If possible, the smear from an abscess or infected wound should be taken directly from the abscess or wound, but it can be taken from a contaminated dressing, provided the area is still moist. If dressings have dried, the smear will probably not be satisfactory.

**Techniques for Staining.** Only two stains are apt to be used in the physician's office — the Gram stain and the Ziehl-Neelsen (acid-fast) stain. (See p. 375.)

GRAM STAIN. A thin film or "smear" of the material to be examined is spread over about 1/2 or 3/4 of the glass microscope slide. The smear is allowed to dry and is then held, smear up, over a flame until it is quite warm but not hot enough to burn the fingers. The heat "fixes" the smear to the slide but does not necessarily kill pathogenic bacteria.

When cool, the smear is covered with a few drops of crystal (or gentian) violet solution (Fig. 22–14). Solutions for the Gram stain are available commercially or can be made up from formulas found in any textbook on microbiology. The violet is allowed to remain on the smear for 20 seconds and is then gently rinsed off with cool water. Gram's or Lugol's iodine solution is then applied for 60 seconds, rinsed off and replaced with 95 per cent ethyl alcohol which is poured off in about 20 seconds and rinsed until all but the thickest parts of the smear have ceased to give off dye. Then a counter stain, usually eosin (other colors may be used if desired) is applied. It is left on for 20 to 60 seconds, depending on the stain used, and then rinsed off. The slide may be left in the air to dry or may be blotted (not rubbed) with soft, clean blotting paper.

A drop of "immersion oil" is put on the smear and it is then ready for examination under the high-power oil-immersion objective of the microscope (Fig. 22–15). Gram-positive organisms appear blue-violet or almost black. Gram-negative organisms appear salmon pink if eosin is used, or they appear whatever color the counter stain is.

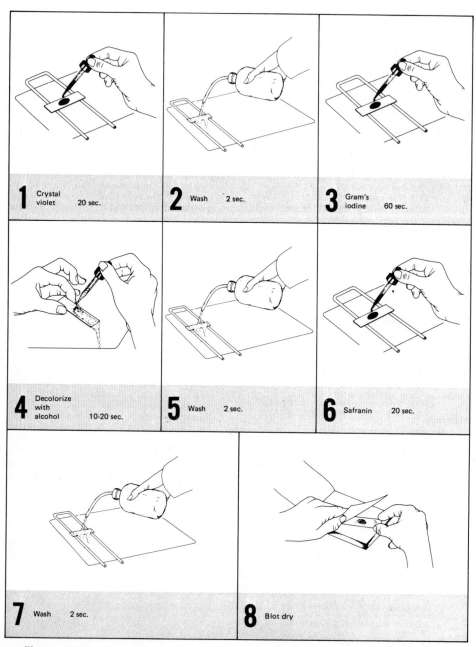

**Figure 22–14** Gram-staining routine. (From Benson, H. J.: *Microbiological Applications*, Dubuque, Iowa, 1973, Wm. C. Brown Co.)

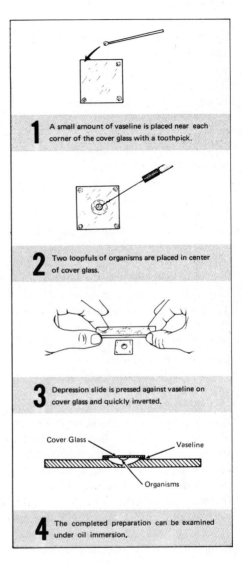

**Figure 22–15** Preparation of slide for microscopic examination: hanging drop slide. (From Benson, H. J.: *Microbiological Applications*, (short edition), Dubuque, Iowa, 1973, Wm. C. Brown Co.)

1  A small amount of vaseline is placed near each corner of the cover glass with a toothpick.

2  Two loopfuls of organisms are placed in center of cover glass.

3  Depression slide is pressed against vaseline on cover glass and quickly inverted.

Cover Glass          Vaseline

Organisms

4  The completed preparation can be examined under oil immersion.

ZIEHL-NEELSEN STAIN.   A smear is prepared as previously described for the Gram stain. The slide is placed on the level cover of a steam bath (about 95° C) and kept flooded drop-wise with a solution of red carbol-fuchsin for four to five minutes. The dye is rinsed off with 95 per cent alcohol containing 10 per cent hydrochloric acid. When all but the thickest portions cease to give off color the slide is then counter stained with methylene blue, brilliant green, or yellow picric acid dye. This is rinsed off with water.

Organisms that tenaciously retain the red dye in spite of the acid alcohol are said to be acid-fast.

The *Mycobacterium tuberculosis*, causing tuberculosis, and the *Mycobacterium leprae*, causing leprosy, are the most pathogenic acid-fast organisms that are seen in the United States and Canada, and the latter is only rarely encountered in the physician's office.

**Cultures.** Microorganisms vary widely in their nutritional needs. Some need only a fluid medium and a few simple chemicals; others require very special substances for growth. However, the majority of pathogenic organisms seen in a physician's office will grow on what might be called "ordinary" culture media. This medium is a combination of agar (to make it solid under culture conditions), partially digested proteins, simple sugars, salt, and water. It is extremely rare for the medical assistant to have to make culture media. If this occurs, a book on laboratory techniques and/or microbiology should be consulted. Most commercial houses furnish various culture media in glass or plastic containers (usually covered dishes called Petri dishes) ready for inoculation.

In some cases blood is added to the media, since certain organisms grow best if blood is present, and differences among organisms can be recognized by this test. For instance, some streptococci hemolyze (destroy) red blood cells and are called hemolytic streptococci; some turn the red blood a greenish color (from partially destroyed hemoglobin) and are known as viridans streptococci; others do not change the blood at all and are known as nonhemolytic streptococci.

The culture is inoculated by passing the contaminated applicator lightly over the medium usually in a streaked form as shown in Figures 22–16 and 22–17. If urine or blood is cultured directly, the culture medium is covered with a thin film of the fluid. The culture is incubated at body temperature (37° C or 98.6° F) for 24 hours unless otherwise ordered. Then a smear is made from the growth and examined.

Blood for a culture is taken in the same manner as for a specimen, but only a small amount (1 or 2 ml) is needed.

Unless the urine is a catheterized specimen taken into a sterile container, special precautions must be observed. For the female patient the vulvovaginal area should be thoroughly washed with soap and water and then rinsed with sterile water, or an antiseptic disposable wash cloth may be used. If there is excessive vaginal secretion, a cotton pledget is placed in the vaginal orifice. The patient is then requested to catch a midstream specimen in a sterile container. With the male patient the penis is washed and rinsed in the same manner and the patient voids a midstream specimen into a sterile container.

CULTURE WITH SENSITIVITY DISCS. In order to ascertain what antiinfective drug will be most effective, sensitivity discs are placed on the culture plate after

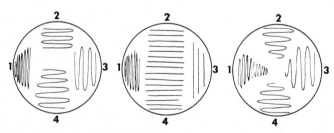

**Figure 22–16** (From Bradshaw, L. J.: *Laboratory Microbiology*, 2nd Ed., Philadelphia, 1973, W. B. Saunders Co.)

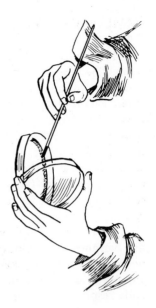

**Figure 22–17** Correct technique for streaking a Petri plate of nutrient agar for isolated colonies. Note the comfortable position of the right hand and the protective angle of the lid held by the left hand. When one sector is completed, the loop is withdrawn and the lid closed. The plate is rotated 90°, and the next sector streaked. (From Bradshaw, L. J.: *Laboratory Microbiology*, 2nd Ed., Philadelphia, 1973, W. B. Saunders Co.)

inoculation and before incubation. These discs are obtained from commercial sources. Each disc contains a minute amount of a common agent such as penicillin, tetracycline, a sulfonamide, and so forth. These are properly identified. After incubation a ring of clear medium indicates that the organism has been killed or cannot grow in the presence of that drug. The size of the ring indicates the effectiveness. Figure 22–18 illustrates inoculation and placing of the discs on the culture medium and the clear zone around certain discs containing an agent that may be effective against that particular organism. The size of the ring indicates the effectiveness. However, if it were found on inquiry that the patient could not take one of the drugs, then another drug must be selected for use.

**Figure 22–18** Chemotherapy and antibiotics. Testing sensitivity of a bacterium to antibiotics or other chemotherapeutic agents by the "disk method." (Courtesy of Linda Kaye Hickey.) In Frobisher, M., and Fuerst, R.: *Microbiology in Health and Disease*, 13th Ed., Philadelphia, 1973, W. B. Saunders Co.

CL-Coly-Mycin
AM-Ampicillin
TE-Terramycin
P-Penicillin
C-Chloramphenicol
PB-Polymyxin B
N-Neomycin
Fd-Nitrofurantoin
T-Tetracycline
K-Kanamycin
LR-Cephaloridine
GM-Garamycin
SSS-Triple Sulfa
CB-Carbenicillin
NA-Nalidixic Acid

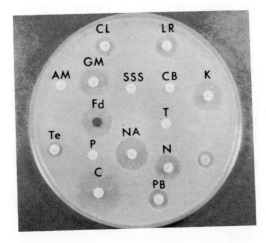

# IMMUNOLOGY—BODY DEFENSES

The lymphatic system and the white blood cells form our internal arma-ment. The lymph circulation is interspersed with lymph nodes, or glands. These trap microorganisms and, unless the microbes win the battle, stop the infection. White blood cells form the next line of defense. The white cell known as a polymorphonuclear cell (called "poly") is phagocytic. A phagocyte is a cell or or-ganism that "eats" other organisms. This is called phagocytosis or the process of destroying other organisms. The reason the exudate from an abscess is so white is partially due to the numerous white blood cells that are trying to destroy the invading bacteria. Of course, the exudate includes other things such as dead cells, dead and live bacteria, interstitial fluid, and if capillaries are injured, blood is also present.

There are several different kinds of white blood cells but the "polys" and the lymphocytes predominate. Antibodies are formed mainly in the lymph nodes, spleen, bone marrow, and lymphoid tissue. Antibodies combine with the antigen to neutralize it. This is called the antigen-antibody reaction. Once the body responds to the invasion and begins to produce antibodies, it can continue to do so for many weeks to several years. Thus, it is possible for immunity to last for many months or years.

Antibodies are carried in the globin protein of the blood. Where the globin contains a number of different antibodies, as it usually does, it has been called gamma globulin. The preferred term now is immune serum globulin. Com-mercial preparations of immune serum globulin are derived from blood serum and are used for prevention and treatment of various infectious diseases. This type of immune serum contains almost all the known antibodies circulating in the blood and provides a passive immunity, usually for about six weeks. Immune. serum globulin, or ISG as it is often designated, is used to prevent development of or to modify the course of a disease which might be serious in a specific case. Suppose a child, ill with rheumatic heart disease, is accidentally exposed to measles for which he had not been immunized. Immune serum globulin could be used during the disease's incubation period. It would either prevent the development of the measles entirely, or if measles did develop it would be a lighter form of the disease.

**Immune Reaction.** The reaction is the union of antigen with antibodies. This reaction is specific; an antigen will react only with an antibody which the antigen itself caused to be formed. Another way of illustrating this concept is the well-known observation that polio vaccine (an antigen) will not protect us against tetanus toxin (another antigen). Each produces its own specific antibodies (anti-polio or tetanus antitoxin). That this reaction has occurred can be observed clini-cally when the patient gets well or when contact with disease-producing antigen produces no disease (resistance). A laboratory test can also be used to detect this reaction. When an antigen is mixed with an antibody in a test tube, clumping (agglutination) may occur, and this can be seen. This is so because the combina-tion of antibody with antigen is insoluble. On the other hand, interaction can occur and not be observed. That something has happened can be demonstrated if the mixture (containing an antigen that by itself can produce disease) is injected into a susceptible animal, and no disease is produced (toxin-antitoxin reaction).

Many other tests have been devised to show whether an antibody-antigen reaction has occurred, but these are beyond the scope of this chapter.

**Interferon.**   In addition to antibodies, the body produces a substance called interferon which is supposed to interfere with the ability of viruses to penetrate the cell membranes and thus cause disease, by inhibiting virus multiplication. It is considered to be nonspecific; that is, it acts against several species of viruses.

The science of immunology is based on a fundamental reaction: antigen + antibody → [antigen-antibody complex] (neutralization). Two very active molecules interact to form an inactive complex. For a long time this process was looked upon as a favorable one; that is, a protective mechanism for animals, and indeed it is. However, more recently scientists have learned that this reaction can backfire and actively produce disease rather than prevent it. This later turn of events is referred to as a "hypersensitive reaction," and the diseases arising from it are called "diseases of hypersensitivity." Among such diseases are those of allergy—hay fever, serum sickness, blood transfusion reactions, and the rejection of transplanted organs. In short, the immune reaction can take one of two turns—a good one or a bad one.

**Antigens.**   These are substances which, upon introduction into the body, result in the production of specific antibodies. Chemically, these substances usually are proteins, polysaccharides, and possibly lipids but almost always are of protein composition. For example, an antigen may be a bacterium, virus, toxin, or a pollen. Drugs and simple chemicals cannot be antigens by themselves, but when combined with proteins, they become antigenic. Actually, the protein portion of the combination is the antigen, but the chemicals change its specificity.

**Immunity.**   Immunity is the resistance of the body to the effects of a harmful agent, such as pathological microorganisms or their toxins. As stated earlier, the immune reaction can occur as follows: antigen + antibody → neutralization of infectivity or toxicity of antigen. The presence of specific antibodies in the body confers immunity. This immunity can be natural or acquired.

NATURAL IMMUNITY.   This is an innate resistance to a disease owing to the presence of antibodies occurring normally in the blood. This natural immunity can be *congenital immunity* that is received from the mother's blood by passage of maternal antibodies through the placenta. This explains the resistance of infants to certain diseases. Unfortunately, like many gifts, this immunity does not last very long. *Inherited immunity* is transmitted from parents through the germ cells. This is a lifelong immunity. Since it is genetically determined, it explains why some animal diseases are not transmissible to humans or why one race is more resistant to some illnesses than other races. This is also known as *species immunity*. An example of this is that cats are not susceptible to some diseases of cows. There are exceptions, as in everything, but they are not common. Already mentioned are some diseases transmitted to man, such as tularemia from rabbits, psittacosis from birds and brucellosis from goats, pigs, or cattle.

ACQUIRED IMMUNITY.   (Also called induced immunity.) This is the result of the formation of antibodies that were not there normally in the body. This immunity may be *naturally acquired* (a result of having had the disease or infection and recovering from it, resulting in the formation of antibodies) and, in some cases, offers future protection against this disease or infection. This protection may be temporary, as in the case of the common cold, or long lasting, as with a case of measles. Active immunity may also be *artificially acquired* by the introduction of various antigens such as vaccines, viral or bacterial, and toxoids into the body. This form of immunization has many advantages:

1. The antibodies are produced by the patient's own body and remain in it rather than being eliminated, which may not be true with foreign antibodies that are introduced into the patient's body by use of immune serums.
2. Artificially acquired active immunization is not likely to make the patient develop the disease. In fact, the patient frequently will have no reaction to the immunization.

There is one disadvantage of active acquired immunization that must be remembered—it takes some time for the body to develop the antibodies that are essential for immunity. The length of time differs with various antigens, but it is usually about six weeks. Thus, for a disease with a short incubation period, active immunization cannot be secured between the exposure time and the time the patient would become ill. It may then be necessary to use passive immunization, or to immunize before exposure. Since artificially acquired immunization is controlled, it may be said that it is man's way of producing or simulating the disease with controlled protection.

Immunizing antigens used to produce active immunity are of various types. A vaccine may contain virus, bacteria, rickettsiae, or toxins that have been killed or attenuated or detoxified or, in some cases, live organisms may be used. The smallpox vaccine is an example of the use of attenuated organisms. The diphtheria toxin has been detoxified and is called alum precipitated toxoid. Vaccines may be mono- or polyvalent; that is, they may contain one or more than one strain or species of a microorganism. Some vaccines are mixed. This means there are several different types of organisms and/or toxoids in the vaccine. The cold vaccine is an example of a mixed vaccine. Undenatured bacterial antigens (UBA) are preparations produced from bacterial cultures by mechanical processes. They contain only antigens of the disease. They appear to be very efficient in producing active immunity quickly; however, the immunity is not so lasting as that secured by other means. Autogenous vaccines are bacterial vaccines prepared from cultures of material derived from a lesion or exudate of the patient to be treated.

PASSIVE IMMUNITY.   The term refers to that immunity received from some outside source. The antibodies are not produced by the individual but are preformed antibodies given to the individual. They are manufactured by an animal or another person, extracted, and then given to the patient. The patient does not manufacture the antibodies. It may be said the patient "passively accepts ready-made antibodies." The protection is immediate but of very short duration. That is because the recipient's body treats these injected antibodies as a foreign substance and removes them by forming antibodies against these antibodies. Thus, antibodies can function as antigens as well. These preformed human antibodies are commercially known as immune serum globulin or gamma globulin.

REVISED SCHEDULE FOR ACTIVE
IMMUNIZATION AND TUBERCULIN
TESTING OF NORMAL INFANTS AND
CHILDREN IN THE UNITED STATES*

| | | |
|---|---|---|
| 2 mo | DTP[1] | TOPV[2] |
| 4 mo. | DTP | TOPV |
| 6 mo. | DTP | TOPV |
| 1 yr. | Measles[3] | Tuberculin Test[4] |
| 1–12 yr. | Rubella[3] | Mumps[3] |
| 1½ yr. | DTP | TOPV |
| 4–6 yr. | DTP | TOPV |
| 14–16 yr. | Td[5] | and thereafter every 10 years |

[1]DTP—diphtheria and tetanus toxoids combined with pertussis vaccine.

[2]TOPV—trivalent oral polio virus vaccine. The above recommendation is suitable for breast-fed as well as bottle-fed infants.

[3]May be given at 1 year as Measles-Rubella or Measles-Mumps-Rubella combined vaccines.

[4]Frequency of repeated tuberculin tests depends on risk of exposure of the child and on the prevalence of tuberculosis in the population group.

[5]Td—combined tetanus and diphtheria toxoids (adult type) for those over six years of age in contrast to diphtheria and tetanus (DT) containing a larger amount of diphtheria antigen.

Tetanus toxoid at time of injury: For clean, minor wounds, no booster dose is needed by a fully immunized child unless more than 10 years have elapsed since the last dose.

For contaminated wounds, a booster dose should be given if more than 5 years have elapsed since the last dose.

Routine smallpox vaccination is no longer recommended.

Approved by the Committee on
Infectious Diseases. October 17, 1971
American Academy of Pediatrics

*From Francis, B. J.: Current concepts in immunization, *Am. J. Nurs.* 73:647 (1973).

Tuberculin testing is done by applying a minute amount of the tuberculin material to the skin, usually of the forearm. The commercial brochure should be consulted for exact details. This test determines if the individual has built up antibodies to tuberculosis, whether or not he has had an active case of the disease. Subclinical tuberculosis is a not uncommon occurrence. If, at the end of 48 hours, there is a red, swollen area lasting several days, the test is positive.

There is a test for susceptibility to diphtheria (the Schick test) which is often used before giving the toxoid to an older child who has not been immunized previously. A minute amount of the toxin is injected intradermally (again in the forearm). If no reaction occurs, it is because the individual has some antibodies (antitoxin) in his blood which neutralize the toxin. He is nonsusceptible. If a wheal occurs there are no antibodies, and the person would probably develop diphtheria upon exposure. He should be given the toxoid.

For anyone contemplating travel in a foreign country, the public health service or a physician should be consulted to see what immunizations are required. Most physicians keep a record for the foreign countries visited most often by their patients. This information can be obtained from the state Department of Health or from the National Communicable Disease Center, Atlanta, Georgia.

## REJECTION OF TRANSPLANTED ORGANS

Unless the organ is transplanted from one simultaneous (identical, homozygous) twin to the other twin, the recipient's body considers the implanted organ to be "foreign protein" and, as such, as something to be eliminated. For this reason, the immunosuppressant drugs are given. These prevent the patient's immune system from producing antibodies against the protein of the new organ. Unfortunately, they also prevent the formation of other antibodies which the patient needs. These patients are very susceptible to any infectious disease, especially those of the respiratory system, such as the common cold or influenza. During the acute postoperative stage in the hospital reverse isolation may be used. However, when the patient is released and allowed to go home, every possible care must be employed to avoid the patient's being exposed to any possible infection. If the patient does develop any symptoms of an upper respiratory disease, immediate and vigorous treatment is indicated. More patients who have had organ transplants die of an intercurrent infection than die from direct organ rejection.

## ALLERGY

The antigen-antibody reactions are varied and complicated. These reactions may be beneficial, as in immunizations against a communicable disease, or they may be harmful in varying degrees, as in an allergy. This allergic, also known as hypersensitivity, reaction is identical, but the interaction of the antigen and antibody is accompanied by harmful effects on the human body. The antigen (allergen) may be bland, such as a pollen or horse serum, but its reaction with the antibodies can produce hay fever in the first case, serum sickness, or even anaphylactic shock in the second instance. The antigen can be harmful in itself (bacteria), but its reaction with antibodies can produce a relatively mild and temporary infection (sore throat) and serious chronic disease (nephritis, rheumatic heart disease, periarteritis nodosa). This antigen-antibody process depends mainly on such factors as the type of antigen (allergen) and the individual's ability to respond to it.

The word allergy was introduced by Von Pirquet in 1906. In its original meaning, it meant a state of altered reactivity. In certain cases there appears to be a genetic lack of some required factor or factors. It is an inherited characteristic. It is found that perhaps 20 to 25 per cent of the population is allergic. However, not all allergic reactions can be classified. The strangeness of this type of sensitivity led to the term "atopy" meaning "out of place," and perhaps a better term for allergy is "atopic hypersensitivity."

The symptoms of an allergy can occur for the first time at any age. The substances that produce an allergic response can be eaten, inhaled, injected, or applied topically to the skin. The response to these allergens bears no relation to the type of material involved. For example, foods may cause either eczema, rhinitis, or asthma. The most common allergies affect the respiratory passages and the skin, although other areas such as the digestive tract, nervous system, joints, kidneys, and blood vessels can be affected. Hay fever symptoms are congested and running nose (rhinitis), spasms of sneezing, itching, and watery eyes. Asthma is an allergy characterized by shortness of breath, coughing and wheezing. The allergies of the skin include urticaria (hives) or itchy swellings and eczema, an itching rash. Contact dermatitis gives a rash similar to eczema and occurs as a result of direct contact of the skin with the allergen. Skin eruptions resulting from insect bites and stings and contact with poisonous plants such as poison ivy, oak, and sumac are also allergic reactions. Emotional factors also play a role in allergy.

The medical assistant will encounter any number of allergic conditions in every type of medical practice, but they will appear more commonly in the office of the internist and family practitioner and, of course, in the specialty office of an allergist. (For further information on Allergy refer to Chapter 30. Physical Examinations.)

The medical assistant must always be alert to the possibility of anaphylactic shock in a patient receiving an injection of a medication that has not been administered previously in the office. These reactions are rare but are very serious when they do occur. Usually, the patient has had the allergen previously and has become "sensitized to it." In other cases there is no history of previous contact with the allergen. Suppose, for instance, the patient is given an injection of penicillin. The patient has been questioned if he ever was given penicillin before and, if so, if he had a reaction to it. The patient does not recall ever having had the medication. He is given the injection of penicillin. In many offices it is customary to have the patient remain in the office for 20 to 30 minutes after an injection of a medication that is new to the patient. If no symptoms occur, the patient is sent home. A few days later he calls and complains of having fever, chills, and headache, but these symptoms are mild and usually no serious effects are anticipated. BUT if the patient complains of feeling "peculiar" and of having an itching of the skin, and possibly some difficulty breathing while waiting in the office, then the medical assistant should notify the physician immediately without any delay. Minutes may mean the difference between life or death in such a situation. Emergency measures should be taken immediately.

Prevention of anaphylactic shock requires a thorough knowledge of the patient's history and various allergies. Any patient who has been given an injection of an animal serum or an antigen should be watched closely for 20 to 30 minutes. The drug most often used to counteract the effects of anaphylactic shock is epinephrine. (See the chapter on Emergencies.)

# Chapter 23

## BEHAVIORAL OBJECTIVES

*The medical office assistant should be able to:*

Read a prescription.

Make out a prescription under the physician's direction.

Order Federal Narcotic Order Blanks and make them out properly for the physician to sign.

Order State Narcotic Prescription Blanks.

Make up a solution by either the per cent or the ratio method of calculation, according to the strength and the type of the solution.

Prepare a part of a drop.

Prepare a dose of a given strength from a tablet of another strength.

Prepare a dose of a given strength from a solution of a specific strength.

Assist the physician to quickly secure information relative to a poison and its antidote.

# Pharmacology and Preparation of Medications

Mary W. Falconer, R.N., M.A.

Drugs are weapons in the doctor's armamentarium for fighting sickness and disease. A drug is defined as a medicinal substance used in the treatment of a disease. The science and study of the effect of drugs is called "pharmacology." Records of pharmacology date back to ancient Egypt.

There are over one thousand drug manufacturers today, and it is estimated that it costs about four million dollars to develop a drug ready for market. Few people fully realize the cost and time involved in the research and manufacture of a drug. About eight out of ten drugs prescribed today were not even on the market ten years ago.

The purchase of a modern drug may save a patient's life; it may be the deciding factor in restoring his health; it will probably help him to return to work much sooner, or he may not need to miss work at all. The consumer must share in the cost of drug research. Although many drugs may at times seem very expensive, if they reduce hospitalization, shorten the illness and return the individual to health and productivity, they may actually result in monetary saving. Their value in terms of human suffering and loss of health, or life itself, cannot be measured.

It is important that every doctor's assistant have a basic understanding of the common drugs used in the professional office. She not only maintains the supply of drugs but often prepares drugs for use or administers them to patients on the physician's directions.

## SOURCES OF DRUGS

Drugs are obtained from four principal sources: animal, vegetable, mineral (natural sources), and the chemist's laboratory (synthetic sources).

**Natural Sources.** Drugs are obtained from the leaf, seed, sap, stem, or root of certain plants. Digitalis is an extract from the leaf of the foxglove, opium comes from the poppy, and quinine is derived from the bark of the cinchona tree.

**Animals** have been the source of therapeutic hormones. Insulin is the hormone extracted from the islet cells of the pancreas; thyroid is obtained from the thyroid gland. Antibiotics are substances secreted or excreted by living organisms (bacteria, yeasts, and molds). Animal fats give us bases for ointments.

**Minerals** are another source of drugs: magnesium sulfate as Epsom salts or sulfur from wells.

**Synthetic Sources.** Most drugs are synthetically produced today by laboratory processes which duplicate a natural process or synthesize a new formula. Oftentimes a synthetic process can virtually eliminate side effects while increasing the potency of a drug. Synthetic drugs can usually be given in lower dosage than similar natural drugs since they contain no extraneous material.

## DRUG NAMES

A drug may bear many different names. The medical assistant should understand the three types of names a drug may have: chemical, generic, and trade.

**Chemical Name.** The chemical name of a drug represents its exact formula and is frequently long, unwieldy, and extremely difficult to understand. For example, the chemical name of Chlor-Trimeton is

2-[p-Chloro-ax-(2-dimethylaminoethyl) benzyl] pyridine maleate.

This name is of no value to the medical assistant.

**Generic Name.** The generic name is the common name of the chemical or drug. This name is not owned by any particular company; it is nonproprietary. A generic name refers to a single substance. "Chlorpheniramine maleate" is the generic name for Chlor-Trimeton.

**Trade Name.** The trade name is the name by which the manufacturer identifies the drug. It is a copyrighted name and cannot be used by another company. The same formula may have several different trade names from several different pharmaceutical companies. Chlor-Trimeton is a trade name of the Schering Corporation; the same product manufactured by Smith, Kline & French is called Teldrin.

There are certain types of preparations of drugs, usually taken by mouth, which have varying rates of releasing the medication within the body. These are also identified by registered trade names. For example, Repetabs by Schering Corporation, Spansules by Smith, Kline & French, Gradumets by Abbott, Extentabs by Robbins. There are many more names used, as there are many more pharmaceutical houses, and each has its own name for time-release action medications.

## USES OF DRUGS

Many people think that drugs are used for therapeutic purposes only — that is, for the treatment of disease or for their curative value. However, drugs are also used for many other purposes. Some of the more important reasons include:

1. Relief of undesirable symptoms of the disease — morphine to relieve pain.

2. Immunizations to prevent disease—vaccine for typhoid fever, toxoid for diphtheria.

3. To aid in the diagnosis of the disease—dyes used as opaque media in x-ray examinations, antigens used for skin testing in allergy.

4. To hasten recovery from illness—usually vitamins, minerals and supplementary food substances, such as amino acids.

5. To give the patient substances his body is not producing (at all or in insufficient amounts)—thyroid extract for hypothyroidism, insulin for diabetes mellitus.

## DRUG STANDARDIZATION

Drugs are standardized in the United States, and two books are recognized as authoritative treatises. These are the *United States Pharmacopeia* (U.S.P.) and the *National Formulary* (N.F.). Both these books are revised every five years under the supervision of physicians, pharmacists, and scientists.

The Council on Drugs of the American Medical Association at intervals publishes books which give up-to-date information on drugs. Originally, these books were called *New and Non-Official Remedies,* but later were entitled *New Drugs.* They were published yearly. The present book is *Drug Evaluation.* It is not published yearly, but as conditions dictate. There are innumerable publications available to the physician for quick reference. Among these are *Modell's Drugs in Current Use, Falconer's Current Drug Handbook,* and *Physician's Desk Reference.* All these publications, and others of the same type, give "thumbnail" information about drugs that are in general use at the time. The first two books listed cover a large number of drugs without respect to their manufacturers. The last gives information on the main drugs manufactured by those pharmaceutical houses supporting the publication. The *Current Drug Handbook* is revised every other year; *Drugs in Current Use* at irregular intervals; and the last, *Physician's Desk Reference,* yearly, with supplements during the year.

Additionally, each box of medications has in it a brochure giving all pertinent information about that particular drug. The assistant will do well to keep an index file of these brochures. It should be kept up to date and be where she and the doctor can reach it easily. This will be the very latest information possible.

## LEGAL REGULATIONS

Drug standards are established and enforced by the United States Food and Drug Administration (F.D.A.), a part of the Department of Health, Education, and Welfare, by authority of the Federal Food, Drug, and Cosmetic Act enacted in 1938. The purpose of the act, as far as drugs are concerned, is to ensure the identity, strength, purity, and quality of drugs shipped in interstate commerce. The first law regulating the sale of foods and drugs was enacted in 1906 and was aimed primarily at the prevention of adulteration of products (the substitution of one product for another—usually a cheaper for a better, more expensive one). This was a rather weak law with many loopholes. The jurisdiction of the

F.D.A. is limited to products that have been involved in interstate commerce. However, this includes practically all drugs with which the doctor's assistant is concerned.

The American Medical Association has had a history of active support of laws which protect the public through pure food and drugs. It is constantly working toward effective controls of quack medicines and devices, cosmetic and food faddism, and quackery in vitamin preparations and dietary foods. The A.M.A. has never hesitated to sponsor or endorse legislation in the health field when it has been indicated.

In 1951 Congress passed the Durham-Humphrey amendment to the Federal Food, Drug, and Cosmetic Act. The main purpose of this amendment was stricter control of the dispensing of dangerous drugs.

**Narcotics.** The Harrison Narcotic Act was passed in 1915 to regulate the manufacture, sale, dispensing, and prescribing of narcotics. This was a federal law under the supervision of the Bureau of Narcotics, United States Treasury Department, making it necessary for every person who prescribed narcotics to register with the Collector of Internal Revenue on or before July 1 of each year and pay a special tax. The possession of narcotics by unauthorized persons is a federal offense and subject to a severe penalty.

In 1970 a new law was enacted covering medications, including narcotics. This was called The Controlled Substance Act of 1970. It became effective in May, 1971; with a few drugs the effective date was January 1, 1972. By this law the Bureau of Narcotics became the Bureau of Narcotics and Dangerous Drugs (BNDD), under the Department of Justice. The Food and Drug Administration, under the Department of Health, Education and Welfare, retained jurisdiction of all foods and those medicinal substances that were not included under The Bureau of Narcotics and Dangerous Drugs. As of 1973 the name of this bureau was changed to the Drug Enforcement Agency (DEA), but was still under the Department of Justice. Narcotics and various other drugs are covered by this agency. The substances that are included in this category are mainly those that tend to be or have been "abused." The drugs are listed in five schedules. A complete list of all drugs included in each schedule can be obtained from the Regional Office of the Agency. The assistant should secure this list for the physician's office and ask that the doctor's name be placed on their mailing list so that as drugs are added, deleted, or moved from one schedule to another, the office list can be kept up to date.

Briefly the drug schedules are:

**Schedule I.** This schedule includes substances which have no accepted medicinal use. The manufacture, importation and sale of these chemicals is prohibited.

EXAMPLES: heroin, marihuana, d-lysergic acid diethylamide (LSD), mescaline, peyote and others.

**Schedule II.** This schedule includes drugs previously known as Class A Narcotics and some non-narcotic medicines. The prescription for these drugs must be entirely hand-written by the physician, usually on special prescription blanks. The states vary from one to another in this matter. Some require only one copy, some duplicates, and some triplicate copies. Where special blanks are required they are obtained from the State Department of Health. The assistant should be sure that there are ample blanks on hand at all times. In any case the physician's narcotic license number must appear on the blank. The non-narcotic drugs listed in Schedule II may be written on the physician's regular blank, but the doctor must write the prescription himself. Preprinted blanks given out by the pharmaceutical houses may not be used.

EXAMPLES:   Narcotics: opium and opium derivatives (morphine, codeine, Percodan, Pantopon, Dilaudid, methadone (Dolophine) and cocaine (not technically a narcotic, but treated here as are the narcotics).

Non-narcotics: amphetamine (Benzedrine and other trade names), methamphetamine (Methedrine and other trade names).

**Schedule III.**   This schedule includes the narcotics previously classified as Class B Narcotics and some non-narcotic drugs. The physician must write the prescription for these as in Schedule II, but his regular prescription form may be used. Preprinted forms from pharmaceutical companies may not be used. Refills, up to five in any six-month period, may be allowed. This must be indicated on the prescription. Telephone requests must be handled by the physician himself.

EXAMPLES:   Narcotics: various combinations of drugs containing codeine, dihydrocodeinone, hydrocodone, and camphorated tincture of opium (Paregoric), previously an "exempt narcotic."

Non-narcotics: glutethimide (Doriden), some barbiturates, such as aprobarbital (Alurate), amobarbital (Amytal), pentobarbital (Nembutal), secobarbital (Seconal), and all the amphetamine compounds not listed in Schedule II.

**Schedules IV and V.**   These two schedules are handled in much the same manner. The prescription may be made out by the assistant, but must be signed by the physician. Refills are the same as for Schedule III, except that requests for refills over the phone may be handled by the assistant under the direction of the doctor.

EXAMPLES:   Schedule IV: Barbiturates not previously listed, some hypnotics, such as chloral hydrate and similar drugs; some muscle relaxants, such as meprobamate (Equanil and other names); and some tranquilizers, such as chlordiazepoxide (Librium).

EXAMPLES:   Schedule V: This schedule includes most cough medications containing codeine and some drugs used for gastrointestinal disorders, such as Donnagel and diphenoxylate (Lomotil).

Canadian assistants will find that Canada has had a similar law for some time. Information as to the schedules there can be obtained from the Provincial or the Dominion Office of the Department of Health and Welfare.

Specific narcotic laws are lengthy, and it is not important that the medical assistant be familiar with them in detail. It is, however, her responsibility to know the provisions of the laws for handling narcotics.

Regulations of the Drug Enforcement Administration governing the purchase and inventory of controlled substances by medical practitioners were outlined in Chapter 5, *Medicine and the Law.*

**Prescriptions for Controlled Substances.**   Although the federal government does not furnish triplicate prescription blanks, many states do require and provide them. These prescription blanks must be used for narcotic prescriptions only. Do not confuse them with the Federal Triplicate Order Forms which are used to order Schedule II drugs for the office or the doctor's bag.

All prescriptions for controlled substances must be dated and signed on the day when issued and must bear the full name and address of the patient, and the name, address and registration number of the physician. The prescription must be written in ink or indelible pencil or typewriter and must be signed by hand by the practitioner. The prescription may be prepared by a nurse or secretary for the signature of the physician, but the prescribing physician is responsible in case the prescription does not conform in all essential respects to the law and regulations.

A written prescription is required for drugs in Schedule II and must be signed by the physician. *The refilling of Schedule II prescriptions is prohibited.* In the case of a bona fide emergency (as defined by the D.E.A.) a physician may telephone a prescription to a pharmacist for a drug in Schedule II. In such a case, the drug prescribed must be limited to the amount needed to treat the patient during the emergency period. The physician must furnish, within 72 hours, a written, signed prescription to the pharmacy for the drug prescribed. The pharmacist is required by law to notify the D.E.A. if he has not received the prescription within 72 hours.

A prescription for drugs in Schedules III, IV, and V may be issued either orally or in writing and may be refilled *if so authorized* on the prescription up to five times within six months after the date of issue. After five refills or after six months, a new prescription is required in either oral or written form from the physician.

**Controlled Substances Records.** As set forth in Chapter 5, *Medicine and the Law*, the physician must keep an accurate record of certain narcotic and non-narcotic drugs which he dispenses to his patients. A special book, kept in a definite place, should be maintained for this purpose. An example of one type of record is shown in Figure 23–1. The record should show:

1. Full name and address of the patient to whom the drug was given.
2. Date drug was given.
3. Character and quantity of drug.
4. Method of dispensing (Rx, dispensing or injection).

The patient's record will show the pathology and purpose for which the drug was given.

**Control of Drug Abuse.** In February 1966, Congress passed the Federal Drug Abuse Control Act, also known as the Harris Bill (HR 2). The purpose of this bill was to stop the flow of illicit drugs, such as stimulants and depressants, as well as certain tranquilizers and hallucinogenic drugs. Most of these drugs are listed in the various schedules given under the Controlled Substances Act.

The laws governing the prescribing of drugs differ somewhat from state to state, but in all states prescriptions may be legally written or telephoned only by the physician; in most states they may be filled only by a registered pharmacist.

The future will bring tighter control of drugs sold over the counter, known as O.T.C. products. The Department of Health, Education, and Welfare has already shown this by the removal of antibiotics from throat lozenges. Pharmacists are becoming more cautious because they are sharing in the legal responsibility of prescriptions. They are pointing out precautions, exposing quackery, and are cautious in recommending O.T.C. items. Pharmacists often ask the patients what

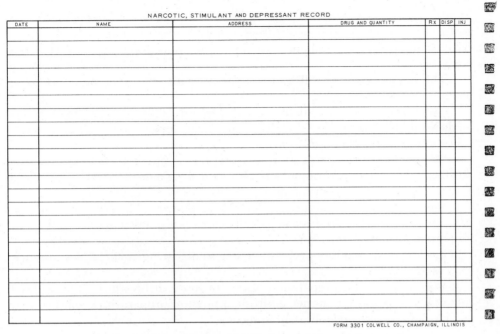

NARCOTIC, STIMULANT AND DEPRESSANT RECORD

| DATE | NAME | ADDRESS | DRUG AND QUANTITY | RX | DISP | INJ |
|------|------|---------|-------------------|----|----|----|
| | | | | | | |
| | | | | | | |
| | | | | | | |
| | | | | | | |
| | | | | | | |
| | | | | | | |
| | | | | | | |
| | | | | | | |
| | | | | | | |
| | | | | | | |
| | | | | | | |
| | | | | | | |
| | | | | | | |
| | | | | | | |
| | | | | | | |
| | | | | | | |
| | | | | | | |
| | | | | | | |
| | | | | | | |
| | | | | | | |
| | | | | | | |
| | | | | | | |

FORM 3301 COLWELL CO., CHAMPAIGN, ILLINOIS

**Figure 23–1**   Page from Narcotic, Stimulant and Depressant Record.

other medications they are taking in an attempt to avoid interactions which can prove serious, and even fatal. Many pharmacies keep personal and family records so as to be able to better advise people concerning the use of the numerous O.T.C. products. This is especially applicable for the family using one pharmacy regularly. So often patients fail to tell the physician of the O.T.C. drugs they are taking. The pharmacist, if he notes a possible interaction or other problem, can consult with the physician before he fills the prescription.

## FORMS OF DRUGS

There are many different ways to classify drugs. One of the most common methods is by their source, as mentioned earlier in this chapter. Another way is by their reaction on the body, or by the part or system of the body they affect. Drugs may also be classified by form.

Drugs are produced in a variety of forms, but they are mainly solids and liquids. The solids are found in powders, in capsules, and in tablet or pill form.

Tablets vary greatly in size, shape, color, and coating. An *enteric-coated* tablet does not dissolve until it has reached the intestinal tract, thereby delaying its action from two to four hours. The coating is insoluble in the stomach. *Sugar-coated* and *chocolate-covered* tablets dissolve in the mouth and have a flavor. *Compressed* tablets have a filler or binding ingredient in them with the medication and have no coating. A *triturate* tablet is a powder which has been moistened with a volatile liquid and then molded into shape; the liquid evaporates and leaves the shaped powder. These tablets dissolve readily in the mouth and are usually mild. Antacid tablets are an example of a triturate tablet. *Hypodermic* tablets are to be dissolved and injected. The diluent is usually sterile distilled water or injectable normal saline.

The following terms will acquaint the assistant with some other forms of drugs:

*Pure Drug.* Any unadulterated powder, crystal, or gum employed as a medicine in the treatment of disease. A pure drug appears in its highest possible concentration. It is chemically pure.

*Saturation.* A solution is saturated when it is impregnated to the greatest possible degree. This saturation is reached when no more of the substance can be dissolved and remain in solution.

*Stock Solution.* Any solution in concentrated form or highly saturated that is kept on hand for the convenience of making up lesser strengths of the same solution at a desired time.

*Tincture.* An alcoholic preparation of a soluble drug or chemical substance, such as iodine.

*Mixture.* A liquid preparation of one or more drugs which unite without chemical action and retain their individual physical properties. A mixture may or may not contain a dissolved substance.

*Elixir.* An aromatic, alcoholic, sweetened preparation usually employed as a vehicle for an active medicine, e.g., elixir of phenobarbital. Elixirs differ from tinctures in that they are sweetened.

*Emulsion.* An oily or resinous substance held in suspension in some liquid such as water or gum acacia. Cod liver oil is usually in emulsion form.

*Syrup.* A solution of sugar and water, usually containing flavoring and medicinal substances, often used as a vehicle. Cough syrups are the most common.

*Diluent.* A substance added to a solid or viscid substance which reduces the strength of the solution or mixture. It is the substance that dilutes. Many injectable medications come in dried or crystalline forms and have a diluent with them to be added prior to administration.

*Suspension.* The diffusion of fine particles of a solid through a liquid. A suspension differs from a solution in that particles do not dissolve but retain their solid form; eventually these particles may sink to the bottom. Such preparations are labeled "Shake well before using."

*Extract.* A preparation obtained by dissolving the medicinal substance in alcohol, ether, or water and evaporating to a prescribed consistency. Extracts are prepared from plant- or animal-derived drugs. Liver extract is an example.

*Suppository.* Mixture of drugs formed into a small mass that is shaped to introduce into a body orifice. Such suppositories are usually formed of a material that melts at body temperature. There are rectal, vaginal, or urethral suppositories.

*Ointment.* A semisolid preparation of a drug in a base, to be applied externally. The base may be wool fat, petroleum, lard, or cholesterol. Creams are similar to ointments, but are water soluble.

*Spirits.* Alcoholic solutions of a volatile substance, easily vaporized. They are also known as essences. An example is aromatic spirits of ammonia.

*Inhalant.* A drug that can be placed in a volatile substance and is capable of being absorbed through the epithelial tissue of the lungs. It has rapid effects. Examples are anesthetics, oxygen, aerosols, ephedrine, and penicillin.

*Vehicle.* A substance, usually medicinally inactive, that is used to carry a medication. Wild cherry syrup is a common vehicle for cough medications. Many pediatric medications, such as penicillin, are in sweet flavored syrups.

## PRESCRIPTIONS

What is a prescription? A prescription is a written order to a pharmacist, by a licensed physician, to supply a particular patient with certain drugs of specific quantity and prepared according to the doctor's direction. These directions may be written in English or Latin. A prescription is a legal document. The prescription will contain:

1. Full name and address of the patient.
2. Date written.
3. Rx symbol, meaning recipe or "take thou."
4. Name and amount of the drug.
5. Instructions to the pharmacist regarding compounding.
6. Instructions to the patient.
7. Signature of the physician.
8. The doctor's name, full address, telephone number, and narcotic registry number.

The formal parts of a prescription are as follows:

A. *Superscription:* Patient's name, address, and the Rx symbol.
B. *Inscription:* Name and quantities of the ingredients.
C. *Subscription:* Directions for compounding.
D. *Signatura:* (or "S" for signa) Directions for the patient.

Prescription writing today is not as complicated as in earlier times, because pharmaceutical manufacturers now prepare most medications ready for administration. It is comparatively rare for a pharmacist to have to compound or mix a medication. A typical prescription is shown in Figure 23–2.

A medical assistant does not write prescriptions, but she will find a knowledge of prescription terms and abbreviations of great value in medical transcription, in taking telephone messages from the pharmacist, and in understanding instructions for administration of medications. Prescription writing is faster and will enable the assistant to take messages more rapidly and more accurately. It is much easier to write "one tab t.i.d.p.c./c aq or p.r.n." than "one tablet three times a day after meals with water or whenever necessary."

Guard all prescription pads well, especially the narcotic forms, lest they be appropriated and used by addicts who may enter the office. It is best to keep prescription forms, both regular and narcotic, in the doctor's desk drawer. If the prescription pad is left on a desk or table top, it is easy for an addict to tear a few pages from the back of the pad while the desk is unattended. In states where the narcotic prescription forms are numbered serially, the medical assistant should regularly check the numbers to see that they are all in sequence. If a number is missing, report this to the physician immediately.

Dr. William MacDonald, in an article which appeared in Medical Economics

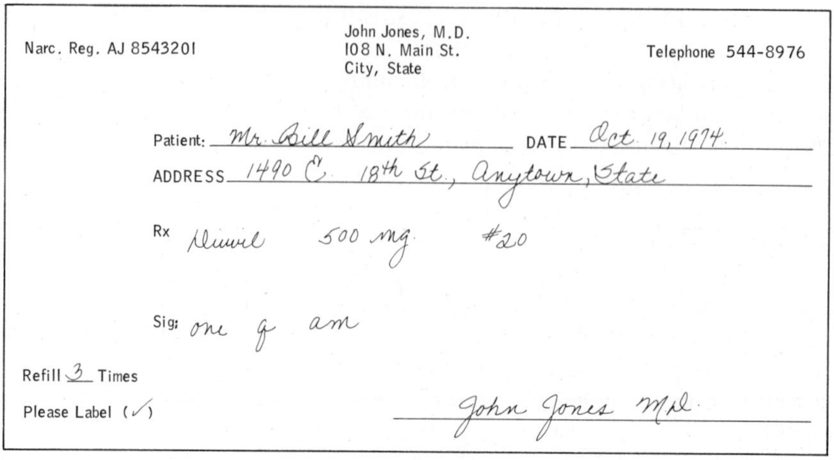

Narc. Reg. AJ 8543201

John Jones, M.D.
108 N. Main St.
City, State

Telephone 544-8976

Patient: Mr. Bill Smith DATE Oct. 19, 1974.

ADDRESS 1490 E. 18th St., Anytown, State

Rx Diuril 500 mg #20

Sig: one q am

Refill 3 Times

Please Label (✓)

John Jones M.D.

**Figure 23–2** A sample prescription.

on "The Law and Your Prescriptions," told of a doctor who used prescription blanks for bridge score pads. "He said he got them free from a local pharmacy," said Dr. MacDonald, "and, from his viewpoint, the blanks could be used as freely as scrap paper." Dr. MacDonald wisely advises doctors and medical assistants to use prescription forms only for the purpose for which they are intended.

Dr. MacDonald also warns doctors to follow narcotic laws to the letter. "Last year, as you know, I moved my office across the street," he writes. "Believe it or not, I got a call from the Collector of Internal Revenue. He said my dollar-a-year stamp authorized me to prescribe narcotics from 28 Maple Street and not from 25 Maple Street. He said I should have notified him *before* I actually moved so that he could amend the tax stamp." Such notifications are the responsibility of the medical assistant.

**Prescription Abbreviations.** The assistant often prepares medications under the doctor's supervision. For this reason she must be familiar with the measuring systems and terminology associated with pharmacology. Symbols and abbreviations widely used in prescription writing and drug dispensing are shown on opposite page.

**Some Frequently Prescribed Drugs and Their Uses.** Table 23–1 shows but a very few common drugs which are prescribed by physicians, drugs that patients will be asking about or reporting about to the physician. The medical assistant should remember that her knowledge of drugs is to aid the physician and help the patient, *not* to advise or prescribe.

**Systems of Measurement.** The metric system of weights and measures is now used throughout the world as the primary system for weight, capacity, and length. In the United States, it is used for scientific work, including most pharmaceuticals, and it may soon be in use for all purposes. However, some physicians still use the apothecaries' system. This necessitates learning both systems and the relationships between the two. A few hints may aid in understanding the system: The metric system is based on the decimal (10), each higher or lower measure is ten times, or 1/10, of the measure at hand. The fraction is always writ-

*(Text continued on page 399.)*

## COMMON PRESCRIPTION ABBREVIATIONS

| | | | |
|---|---|---|---|
| āā | of each | inj. | injection, to be injected |
| a.c. | before meals | kg. | kilogram |
| ad | up to | M. | mix |
| adde | add, let it be added | mcgm. | microgram |
| ad lib. | as much as needed | mg. (mgm.) | milligram |
| agit. | shake, stir | noct. | night |
| alt. dieb. | alternate days | o.h. | every hour |
| alt. hor. | alternate hours | o.m. | every morning |
| alt. noc. | alternate nights | o.n. | every night |
| ante | before | p.c. | after meals |
| a.m. | morning | pil. | pill |
| aq. | water | p.r.n. | whenever necessary |
| aq. bull. | boiling water | pulv. | powder |
| aq. com. | common water, tap water | q.h. | every hour |
| aq. dest. | distilled water | q.i.d. | four times a day (not at night) |
| aq. ferv. | hot water | | |
| aq. frig. | cold water | q.2 h. | every two hours |
| aq. susp. | water suspension | q.4 h. | every four hours |
| b.i.d. | two times a day | q.n.s. | quantity not sufficient |
| /c | with | q.s. | quantity sufficient |
| caps. | capsule | ℞ | take (recipe) |
| comp. | compound | rep. | let it be repeated |
| contra | against | /s | without |
| coq. | boil | sat. | saturated |
| dil. | dilute | sig. | write on label, give directions |
| div. | to be divided | | |
| dos. | doses | sol. | solution |
| elix. | elixir | ss | one-half |
| emul. | emulsion | stat. | immediately |
| et | and | suppos. | suppository |
| ext. | extract | syr. | syrup |
| f. (ft.) | make (let there be made) | tab. | tablet |
| | | t.i.d. | three times a day |
| fl. | fluid | tr. (tinct.) | tincture |
| garg. | gargle | troc. | lozenge |
| gm. | gram | u. | unit |
| gr. | grain | ung. | ointment |
| gt. | drop | M. et sig. | mix and label |
| gtt. | drops | M. et f. pil. | mix and make into pill |
| guttat | drop by drop | | |
| h. | hour | M. et f. pulv. | mix and make into powder |
| h.s. | bedtime (hour of sleep) | | |

**TABLE 23–1**  A FEW REPRESENTATIVE DRUGS WITH THEIR USUAL USES

| *General Category*<br>  *Drug names (generic and*<br>    *proprietary, when indicated)* | *Main Use or Uses*<br>*Specific drug use as*<br>*appropriate* |
|---|---|
| ***Analgesics*** | ***Relief of pain*** |
|   *(Opium alkaloids)* | |
| Codeine phosphate | Mild to moderate pain |
| Morphine sulfate | Moderate to severe pain |
|   *(Synthetic Analgesics)* | |
| Meperidine (Demerol) | Moderate to severe pain |
| Methadone (Dolophine) | Same |
|   *(Minor Analgesics)* | Relief of mild to moderate pain |
| *Aspirin (A.S.A.) | Also used to treat arthritis |
| Acetaminophen (Tylenol) | |
| Propoxyphene (Darvon) | |
| ***Antacids*** | ***Reduce gastric acidity*** |
| Compounds of aluminum, bismuth,<br>  magnesium | Many preparations often combined.<br>  Many proprietary names |
| ***Anti-infectives*** | ***Destroy microorganisms*** |
|   *(Antibiotics)* | |
| Penicillin (many forms) | "Narrow spectrum," active against a<br>  relatively few organisms |
| Streptomycin | As above |
| Tetracyclines (many forms) | "Broad spectrum," active against<br>  many organisms |
|   *(Non-antibiotics — specifics)* | Effective against one or a limited<br>  number of diseases |
| Dapsone (Avlosulfon) | Leprosy |
| Isoniazid (I.N.H.) | Tuberculosis |
| Quinacrine hydrochloride (Atabrine) | Malaria |
| Quinine sulfate | Malaria |
| ***Anticoagulants*** | ***Delay bleeding time (clotting time)*** |
| *Heparin sodium (Liquaemin) | Action rapid, but relatively short |
| Bishydroxycoumarin (Dicumarol) | Action slower, but more prolonged |
| Warfarin sodium (Coumadin, Panwarfin) | As above |
| ***Cathartics and laxatives*** | ***Cause evacuation of intestinal contents*** |
| Agar (from seaweed) | ⎰Hydrophylic — increases content |
| **Psyllium (Betajel, Metamucil) | ⎱Bulk laxatives |
| Bisacodyl (Dulcolax) | Mucosal stimulant |
| Cascara sagrada | Mild intestinal irritant |
| Magnesium sulfate (Epsom Salts) | ⎰Saline cathartics — withdraw fluid |
| Magnesium magma (Milk of Magnesia) | ⎱  from the circulation — help in edema |
| Monosodium phosphate (Sal Hepatica) | |
| Dioctyl sodium sulfosuccinate<br>  (Colace, Doxinate) | Wetting agent |
| ***Diuretics*** | ***Increase the flow of urine*** |
| Ethacrynic acid (Edecrin) | |
| Furosemide (Lasix) | |
| Mercurial compounds | |
| Thiazide compounds | |
| ***Heart (Cardiac) Depressants*** | ***Decrease the rate of heartbeat and aid in<br>  overcoming cardiac arrhythmias*** |
| Procainamide hydrochloride (Pronestyl) | |
| Propranolol (Inderal) | |
| Quinidine (several salts) | |
| ***Heart (other important drugs)*** | ***Varied*** |
| Digitalis (many forms) | Strengthens beat and lengthens rest<br>  period |

**TABLE 23–1**  A FEW REPRESENTATIVE DRUGS WITH THEIR
USUAL USES *(Continued)*

| General Category<br>Drug names (Generic and<br>proprietary, when indicated) | Main Use or Uses<br>Specific drug use as<br>appropriate |
|---|---|
| Nitroglycerin<br>Papaverine | }Relax spasms of the coronary arteries |
| *Iron Compounds* | *Iron deficiency. anemia* |
| Ferrous gluconate (Fergon)<br>Ferrous sulfate (Feosol) | |
| *Muscle Relaxants* | *Relax skeletal muscles* |
| *(Strong)* | |
| Dimethyl tubocuracrine chloride (Mecostrin)<br>Succinylcholine chloride (Anectine,<br>   Sucostrin) | }Used mainly in surgery |
| *(Mild)* | |
| Mephenesin (Tolserol)<br>Meprobamate (Equinal, Miltown) | }Mild relief of tension |
| *(Anticonvulsants)* | |
| Diphenylhydantoin (Dilantin)<br>Paramethadione (Paradione)<br>Phensuximide (Milontin) | }Used mainly in epilepsy |
| *Respiratory Stimulants* | *Used for shock and depressant drug<br>   poisoning* |
| Doxapram (Dopram)<br>Ethamivan (Emivan) | |
| *Sedatives—Hypnotics* | *Light doses produce sedation, heavier<br>   doses cause sleep* |
| *(Barbiturates)*<br>Pentobarbital (Nembutal)<br>Phenobarbital (Luminal)<br>Secobarbital (Seconal) | |
| *(Non-barbiturates)*<br>Chloral hydrate<br>Ethinamate (Valmid)<br>Flurazepan (Dalmane)<br>Glutethemide (Doriden) | As above |
| *Sympathomimetics* | *Stimulate the sympathetic portion of the<br>   autonomic nervous system* |
| Ephedrine sulfate<br>Epinephrine hydrochloride (Adrenalin)<br>Isoproterenol hydrochloride (Isuprel) | Used for the relief of bronchial spasms<br>   and to treat allergy. The drugs in-<br>   crease rate and strength of heart beat<br>   and raise blood pressure.<br>(Ephedrine is used more for main-<br>   tenance, epinephrine in emergencies,<br>   and isoproterenol according to dosage<br>   in both situations) |
| *Tranquilizers* | *Treatment of tension, anxiety, neuroses<br>   and psychoses.* |
| Chlordiazepoxide (Librium)<br>Prochlorperazine (Compazine)<br>Promazine hydrochloride (Sparine)<br>Dimenhydrinate (Dramamine) | Used for motion sickness |
| *Uterine Stimulants* | *Increase the strength of uterine muscle<br>   contraction—initiate labor* |
| Ergonovine maleate (Ergotrate)<br>Oxytocin injection (Pitocin, Syntocinon) | }Also control uterine bleeding |

*Most important drug listed in category.
**Placed here owing to nature of its action.

## ABBREVIATIONS AND SYMBOLS

| Apothecaries' System | | | Metric System | |
|---|---|---|---|---|
| ℞ | min. (m.) | minim | gm. | gram |
| ℈ | scr. | scruple | L. | liter |
| ℨ | dr. | dram | cc. | cubic centimeter |
| fl. ℨ | fl. dr. | fluid dram | ml. | milliliter |
| ℥ | oz. | ounce | | |
| fl. ℥ | fl. oz. | fluid ounce | | |
| O | pt. | pint | | |
| C | gal. | gallon | | |
| | gr. | grain | | |

## TABLE OF WEIGHTS AND MEASURES

| Apothecaries' System | Metric System |
|---|---|
| *Weights* | *Weights* |
| 20 grains = 1 scruple | 1000 milligrams = 1 gram |
| 60 grains = 1 dram | 1000 grams = 1 kilogram |
| 8 drams = 1 ounce | |
| 12 ounces = 1 pound* | |
| *Liquids* | *Liquids* |
| 60 minims = 1 dram | 1000 milliliters = 1 liter |
| 8 drams = 1 ounce | (1 milliliter = 1 cubic centimeter) |
| 16 ounces = 1 pint | |
| 2 pints = 1 quart | |
| 4 quarts = 1 gallon | |

*Avoirdupois weight: 16 ounces = 1 pound.

## CONVERSION FROM ONE SYSTEM TO ANOTHER

| Liquids | | Weights | |
|---|---|---|---|
| *Metric* | *Apothecaries'* | *Metric* | *Apothecaries'* |
| 0.06 cc. = 1 minim | | 0.1 gram = 1½ grains | |
| 1 cc. = 15 minims | | 0.2 gram = 3 grains | |
| 4 cc. = 1 dram | | 0.3 gram = 5 grains | |
| 30 cc. = 1 fluid ounce | | 0.06 gram = 1 grain | |
| 500 cc. = 1 pint | | 0.5 gram = 7½ grains | |
| 1000 cc. = 1 quart | | 1 gram = 15 grains | |
| 4000 cc. = 1 gallon | | 1 kilogram = 2.2 pounds | |

## APPROXIMATE EQUIVALENTS WITHIN SYSTEMS

| Metric | Apothecaries' |
|---|---|
| 0.06 gram = 0.06 cc. | 1 grain = 1 minim |
| 1 gram = 1 cc. | 15 grains = 15 minims |
| 4 grams = 4 cc. | 60 grains = 60 minims |
| 30 grams = 30 cc. | 480 grains = 480 minims (1 oz.) |

HOUSEHOLD MEASUREMENTS AND EQUIVALENTS*

1 minim = 1 drop
1 teaspoon = 1 dram (60 drops)
4 teaspoons = 1 tablespoon (15 cc.)
1 dessert spoon = 2 drams
1 tablespoon = 4 drams
4 tablespoons = 1 wineglass
16 tablespoons = 1 cup
(liquid)
12 tablespoons = 1 cup
(dry)
1 cup = 8 fluid ounces ($1/2$ pint)
1 glass = 8 fluid ounces
1 wineglass = 2 fluid ounces
1 pint = 1 pound
1 tablespoon = 16 cc.
1 ounce = 1 whiskey glass

*These measurements and equivalents are approximate because of the great variation in household measuring devices.

| PERCENTAGE | DECIMAL | FRACTION | RATIO |
|---|---|---|---|
| 25% | .25 | 1/4 | 1:4 |
| 50% | .5 | 1/2 | 1:2 |
| 60% | .6 | 3/5 (6/10) | 3:5 |
| 1/2% (.5%) | .005 | 1/200 | 1:200 |
| 1/10% (0.1%) | .001 | 1/1000 | 1:1000 |
| 85% | .85 | 17/20 | 17:20 |
| 1% | .01 | 1/100 | 1:100 |

ten as a decimal and the number precedes the letters designating the actual measure; thus, one and one-half liter would be written 1.5 L. The letters cc and ml are used interchangeably. The term ml is more accurate, since it is 1/1000 of a liter. Cc refers to cubic centimeters and is a measure of capacity. Under specific conditions of temperature, barometric pressure, and so forth a ml of water will just fill a cubic centimeter (cc) of space. Arabic numerals are used.

With the apothecaries' system either Roman or Arabic numerals are used (although Roman were used exclusively at one time), but not properly in the same prescription. Symbols or abbreviations may be used. One and one-half ounces might be written ℥iss or oz. 1½. The number follows the symbol or abbreviation. The letters ss mean semesis (one-half). Some persons dot the i, but no other letter should be dotted.

## TERMINOLOGY

*Aerosol.* A solution that can be finely atomized and inhaled for producing local respiratory or systemic action. Epinephrine (Adrenalin) is used in an aerosol.

*Analgesic.* A drug to relieve pain by lessening the sensory functions of the brain. It may be taken internally or used topically. Analgesics vary greatly in their ability to quiet pain, from aspirins to the opium derivatives.

*Anesthetic.* A drug used to produce insensibility to pain or the sensation of pain, local or general. *Topical* anesthetics are surface applied and have local action. Other *local* anesthetics are *infiltration* (injected into a nerve), *intraspinal* (spinal fluid withdrawn and an equal amount of anesthetic injected into the spinal canal), and *caudal* (drug injected into base of the spine, used in obstetrics).

*Antibiotic.* An agent which is produced by a living organism and is effective against bacteria. There are several antibiotics on the market today, including penicillin, streptomycin, erythromycin, and tetracycline.

*Antidote.* A substance used to counteract a poison or the effects of a poison.

*Carminative.* A medication which relieves flatulence, aids in the expulsion of gas from the stomach and intestines. Usually contains volatile oils or carbonated beverage.

*Cathartic.* An agent that increases and hastens bowel evacuation (defecation). Commonly called a laxative. Types range from mild laxatives and purgatives to drastic cathartics. Some increase the bulk in the bowel; others irritate the intestinal mucosa.

*Chemotherapeutic Agents.* Chemical substances that are used to inhibit or kill micro-organisms that cause disease. Sulfonamides are chemotherapeutic. There are thousands of different compounds.

*Decongestant.* A drug that relieves local congestion. The most popular of this group are the nasal decongestants, such as ephedrine or phenylephrine (Neo-Synephrine).

*Diaphoretic.* A drug used to induce and increase the secretion of perspiration.

*Digestant.* A drug that promotes the progress of digestion. Enzymes, acids, and bile salts are included in this group.

*Diuretic.* An agent that increases the function of the kidneys and stimulates the flow of urine. Increases the water content of the blood through osmosis or salt action, freeing water from the tissues, reducing edema.

*Emetic.* A drug used to induce vomiting. Mild mustard and plain tepid water are home remedies used as emetics. Ipecac syrup is commonly used.

*Expectorant.* A drug used to increase the secretions and mucus from the bronchial tubes. Makes a cough more productive and breaks up congestion. Some cough medicines are expectorants; some are a combination of antihistamines and expectorants; others are used to decrease flow of mucus.

*Hemostatic.* Drug used to check bleeding, blood coagulants. Absorbable hemostatics are applied directly to the oozing surface, and an artificial clot is formed which gradually absorbs. Gelfoam and Surgicel are examples.

*Hypnotic.* A drug that produces sleep and lessens the activity of the brain. A hypnotic has a sedative action when used in smaller doses. The barbiturates are the most common hypnotics, both oral and injectable: pentobarbital (Nembutal), amobarbital (Amytal), secobarbital and amobarbital (Tuinal).

*Miotic.* Any agent that causes the pupil of the eye to contract, by contraction of the ciliary muscles.

*Mydriatic.* An agent used to dilate the pupil of the eye. Used by ophthalmologists in eye examinations. (Cycloplegics cause loss of accommodation by paralyzing the ciliary muscle of the eye.) Mydriatics have little or no effect on the muscles of accommodation.

*Nutrient.* A substance that supplies nourishment or affects the metabolic rate of the body; a food supplement. Vitamins are considered nutrients.

*Opiate.* Any drug that is derived from or contains opium. It is the oldest known remedy and was used long before the time of Christ. It comes from the opium poppy. There are more than twenty alkaloids from the opium plant, but morphine, codeine, and papaverine are the most common. The synthetic narcotics are similar in action but are not opiates. These synthetics are meperidine (Demerol), methadone (Dolophine), levorphanol tartrate (Levo-Dromoran), and pentazocine (Talwin). They are usually less habit-forming than the opiates.

*Parenteral.* A sterile solution of a medication prepared for injection. A medication given parenterally is given by injection into the body. The various types are: intravenous, intramuscular, subcutaneous, intraspinal, intradermal, intraperitoneal.

*Relaxant.* An antispasmodic; a drug used to reduce or relax muscular spasm, usually skeletal muscle. They are often used with a general anesthetic, as in eye or rectal surgery. Curare (South American arrow poison) produces good muscular relaxation. Uterine relaxants for the nongravid uterus are used to relieve painful menstruation.

*Sedative.* A drug that reduces excitement; a quieting agent, but does not produce sleep as a hypnotic drug does. They are often the same drug, a smaller dose acting as a sedative while a larger dose acts as a hypnotic.

*Stomachic.* An agent used to increase the secretory activity of the stomach and aid in digestion. Not to be confused with a *stomatic*, which pertains to the mouth.

*Tranquilizer.* A calming agent which reduces anxiety and tension without acting as a depressant. Tranquilizers are called "psychotherapeutic" drugs. This group of drugs has increased in large numbers during recent years. Rauwolfia and derivatives are sometimes used. The phenothiazine derivatives are often given. These include chlorpromazine (Thorazine), perphenazine (Trilifon), thioridiazine (Mellaril), and several others.

*Vasoconstrictor.* A drug that causes a blood vessel to constrict, narrows the lumen of a vessel, raises blood pressure, and causes the heart to beat more forcefully. Used to stop superficial bleeding, raise and sustain blood pressure, relieve nasal congestion.

*Vasodilator.* The opposite of a vasoconstrictor, a drug that dilates blood vessels, lowers blood pressure by making blood vessels larger, causing the heart to pump less forcefully. Used in the treatment of hypertension, angina pectoris, and peripheral vascular diseases. Nitroglycerine placed sublingually gives prompt vasodilator action. Aminophylline dilates coronary vessels and bronchial tubes, and is used in asthmatic cases.

# DRUG ACTIONS

There are many different methods, or channels, for administering a medication, either on the body surface in a local area (topical action) or into the body (systemic action).

**Topical Action.**   A topical drug is one applied locally to the skin or mucous membrane, sometimes to the ear or eye. These drugs are usually in the form of a liquid, lotion, emulsion, ointment, or foam. They are used for the treatment of infection, irritation, or an allergic reaction or are given to produce local anesthesia.

*Topical anesthetics* would be applied to produce a lack of feeling or sensation. Cocaine is an example; it paralyzes sensory nerve endings and produces a surface anesthesia. Other topical anesthetics can be in the form of an ointment, such as Surfacaine, Nupercaine, and Tronothane. Some eye medications have a topical anesthetic action, like Butacaine. These are used in the eye prior to testing with the tonometer.

*Astringents* are used to harden or contract tissues. An example is witch hazel in mouthwash.

*Antiseptics* are the best example of local action. When we have a skin abrasion we apply a local antiseptic, such as alcohol, tincture of iodine, Merthiolate, Zephiran.

A local medication can also act as a *counterirritant.* This is an agent that is applied locally to reduce inflammatory reaction in some other part, usually underlying the area where the counterirritant is applied. It relieves a congested organ or an inflamed muscle. Grandmother's mustard plaster is an excellent example.

*Anodynes,* such as oil of clove for toothache or oil of wintergreen for rheumatism, relieve pain but are milder than analgesics. *Irritants* are often applied to produce warmth of the skin. They dilate the blood vessels and usually produce a reddening where applied. *Emollients* have a soothing effect on the skin. They are usually a fatty or oily substance, such as cocoa butter or anhydrous lanolin. Demulcents are similar to emollients but do not contain oil or fat. *Styptics* are applied to a small bleeding area to check the flow of blood. Protective medications, such as Colloidin and Silicone, form a coating on the skin ("new skin"). *Keratolytics* are agents that aid in the loosening of the dry, horny layer of skin such as dandruff or some fungal infections. Selsun and Whitefield's Ointment are keratolytics.

**Systemic Action.**   Systemic actions are also called *general actions.* They occur after absorption of a substance into the circulation, and they may affect the entire body. Effectiveness of a systemic drug depends on how it is introduced into the body. In order to be most effective, it must be able to be absorbed — that is, have the ability to permeate the cells. The drug must be utilized by the specific organ or part of the body for which it is intended, and it must be utilized or be excreted, either unchanged or with other body wastes such as through urine, the lungs, or the skin.

There are many types of systemic actions. When it is intended to increase the activity of a tissue, a *stimulant* is used. Caffeine is a stimulant. In some cases an overdose of a stimulant can give a reverse action and cause depression. *Depressants* cause a decreased activity of the tissues. Bromides and sleeping capsules can be depressants. There are several types of depressants, such as cardiac, cerebral, and respiratory.

Systemic drugs may also cause *irritation* or *stimulation.* These two words are often confused, and understandably so. An irritation causes a slight temporary damage, such as the action of castor oil on the mucous membrane of the intestines. A mild irritation can result in a stimulation, while a prolonged stimulation can produce an irritation.

The words *cumulative action* appear in pharmacologic writings. This means that a drug accumulates in the body; it is eliminated more slowly than it is absorbed. Digitalis, a heart stimulant, is cumulative.

Frequently a physician will say a patient has an *"idiosyncrasy"* to a certain drug. He is referring to the fact that the patient has an unusual response to the drug. An idiosyncrasy may show itself in many different ways, such as a sleeping capsule keeping a person awake, acting as a stimulant to this person. These are abnormal symptoms that cannot always be explained.

*Tolerance* is of major concern to the physician. This is the ability to withstand a quantity of a drug. Often a physician must progressively increase a dosage in order to maintain the desired therapeutic effect. Substances to which people usually develop a tolerance are narcotics, alcohol, and tobacco.

If the patient is taking more than one drug at a time, *interaction* between the drugs may take place. This may or may not be desirable. There are many types of interaction. One drug may enhance the action of another, one may negate another or decrease its action. In some cases, the interaction may produce toxicity. This is one reason why the physician must be aware of *all* drugs being used by the patient, including simple O.T.C. drugs.

## SOLUTIONS

A solution is made up of two parts called the *solute* and the *solvent.* The solute is the substance dissolved and the solvent is the dispersing fluid or the liquid in which the solute is dissolved. The solute may be a solid, gas, or liquid. Most solutions are made of a solid or liquid dissolved or mixed into the solvent. The strength of the solution is the amount of the pure drug or solute in a definite quantity of the solvent. Solute plus solvent equals a solution.

If water is used as a solvent, the result is called an aqueous solution. There are many solvents—for example, alcohol, ether, acids, or oils.

Solutions are spoken of in percentages or ratios. A 5 per cent solution is 5 parts of the solute in 100 parts of solution, or a ratio of 1:20. Many crystals do not displace any appreciable volume so the volume of the solution is practically the same as the quantity of the solvent. Strong solutions are usually given as per cent and weak solutions as ratios.

To make a 5 per cent solution of acetic acid you would measure 5 ml. acetic acid (solute) and add sufficient water (solvent) to make up a total of 100 ml. In other words, you would add 95 ml. water.

The U.S.P. XIV specifies: "When *per cent* is used in prescriptions without qualification, it means: for mixtures of solids, per cent weight in weight; for solutions of solids in liquids, per cent weight in volume; for solutions of liquids, per cent volume in volume; and for solutions of gases in liquid, per cent weight in volume." (See table on page 404.)

TABLE FOR MAKING WEIGHT IN VOLUME
PERCENTAGE SOLUTIONS*

The following table gives the proportion of material to be used with solvent q.s. to make the volume at top of the column. Multiples or fractions of these volumes may be calculated from these figures.

| Strength of Solution | Dissolve the weight specified below in distilled water q.s. to make 100 cc. | Dissolve the weight specified below in distilled water q.s. to make 500 cc. | Dissolve the weight specified below in distilled water q.s. to make 1 fl. oz. | Dissolve the weight specified below in distilled water q.s. to make 1 pint |
|---|---|---|---|---|
| 0.25 per cent | 0.25 gm. | 1.25 gm. | 1.14 gr. | 18¼ gr. |
| 0.5 per cent | 0.5 gm. | 2.5 gm. | 2.28 gr. | 36½ gr. |
| 1 per cent | 1 gm. | 5 gm. | 4.56 gr. | 73 gr. |
| 2 per cent | 2 gm. | 10 gm. | 9.13 gr. | 146 gr. |
| 3 per cent | 3 gm. | 15 gm. | 13.7 gr. | 219 gr. |
| 4 per cent | 4 gm. | 20 gm. | 18.26 gr. | 292 gr. |
| 5 per cent | 5 gm. | 25 gm. | 22.8 gr. | 365 gr. |
| 6 per cent | 6 gm. | 30 gm. | 27.38 gr. | 437 gr. |
| 8 per cent | 8 gm. | 40 gm. | 36.5 gr. | 583 gr. |
| 10 per cent | 10 gm. | 50 gm. | 45.6 gr. | 729 gr. |
| 12.5 per cent | 12.5 gm. | 62.5 gm. | 57 gr. | 913 gr. |
| 15 per cent | 15 gm. | 75 gm. | 68.5 gr. | 1095 gr. |
| 16⅔ per cent | 16.6 gm. | 83.3 gm. | 76 gr. | 1217 gr. |
| 20 per cent | 20 gm. | 100 gm. | 91.28 gr. | 1460 gr. |
| 25 per cent | 25 gm. | 125 gm. | 114 gr. | 1825 gr. |
| 30 per cent | 30 gm. | 150 gm. | 137 gr. | 2187 gr. |
| 33⅓ per cent | 33.3 gm. | 166.6 gm. | 152 gr. | 2433 gr. |
| 50 per cent | 50 gm. | 250 gm. | 228 gr. | 3500 gr. |

437.5 grains = 1 Avoirdupois ounce; 480 grains = Apothecaries' ounce.

*Reprinted from *Current Therapy 1973*, edited by Howard F. Conn, Philadelphia, W. B. Saunders Co., 1973.

## PRACTICAL PROBLEMS IN PREPARING MEDICATIONS

### How to Give a Fraction of a Drop:

Rule:  To one drop of the given solution add sufficient number of drops of water (or solvent) to equal the denominator of your desired fraction, then use the number of drops in the numerator. DILUTE TO THE DENOMINATOR, ADMINISTER THE NUMERATOR.

Examples: (1) Give ⅓ of a drop.
   To the one drop add 2 drops, thus making three drops. Then give one drop, or one third of the original drop.
   (2) Give ¾ of a drop.
   To the one drop add 3 more drops, making a total of four drops. Then give three drops, or three fourths of the original drop.

## How to Give a Fraction of a Hypodermic Tablet:

Rule:  Form a fraction by putting the denominator of the size of tablets you have on hand over the denominator of the size of tablet you want to give. Reduce to the lowest fraction. Do not use less than eight drops to dissolve a tablet.

Examples:  (1)  You have ⅛ gr. tablet and are to give ⅑ gr.

$$\frac{8 \text{ (what you have)}}{9 \text{ (what you want)}}$$  Dissolve tablet in 9 minims of water and give 8 minims.

(2)  You have ⅟₃₀ gr. and you want to give ⅟₄₀ gr.

$$\frac{30 \text{ (what you have)}}{40 \text{ (what you want)}} = \frac{30}{40} = \frac{3}{4}$$

Since you cannot dissolve the tablet in 4 minims you increase the amount three times to ⁹/₁₂. Thus, dissolve in 12 minims and give 9 minims.

(3)  You have an 8 mg. tablet and you want 10 mg.

Since these are whole numbers and not fractions, a different method must be used. Obviously, 10 mg. is more than 8 mg.; therefore, 2 tablets will be required. Two 8 mg. tablets will be $2 \times 8$ or 16 mg. Dissolve the two tablets (8 mg. each) in 16 minims of water and give the patient 10 minims.

## POISON CONTROL CENTERS

Within the last few years over 300 poison control centers have been established around the nation to provide quick and handy sources of information on many chemical products containing potentially injurious substances. These are usually located in major community hospitals or in medical colleges and are often cooperatively set up with local and state health departments, hospitals, and physicians. The medical assistant should post the telephone number of the nearest poison control center in a prominent place in the office so that it will be readily available should the doctor need to secure information fast to help treat a poisoned person.

## BURN CENTERS

The same information should be available for the nearest burn center. So much expensive equipment is used and such specialized personnel needed that the average community hospital is not prepared to care for the severely burned patient. The nearest center should be known and the address and telephone readily available.

# Chapter 24

## CHAPTER OUTLINE

Factors Influencing Dosage
Channels of Administration
    Topical Drugs
    Oral Route
    Parenteral Administration

How to Give an Injection
Precautions Regarding Injections
Changes in Drug Therapy for Various
    Age Groups

## BEHAVIORAL OBJECTIVES

*The medical office assistant should be able to:*

Give medications by any of the methods usually used by paramedical personnel, such as sublingually, orally, subcutaneously, intramuscularly, and intradermally.

Instruct the patient or a relative how to give medications by all of the above methods, except for the last two.

Answer most of the patient's questions concerning the taking of medications prescribed by the physician.

Prepare for, assist with, and clean up after the physician gives a medication intravenously.

Properly care for all office medicines and the equipment used to administer them.

# Administration of
# Medications

Mary W. Falconer, R.N., M.A.

The administration of medications has become one of the most significant functions of the medical world. One of the most important responsibilities which a physician may delegate to a well trained and reliable assistant is the administration of certain medications to his patients. It cannot be said often enough in this book that the doctor relies upon the accuracy and dependability of his assistant far more than the businessman does upon his secretary, for example. Dollars and cents are at stake in the business world—but health and lives are at stake in the medical world. Accuracy is essential! Carelessness is intolerable!

The assistant who is asked to administer medications must have a thorough understanding of the scientific principles of diagnosis and therapy to be able to give them with assurance. She must have certain skills to administer the medications correctly at the doctor's request. She must understand the time element in relation to absorption, tolerance, and so forth of medications. She first should acquaint herself thoroughly with the medications used by her doctor. She should, for example, read all literature enclosed with medications, *not* so that she can treat or diagnose but so that she understands the specific uses, values, limitations, side effects, interaction with other drugs, and dangers of these medications. Additional information about drugs can also be obtained from local pharmacists or drug company representatives.

*No assistant should ever give medications except on the instructions of the doctor or on the basis of his acknowledgment.* If a patient is coming into the office for medication while the doctor is not present, consent should be secured from the doctor beforehand, *not after* the medication has been given.

It is important to observe the patient closely during the administration of any medications. If the assistant has any question, no matter how insignificant, in her mind about administering the medication or the patient's condition, she should immediately check with the doctor. Under no circumstances should she go beyond the doctor's instructions.

**Precautions.**   The administration of medicine must be done with the utmost care. It cannot be said enough: BE CAREFUL . . . BE ACCURATE. If there is ever any doubt, do not give the medication but check with the physician. Always check the patient's chart, making certain it is the correct patient and not just the "patient in the second room." Never use medication from a bottle with a damaged label. Know the medications you are giving.

**407**

No medical assistant need learn all the drugs used or prescribed by her physician, but she should become familiar with the medications that are frequently prescribed and used. An excellent way of acquainting yourself with these medications is to read medical publications, paying particular attention to drug advertisements. Every physician's office receives drug samples. Read the manufacturer's literature which is enclosed with the drug. Read the recommended dosage carefully, the contraindications, side effects, and precautions. Know the actions and uses of the drug. If this enclosed information sheet has been destroyed, consult the office reference books. As mentioned previously, keep a file of the brochures which come with the drugs.

The medical assistant should make a special effort to know the side effects and precautions of commonly prescribed drugs because patients will frequently telephone the office to report on the progress of their illnesses. Since it is not always possible for the patient to speak with the physician, an alert medical assistant may question the patient for more complete information. If she has an understanding of drugs she will know what information should be brought to the physician's attention immediately. This knowledge may aid in preventing a patient from having a drug reaction.

A knowledge of drugs can save many hours in transcribing medical records for the medical assistant who has the name of the drug and the correct spelling at her finger tips. Many drug names sound similar to the untrained ear, but considerable damage can be done through misinterpretation.

The trend toward labeling prescriptions with the name of the drug is helpful in discussing a patient's medication. In case of an emergency, considerable time may be saved by having the name of the drug rather than just a prescription number and a description of the drug's appearance. This also offers a double-check on a medication, because patients can transpose a number when giving it to you over the telephone. There may also be a financial saving to a patient when a similar illness proceeds through several children in a family and the physician prescribes the same medication. However, there is a danger here that must be stressed. The parent must not give a medication ordered for one child to another without the doctor's express order. The assistant must warn the parent if she asks and must confer with the physician before telling the parent that the drug may be used for the second child. Symptoms of various diseases are often very similar, but the cause may be entirely different. As an example, gastroenteritis (plain old "stomach ache") due to dietary indiscretion and acute appendicitis often have the same symptoms—nausea, vomiting and abdominal pain. The drug given for the former would be contraindicated for the latter. Occasionally a physician does not want a patient to know the name of his medication; in this case, the medical assistant must be careful not to give the name of the drug to the patient. If the patient asks for this information, he should be referred to the physician.

**Points to Remember.**   Read each label carefully before administration, not merely the name of the drug but its strength. Medications are prepared in various strengths; this is especially true with injectables. For example, a chorionic gonadotropin hormone comes in three different strengths: 500 I. U. per cc., 1000 I. U. per cc., and 2000 I. U. per cc. The last one is four times the strength of the first.

When recording a medication on a patient's chart, make certain the strength is recorded as well as the amount, how it was given, and where. To write 1 cc. does not tell whether it was 500 I. U. or 2000 I. U. Also, was it given intramuscularly in the deltoid or buttocks?

Check the patient's name again with the physician's orders. Know your patient as well as the medication.

Never use a medication from an unmarked bottle or when the label is not clear and easy to read.

Measure the exact amount. Don't measure air bubbles.

When pouring a solution or medication, pour away from the label. This keeps the solution from running down over the label and damaging it.

If a medication has changed color, or has a precipitation, do not use it. The assistant should examine the label to see if there is an expiration date and be sure that the drug is still usable.

Do not mix medications unless you have been instructed to do so. Some medications are incompatible.

Remain with a patient if there is any question of a possible reaction, or if he feels ill. If there is any doubt, call the physician immediately.

Do not hesitate to admit a mistake! If you have given a patient the wrong medication, tell the physician immediately. This is no time for you to hide your errors; a patient's life may be at stake.

Occasionally newspapers carry stories of tragic accidents that occur when a doctor's assistant, a nurse, or even a physician mistakenly administers the wrong drug to someone. To avoid mistakes, get in the habit of reading every label twice before you administer the medication and once after administration.

## FACTORS INFLUENCING DOSAGE

Insofar as the patient is concerned, there are certain factors to be considered when giving medications. These factors make it necessary on occasion to vary the standard dose: age, weight, sex, previous habits and tolerances, idiosyncrasies and susceptibility, temperament and occupation, condition of the patient, object of medication, time of administration, and channel of administration.

The age of the patient determines the strength of the dose of a medicine to be given. A child or a very aged person may take a smaller dose. Weight is important, too; the lighter the person, the smaller the dose. In some cases, the physician will order the dose on the basis of the patient's optimal weight rather than his actual weight. This is especially true if the patient is very much overweight or underweight.

The average female may be given a smaller dose of the medicine than a male. Concerning previous habits and tolerances, you must consider the patient's medical history. What medicines has he been taking? Does he need more of the drug now than when he started taking it? A "Yes" here indicates tolerance. Remember, to many nonprofessional individuals medicines or medications are substances prescribed by the physician, drugs are illicit agents used by drug addicts, and remedies are things you buy in a drug store without a prescription that make life a little easier. They do not realize that many of these over-the-counter drugs are actually potent medications. Many patients are allergic to certain drugs. Respect any statement they may make as to previous reactions.

Temperament and occupation also influence the amount of a given medicine which can be administered. A nervous person often should take a smaller dose, and a phlegmatic type sometimes will require a heavier dose of certain drugs, such as the antidepressants. Physically active persons may take a larger dose.

The patient's condition is an extremely important factor to consider. What is the intensity of the pain to be stilled, for example? Or, what is the cumulation of the drug in the patient's body? Dyspnea (shortness of breath or labored respiration) may call for smaller, more frequent doses.

It is also necessary to consider what the object of the medication is. For example, in sedation is a deep sleep or rest required? Time of administration also affects the strength of the dose. Is the drug being administered with meals, on an empty stomach, or at bedtime?

Finally, what is the channel of administration?

## Channels of Administration

**Introduction.**  It seems unnecessary to say that medications are administered to people for their benefit. However, medical personnel often become so imbued with the scientific actions of drugs that they overlook this very basic fact. Never forget that it is the patient who is of paramount importance; it is his health which is being restored or maintained. Also remember that it is far better to prevent disease and to keep people healthy than to have to cure them of illnesses.

Medicines are given to patients in a variety of ways. Medical substances may have their main action at the point of contact with the body or in an organ or tissue far removed from the entry area. The former types, as stated in the previous chapter, are called local or topical drugs. These act on the skin and the mucous membranes lining cavities that connect directly with the exterior. The latter kinds are systemic drugs, which must first enter the blood and the lymph circulation in order to be carried to the target area.

*TOPICAL DRUGS (Applied to the Skin)*

The average patient will understand the use of many of the topical drugs perfectly. However, it is important that the physician or his assistant make sure this is true. It is surprising how many patients need a detailed explanation of even the simplest procedure.

The more common forms of topical drugs are ointments, creams (water-soluble preparations similar to ointments), lotions, solutions (wet dressings), sprays, and preparations to be "painted" on. These substances were defined in the previous chapter.

**Ointments and creams** are well understood by most people and will usually require no specific instructions, except perhaps to know whether or not a dressing or other covering should be applied. If the assistant does not know and the prescription does not state the information, the doctor should be consulted to ascertain his wishes in the matter. If the area is to be covered, the type of covering should be explained to the patient.

Though this may not be required information for the assistant, a word of caution concerning ointments may help in an emergency. "Burn ointments" may be used on small, superficial burns. For these injuries they are useful and beneficial. However, *never* put any ointment, cream, or other oily or greasy substance on a deep or extensive burn. Such cases should be taken immediately to the nearest hospital emergency room, burn center, or doctor's office. If any ointment or other oily material has been put on the burn, it will have to be removed, which is often a very painful process, before the burn can be treated. If it is essential to cover the burned area while transporting the patient, a clean cloth may be put over the wound. The inside of folded linen that has been ironed is relatively sterile (it is free from microorganisms, or at least nearly so).

A wet dressing may be used. Water from the hot water heater is also relatively free of bacteria. The dressing should be of saline or drinking water and should be as close in temperature to the surface of the body as possible. The wet dressing should be covered with an impervious material.

**Lotions.** Lotions are often used to control itching. Calamine, with or without phenol, is one such preparation. It should be dabbed on, using a soft cloth or cotton. It should not be rubbed in as this will increase the itching. With this type of medication the area is left uncovered. Lotions are also used to relieve the congestion and pain in muscles and joints—called rheumatism by many individuals. In these cases, the lotion may be rubbed in and is often covered with a thick cloth (wool or other heavy cloth) to retain heat. These lotions dilate the superficial blood vessels, thus drawing the blood to the surface and away from the congested parts below.

**Solution and Wet Dressings.** These can be a real problem, especially if they are to be applied to body parts other than the feet and hands. It is easy to immerse the extremities into a solution, or wrap them in a cloth wet with the solution. If the area to be treated can be covered, plastic wrap can be put over the wet dressing and adhesive put around the edges, thus containing the solution. If this is not practical, plastic may be put under the part and the top left open to the air. If the medication in the solution is a dye, the patient should know about this and be advised to use old bedding and clothing so that if they are stained, it will not be too great a loss.

**Drugs to be Painted on the Skin.** These drugs are frequently used by most individuals. They are common household articles. Included in this category are tinctures (Tr. of Iodine) and nonalcoholic compounds, such as Merbromin (Mercurochrome). The alcoholic solutions are thought by many to be superior to the nonalcoholic types, but they do sting. Iodine should not be put on wet skin or into a deep (punctured) wound, nor should it be covered.

**Sprays.** Sprays are used more for cavities that connect with the exterior than they are for the skin. But they are sometimes used to apply antiseptics to large surfaces. Generally, the same types of drugs are used for sprays as are used for painting on the skin.

The cavities which communicate with the exterior that will be considered here are the ears, eyes, nose, mouth and throat, vagina, and rectum. The bladder, through the urethral opening, also communicates with the exterior, but the patient rarely, if ever, applies medication to the bladder.

*TOPICAL DRUGS (Used in Cavities Which Connect with the Exterior)*

EARS.    Ears are usually treated with ear drops or ointments. If ear drops are ordered, the patient should lie on the unaffected side. The medication is usually supplied in small bottles, with a dropper attached to the cork or cap. The bottle should be held closely in the hand for a few minutes before using, to warm the solution. If any agitation is required, the bottle should be rolled in the hand, never vigorously shaken. The drops should be as close to body surface temperature as possible. Drops too hot or too cold should not be used, as they will increase pain and may cause dizziness. The ear lobe should be pulled slightly downward and backward in the infant and small child, slightly backward in the child and slightly upward and backward in the adult. This procedure straightens the ear canal. The drops should be allowed to flow by gravity down the side of the canal. The patient should lie still for 15 to 30 minutes to allow the medicine to work — to spread over the area and at least partially dry. No ear plug should be used unless specifically ordered. Ointments and creams are often applied by the doctor, but the assistant may do this under his direction. The ointment is applied on a cotton applicator to the side of the canal. Be careful not to go too deep as the tympanic membrane must not be touched. An otoscope will help in locating the portions of the canal needing treatment.

EYES.    The eyes are treated with the same types of medications as the ears, namely, drops and ointments. In giving eye drops, the patient is asked to look up, and the lower lid is gently pulled outward a very little. This makes a cup into which the designated number of drops are placed. Eye solutions also come in dropper bottles. The solution may be at room temperature, but should not be very cold. *Never* drop the medication directly on the sensitive cornea, the covering over the iris (colored portion), or the pupil. Ointments are applied in the same way. Eye ointments come in very small tubes with a minute opening through which the ointment is applied. Be extremely careful never to let the tip of the dropper or the tube touch any portion of the eye or eyelids. A patient can be taught to give himself eye drops and can become very adept at the procedure. The patient is told to hold the head back, open the eyes widely, and let the drops fall into the lower portion of the eye. The assistant can lighten the procedure a bit, if necessary, by telling the patient that his first try may result in a face wash with the drops, but no harm is done except for a small loss of solution.

Tears flow from the upper outer canthus to the inner lower canthus and then drain into the upper portion of the nasal cavity. It may be wise after putting drops into the eyes to place light pressure on the inner canthus for a few minutes to avoid having the drops excrete too rapidly.

NOSE.    In the nose, drops and sprays are the most commonly used forms. To apply nose drops the patient should be lying down, with the head lower than the body, for instance, over the head of the bed, examining table, couch, or so forth. This is to allow the drops to reach the upper nasal cavity, where they are usually needed. Short, rapid breaths (like those of a rabbit) will help spread the solution. With the use of sprays, only one precaution needs to be taken—be sure that the tip of the apparatus is free in the nasal cavity and not against the side of the cavity. For both drops and sprays, one thing must be impressed on the patient: "Do not exceed the amount or frequency for the medication ordered." Usually, these drugs contain a vasoconstrictor—a decongestant. If used too much, the medicine can cause blanching and drying of the mucosa and this can make the condition worse.

Cold sores and other small sores and infections in the openings of the nares are common. They are treated as any skin condition of a similar nature, since there is a small bit of skin lining the outer end of the nares.

ORAL DISORDERS. The care of oral disorders may be the province of the dentist or the physician. Usually, the patient needs few or no directions for mouth care. However, if the throat is affected, instruction may be important. The three most commonly used methods of getting medicines to the throat are painting, spraying, and gargling. Most patients understand the latter process without discussion. If they do not, the directions are simple: the patient takes the medicinal solution into the mouth (not too much at one time); takes a deep, but not a forced breath; holds the head back; opens the mouth and exhales through the fluid. The solution is not swallowed. The procedure is repeated until the prescribed amount has been used.

For painting and spraying it is *absolutely essential* that the person doing the procedure (patient, friend, assistant, or doctor) first look into the mouth and the throat to see where the inflammation is. Many people, professional as well as laymen, fail to do this. They take the applicator or atomizer and blindly dab around in the back of the mouth, frequently touching the posterior pharynx, which is rarely involved in the infection. Often, in this type of procedure, the part most needing treatment is missed entirely. The parts most commonly infected are the tonsils and the pillars at the side of the oropharynx (where the mouth and throat meet). Incidentally, touching the posterior pharynx will cause gagging. One means of producing vomiting is to fluff out the cotton on the tip of an applicator and "tickle" the posterior pharynx.

VAGINA. The vagina is treated with many kinds of medicines in many different ways. Some of these are tampons (cotton or other absorbent material, with a string attached for removal), douches, capsules, ointments, and suppositories.

Tampons are used to apply fluid medications, as well as ointments. They are inserted well into the vaginal canal, left in the prescribed amount of time and then removed. Capsules are usually relatively large. They are lubricated slightly and inserted well into the vaginal canal. If not contraindicated, a plain tampon may be placed at the orifice to aid in the retention of the capsule. Sometimes the capsules are to be inserted at bedtime and remain in place while the patient is asleep. They gradually dissolve and release the medication. Suppositories act in much the same way and are treated like capsules. Douches require little, if any, instruction for the adult female, for whom they are usually ordered. Here a bit of feminine hygiene can be taught. The vaginal secretions are antiseptic in nature, and too frequent douching can remove too much of the secretion, with infection following. The occasional douche is quite all right, but it should not be used too much.

RECTAL. Rectal applications are much the same as those for the vagina. However, by far the most commonly used form is the suppository. The patient must be instructed to insert the suppository well into the rectum. There are two sphincters (a muscle that closes an opening) in the rectum. The suppository must be placed about two inches beyond the second sphincter.

A word of caution here that may seem superfluous, but really is not. Be sure that the patient knows the relationship of the three openings in the vulva (perineal) area. Many patients have inserted a rectal suppository into the vagina and vice versa, or have irrigated the rectum or the bladder when a douche was ordered. This latter mistake could cause a severe infection of the bladder and even of the kidneys.

Another precaution which is essential: be sure that the patient understands that the aluminum foil is removed from the suppository before it is inserted. Many patients have lubricated the foil and inserted the suppository, covering and all. The doctor cannot understand why no results are obtained until a bit of detective work reveals what happened. Suppositories are usually oil based and need little, if any, lubrication, but a little vaseline or a few drops of oil (salad oil is acceptable) may help with the insertion.

## SYSTEMIC DRUGS

The external cavities can be used for giving medications for systemic, as well as for topical, action. This is usually limited to the mouth and rectum.

SUBLINGUAL AND BUCCAL. Medications given by these methods are usually small, readily soluble tablets. Buccal medications are placed in the lower portion of the mouth, at the sides, but outside the teeth. Sublingual (under the tongue) drugs are placed as the name indicates, under the tongue. These areas are richly supplied with blood vessels and the dissolved medication is taken directly into the blood stream. The patient is warned not to eat or drink anything or swallow saliva until the tablet is dissolved and the medicine has disappeared. Of course, the number of drugs that can be given this way is limited. There are several reasons for using this method, such as the following: the drug would be destroyed by the digestive juices; there is no one to give the patient an injection (which is the case in most homes); and the effect of the medicine is needed quickly. The oral route (swallowing) is much slower. Nitroglycerin, a drug used for certain types of heart diseases, is usually given sublingually. It can be given orally, but its action is much slower by that route. Certain enzymes used for biological debridement are given buccally. The digestive juices destroy these enzymes. Drugs given by these methods act almost as quickly as those given subcutaneously (by hypodermic).

RECTAL. Rectally, systemic drugs are given by suppository. The drug is absorbed by the rectal mucosa, which is likewise richly supplied with blood vessels. Unlike the oral route, the rectal route is slow. This may be an advantage, if the physician wants a delayed action. Like the oral procedures just discussed, the rectal method can be used for drugs that the digestive juices destroy. It can also be used when the patient cannot take anything by mouth owing to such conditions as nausea and vomiting.

**Oral Route.** By far the majority of medications are given by the oral route.

Usually no directions other than amount and times of medication need to be given. However, a few hints may be useful.

Cough medications should not be diluted or followed by water. They should be allowed to trickle down, as part of their action is on the throat.

Fluid iron preparations, acids, and certain other minerals should be taken through a straw as they tend to stain the teeth. Rinsing of the mouth following these medications is often advisable.

Capsules are usually easier to swallow than are tablets. Both of these, and pills as well, should be placed on the back of the tongue and swallowed with a little water. Most are best followed with water, but this should be checked, as some are not to be followed by water or any other fluid. Large tablets, especially those that disintegrate quickly, can cause choking. To avoid this, unless contraindicated, tablets can be crushed and put into capsules. This method cannot be used for the various "time-release" medicines, as that would defeat their purpose. However, these tablets are rarely large. The large tablet also may be swallowed with a bolus of soft food, unless contraindicated.

Fluid drugs given to increase the appetite are "bitter." Nothing should be done to disguise the taste, as it is the bitter taste that is wanted. This stimulates the digestive juices and not only makes the patient want to eat more, but also assures that the food will be better digested.

**Inhalation.**   Drugs may be given by inhalation, again either for local or systemic effect. Most drugs given this way are administered by means of a special apparatus. Various inhalators, vaporizers, atomizers, nebulizers, intermittent positive pressure machines, and respirators are used. Each machine has its own rules and the patient must be instructed in the proper way of using the specific equipment ordered. No general rules can be given. The assistant must consult the brochure for each apparatus. Some are for the nose, some for the mouth and some for both. The entire procedure must be carefully explained to the patient. The drug used may be in the form of a fine powder, a fluid, or a gas. If the latter, it is often oxygen or given with oxygen. Usually this is reserved for hospitalized patients, but this is by no means always true. The patient with severe, long-term asthma or heart disease may need oxygen, with or without other medicinal gaseous substances, for months. This would require medication administration in the home. The amount of medicine to be used, in any form, must be carefully measured if it does not come premeasured, as is often the case. If the assistant studies the brochure that comes with the equipment and checks the drug to be used, she should have no difficulty explaining the process to the patient or the member of his family who will be preparing and administering the drug.

It is becoming more and more common for medications to come premeasured and ready for dispensing to the patient. This practice has greatly reduced medication errors. A word here that bears repeating: left-over drugs in the home should be destroyed! They should never be taken by anyone other than the patient, nor should the patient himself take the drugs later for "the same condition," which may or may not in fact be the same. Drugs should never be given to a neighbor when she or he has the "same" disorder. This is not only a highly dangerous practice, it is actually illegal. It constitutes practicing medicine without a license and can be punished by law. Many patients have been made worse and there have been deaths owing to such practices.

An increasing number of drugs are being given by injection. There are many reasons for this trend: topical drugs, applied to the skin, allow very little, if any, absorption, making them very unpredictable; some medicines cannot be given orally; the drug is needed for immediate action, and the oral route would be too slow; and many other reasons. The injection method of administration will be elaborated upon in the next few pages.

## PARENTERAL ADMINISTRATION

The term "parenteral" covers all methods of giving medications (and also fluids, electrolytes and nutrients) by means of a needle or cannula introduced through the skin. The word "hypodermic" is derived from "hypo," meaning "under" and "derm" meaning "skin." Therefore, a hypodermic needle administers a medication beneath the skin. The term hypodermic had been used to designate all parenteral channels, but is now being used mainly in the same manner as subcutaneous (sub—below, cutis—the skin).

**Types of Injections.** The more important forms of parenteral administration with which the assistant will deal are the intramuscular, subcutaneous, intradermal, and intravenous methods. The first three may be administered by the medical assistant under the instruction of the physician. Intravenous injections are always done by the physician with her assistance.

INTRAMUSCULAR. "Intra" means "within" and "muscular" signifies "muscle." Therefore, intramuscular injections are given into the muscle. A moderately long (1 to 2½ inches) and heavier gauge needle (18 to 23 gauge) is used for these injections. This type of injection is used for medications that are irritating to the subcutaneous tissues; the absorption in the muscle is slightly more rapid than in the areolar tissue. Larger doses should be given in the deeper tissues rather than near the surface. The buttocks, thigh, and upper arm, if muscle tissue there is adequate, are the usual sites for an "I.M." injection.

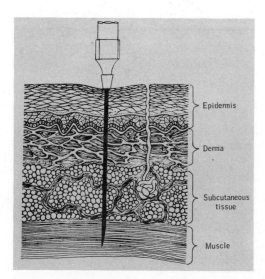

Epidermis

Derma

Subcutaneous tissue

Muscle

**Figure 24–1** Intramuscular injection. (From Falconer et al.: The Drug, The Nurse, The Patient. 4th Ed. Philadelphia, W. B. Saunders Co., 1970.)

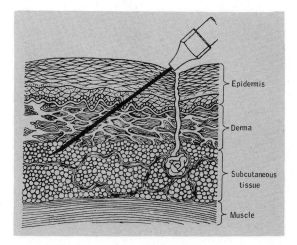

**Figure 24-2** Subcutaneous injection. (From Falconer et al.: The Drug, The Nurse, The Patient. 4th Ed. Philadelphia, W. B. Saunders Co., 1970.)

SUBCUTANEOUS.   "Sub" means "under" and "cutaneous" refers to the skin, so subcutaneous injections are given just under the skin. This type of injection requires a somewhat shorter needle of about ½ to ¾ inch in length, and a finer gauge of needle, i.e., 23 to 25 gauge. This method is used for smaller doses of less irritating drugs. The arm or the thigh is the usual injection site. One type of subcutaneous injection is also called "hypodermoclysis." This is the injection of large amounts of fluid into the subcutaneous tissues in order to supply the body fluids or furnish the body with food in the medium of a fluid.

INTRADERMAL.   "Intra" means "within" and "derm" again indicates "skin." Intradermal injections differ from the subcutaneous type which is given just under the skin; intradermal injections are given within the skin. A very short needle of a small gauge is used for this type of injection, i.e., ½ to ¼ inch in length and 25 to 27 gauge with a special bevel. This method is used to introduce minute amounts of medications for diagnostic as well as for therapeutic pur-

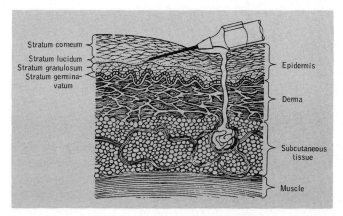

**Figure 24-3**   Intradermal injection. (From Falconer et al. The Drug, The Nurse, The Patient. 4th Ed. Philadelphia, W. B. Saunders Co., 1970.)

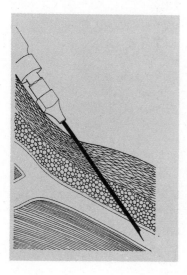

**Figure 24–4.** Intravenous injection. (From Falconer et al.: The Drug, The Nurse, The Patient. 4th Ed. Philadelphia, W. B. Saunders Co., 1970.)

poses. A small wheal or elevation is raised on the skin when a good intradermal injection is given (see Fig. 24–3, p. 417).

INTRAVENOUS. This type of injection is given directly into the veins, the blood, and the circulatory system.

**Areas of Injections.** Hypodermic injections may be given almost anywhere on the body, but not too near bone or blood vessels. Injections should never be given into an area where there is scar tissue, change in the skin pigmentation, change in skin texture, or excess tissue growth such as a mole or wart. The point of injection should be as far as possible from a major nerve. The selected site should be capable of holding the amount of medication that is injected. Many malpractice suits have resulted because these facts have not been carefully taken into consideration.

*Intramuscular* or intragluteal injections are usually given in the upper outer quadrant of the buttocks into the gluteus medius muscle. Great care should be taken to remain in this area and not enter into the other quadrants. The lower inner portion of the buttocks contains the great sciatic nerve and the major blood vessels. The quadrants of a buttock are measured from the crest of the ilium (top of the hip bone) to the lower portion of the "cheek" of the buttock. Some physicians prefer the ventrogluteal site. This area is immediately below the crest of the ilium on the side of the hip and is the farthest from all major nerves and blood vessels. The subcutaneous fat is thinner and the tissue easy to puncture. It is especially good for bedridden patients, patients who have frequent injections, or patients with extremely obese buttock "cheeks." Another site used frequently is the thigh into the vastus lateralis muscle. The area for injection is a narrow band extending from a hand breadth below the greater trochanter, the head of the femur or thigh bone, to the same distance from the knee. There are no important nerves or blood vessels in this area. This area does not offer the absorption of the gluteal area.

The thigh or ventrogluteal sites, as well as the deltoid muscle, are frequently the choice for injections in a small child. The deltoid muscle is often used in adults, although it is a little more painful than the other muscular areas. Patients often pull up their sleeves without exposing the deltoid muscle adequately; the injection enters the triceps and is too close to the radial nerve. It is always best to ask the patient to remove the clothing over this area. A sleeve pulled tightly over the upper arm will also act as a tourniquet and increase bleeding from the site of the puncture. The deltoid muscle should be used only if there is sufficient muscle tissue to absorb the drug readily. It should be avoided in the elderly patient or a patient who has had a mastectomy or any lymphatic excision.

For an injection into the buttocks, the patient is usually lying in a prone (face down) position on the examining table. The toes should be turned inward and the arms hanging over the sides of the table. With the toes turned inward, the gluteal muscles are relaxed and the medication will remain in the muscle and not be forced back along the tract of the needle into the subcutaneous tissue. Occasionally a patient will prefer to receive the injection in a standing position. In this case, the patient should stand on the leg opposite the side the injection is given, or be asked to place the feet with the toes turned sharply in, in a pigeon-toed position. The buttocks should always be fully exposed to aid in the correct selection of the site. Tight underclothing should not be only half raised or lowered, because this forces fatty tissue up, thus causing the medication to be placed in obese tissue, in which necrotizing lesions have a greater tendency to form.

*Subcutaneous* injections are usually administered into the upper arm below the deltoid muscle. The thigh or abdomen is also used. The syringe is held at a 60 degree angle and the needle is inserted approximately $1/2$ inch so that the medication is introduced just beneath the skin.

*Intradermal* injections are usually given into the arm, either the upper arm or inner surface of the forearm. Many intradermal injections are given for diagnostic purposes, with the possibility of an allergic reaction, and the arm makes it possible to apply a tourniquet. Considerable control is necessary when giving an intradermal injection to prevent going too deep into the skin. A correct intradermal injection will raise a small wheal.

In administering injections to infants, it is helpful for the mother or the assistant to hold the infant in a suitable position, as shown in Figure 24–5.

## HOW TO GIVE AN INJECTION

When giving medications by injection great care should be taken. Never at any time become lax in your technique. The procedure may become easy and even automatic, but never relax precautions. As stated before, and stressed often, always follow the physician's orders. Do not vary in the slightest degree, and, if you do not understand, recheck your orders before administering the medication.

Make certain that all materials are ready for use. Many offices have a central room where medications are prepared and then taken to the waiting patient in another room. This has many advantages, but care must be taken that the syringe and needle are transported to the other area with sterile technique. Always cover the needle; the sheath covering disposable needles is an excellent protector. When carrying a syringe and needle, hold it horizontal and parallel to your body. If

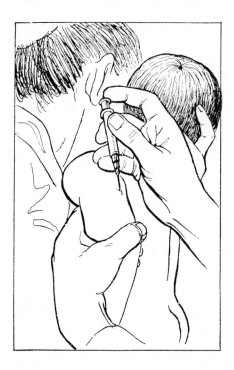

**Figure 24–5** Injection of an infant.

you are preparing the medication, but not giving the injection, place the vial or ampule of medication beside the filled syringe with the needle protected. This shows what medication is in the syringe and offers the physician a double check. Acquire the habit taught to all medical personnel: READ THE LABEL OF A MEDICA-TION THREE TIMES. *Never* depend on shape or color, or where it was stored, as a means of identifying a medication. If the medication is dated, check the expiration date and also examine the contents for any possible deterioration. Before withdrawing the medication it is a good idea to make certain there is sufficient quantity. If you practice good management, you will have ordered another supply when you find it becoming low.

If the medications are prepared in a central room, great care must be exercised to be sure the medication is given to the right patient. *Never* take more than one drug at a time, unless two or more are for the same patient. Check the patient's name and room number three times, as with the medication, before you prepare the injection, before you leave the central room, and with the patient's chart in the examining room. Incidentally, do not put more than one drug in a syringe unless specifically ordered to do so by the physician. Many law suits have occurred and been won because a patient received the wrong medicine or did not receive a drug ordered for him.

**Filling a Syringe From a Vial.** A vial is usually a multidose medication container that has a rubber stopper to facilitate multiple entries. Vials vary greatly in size, from one or two doses to 50 or more doses. Because they are entered more than once, extreme caution must be taken every time a needle is inserted into the medication. Contamination of the contents could be very serious. If at any time an error is made and there is danger of possible contamination, the medication should be discarded. Avoid the danger of an infection; no medication is more valuable than a patient's life. READ THE LABEL THREE TIMES. Make certain it is the correct patient, the correct medication, and you understand the dosage the physician has prescribed.

1. Cleanse the stopper of the vial thoroughly. (Many vials are manufactured with a "dust cap" on the top that must first be removed. This cap is usually of a soft metal that is easily torn off. If the cap can be replaced after initial removal it will aid in keeping the top clean.)

2. You can leave the cleansing sponge on the top while you now assemble the syringe and needle.

3. Draw as much air into the syringe as the amount of medication you plan to remove from the vial. This air-medication exchange prevents a vacuum from forming in the vial and permits the entire amount of medication to be used.

4. Insert the needle through the center of the rubber stopper in the vial by holding the vial in an inverted position (Fig. 24–6). Use a steady push, taking care not to bend the needle in any way. The needle should be inserted just far enough to facilitate withdrawal of the medication.

5. Gently push in the plunger of the syringe and inject the air into the vial. Now withdraw the medication by pulling down on the plunger gently. Keep the vial and syringe unit in a perpendicular position. If air has entered the syringe, gently push the plunger back up and force the air back into the vial. During this time be very careful not to touch the top of the vial or the needle.

6. After the correct amount of medication has been withdrawn into the syringe, guard the plunger of the syringe against slipping as shown in Figure 24–6 and remove the vial from the needle.

7. Check the label on the medication again.

8. It is good practice to use one needle to enter the vial and remove the medication, then place the needle size on that is desired for the injection. By

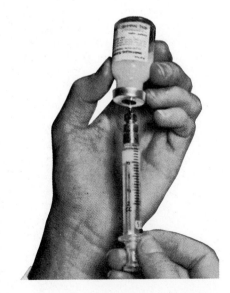

**Figure 24–6**  Filling a syringe for injection.

making this change of needles, a larger needle can be used to remove the medication. This is strongly recommended in medications that are irritating to the cutaneous tissue. When placing the needle on that will be used for the injection, take care that the medication is not pushed up into the needle.

9. If the medication is not to be administered immediately, place the vial next to the syringe unit and protect the needle with a sterile cover.

10. Some busy offices prepare several medications at a time so they can be injected at a later hour. This is a dangerous practice that can lead to errors in medication and dosage as well as to contamination.

**Filling a Syringe From an Ampule.**    Many medications are prepared in small single-dose glass ampules. READ THE LABEL THREE TIMES, making certain it contains the medication and dosage that has been prescribed.

1. Cleanse the neck of the ampule with an antiseptic solution. (If the ampule does not have a band around the neck and it is necessary to file the neck to facilitate breaking, file before cleansing.)

2. By holding both ends of the ampule as shown in Figure 24–7, "bend" the ampule until it snaps.

3. Insert the needle into the ampule and withdraw the medication. There should be no air in the syringe before it enters the ampule.

4. Gently withdraw the syringe plunger and fill the syringe.' After all the medication has been drawn into the syringe, hold the syringe in a perpendicular position and expel the air.

5. Check the amount of dosage and the label again.

6. If the medication is not to be administered immediately, replace the needle in the empty ampule or in the sheath of the needle, if a disposable needle is used. Both of these are sterile and are safe for temporary storage.

7. Place the empty ampule next to the syringe for identification.

**Giving the Injection.**    Explain to the patient what area is desired for the site of the injection and prepare him. The site must be fully exposed to facilitate correct selection. Clothing too near the site can also be a source of contamination, or the clothing may slip during the injection and interfere.

1. Wash your hands. Select the sterile syringe and needle of the correct size. Check the label on the medication.

2. Cleanse the stopper of a multiple-dose vial or open the ampule.

3. Withdraw the desired medication into the syringe. If a multiple-dose

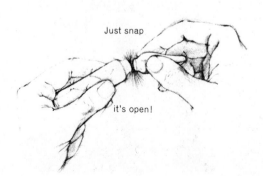

Just snap

it's open!

**Figure 24–7**   Opening an ampule.

vial is used, make certain to inject air into the vial equal to the amount of medication withdrawn.

4. Cleanse the site of injection thoroughly with a sterile sponge soaked with disinfectant solution; 70 per cent alcohol is usually used but other solutions are equally good. It is recommended that sterile dressings be used to swab the disinfectant solution on the skin, instead of cotton, because a minute amount of lint may be caught up by the needle and injected into the skin, where it can cause the formation of an abscess. If the injection is not administered immediately, the needle should be placed in a sterile container until ready for use. It is not advisable to wrap a sterile sponge around it because of the lint, nor is an alcohol-soaked sponge advisable because the medication may tend to draw up some of the alcohol from the sponge.

5. Hold the syringe and needle with the injecting hand and with the other hand, which has cleansed the skin, draw the skin to make it taut. The skin may be spread apart or squeezed up, whichever method is preferred. This usually depends on the site of injection. If the skin is spread to be made taut, make certain that the fingers do not rub over the area that has been cleansed for the injection. If the skin is not made firm at the point of injection, the needle will not penetrate readily and some pain may be felt. Also, the gentle tautening of the skin distracts from the actual injection.

6. Hold the syringe between the thumb and fingers and, with the wrist relaxed, insert the needle with a short, quick, darting motion. In intramuscular injections the needle is inserted the full length to about $\frac{1}{8}$ inch from the hub. It is best to never insert a needle completely to the hub; in case it breaks off, the small amount exposed makes removal comparatively easy. (A broken needle is extremely rare and practically never happens if proper technique has been used.)

7. All intramuscular and subcutaneous injections should be aspirated. This precaution should never be omitted. Although it is very rare, there is always the danger of the tip of the needle being introduced into a blood vessel. To aspirate, the plunger of the syringe is drawn back slightly. If the tip of the needle is in a blood vessel, blood will appear in the tip of the syringe. Take care that the position of the needle does not change during aspiration or after aspiration, because the change of location of the needle may place it in a vessel. If blood is aspirated, *do not inject into this area;* withdraw the needle and inject about an inch from the original site. It is preferred that another needle be placed on the syringe as a general precaution. Be certain to aspirate again at the new site of injection. If you are not in a blood vessel, about 0.2 cc. of air will appear in the syringe. This air aids in the diffusion of the medication, minimizes the pain, and prevents the leakage of the medication along the puncture canal.

8. As you start injecting the medication, release your hand that is holding the tissue slightly to facilitate entrance of the medication into the tissue. Inject the medication at a moderately slow speed to allow time for distention of the tissue and avoid pain from the pressure of the entering medication. Most medications can be injected by placing the index finger on the plunger of the syringe and gently pressing. Take extreme care not to move the syringe about while aspirating and injecting, because there will be equal movement of the needle within the tissue and you will cause pain as well as destroy tissue.

9. After all the medication has been injected, withdraw the needle quickly in

the same path as it was injected. If a slight clicking sound is heard on removal it may mean that the syringe was not brought up along the same line on which it was inserted. This will cause pain to the patient, as well as increase the size of the canal through which the needle passed into the tissue.

10. Immediately after removal of the needle place a sterile sponge that is saturated with disinfectant over the site of injection. Massage the site gently but firmly. Most beginners tend just to rub the skin surface rather than massage. There are some medications that state "Do not massage site of injection"; in these cases a sterile sponge should be held over the site with slight pressure for a few moments. If the injected area is exposed or shows signs of bleeding, a small dressing should be placed over it.

11. Assist the patient from the examining table. Some patients may need assistance in dressing. If the medication was painful or the patient is apprehensive of injections, it may be best to allow him to rest for a few minutes.

12. If the syringe and needle are reusable, rinse them immediately in running tap water. If a disposable syringe and needle were used, make certain the needle is broken and the syringe is destroyed. Manufacturers of disposable syringes and needles are now marketing small units that destroy these items and are then safe for the trash.

13. Record the medication given, the strength of the medication, and the site of the injection.

**"Z-tract" Method of Intramuscular Injection.** Some medications are absorbed more rapidly into the muscle than in the subcutaneous tissue. Because of poor absorption and possible irritation in the subcutaneous tissue, the injection must be given in such a method as to prevent any leakage back from the deep muscle into the upper subcutaneous tissue. These medications are always given into the gluteal muscle of the buttocks and never given into the deltoid or other less deep areas. For these medications the "Z-tract" method is used for injection and a longer needle than usual is employed. This method of injection displaces the upper tissue laterally before the needle is inserted.

1. Prepare the skin for injection as previously instructed.

2. Before the needle is inserted, pull skin to one side and hold firmly in place. If the skin is slippery from the cleansing solution, the cleansing gauze will aid in holding the skin in place.

3. Insert the needle, making certain you are deep in the muscle and not in adipose or cutaneous tissue. DO NOT RELEASE THE SKIN.

4. You may aspirate by using the first and second fingers of the syringe hand to pull upwards on the plunger.

5. If the needle tip is in the correct area, inject the medication slowly. Some medications will carry the instruction to inject 0.5 cc. of air following injection of the medication. This air will clear the needle of the medication and prevent it from following along the tract of injection. This air can be pulled into the syringe after the medication has been drawn in. Because the patient is in a prone position the air will be the last to enter the tissue.

6. Wait a few seconds before withdrawing the needle. Immediately upon withdrawal of the needle release the skin.

7. Check the instructions accompanying the medication. Many medications

that require the "Z-tract" method of injection should not be massaged after injection; just hold a sterile sponge over the area for a few moments.

8. Walking will not hurt but will help in the absorption. Avoid pulling a tight girdle over the site of injection. Use alternate buttocks for injections.

## PRECAUTIONS REGARDING INJECTIONS

1. Administer medications only on a physician's orders.
2. Administer exactly as ordered.
3. Select the site of injection carefully.
4. Be sure the patient is relaxed for proper absorption of the medication.
5. Cleanse the skin thoroughly.
6. Do not touch the site of injection after it has been cleansed.
7. Know the points of contamination on a syringe and needle.
8. ALWAYS ASPIRATE ON INTRAMUSCULAR INJECTIONS.
9. Inject moderately slowly.
10. Have nervous or very ill patients rest for a few moments after an injection.
11. Record immediately and be accurate and complete.

## CHANGES IN DRUG THERAPY FOR VARIOUS AGE GROUPS

Previously it was mentioned that the dosage of drugs for the infant, child, and older patient must be adjusted since the adult dose would in most cases be too great. There are other changes in medications for these groups.

**Infants.** With infants, the medication must be in liquid form. It can often be given with the formula, orange juice, or water. The physician should designate what media is to be used. It is best to put the medicine in a small amount of liquid, giving additional formula or orange juice afterward if needed. If the drug is put into too much fluid, the infant may not take all of the fluid and some of the medicine would be lost. The giving of parenteral medicines to the infant and small child has already been discussed.

**The Small Child.** For the small child, liquid drugs are used, as are candy-like preparations (chewables). *Never* disguise medications for the child in his food or drinks. This is one way to produce a feeding problem, for sooner or later he will realize that something has been added to his food. *Never* lie to the child as he will find out and will never trust you again. Expect the child to take his medicine as an adult would and he will usually respond.

**Older Children.** As the child grows older he becomes more and more mature and can be treated accordingly. Do not underestimate the knowledge of the child or "teenager." Never talk down to them—or to anyone else, for that matter. You also may have vastly more medical knowledge than the patient has, but it is the mark of an intelligent person to talk in the language and in the way that the people spoken to know. In other words, use simple English words with children, not medical terms. Of course, there is the possibility that the child has considerable misinformation. The assistant should be able to correct such misinformation. As with almost any patient, she may have to "interpret" what the doctor has told the patient. Children and adults alike hesitate to ask the doctor to explain, but have no such feeling with the assistant.

**Elderly Patients.** Physically, the older patient usually has relatively less adequate intestinal absorption than does the healthy adult. If the drug given orally does not seem to be securing the results desired, poor absorption should be investigated. Hard coated pills or tablets may pass through the intestinal tract unchanged and appear in the stools. The difficulty with large tablets was discussed previously. The older person is especially prone to choking and is in great fear of choking to death. This increases the possibility of trouble.

Parenteral drugs pose several problems. The older person rarely has the same amount of muscle tissue as the younger individual. It is therefore often difficult to give the older person intramuscular medications, especially if they are to be given frequently. Older persons tend to be edematous, emaciated or obese, and in each case the intramuscular or the subcutaneous administration of drugs presents difficulties. Ecchymosis and sterile abscesses are more frequent than in the individual with normal tissue turgor. If there is a tendency to dependent edema, the buttock (inner angle of the upper outer quadrant), often used for the younger person, is not an advisable site of injection since absorption may be slow and incomplete.

Emotional factors play a large part in the psychology of the older individual. The factors are manifold and cannot be discussed in detail here. However, a few points may help the assistant understand her patients better. Most older people have been taking medicines for a long time whether or not they were ordered to by the doctor. Self-medication is a national habit of immense proportions. It is not limited to the older person by any means, but is common to all ages. One problem that is not often realized is that the patient may not know that the same drug can come in several different forms. Company A puts their drug in a capsule, company B's is a tablet which is white, and Company C's is green. To the patient there are three different drugs. Occasionally this can be used to advantage. The patient complains that the medicine is not helping him. The physician has the pharmacist give the same drug, but from another company. The patient thinks it is a new drug, and believes it does a lot more than the old one. Older people are more creatures of habit than younger persons. They have had more time for the habit to become established. The assistant may need to explain in detail why the new medicine should be taken at a different time or in a different way than the old one.

In most cases, not only the form of the drug, but the type of drug may have to be changed for the older person. For instance, they can usually take less of the depressant drugs and digitalis preparations than the younger adult. There are many other similar conditions.

## A Few General Rules That May Prove Helpful

If oral medications are given in the physician's office, the same precautions should be used as for injections: check the medication, dosage, patient's name, and room number three times — once before measuring and preparing the medicine, again before leaving the central supply or after preparation, and last with the patient's chart before giving it to the patient. Again, take only one drug at a time unless the patient is to have two or more medicines at the same time. *Never* leave until the patient has taken the drug. If the patient seems at all ill, stay with him until this has cleared, or if it persists call the physician.

If the physician is to give a medication intravenously, the assistant will be expected to prepare the medicine and the equipment and to assist with the procedure. The same precautions as for any other medication prevail. In general, the equipment is the same or similar to that for an intramuscular injection. Some form of tourniquet will be needed. The blood pressure cuff is often used, as is a wide piece of rubber which can be placed around the extremity, usually the arm. The assistant should have everything ready for the doctor. She will be expected to apply the tourniquet and to release it at the time the physician indicates. Patients are often very fearful of such a procedure and the assistant can do much to relieve this anxiety by her manner, as well as by reassuring words. If the assistant appears unhurried, is willing to listen to the patient and to offer reassurance as needed, she will do much to make the procedure easier for the patient. (Remember, actions speak louder than words.) Such procedures become very routine for the assistant; however, they are anything but routine for the patient. Of course, the assistant will be expected to complete the procedure, that is, examination room cleanup, charts, and so forth. When the procedure is completed it may be wise with some patients to stay with them for a few minutes.

The assistant will often need to instruct the patient or his family about any drugs to be taken at home. If the doctor has done this, she may have to explain what the physician meant by this or that statement. She must be sure that what is to be done is clearly understood, such as the form of the medicine, how it is to be taken, and the time sequence. This last can be easily misunderstood. For instance, the order may state to take medication "every four hours." Does this mean night and day or day only? Again, it may be "four times a day." Does this mean four times in 24 hours or four times during the waking hours? If the order is for three times a day, does this mean before, during or after meals or between meals? There can be much confusion about such orders. The assistant should ask, if she does not already know, just what the doctor wants and explain this to the patient.

There are other things to be explained, as well. Is the drug to be taken with water, with food or without any dilutant? Some medicines must not be taken with milk, others not with food. These are things the patient must understand. In the case of milk, does this mean no milk or milk products at all, or just for a time before and after taking the medicine? With food, how long should there be between taking food and taking the medicine?

It is not possible to cover all the varied conditions the assistant will encounter. However, if she is interested in people, wants to help them, understands the drugs commonly used and where to get information about those she does not know, she will find her explanations to her patients a very satisfying part of her official duties.

# Chapter 25

**BEHAVIORAL OBJECTIVES**

*The medical office assistant should be able to:*

Identify the most commonly used
    surgical instruments.
Protect instruments through correct
    usage and storage.

Correctly sterilize instruments.
Correctly sterilize syringes.
Clean, sharpen, and sterilize
    hypodermic needles.

# Instruments, Syringes, and Needles

Surgical instruments, their identification, and care, are often the core of clinical procedures in the physician's office. A clinical assistant must have a knowledge of instruments, how they are used, and their specific place in a setup. She must know how to care for them and how to sterilize them correctly. An administrative assistant must recognize the names of instruments so as to aid in transcribing the physician's dictation. This knowledge is also necessary for the correct purchasing and inventory of instruments.

George D. Wolf, M.D., says, "The artist and the surgeon alike require special tools for the delicate techniques they have developed." Medical instruments are precision instruments and are very expensive. For this reason a chapter has been devoted to their identification, use, and care. Special instrument setups are covered in the chapters on Physical Examinations and Minor Surgery. This chapter will cover briefly those instruments found in the physician's office. Since this is not a book on surgical instruments, the most frequently used nomenclature will be used to identify the instrument and its purpose. There are thousands of surgical instruments cataloged in books, and there are great variations in names. The same instruments may carry two or three different names depending on the physician, hospital, or geographic location in which they are found.

## LEARNING SURGICAL INSTRUMENTS

If you have looked through a surgical or medical catalog, you have seen many strange and confusing names. The medical assistant is not confronted with the instruments a hospital central supply person would encounter or those the operating room nurse must know, but she must know the basic instruments. Train yourself to look at each instrument carefully and recognize the distinctive parts. For example, compare the mosquito hemostatic forceps and the physician's splinter forceps. They are both the same size and at first glance may appear to be identical. More careful inspection reveals that the hemostatic forceps has ratchets, and that the splinter forceps does not. Both have serrations, but the splinter forceps has a much sharper tip, as is common with all splinter forceps. Another example is the 6-inch dressing forceps and the 6-inch tissue forceps. They are both thumb forceps, but the tissue forceps has teeth.

There are many methods of classification of instruments, but basically, there are those instruments that are used for *general purposes* and those that have only one *specific* use. An example of a general purpose instrument would be the general operating, or surgical, scissors that can be used to cut tissue, soft sutures, or delicate fabrics. An example of the second classification would be the Michel skin clip forceps which can be used only to apply or remove skin clips. Another method of naming an instrument is by its use—cutting, draining, scraping, puncturing, or holding. Along with these usage names there may be a specific name taken from the surgeon who designed it or the hospital or clinic where the procedure was first done. Sometimes a manufacturer's name is given to an instrument. Many general instruments will be further identified by the part of the body where they are used such as a rectal speculum, a vaginal speculum and a nasal speculum. Hemostatic forceps often carry the proper name of some renowned surgeon such as Allis, Cushing, Ochsner, or Sims.

To start learning instruments, study the instrument catalogs. Look carefully at each instrument, identify its length, handle, serrations, ratchets, and movable parts. Then look at the instruments in your office and handle them, visualizing how they are used. As you study instruments you will be able to pick up an instrument that you have never seen before and at least identify its purpose. For example, the many different retractors all have one thing in common—they hold back tissue and retract or pull away from the area in order to facilitate better vision. Often the length of an instrument will aid in its identification. The uterine vulsellum and the Bozeman uterine dressing forceps are designed with long handles to reach through the vaginal speculum to the uterine cervical area. Apply these observations to the identification of all instruments, both therapeutic and diagnostic.

## Identifying Parts of Instruments

Most instruments have either a ring handle (Fig. 25–1A) or a spring handle, called "thumb handle," as shown in Figure 25–1B. Forceps of the ring handle type are usually made with a ratchet catch (Fig. 25–1C) and a box lock (Fig. 25–1D). The ratchets may be closed at any one of three or more positions; the more teeth engaged, the tighter the grip of the instrument. The box lock is composed of two parts which are riveted together, giving the instrument permanent strength.

The inner surfaces of the jaws on some instruments have sawlike teeth called serrations (Fig. 25–1E). Hemostats have serrations; both ring handled and thumb type instruments may have serrations. These serrations may be crisscross, horizontal, or lengthwise (Fig. 25–1E). They may be on plain tipped or mouse-toothed instruments. Serrations prevent small blood vessels from slipping out of the jaws of the instrument.

The tooth ends on instrument jaws are called mouse toothed, and sometimes rat toothed (Fig. 25–1F). They are found on ring handled and thumb type, on plain and serrated jaws. Usually one jaw has one more tooth than its partner to prevent a sharp edge from being exposed. Toothed instruments are usually called tissue forceps and are identified by the number of intermeshing teeth—

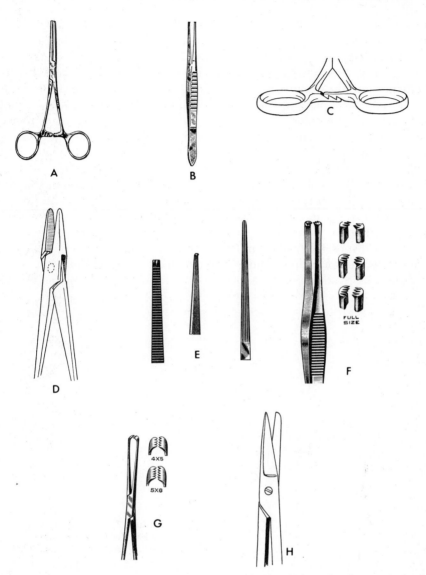

**Figure 25–1**   Identifying parts of instruments. A. Ring handle. B. Thumb type. C. Ratchets. D. Box lock. E. Serrations: horizontal, crisscross, and longitudinal. F. Mouse-toothed. G. Allis tissure. H. Scissors.

$1 \times 2$, $2 \times 3$, $3 \times 4$, and so forth. Similar to the mouse toothed is the soft tissue forceps, which also has teeth of lesser depth and sharpness, as shown in the Allis forceps in Figure 25–1G. These teeth are finer and slightly rounded, and there is usually a greater number of them. Their grip is also closed by ratchets, as on the hemostat, but they are used for a delicate grip that provides a secure hold with a minimum of injury to the tissue.

Other teeth that may be seen are the rather long single or double teeth of the tenaculum and vulsellum. Usually the tenaculum has a single sharp tooth on each jaw (Figure 25–7, #4), while the vulsellum (Fig. 25–7, #3) has a double tooth which resembles the fangs of a snake. Both the tenaculum and the vulsellum are tissue seizing instruments and are locked into position by ratchets.

**Surgical Scissors.**   Figure 25–1H shows a pair of scissors, its two parts joined by a screw lock or screw joint. When a pair of scissors is completely closed and held to the light, the two blades will be seen to touch at the tips. As the instrument closes, this meeting place travels from the joint to the tip, giving the shearing action. Scissors are identified as straight (str.) or curved (cvd.). The blade points are sharp or blunt. They are described as sharp-sharp (s/s), sharp-blunt (s/b), or blunt-blunt (b/b).

**Knives.**   Surgical knives (scalpels) are used to make incisions. Most knives now are disposable or have disposable blades furnished in different shapes and sizes as shown in Figure 25–2. The three standard handles are #3L (long), #3 and #7. Number 3 is most commonly used, and #3L is the same as #3 except for its increased length. Number 7 is more delicate for use in narrower places. Combinations of disposable blades and handles are available in various blade sizes. Some of the reusable handles now have a "flip off" spring for ease in removing the blade.

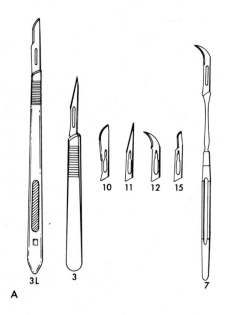

**Figure 25–2**   A. Bard-Parker operating knives (handles with various disposable blades). B. Disposable blade and handle.

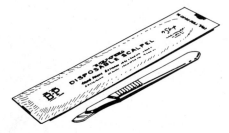

**Splinter Forceps.** The four types of splinter forceps shown in Figure 25–3, numbers 1 to 4, are quite different in construction. They are all used, however, to grasp foreign bodies embedded in the skin or under fingernails. The fine tips lend themselves particularly to the retrieving of splinters.

**Towel Clamps.** Three popular styles of towel clamps are shown (Fig. 25–3, numbers 5, 6, and 7) and are used to place sterile drapes around the site of the

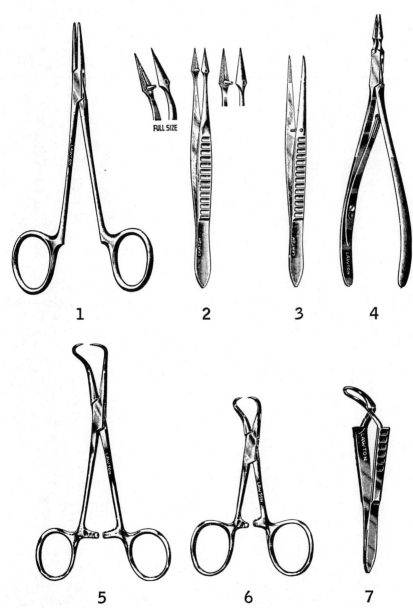

**Figure 25–3** 1. Physicians' splinter forceps (ring handle), 5½". 2. Hunter splinter forceps (thumb or spring handle), straight or curved. 3. Plain splinter forceps, 3½" or 4¼". 4. Virtus splinter forceps, 5¾". 5. Backhaus towel clamp 5¼". 6. Backhaus towel clamp, 3½". 7. Jones towel clamp (spring handle), 3".

operation. In minor (office) surgery the towel clamp holds various layers of drapings or towels in place. All towel clamps have sharp points which are used occasionally to hold the drape to the edge of the incision. The curved tips allow them to hang freely without interfering with the line of vision.

**Hemostatic Forceps.** Figure 25–4, numbers 1, 2, and 3, shows three of the more commonly used hemostats. These instruments are employed to clamp off smaller blood vessels and bleeders. They effect hemostasis until the doctor can tie off the bleeder with a suture. In hospitals a greater variety of hemostats is used, but the most usual patterns have either a fully serrated (grooved) jaw, a jaw serrated half way, or a jaw with serrations and teeth. The size and length of the jaw vary according to the need. They may be straight or curved.

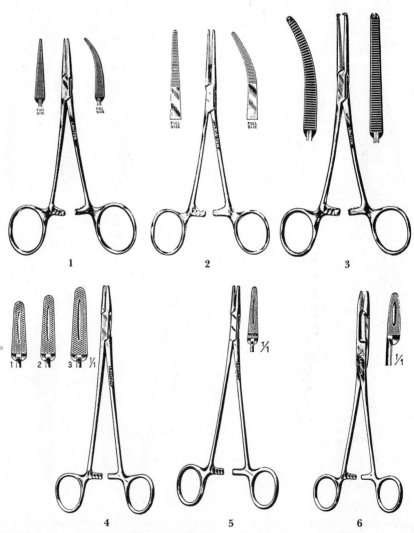

**Figure 25–4** 1. Halsted mosquito hemostat, straight or curved, 5″. 2. Kelly hemostat, straight or curved, 5½″. 3. Rochester-Ochsner hemostat, straight or curved, 6¼″. 4. Mayo-Hegar needle holder, 6″, 7″, or 8″. 5. Crile-Wood needle holder 6″. 6. Olsen-Hegar needle holder, 5½″.

**Needle Holders.** Numbers 4, 5, and 6, show some commonly used needle holders. A needle holder as used in the office is employed to grasp firmly a needle which is then passed through the skin flaps adjoining the incision. A needle holder with a thin jaw may be advantageous for fine needles as used in plastic surgery or eye surgery. A needle holder (6), in addition to having a needle grasping surface, has a scissors feature. Since needle holders wear smooth at the jaws after continued use, most are now available with a carbide jaw insert to be sure the needle will not twist.

**Other Instruments.** Numbers 1 through 10 of Figure 25–5 show a number of instruments one is likely to see in every doctor's office.

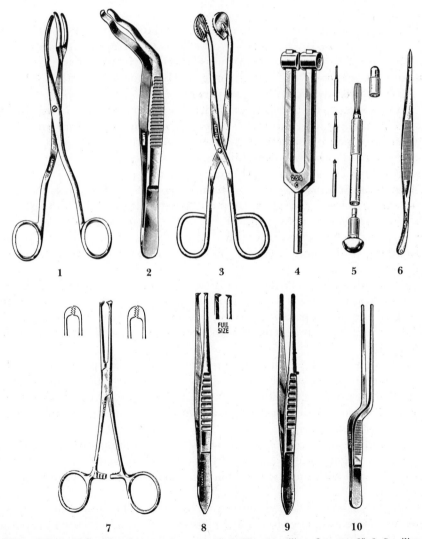

**Figure 25–5** 1. Sterilizer forceps, 3 prong, 8″. 2. Hypo sterilizer forceps, 6″. 3. Sterilizer forceps, 8″. 4. Tuning fork. 5. Fingernail drill. 6. Comedo extractor, double end. 7. Allis tissue forceps, 6¼″. 8. Plain tissue forceps, 5½″. 9. Plain thumb forceps, 5½″. 10. Lucae bayonet forceps, 5½″.

STERILIZER FORCEPS.   The three illustrated types of sterilizer forceps (1, 2, and 3) are used to retrieve sterile instruments, syringes, needles, etc., from sterilizer or autoclave. The types shown all have curved jaw surfaces which facilitate the holding of syringes.

TUNING FORK.   The tuning fork (4) is used to test audioperception. The forks come in a variety of frequencies (wave lengths). It is held by the single end and gently tapped on the examiner's knuckle or plucked between the thumb and index finger. It is not advisable to rap it on a hard surface and then hold it near the patient's head.

FINGERNAIL DRILLS.   Fingernail drills (5) are used to perforate the nail under which a blood clot or infection has formed.

EXTRACTORS.   Comedo extractors (6) come in various sizes and styles. The Saalfeld type shown has a lance end as well as a blunt end to press out foreign matter (e.g., blackheads).

FORCEPS.   The Allis tissue forceps (7) is used to grasp tissue such as muscle tissue or epithelium. In the doctor's office it is also frequently used to grasp sponge or bandage. The same function is served by the plain tissue forceps (8). These are made from 4″ up to 12″ in length. The number of teeth (1 × 2, 1 × 3, etc.) may vary greatly, depending on preference.

Thumb forceps (9) are primarily dressing instruments. Thumb dressing forceps are made from 4″ up to 12″ in length with finely serrated tips.

Lucae bayonet forceps (10) is a simple angled thumb forceps. It is used to best advantage in the nose or ear. The bayonet shape provides for a better field of vision. These are made in lengths up to 8½″.

**All-purpose Scissors.**   Figure 25–6, numbers 1, 2, and 3, shows the all-purpose operating scissors. The most frequently used pattern is 5½″ in length. They are made in half-inch lengths from 4½″ to 6½″, either straight or curved. As the name implies, these scissors are handy to cut lengths of fine sutures and tissue. As circumstances demand, they can be used with two sharp, two blunt or one sharp, one blunt tip.

In blunt dissecting, frequently a dissecting scissors (4) is used. This is the process of exposing vessels from surrounding tissue, or perhaps exposing bone or cartilage and also separating layers of tissue. The Mayo style scissors shown has a beveled blade. It is also made with a completely round blade and in a 5½″ length as well.

The Lister scissors (5) is used to remove bandages. The probe pointed blade can easily be inserted under the bandage with relatively little discomfort to the patient. Also, a probe point is less likely to puncture the skin. The gauze shears (6) are used to cut to size not only gauze but also such things as rubber sheets, tubing, and adhesive strips.

The Littauer stitch scissors (7) is one of several popular styles employing a beak or hook to get under a suture. When an incision is sufficiently healed, the suture is severed with these scissors and the ends pulled out with a thumb forceps.

The iris scissors (8) shown here was originally used in eye surgery. Many physicians, however, prefer it to a stitch scissors or in some cases to the operating scissors. The usual length is about 4″, although longer and shorter patterns are

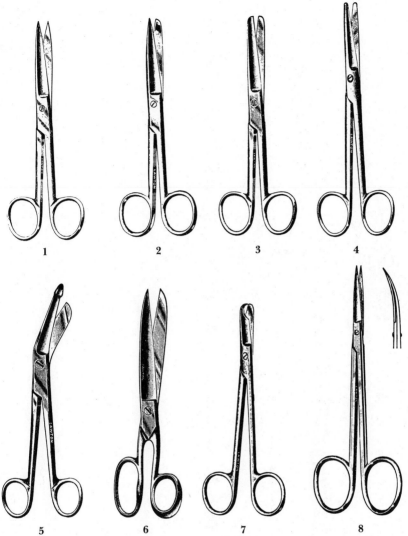

**Figure 25–6** 1. Operating scissors, straight or curved. Sharp-sharp. 2. Blunt-sharp. 3. Blunt-blunt. 4. Mayo dissecting scissors, straight or curved. 6¾". 5. Lister bandage scissors, 5½". 6. Gauze shears, U.S.A. style, 7½". 7. Littauer stitch scissors, 5½". 8. Iris (eye) scissors, straight or curved, 4⅛".

made. The tips may also be varied as on the operating scissors—e.g., blunt and sharp.

**Gynecologic Instruments** (Figure 25–7).   The Sims curette (1) is one of six sizes frequently used. They are used to remove minor polyps, secretions, bits of afterbirth (placental matter) and to obtain specimens from the uterus. Identical sizes are also made with dull blades. The Bozeman dressing forceps (2) is used to reach the cervix, uterus, and vagina. Employed to hold sponge or dressing, it can also be handy in the application of medication. The curved handle allows for better visibility. The Schroeder vulsellum (3) and tenaculum forceps (4) are used to

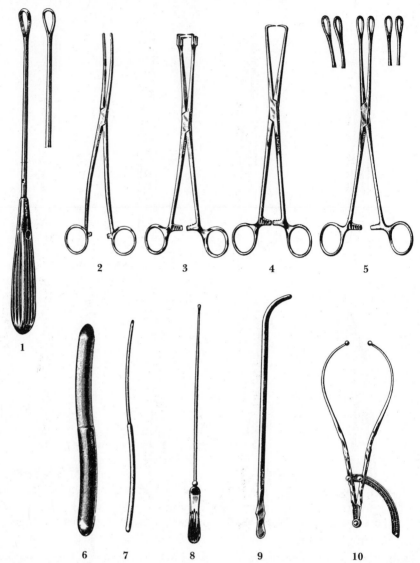

**Figure 25–7** 1. Sims uterine curette, sharp or blunt, 12″. 2. Bozeman uterine dressing forceps, 10″. 3. Schroeder uterine vulsellum forceps, straight, 9″. 4. Schroeder uterine tenaculum forceps, 9″. 5. Foerster sponge forceps (uterine sponge forceps), straight or curved, 9½″. 6. Hegar uterine dilator, double-ended, largest. 7. Hegar uterine dilator, double-ended, smallest. 8. Sims uterine sound. 9. Van Buren urethral sound. 10. Martin pelvimeter.

hold tissue, such as that on the cervix during the obtaining of a specimen or biopsy. The Foerster sponge forceps (5) may be used in lieu of the Bozeman for dressing purposes.

The Hegar dilators, of which the largest (6) and smallest (7) sizes are shown, come in sets of eight sizes. These are double-ended so that there are actually 16 different sizes. These are used to dilate the cervix for examination purposes and also prior to dilation and curettage.

The Sims uterine sound and the Van Buren urethral sound (8 and 9) are needed by the physician to ascertain the size and shape of either the uterus or the urethra. The Martin pelvimeter (10) is used to measure the female pelvis. This lets the doctor know whether a baby will be born normally or whether perhaps a cesarean section may be necessary.

**Eye, Ear, Nose, and Throat Instruments** (Figure 25–8). The Krause nasal snare (1) has a wire loop which, when tightened, may be used to remove polyps from the nostrils. A similar snare, smaller in size, is available for use in the ear. The Hartman "alligator" forceps shown here (2) has a 3½″ shaft. It is so called because of the jaw which moves in an alligator-type action. It is employed through a speculum either in the ear or nose for removal of foreign bodies. The alligator jaw is made in a variety of styles (e.g., cup jaw, with teeth, etc.) so that it can be used on foreign bodies or polyps with different shapes.

The Weider tongue depressor (3) fits comfortably into the doctor's hand during throat, postnasal, and mouth examinations. Inset shows actual size of the blade.

The doctor is frequently called upon to remove foreign bodies from the eye. Deeply embedded splinters are, of course, handled by the specialist; however, the Dix spud (flat end) (4) is helpful in office procedures, as is the golf-club-shaped end of the La Force spud (5).

Ear curettes (Buck's) (6) are used to remove matter from the ear canals. Usually this is an accumulation of wax. They are made with sharp scraper ends or a blunt ring and can be obtained in a variety of sizes.

The Freer dissector and elevator (7), one end of which is sharp and the other dull, aids in separating tissue from bone or cartilage. This is its dissecting function. As an elevator it is used to lift tissue away, either to permit improved examination or to facilitate dissection.

The Hartman eustachian catheter (8) is used to blow air into the eustachian canal which connects the nasopharynx to the cavity of the middle ear.

The Senn retractor (9) is a double-ended instrument, 6½″ in length, one side of which has three sharp prongs and the other a flat blade. This is used to hold open small incisions by retracting their edges.

A trocar (10), such as the nested set of three sizes illustrated, is used to withdraw fluids from cavities. It consists of a cannula (outer tube) and a sharp pointed stylette. Once the trocar is inserted, the stylette is withdrawn. Another variety is the Ochsner trocar with drain (11).

The Reiner syringe (12) shown here happens to be made completely of metal. Similar models are available in glass and some in part rubber or plastic. All types are fitted with a piston by means of which a stream of fluid is forcibly injected into the ear canal for cerumen removal and ear irrigations. A small splash shield has been mounted behind the tip to help collect the wash-back in a basin usually used during this procedure. The three-ring control-type handle facilitates a firm grip.

**Specula** (Figure 25–9). Among the important aids to the visual examination of the body orifices are the instruments known as specula. A speculum is an instrument for opening or distending a body orifice or cavity to permit visual inspection. A bivalve speculum is one with two valves or parts, sometimes referred to as blades or bills. These valves are spread apart, thus dilating the

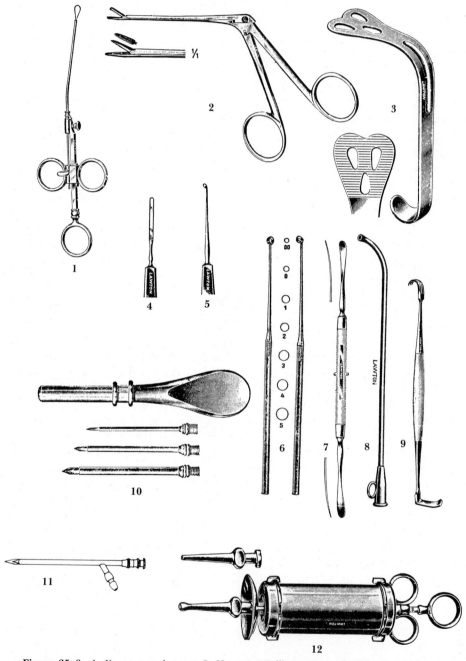

**Figure 25-8** 1. Krause nasal snare. 2. Hartman ("alligator") ear forceps. 3. Weider tongue depressor. 4. Dix eye spud (flat end). 5. La Force ("golf club") foreign body spud. 6. Buck ear curette. 7. Freer dissector and elevator. 8. Hartman eustachian catheter. 9. Senn retractor. 10. Nested trocars, set of three. 11. Ochsner trocar. 12. Reiner ear syringe with shield and control handle.

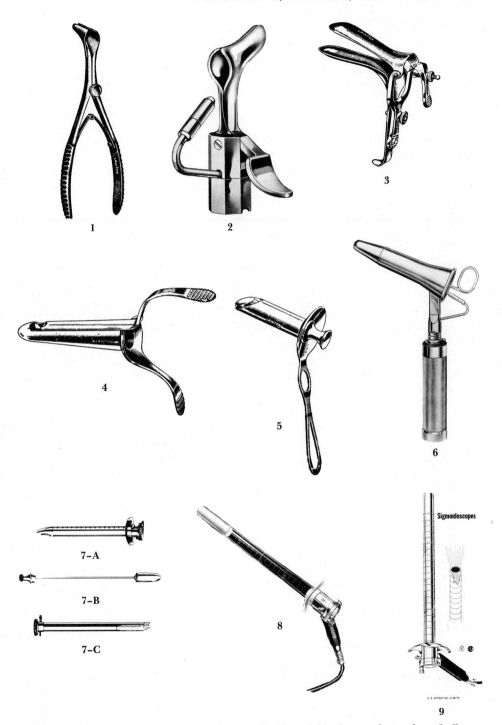

**Figure 25–9**  1. Vienna nasal speculum. 2. Illuminated bi-valve nasal speculum. 3. Graves vaginal speculum. 4. Brinkerhoff rectal speculum. 5. Hirschmann anoscope. 6. Illuminated anoscope. 7–A. Plain proctoscope with obturator (7–B) and light carrier (7–C). 8. Fiber-optic disposable sigmoidoscope. 9. Sigmoidoscope. (Figures 2, 6, 8, and 9 courtesy of Welch Allyn, Incorporated, Skaneateles Falls, N.Y.)

opening. The Vienna speculum shown in (1) and the illuminated nasal speculum (2) are used to spread the naris for examination of the nasal cavity. By spreading the valves the physician can examine for nasal polyps or sources of irritation and be aided in the introduction of applicators and snares into the naris. The Graves vaginal speculum (3) is also made in different sizes and is used in a vaginal examination. The Brinkerhoff rectal speculum (4) is used in examination of the rectal wall.

**Scopes.** The term "scope" is usually applied to a viewing instrument that is equipped with a light source. Generally a "scope" does not have a movable part that would increase dilation after the instrument has been inserted, as found in the Graves vaginal speculum or the Vienna nasal speculum. Examples of some "scopes" are found in numbers 5 through 9.

The anoscope (5 and 6) is approximately (8.9 cm) 3.5 inches in length and enables the examination of the anal area and lower rectum. Because of its limited length, an anoscope may not be illuminated. The proctoscope (7) is approximately 15 cm (6 inches) in length and facilitates examination of the rectum above the limits of the anoscope. The sigmoidoscope (8 and 9) is approximately 25 cm (10 inches) in length and permits examination of the sigmoid bowel area. Both the proctoscope and the sigmoidoscope must have some form of illumination as shown in the light carrier for the proctoscope. Number 7–B illustrates the obturator used to ease insertion of the sigmoidoscope.

**Obturators.** An obturator is the part of an instrument that closes a lumen (opening) of the instrument in order to facilitate the insertion of the instrument into a body cavity. These obturators are usually removed after the initial insertion of the instrument has been made. The obturators of the rectal scopes are rounded and smooth to ease the insertion of the instrument through the anal sphincter muscle. Some obturators are sharp in order to aid in puncturing tissue. An example of this is the sharp tipped obturator of the trocar that must be inserted through the skin.

**Applicators, Probes, and Directors** (Figure 25–10). The ear and/or nose applicators shown all have the same function. Cotton is twisted around the end, and to this medication is then applied. The style with the six-sided handle (1) is called a Buck applicator and measures 7½". It is made with either a triangular, twisted, or roughened end.

The Brown applicators (2) with the oval handle are 6" in length and are frequently made of copper or nickeloid material. This adds to their flexibility.

Numbers 3 and 4 show two grooved directors. The grooved director is employed to guide a cutting instrument, such as a scalpel. Notice that the director shown in 4 has a probe point. This point is used to explore the direction and depth of wounds. Probes and directors come in lengths ranging from 4½" to 12". The Larry probe (5) is used for rectal examinations for which its slender construction makes it more suitable. The pointed probe (6) is useful for exploring subcutaneous foreign bodies.

The long curved applicator (7) is called an Ivan laryngeal applicator. It has a length of 9" and the curve lends itself to use in the throat and postnasal area. Finally, the laryngeal mirror (8) is used for visual examinations of the larynx and postnasal area. These, too, are made in a variety of sizes and are often made so that the mirror surfaces will not fog.

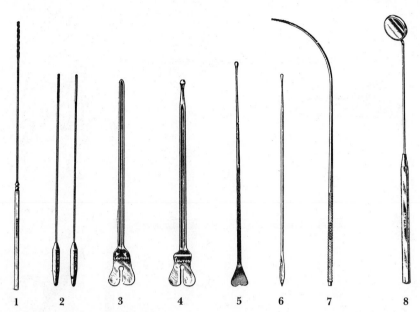

**Figure 25–10** 1. Buck applicator. 2. Brown applicator, 6″. 3. Grooved director. 4. Grooved director, probe point. 5. Larry probe. 6. Pointed probe. 7. Ivan laryngeal applicator. 8. Laryngeal mirror.

**Biopsies.** The instruments illustrated in Figure 25–11, numbers 1 to 4, show a number of styles used for getting specimens for biopsy. This is most usually done to ascertain the presence of cancer cells. The rectal biopsy punch (1) is used through a proctoscope and is made so that stems can be interchanged. These have different lengths and are made with cupped, basket type, straight or angled jaws. The tooth style affords a better grip on tissue. The inset shows a different jaw. The ring-handled biopsy punch is called a Wittner biopsy punch (2). It is one of several styles of instruments used for cervical biopsies.

A different technique (for obtaining cells to be used in the Papanicolaou test) involves the use of a curette. To the Novak biopsy curette (3) a suction machine is attached which collects the cells as they are dislodged by the curette. A still different system to gather cells uses a long scraping instrument. It is quite similar to a spatula. The type pictured here is known as an Eisenstein cervical spatula (4).

**Syringe.** An Asepto irrigation syringe with tip is shown in number 5.

**Hammer.** Number 6 shows a neurological hammer with pin and brush. The sharp pin and brush are for testing the quality of nerve reflexes. The Taylor percussion hammer (7) is used to test muscular reflexes.

The illuminated diagnostic set in Figure 25–12 consists of several different attachments for the battery handle (A) that is the source of power for the light. Popular attachments include the two otoscopes. The diagnostic otoscope (B) provides a large magnifying lens but restricts the area in which an applicator may be passed through the speculum. The operating otoscope (C) has a smaller magnifying lens but affords a broader area for working past the light source into the ear canal. The fiber optics otoscope (D) gives an increased level of illumination

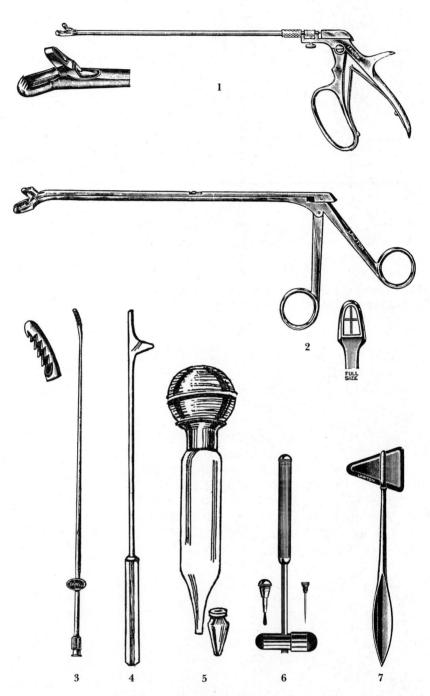

**Figure 25–11** 1. Rectal biopsy punch. 2. Wittner biopsy punch. 3. Novak biopsy curette. 4. Eisenstein cervical spatula. 5. Asepto irrigation syringe with tip. 6. Neurological hammer with pin and brush. 7. Taylor percussion hammer.

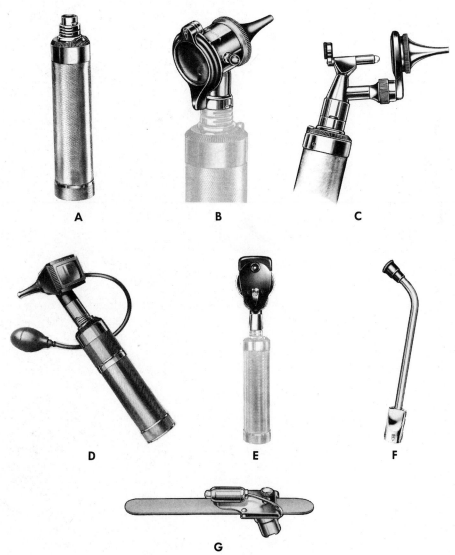

**Figure 25–12**   Illuminating instruments. A. Battery handle. B. Diagnostic otoscope. C. Operating otoscope. D. Fiber-optic otoscope. E. Ophthalmoscope. F. Curved transilluminator. G. Illuminated tongue blade holder. (Courtesy of Welch Allyn Incorporated, Skaneateles Falls, N.Y.)

and allows for the injection of air pressure into the ear canal. Different size specula may be interchanged on these otoscopes. The ophthalmoscope (E) is used to determine general physical health by allowing the physical examination of the optic nerve, retina, and blood vessels of the interior of the eye. The transilluminator (F) allows the light to be passed through an area such as the sinuses or breasts. The flexible rotating or curved transilluminator is adjustable for viewing the throat. A wooden tongue depressor may be inserted into a holder (G) for viewing the oral cavity. The illuminated battery handle may also be used as the light power source for an anoscope, proctoscope, or sigmoidoscope.

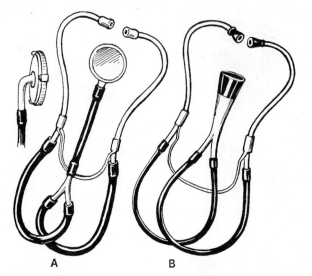

**Figure 25-13** Stethoscopes. A. Bowles stethoscope with disk-shaped chest end. B. Ford stethoscope with bell-shaped end.

**Stethoscopes.** These instruments are used in auscultation to convey to the examiner's ear the sounds produced within the body, especially the sounds of the heart and lungs (Figure 25–13). Most stethoscopes are biaural with two earpieces and a flexible tube leading to the end that is placed on the patient. The flat, disc-shaped tip is a Bowles stethoscope, while the one with a bell-shaped end is a Ford. There are several variations of these as well as a dual tip stethoscope with both disc and cone ends.

**Tonometer** (Figure 25–14). The tonometer is an instrument used for measuring intraocular tension. Glaucoma is second only to cataracts as a cause of blindness. All ophthalmologists routinely check their patients for glaucoma, but now many general practitioners are also checking their patients for glaucoma. In a survey made by the American Academy of General Practice in 1971, 41 per cent said they performed tonometry, and 65 per cent of these said they do the test at least three times a week. The tonometer is an expensive instrument and extremely delicate, and it *must* be cared for properly. This care includes proper storage that supports the delicate balances when it is not in use. It is usually sterilized by ether and distilled water. It should be disassembled and very carefully cleaned about once a year. Since these instruments are so finely calibrated, they should be sent to an authorized checking station periodically. It is advisable to purchase the proper stand and support for the instrument for the purpose of correct storage.

## CARE OF INSTRUMENTS

Since instruments are expensive, and a physician's skill is somewhat dependent on these "tools of the trade," the medical assistant must not only be able to identify them and know their uses, but must also be able to care for them properly in order to extend the life of the instrument and enable it to be used as it was intended.

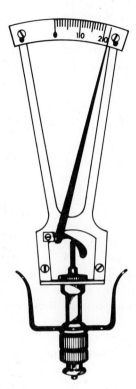

**Figure 25-14**  Tonometer.

Most instruments are made of fine grade stainless steel. The proper hardness and flexibility is important. Inexpensive instruments may be too brittle, easily stained and not able to function properly. Mistreatment of a chrome plated instrument can cause minute breaks in the finish which may become a source of contamination and may also tear the surgeon's glove.

Instruments should be carefully examined when they are first received from the supplier. Scissors should be tested to see if they shear the full length of the blades, clear to the tip. This can be checked by cutting a piece of cotton. If the scissors cut cleanly and do not chew at any point, even at the tip, then they are functioning correctly. Teeth and serrations are checked to see if they intermesh completely, and if the jaws are even on the sides and tip. Each instrument should be felt over its entire surface for any rough areas that may tear or snag the surgeon's glove. Box-locks and hinges must work freely but not be too loose. Thumb and spring handled instruments must have the correct tension and meet evenly at the tips.

Under no circumstances should instruments ever be bunched together or be allowed to become entangled. If an instrument is accidentally dropped, it may be permanently damaged. If scissors are dropped while the blades are partially open there will be a nick at the point the blades are crossed. Do not leave ratchets tightly closed or leave a hemostat clamped onto thick material such as a drape or gauze. Use a towel clamp or dressing forceps for this.

Reserve a special place during a surgical procedure to receive contaminated instruments. This is usually a basin of disinfectant solution placed in the sink or within reach of the assistant. If a metal basin is used it is advisable to place a small towel in the bottom of the basin in order to prevent damage to the instruments as they are dropped into the solution. Never allow blood or other coagulable substances to dry on an instrument. If immediate cleaning is not possible, then they should be rinsed well and placed in a cold water solution of a blood solvent and a mild detergent. The detergent increases the wetting ability of the water, allowing the instrument's surface to be better exposed to the solution. Each manufacturer of the various disinfectants and blood solvents will recommend the correct dilution and time of immersion for its product. Read the label. Upon completion of the surgical procedure, the receiving basin for the instruments can then be removed from the area and taken to the cleaning and sterilization room. This will also get it out of sight of the patient.

Separate the various types of instruments. Sharp instruments should be separated in order to prevent damage to the cutting edges as well as possible injury to the person sanitizing them. Rubber and plastic items puncture easily and often discolor metals. Some plastic and rubber goods should not be soaked too long because they will discolor. Plastics may become porous and lose their glossy surface. Many of these are best sanitized by cleaning in the usual way without soaking, or wiped with alcohol and dried. This method is not sufficient for instruments that will penetrate the body tissues, since it does not sterilize them.

**Sanitization.** All instruments and other items used in office surgery, examination, or treatment must be carefully cleaned *before* sterilization or disinfection. Sanitization is sometimes incorrectly called disinfection, but sanitization comes before disinfection as well as before sterilization. It is a very important step and cannot be overlooked or done carelessly. Stainless steel instruments that are not cleaned immediately after use may acquire a tarnish that is difficult to remove. Plated instruments may rust in minute breaks in the plating and thus, be a source of bacterial deposits.

If instruments were not rinsed thoroughly immediately after use but were received in a solution basin, then the solution should be drained off after the desired time of immersion and rinsed well in running water. Open all hinges and scrub serrations and ratchets with a small scrub brush or toothbrush. This step must not be skipped, because sterilization cannot penetrate to the instrument's surface through coagulable substances. At this time check the instruments carefully for proper workability.

Boiled instruments should not be considered sterile, because boiling only eliminates the organisms that are killed at 212° F or less. Boiling is used to disinfect the instruments after they have been sanitized. The boiling water cannot reach the instrument's surface unless all foreign substances have been removed. The boiling method of disinfection is sometimes used for instruments that do not penetrate the body tissues and need not be sterile, such as nasal and ear specula. The efficiency of boiling water may be increased by the addition of enough sodium carbonate to make a 2 per cent solution. This increases the disinfecting power of the boiling water and decreases the corrosive action on metals. John J. Perkins states, "Bacterial spores in water resisted boiling for about 10 hours, but they are destroyed in a 2 per cent soda solution at 208° F (98° C) in 10 to 30 minutes. Other workers employing a similar technic demonstrated that when contaminated and oiled instruments were boiled in a 2 per cent soda solution, a period of 10 minutes' boiling was necessary to produce sterilization. Boiling water to which alkali has been added in the above-mentioned concentrations is adequate for destruction of most spores in an exposure period of 15 minutes."*

If instruments are to be disinfected by boiling they should have all the surfaces exposed by opening hinges and ratchets and then be placed on the tray of the boiler and protected from hitting each other. The water should be of sufficient level to completely cover the instruments when the tray is immersed. Instruments are usually boiled for 15 to 20 minutes. Do not start the timing until the water is at a rolling boil.

Chemical sterilization is recommended for instruments that are not thermally stable or that may be dulled by heat sterilization methods. Read the manufacturer's instructions on the bottle carefully. Many of these chemicals are disinfectants and not sterilizing agents. Gas is a new accepted method of sterilization but has limitations in an individual physician's office. (See the chapter on Sterilization for further information on gas sterilization.) Both chemical and gas sterilization methods may require that an instrument be rinsed with sterile distilled water before use in order to remove any residual chemical that is not compatible with body tissue.

HANDLING STERILE INSTRUMENTS. If instruments have been chemically sterilized by immersion in a chemical or boiled for the correct length of time, they are removed by sterile forceps from the container or boiler. If the sterilizing chemical is strong enough to damage contacted tissue, the instrument must be rinsed with sterile distilled water. The instruments are then placed on a sterile field that has a barrier drape to prevent moisture from drawing any contamination from the surface below the drape. Do not touch the instrument with your hands or allow any contaminated materials to come in contact with the field. This method of handling instruments is not satisfactory unless the instruments are used immediately. It is very difficult to dry, wrap, and label them for storage and still maintain sterility.

Instruments that need not be stored sterile should be removed from the solution with sterile forceps, but they can be rinsed under hot running water to remove the solution that could damage the instrument during storage. Dry it very carefully, since moisture is the main enemy of an instrument. Instruments may be wiped with an oiled cloth if they are to be placed in storage for any length of time, but remember, this oil must be removed before they are sterilized at a later date.

LOADING THE STERILIZER. Here is an important rule to remember which applies to use of the autoclave and the dry heat oven. When loading the sterilizer, prepare all packs and arrange the load in such a manner to present the least amount of resistance to the flow of steam and heat (Fig. 25–15). Articles should be placed so that they rest on their edges rather than on their flat sides in order to permit proper permeation of the materials with moisture and heat. Tiers should be placed alternately. Under no conditions permit crowding of

---

*Perkins, J. J.: *Principles and Methods of Sterilization in Health Sciences,* 2nd Ed., St. Louis, Charles C Thomas, 1970.

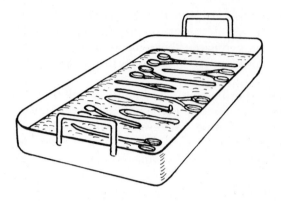

**Figure 25–15** Place instruments in their proper place on a soft fabric in the autoclave tray. A perforated bottom tray is necessary for effective steam flow. Then cover the tray with a towel to protect against contamination after removal from the autoclave and also to increase drying speed.

packs into tight masses. Jars and containers should be placed on their sides. When the container is right side up, even with the cover removed, air is trapped within the container and there is no flow. The perforated trays supplied with many autoclaves serve ideally for routine sterilization of instruments. Place a layer of muslin under and over the instrument to facilitate drying and prevent contamination when removing from the autoclave. Because steam will not penetrate oil, all oil should be removed from the materials and instruments to be sterilized.

STERILIZATION IN AN EMERGENCY. It is occasionally necessary to sterilize instruments in a great hurry or in places where there are no facilities for proper sterilization. In such cases, the instrument may be dipped in alcohol or gasoline and then ignited. As soon as the object is dry, it is considered sterile. These are emergency methods only, though sometimes necessary, and are not recommended, as the process is very hard on good instruments. The tip of an instrument may be dipped into tincture of iodine, Zephiran or Merthiolate for a few minutes for emergency use, but these solutions are hard on the metal surfaces of the instrument.

If an instrument is in need of oiling in order to make it work properly, use a small amount of water-soluble grinding or lapping (polishing) compound and work the compound into the area by opening and closing the instrument several times until it moves freely. Rinse well and sterilize.

Very seldom nowadays it is necessary to sharpen an instrument, since most knife blades are disposable. However, many scissors are reusable and may need sharpening and adjusting. It is advisable to send the scissors to a competent instrument repair service. Your surgical supply representative may be able to suggest where you can get this repair service.

## CARE OF SYRINGES AND NEEDLES

Although reusable syringes and needles are not used as frequently as in the past, there are some specialty syringes and needles that require special care. Often these specialty items are expensive, and extra care will extend the life of the syringe or needle. The most important rule to remember in caring for a syringe and needle is to rinse the unit under cool running water immediately after use. This practice is especially important if the syringe has been used for any blood work or for a medication that can form a film on the inside of the syringe and needle.

Rinse the syringe well by first separating the unit and allowing the water to run over both parts. Then reassemble the unit, draw the water into the barrel, and force it gently through. Repeat this process several times. If a reusable needle was used, attach the needle to the tip of the syringe and force the water through. Grip the unit well with your hand, and place your forefinger on the hub of the needle in order to prevent the needle's being forced off.

**Removing Substances from Syringes.** If the syringe has sediment in it, scrub it with a small bottle brush. There are special brushes for syringe cleaning that have a smaller brush attached for cleaning the hub of a needle and a stiff plastic stylus that is used to clear out the syringe tip. An oily substance can be cleaned from a syringe by rinsing with ether, acetone, or alcohol. Then, wash the unit well with a detergent and rinse with distilled or demineralized water. Syringe barrels and plungers should remain separated until they are ready for use again. Alkali deposits may be removed by 10 per cent nitric acid solution. This solution will also remove gentian violet and blood stains. Iron stains may be removed by a 10 per cent hydrochloric acid solution. It is not advisable to soak the syringe in an acid solution, because it will remove the markings and will erode any metal such as a Luer-lok tip. It is best to saturate a cotton applicator and swab out the syringe, rinsing well afterwards. Take care that the acid solution does not come in contact with the metal. There are also excellent commercial cleaning products on the market.

Because reusable syringes are individually made by expert glass blowers, the surfaces must not be allowed to collect deposits. Some syringes are made with matching barrel and plunger. These units will bear a matching number on the barrel and plunger, and the numbers must match in order for the unit to be usable. The parts of these numbered units are not interchangeable with other syringes. Many reusable syringes are now Multifit* syringes. These plungers and barrels are interchangeable with other units. In case of breakage, unbroken parts may be used with other remaining parts.

Disposable syringes are made of plastic or other synthetic materials. These syringes are unbreakable and very sturdy. Disposable syringes are individually packaged and are color coded for easy identification. The use of disposable units absolutely prevents cross infection of patients. It also eliminates the time lost in cleaning and sterilizing reusables. Disposable units are supplied in a wide range of types and sizes. Sterile disposable needles are used almost exclusively, with the exception of some special needles. These are also color coded by the hub for easy identification. Remember, ALWAYS BREAK AND DESTROY A DISPOSABLE NEEDLE AND SYRINGE BEFORE DISCARDING. This is safe and easy with some of the cutting units now available (Fig. 25–16 and 25–17). This method prevents the medical assistant or the physician from accidentally puncturing himself and possibly becoming infected. Never give a child a syringe as a toy or reward.

---

*Becton-Dickinson Company

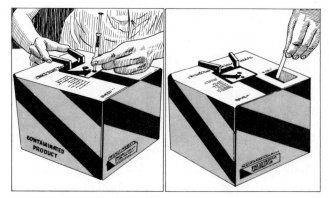

**Figure 25–16**   Disposal carton for syringes.

**Destruction of Used Hypodermic Syringes and Needles.**   Used syringes and needles must be disposed of safely. There are numerous destruction units on the market, but many are not practical for the physician's office. The unit in Figure 25–16 cuts off the needle and the syringe tip and provides a place for storage of the destroyed unit. In Figure 25–17 the unit is smaller, and it destroys the needle and the syringe tip. It is of vital importance to destroy needles and syringes before discarding them.

Some states have rather severe fines and/or penalties for discarding needles that have not been rendered unusable.

**How to Open a Stuck Syringe.**   Sometimes, even with careful handling, a syringe becomes stuck. If this happens, fill the air space of the stuck syringe with warm water by using another syringe and needle and injecting water through the tip. Then, allow the syringe to soak for some time. This, however, will not loosen a tightly stuck syringe.

Boiling the syringe in a 25 per cent aqueous solution of glycerine is sometimes successful in separating stuck syringes. This method often makes it possible to remove the plunger by rotating it with a circular motion while it is hot. It may help to immerse the syringe in cold water for ten minutes and then plunge it

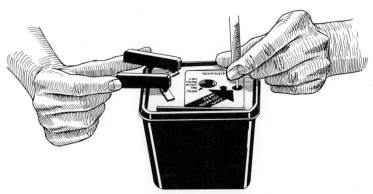

**Figure 25–17**   Cutting device for disposable syringes.

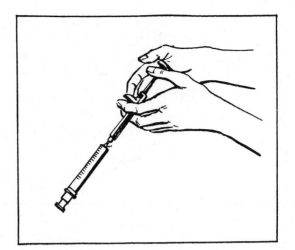

into boiling water for a few seconds. This heats the barrel and causes it to expand, while the plunger remains cool and contracted.

The most satisfactory method is the use of the B-D Syringe Opener No. 26, as shown in Figure 25–18.

**Sterilization of Syringes.**   Sterilization by autoclaving or dry heat is the most widely accepted method. To prepare the syringe, sanitize it as mentioned previously. Sterilization envelopes or small bags are the most satisfactory method of wrapping syringes for autoclaving. These syringe bags have a sterilizer indicator on the bag (Fig. 25–20). The syringe parts are separated and placed in the bag with the barrel flange and the thumb rest of the plunger toward the open

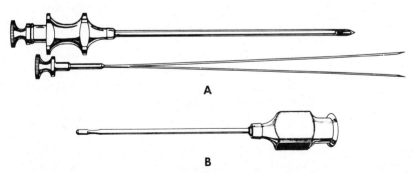

A

B

**Figure 25–19**  A. Silverman Biopsy Needle: 14G cannula with fitted stylus (inserted here). Split inner cannula for biopsy retention. The biopsy needle is used to obtain a specimen from an internal organ or underlying soft tissue. With the needle stylus in place the needle is inserted through the body wall to the depth desired. The stylus is then removed, and the split inner cannula is inserted. The tissue specimen is picked up by the inner cannula. A needle biopsy is frequently preferred to an incisional biopsy for soft tissue biopsies. B. Abscess cannula 18G, 1¼″ with bulbous point and flexible cannula. The abscess needle is attached to a syringe and is used to withdraw fluid or pus from an abscess or cyst.

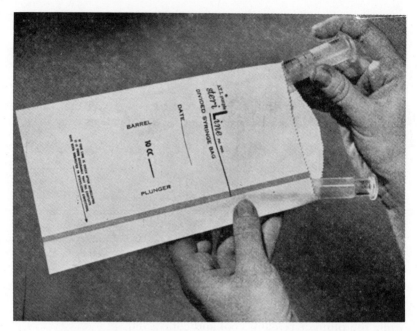

**Figure 25-20**  Envelope for sterilization and storage of syringe.

end. This makes it easier to assemble the unit without contamination when the sealed end is torn open. The bag should be clearly labeled with the size of the syringe and the date of sterilization. If several persons are cleaning and autoclaving syringes, it is advisable to initial the bags. Syringes may also be autoclaved in muslin wraps (Fig. 25–21). The syringe parts are separated and wrapped together with a piece of gauze between the plunger and barrel. This muslin pack may be secured with string or sterilizer tape. Syringes may also be autoclaved in test tubes (Figure 25–22). Assemble the syringe after a thorough sanitizing and place it in a Pyrex test tube. The syringe does not have to be completely dry, but do not leave too much moisture on it. The tube is of large enough diameter to allow the syringe, but not the flange of the syringe, to drop in. This prevents the tip of the needle from touching the butt of the test tube. Cover the exposed plunger with muslin or sterilizer paper and secure with a string or rubber band. When sterilizing by this method, there is no need to label. The date of sterilization is sufficient. This method is useful if the unit may receive a little rough handling, as in a physician's bag. These units are autoclaved for 20 minutes at 250° F.

DRY HEAT.  This method of sterilizing syringes is used, because all the moisture is eliminated and the sterilizing can be done in a regular oven, if necessary. The syringe is prepared in the same manner as for autoclaving. The exposure time is one hour at 320° F (160° C.) Do not overload the oven; this prevents circulation of the air.

BOILING.  The syringes are sanitized in the same manner as for sterilization by steam pressure or hot air. There are advantages to using distilled or demineralized water in the boiler, although using such water does increase the expense

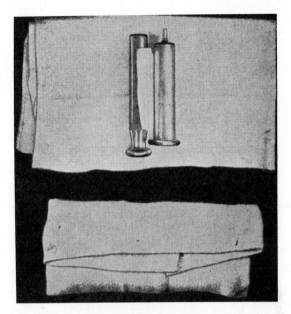

**Figure 25–21** Preparation of syringes for autoclaving.

and is sometimes inconvenient. Hard water erodes the glass and leaves an alkali deposit which causes a syringe to stick. Boiling in hard water shortens the life of a syringe. The use of bicarbonate of soda or alkalizing sterilizer tablets is not recommended.

If hard water is used for boiling syringes, the barrel and plunger should be assembled with the plunger pushed completely into the barrel. If distilled or demineralized water is used, then the syringes are separated. Arrange all syringes in the boiler parallel to one another and all pointing in the same direction; do not crowd them. Boil for 15 to 20 minutes at a rolling boil. Do not overboil, since this shortens the life of the syringe.

Since boiling is effective against some organisms but not against all spores or viruses, like that of infectious hepatitis, boiling is not recommended as a method of sterilization.

## Care of Hypodermic Needles

A good hypodermic needle is absolutely essential. No one likes to use a dull needle or one with a fish hook on the point. Most needles used for injections today are disposable. Do not attempt to cut expenses by purchasing inferior or unknown brands of needles or syringes. This is truly an example of false economy and may even lead to injury of a patient and a lawsuit. Good disposable needles are made with exacting precision and are appreciated by the patient as well as by the medical assistant.

**Construction of Needles.** Figure 25–23 shows the construction of the various hypodermic needle points. As you can see, the Huber point has a "closed" point. This is to prevent tissue plugs from forming when the needle is

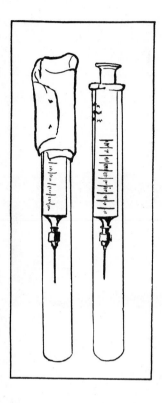

**Figure 25-22** Preparation for autoclaving syringes in a test tube.

inserted. The Huber point gives a smooth sliding action through the tissues, thus reducing the danger of such plugs. The short and intradermal bevels are preferred when medication is injected into the outer layer of the skin and only the bevel of the needle needs to be inserted. Figure 25-23 illustrates some specialty needles. These needles are reusable and must be carefully cleaned and sterilized. The points should be protected when they are in storage.

There are some facts to remember about the construction of a hypodermic needle. This statement was prepared by the Becton-Dickinson Company.

> The size of the needle is governed by four factors: safety, rate of flow, comfort of the patient, and depth of penetration. There are three standard dimensions: length, outside diameter of the cannula, and wall thickness. Regular needles are measured for length from where the cannula joins the hub to the tip of the point (hub not included). The outside diameter or "gauge" of a needle is measured by a Stubb's English wire gauge, standard throughout the United States. The diameter sizes are indicated by gauge numbers running from 13 to 27. The larger the gauge number the smaller the needle. Gauge numbers are often stamped on the flat surface of the hub for ready use.

**How to Clean Needles.** Although most of the needles used in physicians' offices are disposable, an occasional reusable needle must be cleaned and sterilized. These reusable needles may also need to be sharpened on occasion (Fig. 25-25).

Clean the needle immediately after use, while it is still attached to the

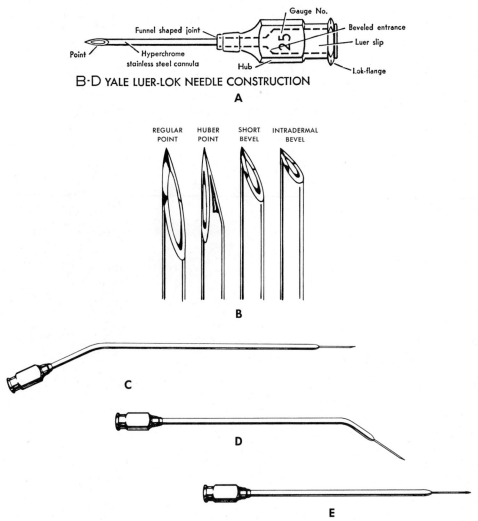

**Figure 25–23**    Construction and types of hypodermic needles. A. Components of hypodermic needles. (Courtesy of Becton-Dickinson and Co.) B. Variety of points. C. Hemorrhoid needle. D. Curved tonsil needle. E. Straight tonsil needle.

syringe, by forcing water through it several times. Then remove the needle from the syringe and rinse it under running water. Push a stylet through the needle to make certain the cannula is clean. Always insert the stylet from the hub end, not from the point. Clean the inside of the hub with a cotton applicator. Take care never to touch the point of the needle to anything. Needles become dull or have fish hooks only through misuse or abuse.

**How to Remove a Stuck Needle.**    Sometimes a hypodermic needle becomes stuck on a syringe. If this happens, grasp the hub of the needle with a forceps, as shown in Figure 25–26, and turn the syringe counterclockwise. This should loosen the needle. Do not twist the needle or wiggle the syringe, since breakage may occur.

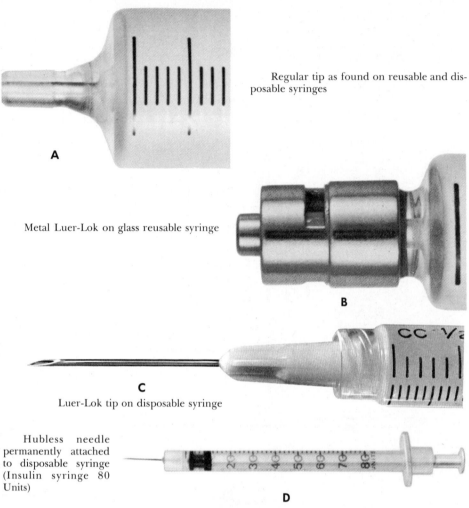

Regular tip as found on reusable and disposable syringes

A

Metal Luer-Lok on glass reusable syringe

B

Luer-Lok tip on disposable syringe

C

Hubless needle permanently attached to disposable syringe (Insulin syringe 80 Units)

D

Figure 25–24  Types of syringe tips.

**How to Sharpen a Hypodermic Needle.**  Needles should be kept sharp and smooth. Trauma, pain, and seepage are greatly reduced by eliminating burrs and fish hooks. Needles should always be inspected prior to each sterilization, and those needles requiring sharpening should be placed aside.

Instructions for sharpening hypodermic needles are given by the Becton-Dickinson Company as follows.

Use a magnifying glass to detect burrs, fishhooks, and dull, broken, and misshapen points. To remove burrs from the inside edges use a pointed stylet, trocar, or discarded needle. Use a smooth (Arkansas Stone) oil stone. A light mineral oil on the stone hastens sharpening and gives a smoother finish. To hold the needle more rigidly, attach a small syringe if desired. Use the index finger of the other hand for gentle pressure. Place the needle bevel flush on the stone at the proper angle (see Figure 25–25) and sharpen by sliding forwards and backwards, and also by moving laterally across the stone to prevent wearing grooves in the stone. In sharpening a needle with a fitted stylet, keep the stylet in place so that perfectly matched bevels are maintained.

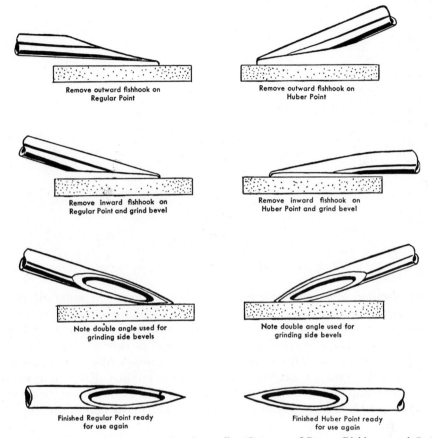

Remove outward fishhook on
Regular Point

Remove outward fishhook on
Huber Point

Remove inward fishhook on
Regular Point and grind bevel

Remove inward fishhook on
Huber Point and grind bevel

Note double angle used for
grinding side bevels

Note double angle used for
grinding side bevels

Finished Regular Point ready
for use again

Finished Huber Point ready
for use again

**Figure 25–25**  Sharpening a hypodermic needle. (Courtesy of Becton-Dickinson and Co.)

**Figure 25–26**  Removing a stuck
hypodermic needle.

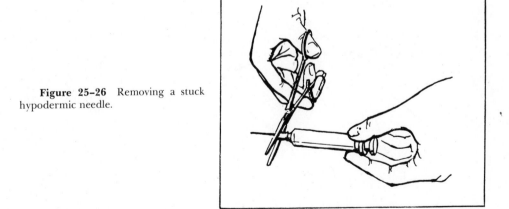

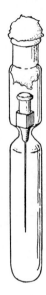

**Figure 25–27**   Constriction tube.

**Sterilization of Hypodermic Needles.**   Like syringes, hypodermic needles are sterilized by autoclaving or hot air methods. Boiling is not recommended, because sterilization is not assured. Chemical sterilization may be used, but it is unsatisfactory because the sterilizing chemical must be rinsed off with sterile distilled water before use. This extra step is often a source of contamination. Autoclaving is the most satisfactory and convenient method. Extra long needles, such as tonsil and hemorrhoid needles, may be placed in glass tubes for autoclaving. About one-half inch of cotton should be placed in the butt of the tube; then

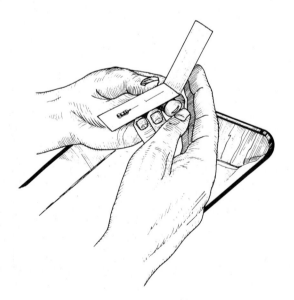

**Figure    25–28**   Paper    needle holder for autoclaving.

insert the needle into the tube, point first. Cover the end of the tube with gauze or sterilizer paper and date the package.

Constriction tubes (Fig. 25–27) are excellent for sterilizing regular needles because they prevent the point of the needle from touching anything by means of the constricture in the tube that holds the needle by the hub. Use a cotton plug (not too tight) or gauze or paper over the end. Do not use a rubber stopper because steam cannot penetrate it. It is a good idea to insert a sterilizer indicator, such as Diack, in one tube of each batch to be sterilized. There are also paper holders that protect the point of the needle and permit a needle to be placed in an envelope with a syringe without the danger of the needle puncturing the envelope (Fig. 25–28).

# Chapter 26

**BEHAVIORAL OBJECTIVES**

*The medical office assistant should be able to:*

Define the listed terms applicable to
   sterilization and disinfection
Compare the requirements for
   sanitation, disinfection, and
   sterilization
Prepare items for sterilization and
   disinfection
Operate the equipment described in
   this chapter

Select the appropriate technique for a
   given item
Perform sterilization and disinfection
   procedures
Recognize failures in technique
Protect sterilized items from
   contamination

# Sterilization Techniques

Sterilization and the attempts to reach and understand sterility are as old as recorded history. Many practices and theories have been tried and then discarded, but with each something has been added to the total knowledge.

Cremation was known to man centuries ago. Man has also known that desiccation sometimes preserves body tissue, and prevents the spread of sepsis. Moses, in about 1250 B.C., gave the ancient Hebrews the first recorded sanitation laws. In a sense, Moses was our first "public health officer." The ancient Greeks used forms of fumigation to combat epidemics. Hippocrates (460–370 B.C.), who separated philosophy and medicine, realized the value of boiling water, washing hands, and using certain medications while dressing an infected wound. The next contribution of significance was the discovery of bacteria in 1683, chiefly by Anton van Leeuwenhoek. Then Joseph Lister (1827–1912), Louis Pasteur (1822–1895), and others started the world on the miraculous path of sterilization. Pasteur said on April 30, 1878, in a lecture to the Academie de Medecine:

> If I had the honor of being a surgeon, convinced as I am of the dangers caused by germs of microbes scattered on the surface of every object, particularly in hospitals, not only would I use absolutely clean instruments, but, after cleansing my hands with great care and putting them quickly through a flame (an easy thing to do with a little practice), I would only make use of charpie, bandages, and sponges which had previously been raised to a heat of 130° C. to 150° C.; I would only employ water which had been heated to a temperature of 110° C. to 120° C. All that is easy in practice, and, in that way, I would still have to fear the germ suspended in the atmosphere surrounding the bed of the patient; but observation shows us every day that the number of those germs is almost insignificant compared to that of those which lie scattered on the surface of objects, or in the clearest ordinary water.

Joseph Lister was the first surgeon to use chemical disinfection. One of his principles, which was the basis for antisepsis, was that "all instruments, dressings and everything else in contact with operations, including the hands of the surgeon and the assistant, should be rendered antiseptic." Lord Lister has been given full honor for introducing the sterile instruments, dressings, and glassware used in the operating room. He gave this advice to his fellow surgeons:

> In order, gentlemen, that you may get satisfactory results from this sort of treatment, you must be able to see with your mental eye the septic ferments as distinctly as we see flies or other insects with the corporeal eye. If you can really see them in

**463**

this distinct way with your intellectual eye, you can be properly on your guard against them; if you do not see them you will be constantly liable to relax in your precautions.

We all give thanks to these gentlemen and many others who contributed to the knowledge of sterility and sterile technique.

## Basic Terms Defined

**Antiseptics.** Substances which, when applied to microorganisms, will render them harmless either by killing them or by preventing their growth, according to the agent or the method of application. Antiseptics are agents made especially for application to the living tissue. If the substance only prevents the growth of bacteria it may then be referred to as a bacteriostatic agent. The term antiseptic is sometimes used to include disinfectants, although disinfectants are usually too strong to be applied to living tissue. Antiseptics are used in the treatment of wounds and infections, and are applied to the skin before surgery. Antibiotics are not included as antiseptics because they are taken internally.

**Asepsis.** The absence or prevention of access of microorganisms to materials. Medical asepsis refers to destruction of organisms after they leave the body. This technique is used in the care of patients with infectious diseases, to prevent re-infection from person to person. This is achieved by the isolation technique. Surgical asepsis refers to the destruction of organisms before they enter the body. In surgical asepsis an object is either sterile or nonsterile. Measures that can be taken to provide surgical asepsis include absolute sterilization of all instruments, linens, and other inanimate objects that come in contact with the surgical wound.

**Aseptic Technique.** The process designed to exclude or avoid all germs. This technique is used in the operating area and in handling infectious diseases.

**Concurrent Disinfection.** Immediate disinfection and disposal of body discharges and infective matter through which a disease may be passed during the course of its progression. This process is being carried on constantly in professional offices and hospitals.

**Contamination.** Describes the state of an article or surface that may have become soiled through contact with non-sterile material, especially with the introduction of disease-producing or infectious organisms. If an object is not sterile it is then considered to be contaminated.

**Disinfection.** The destruction of pathogenic organisms by chemical or physical means, but commonly reserved for use only with chemical agents. A disinfectant is an agent that destroys infectious organisms. As ordinarily employed, the disinfection process may or may not be adequate for the destruction of all pathogens, such as the tubercle bacilli, spores, or certain viruses. Disinfectants should be used only on inanimate objects, and should not be confused with antiseptics that are applied to living tissue.

**Fumigation.** The process by which microorganisms or insects and vectors of infection are destroyed, usually by the use of gaseous agents; also defined as exposure to disinfecting fumes.

**Fungicide.** An agent that destroys fungi (has fungicidal action).

**Germicide.** An agent that destroys pathogenic organisms. Common usage involves the application of chemical agents to kill disease-producing germs, but not necessarily bacterial spores. Germicides are applied to living tissues, as well as to inanimate objects. Another commonly used term, with similar definition, is bacteriocide.

**Sanitization.** The act of making sanitary, an important step toward sterilization and disinfection. Sanitizing agents are usually water and detergents, utilized by scrubbing and soaking. Under no circumstances does sanitizing replace or substitute for sterilization. Sanitizing only reduces the number of bacteria on an item and removes certain protein substances so sterilization may be obtained. *Sanitization* is a less precise term than *disinfection* since it is more of a cleaning process.

**Sterilization.** The complete destruction of *all* forms of microbial life. An object which is free of all living organisms may be called *sterile.* Technically, there is no such thing as nearly sterile or partially sterile. An object is either sterile or it is contaminated.

**Vermicide.** An agent that destroys parasitic worms or intestinal animal parasites.

## Preparation for Sterilization

In the physician's office cleanliness takes the extreme form of sterilization. Sterilization reduces the perpetual threat of contamination to patients, to the physician, and to the medical assistant.

To assure proper sterilization, a definite area should be set aside in each office for just this purpose. This area should be divided into two sections. One section is used for receiving contaminated materials. This area should have a sink, as well as receiving basins, proper cleaning agents, brushes, sterilizer wrapping paper and envelopes, and indicators. The other section should be reserved for receiving the sterile items after they are removed from the sterilizer. Clear, clean plastic bags in which to store sterile packs may be kept in the sterile area.

Both areas should be spotlessly clean and well organized. If highly contaminated materials are to be handled, or if the medical assistant has an open cut or wound on her hands, she should wear disposable gloves in handling the contaminated items.

## CLASSIFICATION OF METHODS OF STERILIZATION AND DISINFECTION

There are many methods of sterilization and disinfection with varying degrees of value. It is extremely important to understand these methods, their advantages and disadvantages, the possible sources of error, and the proper technique of application.

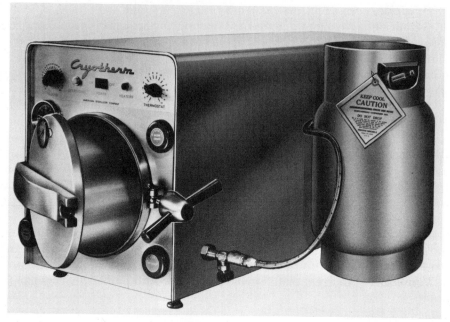

Gas sterilizer utilizing ethylene oxide. (Courtesy of American Sterilizer Company.)

## Physical Methods

### Radiation

ULTRAVIOLET. These rays, found in sunlight and ultraviolet lamps, are used to prevent airborne bacteria from spreading in operating rooms, classrooms, and bacteriological laboratories. Beauty salons and barber shops use ultraviolet rays in their cabinets. These rays are sometimes used in the preparation of certain vaccines. The cidal value of the ultraviolet ray varies greatly with the distance from the source, the air it passes through, and the surface of the article it hits. This form of radiation is not considered a method of sterilization because of its limitations and its lack of penetrating power.

X-RAYS. The x-ray, or roentgen ray, is known to have lethal power. These rays penetrate deeply and rapidly. Many authorities feel that the rays will be used for sterilization in the near future, but techniques must still be perfected. Their uses in a medical office are limited.

### Ultrasonics.
Ultrasonics are vibratory sound waves of such high frequency that they cannot be heard by the human ear. To date, these sound waves are used mainly for sanitization of instruments prior to their sterilization by placing the instruments in a bath and then passing the sound waves through it. This forms microscopic bubbles which create a terrific suction and pulling action on the materials attached to the instrument but does not damage even the most delicate of instruments.

### Refrigeration.
A few species of bacteria are killed by freezing temperatures, but a large majority of them survive even subzero temperatures. This method is not used for sterilization but rather for the preservation of foods. It

prevents the growth of bacteria. Upon thawing, growth and multiplication can resume, and often foods spoil more quickly.

**Filtration.**   When fluid substances cannot be subjected to heat without causing injury to them, they are filtered through unglazed porcelain with pores so minute that most of the bacteria are held back while the fluid passes through. This method is used for the sterilization of some drugs, bacterial toxins, antitoxins, and certain culture media. Viruses and rickettsiae which pass through these filters are known as filterable organisms. The most commonly used laboratory filter for this is the Berkfeld filter. The water supply of some cities is purified by the filtration method.

**Desiccation.**   Desiccation, or drying, is used to inhibit or preserve, especially bacterial cultures and foods. Often freezing and drying are performed rapidly for preservation. Spores are extremely resistant to this method. Desiccation is extremely limited for sterilization.

**Heat.**   Heat is the most widely used method of sterilization and disinfection in medical offices. The average organism is killed by heat of 145° F (65° C). The temperature at which an organism is killed is known as the *thermal death point.* This point of death is not a fixed temperature because of some variables, such as the time involved to reach this temperature, and the exposure time, as well as the surrounding environment. This is evident in the fact that if the temperature is increased the time may be decreased, or the reverse. In other words, the thermal death point is reached by a temperature and time formula. Other factors are also considered in this formula, such as toxins that are formed by the organism and pH changes.

DRY HEAT.   Dry heat can be produced by direct flame or ovens.

Incineration or burning by direct flame destroys an organism immediately. Bacteriological loops are flamed until the wire glows. For years, mothers have flamed needles for the removal of splinters. Incineration is used to destroy disposable items, as well as contaminated dressings, swabs, sputum cups, and so on. Ironing is a form of burning and is used in the home by ironing dressings just to the scorching point.

The use of dry heat ovens is a preferred method when direct contact with saturated steam is impractical. Dry heat penetrates slowly and unevenly, so longer exposure time is required. Most dry heat sterilizers are electrically heated and heavily insulated ovens with blowers to force air for even distribution of heat. These ovens should not be overloaded. Glassware should not touch other objects. Items should be kept away from the sides of the oven so air can circulate freely. It is advisable to heat the oven and cool it slowly. There are many variations of temperature and time, depending on the load, but the following are suggested:

340° F (170° C) for one hour
320° F (160° C) for two hours
250° F (121° C) for six hours

The great variance found in temperature and time is influenced by the type of substances being sterilized. For example, the destruction of some spores in anhydrous oil requires 320° F for 160 minutes, but with a very small amount of water added, less than 0.5 per cent, sterilization can be reached in 20 minutes at 320° F.

Some offices have attempted to use the autoclave as a dry heat oven, but it is not the most satisfactory method of sterilization. An autoclave equipped with a steam jacket and manual controls must be used in order to prevent the steam from automatically being transferred to the chamber. If jacket pressure is maintained around 15 to 18 pounds, the chamber walls are heated to about 250° F. This is very difficult to gauge, however, because the chamber thermometer gives an accurate reading only when steam is in the chamber. Sterilization by this method would require six hours, and this would be very difficult to accomplish. It is best to use this as a heating and drying source and NOT as a method of sterilization.

MOIST HEAT. The forms of moist heat are boiling water, free-flowing steam, and steam under pressure.

*Boiling water* (212° F or 100° C) kills most vegetative forms of pathogenic bacteria, but bacterial spores and some viruses associated with infectious hepatitis are resistant to boiling. Because of these limitations, boiling is discouraged as a means of sterilization, and is used for disinfection only.

No matter how much heat is applied or how vigorous the boil, water will reach only 212° F at sea level. The higher the elevation, the lower the temperature required to obtain a boil. For example, in Denver, Colorado, water boils at 202° F. Water in a boiler should first be taken to a brisk boil and then the heat turned down to produce a mild roll. Whenever bubbles are regularly formed, the water has reached the boiling temperature. All a violent boil does is to increase the amount of steam and the loss of water through evaporation. Boiling water is a very poor substitute for steam under pressure.

The addition of 2 per cent soda solution greatly increases the killing power of boiling water, as well as dissolves dried blood and other coagulable substances, but it is harmful to glass and rubber goods. Objects must be completely immersed and the timing started only after the water shows a rolling boil.

*Free-flowing steam* reaches the same temperature as boiling water. It is used for materials which would be harmed by higher temperatures and which cannot be immersed in water or subjected to dry heat. The fractional or intermittent method is used, *i.e.,* materials are exposed to flowing steam for 30 minutes on three successive days. The Arnold Sterilizer is used for this purpose. This fractional method is seldom employed in a medical office because of the time involved, but it is used in laboratories.

*Steam under pressure* as represented in the autoclave (Fig. 26–1) is the best and most accepted method of sterilization used to date in the medical office. It is fast, convenient, and dependable if certain rules of technique are followed. *Steam under pressure is used for the sole purpose of obtaining a higher moist heat.* The increased pressure alone offers no advantage. It is the higher heat plus the moisture of the steam that is more effective, with the moisture playing a very important part. The two factors of heat *and* moisture must be present to be effective. When steam is admitted into the autoclave chamber it condenses on the cold objects, simultaneously heating and wetting the object, coagulating proteins, and destroying all living organisms. *All* surfaces must be contacted by this moisture. Steam under pressure is capable of much faster penetration of fabrics and textiles than dry head BUT it has definite limitations if the rules are not followed.

Incorrect operation of an autoclave may result in superheated steam. When

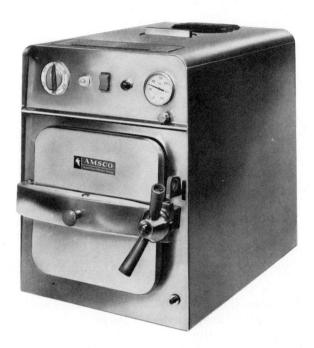

**Figure 26-1** Medical office autoclave. (Courtesy AMSCO American Sterilizer Company, Erie, Pa.)

the steam is brought to a higher temperature, it is literally dried out and the advantage of a higher heat is diminished. It then acts more as hot air, with less penetrative ability, and possibly is ineffective as sterilization. Wet steam is another cause of incomplete sterilization. This presents a particularly difficult problem with fabric packs because the packs are soaked with moisture and the steam becomes ineffective. Moreover, it is extremely difficult to dry the packs during the drying cycle. A wet pack literally sucks up bacteria from the air and any surface it is placed upon.

Wet steam may result from failing to pre-heat the chamber, resulting in excessive condensation in the interior of the chamber. It can be compared to taking a hot shower in a cold bathroom, which results in heavily steamed mirrors and tile walls. Cold instruments placed in a hot chamber will also increase condensation. A little condensation is helpful, but excessive moisture is not. Other causes of a wet load are opening the door too wide during the drying cycle and allowing a rush of cold air into the chamber; also, over-filling the water reservoir may produce a wet load.

The main cause for incomplete sterilization in the autoclave is the presence of residual air. Without the complete elimination of air, an adequately high temperature cannot be reached. *Air and steam do not mix.* Since air is heavier than steam it will pool wherever possible. One-tenth of 1 per cent residual air trapped in the chamber will prevent complete sterilization. This is especially dangerous in older autoclaves that do not have a chamber thermometer separate from the temperature marks on the same gauge as the pounds pressure. *Fifteen pounds pressure does not guarantee 250° F.*

All escape valves and discharge lines must be kept clean and free from dirt and lint. Air will flow out of jars, cans, bottles, and containers, as water would flow out, if they are properly placed on their sides. If the operator mentally visu-

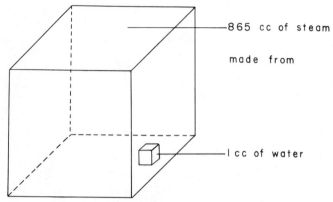

**Figure 26-2** Quantitative aspects of water and steam.

alizes water for air she can then visualize this air flowing out as water would flow out by gravity. One cubic centimeter of water will provide 865 cubic centimeters of steam (Fig, 26–2), so containers that cannot be placed on their sides should have a few drops of water placed in them before loading; the steam forming will force out the air that would otherwise be trapped in the container.

Many autoclaves consist of a sterilizing chamber surrounded by an outer jacket. (Because there are so many different models used in medical offices, the authors will discuss general principles only). Steam is admitted in the bottom of the jacket from the water reservoir as the water boils and forms steam. The connection into the chamber is closed until the jacket pressure is sufficient to transfer into the chamber. This connection is opened manually or automatically, depending on the model. The steam then flows from the jacket into the chamber from the upper rear of the chamber (Fig. 26–3). This flow of steam from the upper rear drives the air in the chamber down, forward, and out the air exhaust valve. Remember, air is heavier than steam and will flow out, if not trapped, like water flowing out of a sink. When the air in the chamber has been driven out and the temperature starts to rise, the thermostatic valve will automatically close, sealing off the chamber at the air exhaust valve. Autoclaves have numerous gauges: one indicates the jacket pressure; one indicates the chamber pressure, and another indicates the chamber temperature. Some of the older models have the temperature marking on the same gauge as the chamber pressure. As stated before, pressure gives no guarantee of temperature. When the pressure in the chamber starts to rise, you then should watch the chamber temperature gauge. You *do not* start your timing of the load until the desired temperature has been reached. Then adjust the heat control to maintain the temperature and set the time clock.

The autoclave chamber must be cleaned before each loading. If there has been any ebullition of solutions, the water reservoir must be drained and thoroughly cleaned and rinsed. On many models there is no access to the reservoir and it must be cleaned by a professional serviceman. Check the manufacturer's instructions carefully and do not use a commercial cleaner unless advised by the manufacturer. A mild detergent may be used in the chamber but make

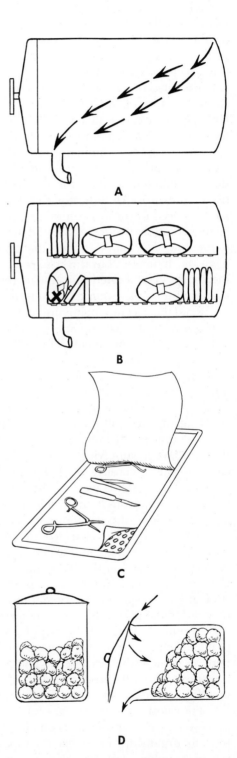

**Figure 26–3** A. Cross section of a cylinder type autoclave. Arrows indicate the direction of the flow of steam and air elimination.

B. The X marks the placement of an indicator near the exhaust outlet. Note the jar is placed on the side with the lid opened and the glove envelopes are on end. The packs are not crowded and there is space between top and bottom shelf.

C. Instruments are placed on a thin towel on a tray and covered with a layer of towel. All jointed instruments are opened to permit steam to all surfaces. All trays used should be perforated.

D. Shows the flow of steam into the right container but not into the left one. An indicator should be placed in the lower back of the container on the right.

certain it is very thoroughly rinsed after using any type of cleaner. Many manufacturers will not honor a guarantee if anything other than distilled water is used or if any type of cleaner has been put through the reservoir tank.

The trays must also be kept clean and free of lint. Do not remove the bottom tray except to clean. It must be in place for proper steam circulation. The air exhaust valve is one of the most important parts of the autoclave and must be clean and free of lint, otherwise the air will not exhaust from the chamber. Unless proper care is taken of the autoclave, the dressings and instruments will have been *well heated* but not *sterilized.*

*Indicators.* To eliminate the constant doubt of complete sterilization, indicators should be used. These indicators show, by melting or by changing color, that a certain temperature for a given period of time has been reached, irrespective of pressure. An indicator should be placed with each load, buried deep in packs, placed in constriction tubes, put in the bottoms of containers that cannot be turned on their sides, or located in any other places that might be inaccessible to the flow of steam. Many feel that an indicator is not necessary if the chamber has a thermometer, but this tells you the temperature only where the tip of the thermometer is located and not in the above-mentioned places. An indicator should also be placed in the lower front near the air exhaust valve.

Read the accompanying instructions for the indicator you use. The dangers of incomplete sterilization are too great for you to be lax in your technique or in the care of the equipment. The A.T.I. Steam-Clox indicator will give you an extra check on your sterilization. It consists of a small piece of paper with four spots on it that change color from purple to green. The different spots indicate different times during the sterilization procedure and show the operator the progress of sterilization. These spots change color only in the presence of heat AND steam; they will not change in the presence of heat alone.

To illustrate: If only spot No. 1 changes color, there is a definite failure of the autoclave in supplying steam or eliminating air from the chamber. This spot changes after exposure of 250° F for two minutes, which is not enough for sterilization. Spot 2 is used to check the sterility of rubber goods, instruments, and other nonporous items which can be thoroughly cleaned before sterilization. This spot allows the minimum exposure time and temperature (250° F in 10 minutes) for such hard-surfaced items. Spot 3 is recommended for use when packs of gauze sponges and dressings are to be sterilized. These items may have bacteria imbedded in the fibers that revert to more resistant spores. This spot changes color after 15 minutes exposure at 250° F. Spot 4 is in the center and is circular. If this spot turns green it indicates needlessly long exposure, resulting in wasted time and unnecessary deterioration of materials.

Another indicator that is popular and has proved useful is the small, hermetically sealed glass tube that contains a tiny pellet which requires only five to eight minutes to melt when exposed to 250° F. At a slightly lower temperature (245° F) it requires 20 to 30 minutes to melt. These sealed glass indicators may be placed in a fluid without damage to themselves or to the fluid.

The most accepted means of determining the efficiency of sterilization processes is the indicator that contains dried bacterial spores of established, heat-resistant organisms. These bacterial spore strips are available commercially from reliable suppliers, but the indicators are not always practical for a physician's of-

**TABLE 26–1**  TIPS FOR IMPROVING YOUR AUTOCLAVING
TECHNIQUES

---

### LINENS
#### Too Damp

| *Probable Cause* | *Correction* |
|---|---|
| Clogged chamber drain. | Remove strainer; free openings of lint. |
| Goods removed from chamber too soon following cycle. | Allow goods to remain in sterilizer an additional 15 minutes with door slightly open. |
| Improper loading. | Place packs on edge; arrange for least possible resistance to flow of steam and air. |

| *Stained* | |
|---|---|
| Dirty chamber. | Clean chamber with Calgonite solution. Never use strong abrasives, steel wool, and so forth. |
| | Rinse thoroughly after cleaning. |

### INSTRUMENTS
#### Corroded

| | |
|---|---|
| Poor cleaning; residual soil. | Improve cleaning. Do not allow soil to dry on instruments. Sanitize first. |
| Exposure to hard chemicals (iodine, salt, acids, and so on). | Do not expose instruments to these chemicals. If exposure occurs, rinse immediately. |
| Inferior instruments. | Use only top quality instruments. |

#### Spotted or Stained

| | |
|---|---|
| Mineral deposits on instruments. | Wash with soft soap and detergent with good wetting properties. |
| Residual detergents from cleaning. | Rinse instruments thoroughly. |
| Mineral deposits from tap water. | Rinse with distilled water. |

#### Stiff Hinges or Joints

| | |
|---|---|
| Corrosion or soil in joint. | Clean with warm, weak acid solution (10% nitric acid solution). Rinse thoroughly after. |
| Jaws and shanks out of alignment. | Realignment by qualified instrument repairman. |

### SOLUTIONS
#### Ebullition or Caps Blow Off

| | |
|---|---|
| Exhausting chamber too rapidly. | Use slow exhaust, cool liquids, or turn autoclave off and let cool at its own speed. That is, let the pressure decrease at its own rate. |

### MECHANICAL
#### Steam Leakage

| | |
|---|---|
| Worn gasket. | Replace |
| Door closes improperly. | Re-open door and shut carefully. Have serviced if unable to close door properly. |

#### Chamber Door Will Not Open

| | |
|---|---|
| Vacuum in chamber (check chamber pressure gauge). | Turn on controls to starting steam pressure and wait until equalized, then vent and open door. |

---

*(Adapted from *Tips for Improving Your Sterilizing Techniques*. Prepared by the Education and Research Departments of AMSCO (American Sterilizer Company), Erie, Pennsylvania.)

fice because the strip, after autoclaving, must be sent to a bacteriological laboratory for sterility testing.

Autoclave or sterilizer tapes frequently have some form of indicator on them that changes after exposure to sterilization procedures. These tapes are excellent for securing packages and bags, but they are not to be used as sterilizer indicators. They never were intended for this purpose; they only indicate that the package has been processed, not that sterility has been reached.

Sterilization indicator bags are also very convenient. They are made of disposable paper or glassine paper in which syringes, tubing and many other items can be sterilized and stored. The paper or glassine is permeable to steam and provides a barrier against airborne bacteria during storage. Each bag has an indicator printed on it, similar to the sterilizer tape. It shows that the bag has been autoclaved but does not prove it is sterile.

*Wrapping Materials.* The maintenance of sterility is completely dependent upon the wrapper and its porosity, as well as on the method of wrapping. The wrapping material must be permeable to steam but impervious to contaminants such as dust and insects. Muslin should be of 140-thread count and a double thickness used. Canvas or duck fabric is not advisable because steam cannot penetrate it properly. Paper is the most popular wrap in the physician's office. It should be permeable to steam, resistant to contamination, but able to withstand

**TABLE 26–2** STERILIZATION CHART

| Article | Method | Temperature | Time |
|---|---|---|---|
| Gauze, small, loosely packed | Autoclave | 250 F | 30 minutes |
| Gauze, large, loosely packed | Autoclave | 270°F | 30 minutes |
| Gauze, small, tightly packed | Autoclave | 250°F | 40 minutes |
| Gauze, large, lightly packed | Autoclave | 270°F | 40 minutes |
| Gauze, tightly packed | Dry heat | 320°F | 3 hours |
| Gauze, loosely packed | Dry heat | 320°F | 2 hours |
| Glass syringes in tubes | Autoclave | 250°F | 30 minutes |
| Glass syringe and needle in muslin | Autoclave | 250°F | 30 minutes |
| Glass syringe in muslin | Dry heat | 320°F | 1 hour |
| Hypodermic needle in muslin | Dry heat | 320°F | 2 hours |
| Instruments on tray, muslin under and over | Dry heat | 320°F | 1 hour |
| Instruments on tray, muslin under and over | Autoclave | 250°F | 15 minutes |
| Rubber gloves in glove envelopes | Autoclave | 250°F | 15 minutes |
| Solutions in flasks with gauze plug | Autoclave | 250°F | 30 minutes |
| Glassware unwrapped | Dry heat | 320°F | 1 hour |
| Glassware wrapped | Autoclave | 250°F | 30 minutes |
| Petroleum jel, 1 oz. jar | Dry heat | 340°F | 1 hour |
| Petroleum jel, 1 oz. jar | Dry heat | 320°F | 2 hours |
| Petroleum gauze in instrument tray | Dry heat | 320°F | 150 minutes |
| Powder, 1 oz. jar | Dry heat | 320°F | 2 hours |
| Powder, small glove packs | Autoclave | 250°F | 15 minutes |

Remember to always place an indicator in areas where there is doubt that the steam will penetrate.

DO NOT MEASURE BY CHAMBER POUNDS. A THERMOMETER AND INDICATOR ARE THE RELIABLE METHODS OF JUDGING A KILLING TEMPERATURE.

the moisture of steam without disintegrating. The paper must be of a quality that will not become brittle with heat or storage. There are several manufacturers of "sterilizer paper," such as Dennison and Kraft. Paper lends itself well to autoclaving but tends to become brittle with dry heat. This can happen with autoclaving if the drying cycle is too long. For this reason, it is not advisable to autoclave muslin wraps with paper wraps because of the difference in the drying cycle time. Glassine bags also tend to become brittle and may stick to a metal surface, but they are transparent and allow easy visibility of contents. Aluminum foil is used only for dry heat sterilization. Cellophane may be autoclaved but should not be subjected to dry heat sterilization. Plastics should not be used as wrappers unless specifically recommended.

There is great diversity in the length of time supplies may be considered to remain sterile. If the storage area is dust free and has very limited air circulation, if the packs are not handled and are covered with clean plastic bags, then it is generally felt they will remain sterile for at least 30 days. When an item is resterilized it must be completely reprocessed with a new wrapper. Any time a package seal is broken or damaged in any way, it is considered contaminated.

## Causes of Incomplete Sterilization

1. Inadequate sanitation
2. Incorrect loading of autoclave chamber
   a. overloading
   b. placing jars in upright position
   c. allowing small trays to act as barriers
   d. placing articles horizontally and not vertically
   e. removing bottom tray and placing items on autoclave floor
3. Dirty or clogged discharge air exhaust line
4. Reading pressure rather than temperature
5. Improper placement of indicators
6. Inadequate drying during drying cycle
7. Incorrect wrapping
8. Using nonpermeable wrapping material
9. Failure to maintain full correct temperature during entire cycle
10. Starting timing before correct temperature is reached
11. Failure to pre-heat chamber for first load

## Chemical Disinfection

Remember the term "sterilization" means the complete destruction of all living organisms. This is an absolute term and cannot be used with such words as "almost or "partially." The Council on Pharmacology and Chemistry of the American Medical Association has reported:

The Council on Pharmacology and Chemistry has formally gone on record as disapproving of the use of the terms "sterilize," "sterile" and "sterilization" in a bacteriological sense other than in their correct scientific significance; i.e., meaning the absence or destruction of all microorganisms. These terms are not relative and to permit their use in a relative sense not only is incorrect but opens the way to abuse and misunderstanding.

The term "disinfection" is therefore preferred when discussing chemical means of killing organisms. Chemical disinfection has certain limitations and is very difficult to verify since there are no convenient indicators such as those used for steam pressure sterilization. Most commercial promotions of disinfectants are directed toward the killing of staphylococci. Some claim cidal powers on tubercle bacilli, fungi, and even spores and viruses. Because physicians and medical assistants are not familiar with chemical disinfectants, they can only rely upon established, ethical manufacturers who have rigid tests and standardization of their products and do not make false advertising claims.

Disinfectants are used because they are convenient and are often the agent of choice because some materials are damaged by heat; e.g., fine cutting edges, lensed instruments, and synthetics that are not thermostable.

A good disinfectant and antiseptic should be effective in a moderately low concentration; it should not irritate tissue (this applies to antiseptics more than to disinfectants); it should retain its potency in the presence of some dead organic matter; it should not be too volatile with a high evaporation; and it should be effective within a reasonable length of time. Often a disinfectant solution is not effective because (1) it is left in an open container where evaporation changes its consistency; (2) sanitized instruments are not dried, and the wet instruments, when placed in the solution, dilute it beyond the manufacturer's recommendation; or (3) items are not thoroughly sanitized before being placed in the solution, and the attached organic matter changes the action of the disinfectant.

Fabrics placed in the bottom of a container or instrument tray are often the cause of weakening a solution because chemicals are trapped in the fibers and are not in solution. The solution in containers with fabric in the bottom should be changed more frequently than should the solution in containers without fabric pads.

Destruction of organisms by chemical means varies greatly, depending upon the type of chemical used. No chemical can kill unless it reaches the instrument's surface; therefore, complete sanitization is absolutely necessary. Very strong agents will kill in a short time but they are usually very hard on an instrument. Time and strength cannot be separated. Temperature is somewhat of a factor, although most agents are used at room temperature. The effectiveness of some agents is increased by adding to boiling water; others are less effective if chilled. Reliable manufacturers will state the organisms that can be expected to be killed by the solution in a specified dilution, for a specified time. They will also state which organisms will not be killed.

## Commonly Used Chemicals

**Soap.**  For many years soap was considered the "all-purpose" disinfectant but studies have shown that soap has very limited killing power. It is the scrubbing action and the running water that have real value, as in handwashing and sanitizing. The average household soap has limited effect, but since soap is not a single chemical there are additives that do have cidal power. Although there is considerable controversy on "germicidal" or "surgical" soaps, there are some germicidal soaps that do kill organisms, mainly staphylococci, which are the greatest offenders on our skin. These germicidal soaps leave a film of disinfectant on the skin that will last for several hours. Hexachlorophene is virtually insoluble in water but soluble in alcohol, so it will remain on the skin and not be removed by a routine handwash, but it is removed if the hands are rinsed in alcohol.

**Detergents.**     These are mainly wetting agents to increase penetrating and wetting power; they are sometimes called "soapless" soap. Because of their ability to emulsify fats and oils, they aid in the mechanical removal of bacteria, especially from the skin. Detergents that are very alkaline are corrosive to aluminum and will also attack ground glass surfaces, such as syringes. Strong alkaline detergents are also harmful to rubber. Most detergents are slightly alkaline and may be used for general purposes but it is best to use detergents that are manufactured for cleaning glassware and rubber goods.

**Alcohol.**     Alcohol is the most widely used disinfectant. Absolute alcohol has very limited germicidal action, but it is markedly increased in effect when in a 70 per cent dilution. Ethyl alcohol had been widely used in the past, but isopropyl alcohol has become more frequently used. It exhibits slightly greater germicidal action than ethyl alcohol. It is an excellent fat solvent and therefore good for cleansing the skin, but continued use is hard on the hands. Iodine and other chemicals are sometimes added to alcohol to increase its cidal powers. Alcohol may be used to disinfect delicate instruments but it tends to rust them. Care should be used in cleansing lensed instruments with alcohol because it may dissolve the cement around the lenses. It is a good cleanser but any excess should be wiped off or allowed to evaporate before using the instruments.

**Acids.**     Acids in concentrated form are excellent germicides but are corrosive. The more they are diluted to decrease these hazards, the less valuable they are as disinfectants. Boric acid is a very weak antiseptic even in saturated solutions. On the other hand, nitric acid is extremely caustic and is still used in treating bites of animals.

**Phenol.**     Phenol (carbolic acid) was first used as an antiseptic in 1865 by Joseph Lister. It is toxic to tissues in strong dilutions but is often added to other agents. Pure phenol is used as a standard for testing disinfectants. This standardization is the cidal action of an agent as compared to phenol acting for the same length of time, on the same organisms and at the same dilutions. This procedure is useful but has limitations because of the various requirements an antiseptic should meet. These comparisons are carefully set according to the specifications of the United States Food and Drug Administration. Hexachlorophene is a phenolic derivative.

**Alkalines.**     These include lye and quicklime. They are extremely corrosive and are used mainly for sanitation of barns, chicken houses, and so on. A pasty mixture is called "milk of lime" and a thin dilution is known as "whitewash."

**Formaldehyde.**     Formaldehyde (formalin) has strong disinfectant properties and is used as a preservative of tissue (10 per cent solution). A 5 per cent solution is actively germicidal and sporicidal in the presence of organic matter. It is irritating to tissue, and any instrument disinfected with it must be thoroughly rinsed with sterile water before use. It should be used at room temperature because cooling reduces its cidal power.

**Metals.** Certain metals are used in antiseptics and are very effective. Silver is used as silver nitrate ($AgNO_3$) in many different percentages, and as argyrol in 5 to 20 per cent aqueous solutions. Mercury is used as bichloride of mercury, mercurochrome, and merthiolate. Arsenic and zinc are also used.

**Oxidizing Agents.** Oxidizing agents such as hydrogen peroxide ($H_2O_2$) are used for bacteria that are anaerobic—that is, they cannot exist in the presence of free oxygen. These agents are usually not stable and are considered only mildly antiseptic but are used to irrigate cuts and minor wounds.

**Dyes.** Dyes are sometimes used as germicides, but they are considered mild. With the discovery of sulfonamides, dyes are not used as much today. They are more bacteriostatic and fungicidal than antiseptic. Some of the dyes used are crystal violet, carbol fuchsin, and brilliant green.

**Oils.** Oils have a weak germicidal effect. They are used more for their pleasant odor and mild astringent effect than for antisepsis. Some of the oils used are cloves, pine, wintergreen, thyme, and peppermint.

**Iodine.** As tincture of iodine, an alcoholic solution, this is the traditional agent for cuts and abrasions, and for preoperative preparation of the skin. A 1 or 2 per cent solution dissolved in 70 per cent alcohol is an excellent skin antiseptic. It may be irritating to the tissues. A 2 per cent aqueous iodine solution is often used as an instrument disinfectant in emergency situations. However, because it is a tincture, it tends to evaporate and become stronger, burning the skin and having less antiseptic power. There are many commercial iodine compounds that are less dangerous to use and are stable. It is generally considered to be more of an antiseptic than a disinfectant.

**Quaternary Ammonium Compounds.** These are very popular. Zephiran is an example. They are highly stable and nonirritating when used as directed. They are in tincture solutions for skin antisepsis and in aqueous solutions for instrument disinfection.

**Gas.** Using gas for sterilization is both old and new. Fumigation is an old method used for many years, but new products that are destroyed by heat, moisture, or chemicals have required newer methods. Formaldehyde was used over 50 years ago to fumigate sickrooms and laboratories. It was adequate for large areas but was effective only on exposed surfaces and required considerable airing before the area was tolerable. Gas sterilizers using moderately heated mixtures of ethylene oxide with low humidity are useful for such materials as leather, fabrics, and paper goods and are especially good for delicate cutting instruments and lensed instruments.

The chief advantage of gas is its ability to sterilize materials that would otherwise be destroyed by heat and moisture. Its disadvantages are the longer exposure periods required, which range from 6 to 16 hours. Liquid ethylene oxide acts as a solvent to some acrylic plastics. It may crack, or "spiderweb," or give plastics a "milky" appearance. There may be residual gas in rubber goods, leather, and plastics; these materials require several hours of airing before they are free of the gas.

The preparation of articles to be sterilized by this method is the same as with the steam pressure method, making certain the wrappings are permeable to the gas. There are excellent indicators available for gas sterilization so the operator can tell if complete sterilization has taken place.

IT IS EXTREMELY IMPORTANT THAT YOU READ THE LABELS CAREFULLY ON ALL CHEMICAL ANTISEPTIC AGENTS. Many times the anxious salesman may mislead you or try to save you a few pennies. Read to see if a solution is a *sporicide*, a *tuberculocide*, or an *antiseptic*.

## Sterilization of Items Used in the Physician's Office

**Dressings.** There are as many different designs of surgical dressings as there are surgical techniques. The American Medical Association has found about 5000 different styles in use. Frequently the same dressing has several different names.

Some medical offices make their own dressings, but usually the machine-made dressings are less expensive, are more uniform in size and shape, and save considerable time for the medical assistant as well. These dressings may be purchased in large bulk nonsterile packages and rewrapped in smaller packs for autoclaving. Pre-sterilized individual packaging increases the cost considerably for materials that are used in quantity.

Most dressings and gauze sponges are made of cotton, but some are made of silk, wool, or wood fibers (cellulose). They are folded in various sizes and shapes, with all raw edges carefully placed inside the folds. Ravelings from raw edges could cling to a wound and act as a foreign body. Some dressings have a thin layer of synthetic material that will not adhere to a wound.

Dressings should be sterilized in the autoclave or by dry heat. Wrap them in small packets with a double layer of muslin or with sterilizer paper. Muslin wraps may be reused but must be washed, and checked for holes and lint. Muslin will discolor with repeated heating. Each packet should be firm enough to hold together during normal handling but not too tightly packed to permit the flow of steam and heat. The packets are sealed with sterilizer tape, labeled, and dated. Pins are not too satisfactory because they leave holes. Pins should be completely embedded in the pack except for the head; otherwise, when the pin is removed the unsterile areas of the pin will be drawn through the sterile dressing. The use of sterilizer tape can serve several purposes: to fasten a package, identify the contents, and indicate the pack has been sterilized. Do not crowd the packs too closely together in the chamber, as this would prevent complete circulation of steam and heat.

If your office does not have an autoclave and you need sterile dressings, make up several small packs, place them in a pillow case and send them to your doctor's hospital for sterilization. Make certain the package is well marked with the doctor's name, the date, the contents, and the manner in which you wish the dressings to be sterilized. Most hospitals are very cooperative, but they should be allowed ample time to complete the work. These extra packs are put into the autoclaves at odd hours whenever time permits.

Remember that a six-inch pack takes twice as long to penetrate as a three-inch pack. An indicator should be placed in the thickest part of a pack. It is inad-

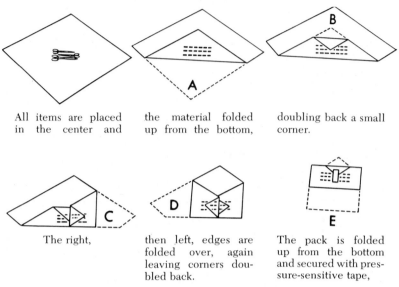

All items are placed in the center and

the material folded up from the bottom,

doubling back a small corner.

The right,

then left, edges are folded over, again leaving corners doubled back.

The pack is folded up from the bottom and secured with pressure-sensitive tape,

**Figure 26–4**   Steps in wrapping dressings for sterilizing.

visable to mix dressings and instruments in the same load because the timing must be set for the longest time that is required for the dressings, and this increased time is hard on the instruments.

**Jars, Bottles, and Trays.**   Jars, bottles and trays must be wrapped and placed on their sides to be autoclaved. The wraps should be secured with string and not with rubber bands if sterilized by dry heat. If these items are not to be stored sterile they need not be wrapped. Covers on jars and containers should never be put in place, but put on one side or slightly ajar, otherwise steam cannot circulate

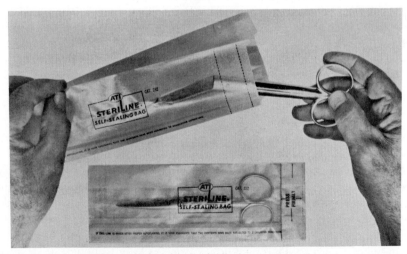

**Figure 26–5**   Instruments autoclaved individually for easy identification and storage. (Courtesy Aseptic-Thermo Indicator Co.)

inside and drive out trapped air. These caps and lids are replaced before being removed from the chamber, taking care not to contaminate them.

**Oils and Ointments.**    The sterilization of oils and ointments presents a different problem. Because steam cannot penetrate oils, it is best to sterilize oily substances by dry heat, usually for one hour at 320° F for a one-ounce jar. A four-ounce jar would require 100 minutes for sterilization by dry heat.

The most common item in this group would be gauze dressings impregnated with petroleum jelly (vaseline). These are sterilized in glass jars or metal instrument boats. Once the container has been opened and some contents removed it is considered to be contaminated. For this reason, it is best to sterilize small amounts at a time. Use heat resistant glassware and metals and do not place the cover directly over the top but tilt it slightly. Autoclave these items the same as you would a fluid (petroleum jelly is the same as mineral oil when heated.) Be very careful not to decrease the pressure rapidly or there will be ebullition, which could possibly require a professional service cleaning of the autoclave. Read the manufacturer's instructions. Some guarantees are void if oils and solutions have been processed in the autoclave. The use of dry heat is suggested for these substances.

**Solutions.**    Some medical offices wish to keep bottles of sterile distilled water or normal saline on hand for irrigating and rinsing purposes. (These solutions are not to be used as injectables). Sterilization of irrigating and rinsing solutions may be done in an autoclave that has a "Fluids Vent" cycle; otherwise, there will be an ebullition of the solution.

To prepare these solutions for autoclaving, use a Pyrex container. Fill the container about two-thirds full, no more, and place a hermetically sealed glass tube indicator in the solution. Make a plug by covering a couple of cotton balls with gauze and secure with a rubber band. Do not make the plug too large or too tight in the neck of the container, because steam must circulate through. Do not use cotton alone because it will leave lint on the inside neck of the container. Next, cover the top of the container with a double layer of muslin or paper wrap, secure with a rubber band. This will keep the lips of the container sterile for pouring purposes. Now date and label the contents (see Fig. 26–6).

**Powders.**    Powders are best sterilized by dry heat. They are prepared the same as oils. The timing is two hours for a one-ounce jar at 320° F or one

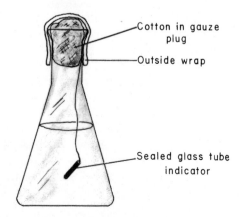

**Figure 26–6**    Preparation of solution for sterilizing.

hour at 430° F. Some powders, such as sulfonamides, should be run at a lower temperature of 285° F for three hours. Talcum to be used with gloves may be run at 320° F for 55 minutes in small packets of about two tablespoons each. Always check first to make certain a powder may be sterilized by a heat method.

**Tubing.**   Wash and clean well and rinse with distilled water. Shake out the excess water, leaving a small amount of moisture which will form steam and drive out the trapped air. Steam pressure sterilization is best for tubing that can withstand the heat; therefore, follow the manufacturer's recommendations. If chemical disinfection is indicated, use 70 per cent isopropyl alcohol for 15 minutes, or other recommended agents. Then rinse again with sterile water before use. Nylons have excellent chemical resistance, except some may be soluble in alcohol and/or phenols. Also, some synthetics absorb chemicals if they are soaked too long.

**Rubber Goods.**   Too much heat, light, moisture, or exposure to certain chemicals destroys many rubbers. These items are sterilized separately, not only because they require a different sterilization time but also because they discolor metals and may stick to them. Improper handling of rubber can destroy it.

Here are general instructions for handling rubber goods. Always rinse rubber in cool running water immediately after use. If necessary, such items should be placed in a basin of disinfectant, then washed well in warm water and cleansing agents, such as soap. Do not use detergents, scouring powders, ammonia compounds or bleaches on rubber. Open all pockets and folds while cleaning and remove metal clips. Rinse well in warm water and towel dry as thoroughly as possible. Powder with a glove talcum to prevent sticking. Hot water bottles and ice bags should be drained by hanging upside down. When they are dry, they should be inflated and capped. The inside surfaces of rubber should not be allowed to touch. Tubing should be hung over two pegs to prevent sharp turns in rubber which may crack. Do not soak rubber too long. All rubber goods should be dusted with powder and wrapped if placed in storage.

Methods of sterilization of rubber goods include autoclaving and some chemicals. Boiling and other chemicals are used for disinfection. Rubber goods that are to be boiled should be sanitized as previously described and wrapped lightly in gauze before being placed in the boiler, to prevent them from contacting the metal tray and sides of the boiler. Make certain all air pockets are eliminated. It is sometimes necessary to place a weight on the articles to keep them completely immersed. Boil about 15 to 20 minutes but do not overboil. Remove them with sterile tongs and place them on a clean or sterile field that has a barrier back to prevent contamination from the under side. They may be dusted with sterile powder, wrapped and labeled. Rubber goods should be considered disinfected but not sterile.

Rubber goods are prepared for chemical disinfection in the same manner as for boiling, but will have to be rinsed with sterile water after being removed from the disinfectant solution.

**Autoclaving.**   Rubber gloves are the most common rubber materials which require sterilization. Although most offices now use disposable gloves, some may wish to have reusable gloves on hand. Gloves should never be autoclaved atop each other because the pressure will prevent the proper flow of steam into the

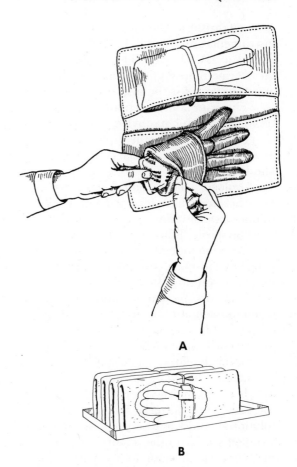

**Figure 26–7** A, Method of preparing gloves for autoclaving. B, Packs of glove envelopes.

A

B

fingers. They should be placed in glove envelopes with the thumbs up, as shown in Figure 26–7A.

As with all rubber goods, steam must contact all surfaces of the glove in order to effect complete sterilization. After the glove has been carefully sanitized it is towel dried. Gauze may be placed in the palm of the glove but this should be large enough to allow for the flow of steam into the fingers and permit easy removal without contamination to the outside of the glove. The cuff is then folded down over another layer of gauze (Fig. 26–7B). Place in the glove envelope with the thumbs toward the outside folds. Load the packs in the autoclave with the thumbs up to allow the air to flow out. The usual grade of good rubber can not withstand autoclaving of more than 15 to 20 minutes.

Remember that all wrapped and autoclaved items must be properly labeled and dated.

## Sterilization Problems in Specialty Offices

**Obstetrics and Gynecology.** Routine examination equipment, such as vaginal specula and uterine dressing forceps, is sometimes carelessly cleaned and "rushed through" chemical disinfectants. More offices are now autoclaving these instruments and storing them in clean toweling. Any instrument that penetrates the tissue MUST BE STERILIZED and stored sterile. Some examples include the uterine biopsy punch, uterine tenaculum, cervical dilators and sounds, and any item used for the insertion of an IUD.

The common infections in the OB/Gyn office are VD, monilia, *E. Coli*, trichomonas and staphylococci from the perineal area and from vaginal discharges. Be very careful while handling contaminated items, especially from a gonorrhea infection, which could result in gonorrheal conjunctivitis and possible blindness.

**Urology.** These offices have many problems that are unique to urology. Such problems have lessened with the use of disposable syringes, catheters, and solution bowls. Items used for insertion into the urethra and bladder instillation must be sterile. Reusable catheters are a major source of contamination and are not recommended. Office-sterilized instillation medications may contain pyogenic substances even if they are sterile. It is best to use reliable commercially prepared solutions.

If cystoscopic examinations are done in the office, extreme care must be taken to maintain sterility. A majority of these procedures are now done in the hospital. Office vasectomies must be done with sterile operating room techniques to prevent contamination.

**Ophthalmology.** The major concern here is in the careless use of eyedrops and careless handling of the medicine dropper. The use of stock solutions has long been discouraged because of the dangers of the solution becoming a culture for pathogenic bacteria. Eye ointments present a similar problem. Only sterile solutions should be used if there is a laceration or ulceration in the eye. Instruments used for the removal of a foreign body should be sterile. It is advisable to reserve a medication for the patient for whom it is prescribed and not use it on other patients.

**Ear, Nose and Throat.** Routine examination instruments are sterilized after use and stored in a clean area. The main danger here is in the changing of dressings, placing of packs, and in performing minor surgery. Dressing forceps are often returned to a disinfectant solution and used again before the time lapse required to disinfect. There is frequently some carelessness in handling such items as tracheotomy tubes.

**Neurology.** Most neurological offices do not use many items that puncture the skin so sterilization technique may become lax or is never practiced. The most crucial technique done in the neurological office may be a spinal puncture, but this is rare nowadays since most physicians prefer to use the hospital for this procedure. Surveys have shown that on rare occasions spinal needles which have been carefully cleaned and autoclaved have caused aseptic meningitis as a result of pyogens in the distilled water. This can be avoided by using disposable needles that have been sterilized by dry heat or gas sterilization.

**Pediatrics.** It has been known for many years that the main source of cross infection in pediatrics has been the fever thermometer. Because it is used so frequently, the thermometer does not have time to disinfect between uses. Often there is some carelessness in rinsing and wiping the thermometer before returning it to the disinfectant. The disinfecting solution may not be changed or the container sterilized as frequently as it should be. Usually alcohol is used in the container and this solution is not a tuberculocide or virucide, especially for hepatitis virus. Thermometers used by patients with hepatitis should be discarded and not used again.

There is also carelessness involved in removing small foreign objects from the skin, such as splinters. Sterile procedure and sterile instruments must always be used when entering the skin, regardless of how uncooperative the patient may be.

**Thoracic Medicine.**   The most common source of contamination here is in the use of the pulmonary function test equipment. These machines are difficult to sterilize and asepsis is frequently ignored. The interior of the apparatus is not accessible and cannot be sterilized except by gas sterilization. The parts that are nearest the patient should be autoclaved or carefully disinfected. Disposable parts such as mouthpieces and tubes are available.

## REFERENCES

Perkins, J. J., *Principles and Methods of Sterilization in Health Sciences* (2nd Ed.), Charles C Thomas Publishers, Springfield, Ill., 1970.

Seedor, M. M., *Introduction to Asepsis;* A Programmed Unit in Fundamentals of Nursing (Revised Ed.), Bureau of Publications, Teachers College, Columbia University.

# Chapter 27

**BEHAVIORAL OBJECTIVES**

*The medical office assistant should be able to:*

Identify the need for accuracy and care in collection, labeling, and handling of specimens in the medical office.

Describe routine procedures involved in the examination and testing of urine, blood, sputum, feces, and other laboratory specimens.

Identify the variety of radiographic techniques introduced in this chapter, as well as the indications for their use in special circumstances.

# Diagnostic Laboratory Procedures and Instructions

Because laboratory tests and x-rays are an essential part of a medical diagnosis, an aid to treatment, and frequently a control of medication, it is important that the medical assistant have an understanding of these auxiliary services. This understanding should include the various tests available for the special needs of the physician, the preparations the patient should be instructed to follow, and how the specimens are collected and sent to the laboratory.

This knowledge and understanding will enable the medical assistant to know the patient as a person with medical needs. There must be good communication between the patient, the physician's office, and the x-ray or laboratory departments. This communication can only exist with the understanding of the needs of each area in aiding the others with better patient care and testing. Remember, the medical assistant is usually the link among these services, and her knowledge and accuracy are essential.

It is frequently the medical assistant's attitude toward these services that determines whether the patient realizes the importance of cooperating and carefully following instructions in preparation for the tests. It can be helpful if the medical assistant has a basic knowledge of the equipment used or of the steps of the particular procedure in order to ease the patient's apprehensions or fears. To a degree she will be called upon to teach the patient in preparation for some tests; therefore, she must be informed in order to be accurate in her teaching.

As well as possessing knowledge of the various tests requested by the physician, the medical assistant should know the normal ranges for these tests. This is essential when an abnormal report that should be brought to the physician's attention immediately is received in the office. No report should be filed in a patient's medical record until it has been shown to the physician. It may be a good idea to have the physician initial each report *before* it is filed. Many pathologists and roentgenologists will telephone the referring physician if there is an abnormal result that may require immediate care. These calls should be put through to the physician immediately.

Accuracy in reporting cannot be stressed enough. It is a dangerous practice to retype or copy a report onto the patient's medical record. Most offices have some method of entering the laboratory or x-ray form directly in the patient's file. An illustration of laboratory forms in a patient's record is shown in Figure 13–2 in Medical Records. Most laboratories require the technicians to sign or initial their reports. This practice is helpful if the referring physician has any questions. If it is necessary to retype or copy a report onto the patient's record, then be very careful to copy it exactly as it is written. Do not destroy the original report, but file it with other reports from the laboratory. A carelessly misplaced decimal point could be extremely dangerous, and so could an error such as typing "gm." for "mg." Some medical assistants will underline with colored pencil any abnormal results. This is helpful if the forms are small and rather difficult to read. This can also be done with lengthy x-ray reports or summaries.

If the physician requests, the medical assistant should note on the laboratory or x-ray request form any medication the patient may be taking that could make changes or cause a possible interference in the results. A clinician's interpretations may also be sharpened by a brief note dictated by the physician or taken from the patient's medical record that would alert the pathologist or roentgenologist to a possible or tentative diagnosis.

No attempt is made in this book to give detailed instructions for the techniques of doing the tests but only to alert the medical assistant to the various tests requested by the physician. She must know how to collect the specimens, know what special instructions to give to the patient, and know the normal ranges for these tests. With this knowledge, she can enhance patient care and increase her value to the clinical laboratory and radiology departments. This knowledge will also enable her to answer some of the questions from patients and to alert the physician if time is an important factor.

## SPECIMEN COLLECTION

The importance of accurate specimen collection cannot be overemphasized. If this is not done correctly it can easily lead to inaccurate results. Be careful while collecting and handling a specimen in order to prevent contamination of the specimen or of yourself.

Use only the correct containers. Never use a preservative or disinfectant unless you have been so instructed. Check whether the specimen needs to be kept warm or cool.

### Labeling of Specimens

All specimens must be labeled accurately and neatly. It is best to type a label whenever possible. If it must be handwritten, then use a ball point pen and write legibly and firmly enough to be read through all carbon copies. Include the following information:
1. Patient's full name, surname first.
2. Patient's age and sex.
3. Patient's address. This is important if the specimen is sent out of the office or if the results may be reportable, such as a contagious disease or a positive venereal disease.
4. The physician's full name. This is important if the specimen is sent to an outside laboratory or if there are several physicians in the office.

5. The date the specimen was collected as well as the date it was sent to the laboratory. Some specimens may require the hour of the day they were collected. Time is important in many tests.
6. Source of the specimen. Many times it is not obvious whether it is a sputum or a gastric specimen, an exudate from an abscess, or a throat smear.
7. The specific test requested. There are many different tests that can be done on a urine specimen alone. State whether the physician wants a routine urinalysis, bacteriological examination, special chemistry test, and so forth. Be specific.
8. Possible diagnosis. Many times this is only a tentative diagnosis, but it will give the pathologist or technologist a lead and alert him to watch for specifics.
9. Any other information that may be of importance, such as whether the patient has had any special medication or treatment that may interfere with the test. It is very important in some cases to state whether it is a new diagnosis or a treated case.

## SPECIFIC EXAMINATIONS

### Urine Examination

**Collection of Urine Specimen.** A specimen for a routine urinalysis should be collected in a clean, dry container, and the specimen should be fresh. A specimen over two hours old may not give accurate test results. If it is necessary to keep a urine specimen over two hours it should then be refrigerated and the time of collection written on the label. It is best to collect the specimen in the office or the laboratory for immediate examination. Provide the patient with a wide-mouthed container that has a secure lid and is properly labeled. If the specimen is collected at home, the patient is instructed to bring it to the laboratory as soon as possible after voiding. It is advisable to provide the patient with a container that can be used at home. Do not allow the patient to use a container which has had perfume, hair oil, or any other contaminants in it, because these interfere with the examination. There are two ways to collect a urine specimen—a freely voided specimen and a catheterized specimen. The freely voided specimen is the most frequently used and is satisfactory if correctly collected. Catheterization is necessary for some bacteriological cultures, but it is an unpleasant procedure for the patient and does involve some degree of risk.

The first voiding in the morning is usually used because it is more concentrated, except in possible diabetes mellitus or orthostatic albuminuria. A freely voided specimen in the male is easy but a specimen from the female may present a problem, especially if the patient has a vaginal discharge. The medical assistant should instruct her in the collection of an uncontaminated voided specimen.

COLLECTING A VOIDED FEMALE URINE SPECIMEN. The patient is instructed to stand astride the toilet bowl. With the labia minora spread apart she is to thoroughly cleanse the area around the urethral opening with a disposable disinfectant cleansing tissue. While still keeping the labia spread she should void forcibly, allow the initial urine stream to drain into the toilet, and then collect the midstream specimen in the wide-mouthed container. This technique is especially necessary during menstruation. If the menstrual flow is heavy a tampon should be inserted in the vagina and the area cleansed very carefully.

**Routine Urinalysis.** This includes several tests.

APPEARANCE. The color of the specimen may be influenced by various drugs, foods, and diseases. The clarity or turbidity is also influenced by these.

THE pH (ACIDITY OR ALKALINITY). This information is important only if the specimen is freshly voided. The pH determines whether certain elements are preserved or destroyed for microscopic examination. An example of this would be urinary casts that are highly diagnostic and are destroyed in an alkaline pH. Normal urine has a pH range of 4.5 to 7.5.

SPECIFIC GRAVITY. Specific gravity is the weight of a substance or a liquid. It is a convenient way to measure the dilution or concentration of the urine. A highly concentrated urine may imply that the patient is dehydrated. The normal range is 1.010 to 1.025.

ODOR. This is not routinely checked unless it is noticeably different from that of normal urine.

Chemical analysis of urine includes the following. *Protein (albumin)* is not a normal constituent in urine. It may be found in a specimen that has not been collected properly, especially in women with a vaginal discharge, and thus give misleading results. True proteinuria indicates some abnormality in the urinary system. Persistent proteinuria is due to renal disease, and its cause should be investigated. Transient proteinuria may be of little account. Positive protein is reported as trace, 1+, 2+, 3+ and 4+, *Glucose.* Ordinarily the presence of glucose in urine indicates diabetes mellitus, but this is not always true. Some persons may have a low renal threshold, i.e., the blood sugar level at which glucose is spilled over into the urine. These persons will give a positive glucose reaction but have no intrinsic disease. A positive glucose reaction is also found in a majority of healthy women during pregnancy and during the postpartum period. The presence of glucose in the urine warrants further investigation and is considered abnormal. *Ketone bodies* found in the urine are also considered to be abnormal. These are often referred to as "acetone" on the laboratory forms. Ketonuria is usually associated with diabetic acidosis, but it may be found in cases of severe starvation and body wasting (cachexia). *Bilirubin* (bile) may appear in urine when there is partial or complete obstruction of the extrahepatic biliary system. It may also appear in the urine in patients with hepatitis or liver damage. The presence of bile in the urine facilitates an early diagnosis of a hepatic disorder because it may appear in the urine before the patient's skin appears jaundiced. *Occult blood* refers to blood that is hidden and not seen macroscopically when checking the urine's color; nor are red blood cells always seen microscopically because they may have been dissolved owing to the urine hypotonic state. *Red blood cells* are not normal in the urine but may be the result of contamination from menstrual blood or a slight injury to the tissue during catheterization. *White blood cells*, sometimes called "pus cells" on the laboratory forms, are usually present in voided specimens, especially in the female. They are reported by how many are seen per the high-power field on the microscope. Normally 0 to 5 cells may be found. An excess of this number is usually checked to make certain it is not from external contamination of a voided specimen. *Epithelial cells* are also found in the urine.

They are usually of three types: renal cells that are found in excess if there is renal damage; transitional cells that are from the pelvis of the kidney, ureters, and bladder and are present when pathological conditions exist in these areas; and last, squamous cells that are from the urethra and vagina. They are the most numerous and are continually being sloughed off from time to time. They are not considered pathological. Cells are reported by how many there are per low-power field on the microscope. If there are too many to count, then they are reported from 1+ to 4+.

As mentioned earlier, *urinary casts* are highly diagnostic. They are molds of the urinary tubules and are made up of protein-plasma gel and/or cells. They are seen in urines with a pH of 6.0 or less and with a high salt concentration (hypertonic). Casts are named usually for the element contained in them, such as pus casts, blood casts, granular (containing crystals) casts, etc. Hyaline casts are seen in cases of renal disease, heart failure, high fevers, shock, or excessive exercise. Casts are reported by how many are seen per field under the microscope.

Crystals are often seen in urinary sediment but are of limited diagnostic interest unless associated with the administration of drugs, such as sulfonamides, or with protein breakdown. Crystals are noted if there is a tendency to form renal calculi. Crystals commonly seen are classed by the pH of the urine. The acid urine crystals are amorphous urates, uric acid, and calcium oxalate. Those seen in the alkaline urine are amorphous phosphates, triple phosphates, calcium diphosphates, and ammonium biurate crystals.

Other elements such as cotton fibers (lint) are not reported but are from clothing or container contamination. Bacteria seen are of limited value, especially in a voided specimen or one that is not fresh. In a catheterized specimen, bacteria are significant and should be reported and further investigated. Spermatozoa are seen in the urine and are not highly significant but are reported. Parasites, such as *Trichomonas vaginalis,* may be present and are also reported. These are from vaginal secretions.

### Some Special Urine Examinations

ADDIS COUNT.   This is done to find the patient's urinary output for a given period of time, 12 or 24 hours. During the time of the test, the patient is allowed no fluids and he is to collect all the urine voided. The volume of the output is measured and examined for protein. The amount of fluid taken in for approximately 16 hours prior to the test is restricted or eliminated. This test is a diagnostic and prognostic aid in the treatment of renal disease.

PREGNANCY TESTS.   There are many types of pregnancy tests now available. The most common ones are based on measuring the chorionic gonadotropin hormone present. There are two types of tests used, the biological tests in which animals (rabbits and frogs) are used and the immunological tests that are based on antigen-antibody reactions involving agglutination. Some of the biological tests are Ascheim-Zondek, Friedman, Wiltberger-Miller, Hogben, and Magnini. The immunological tests include Pregnosticon (Organon, Inc.), UCG (Wampole Laboratories), and Gravindex (Ortho Pharmaceutical Company).

Fluids are avoided after the evening meal and the morning urine specimen is collected. It should be collected without vaginal contamination. At least 2 ounces is required. The specimen is delivered to the laboratory as soon as possible after collection. The patient should be instructed to discontinue any sedatives

# CRYSTALS FOUND IN ACID URINE 400 X

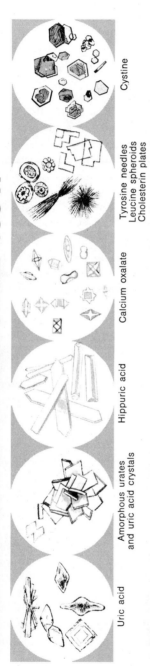

Uric acid — Amorphous urates and uric acid crystals — Hippuric acid — Calcium oxalate — Tyrosine needles / Leucine spheroids / Cholesterin plates — Cystine

# CRYSTALS FOUND IN ALKALINE URINE 400 X

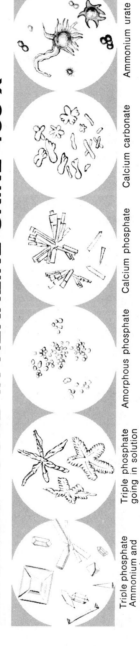

Triple phosphate Ammonium and magnesium — Triple phosphate going in solution — Amorphous phosphate — Calcium phosphate — Calcium carbonate — Ammonium urate

# SULFA CRYSTALS

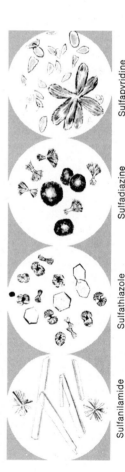

Sulfanilamide — Sulfathiazole — Sulfadiazine — Sulfapyridine

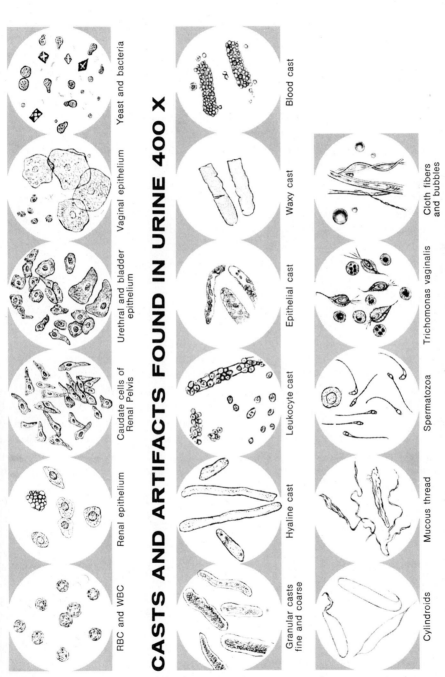

**Figure 27–1**   Ames Atlas of Urine Sediment. (Courtesy of Ames Company, Inc., Elkhart, Indiana.)

or analgesics for 24 hours prior to the test if an animal test is to be done because it may kill the animal. The patient should be three to four weeks pregnant, 10 to 14 days past her menstrual period for the test to be most accurate. The patient's blood may also be used for some pregnancy tests; about 1.5 to 2 cc. serum is needed.

ROUTINE BACTERIOLOGICAL URINE CULTURES.   If a urine specimen is to be sent to the laboratory for a bacteriological culture, it must be collected and handled with sterile technique. Of course, a catheterized specimen is preferred, but this is not always possible or advisable. A voided specimen can be used for culturing if the patient follows these instructions carefully.

Instructions for the female patient:
1. Clean the entire vulvar area with soap and water, then follow with a thorough cleansing with Zephiran Chloride. If the Zephiran Towelettes are used, instruct the patient to use several.
2. With the labia still held apart, have the patient void forcibly a small amount and then collect the midstream in a sterile bottle.
3. Cap the bottle immediately with a sterile cap.
4. Take the specimen directly to the laboratory.

Instructions for the male patient:
1. Clean the urethral meatus and glans well with soap and water and follow with Zephiran Chloride.
2. Have the patient void a small amount. Then collect the midstream portion of the urine in a sterile bottle.
3. Cap with sterile cap and send immediately to the laboratory.

COLLECTING URINE SPECIMENS FROM INFANTS.   The male infant presents very few problems because a test tube or a plastic birdseed cup may be lightly taped to the penis. This birdseed cup may also be used for the female infant. Some offices have found that a disposable ileostomy drainage bag may also be used. The ileostomy adhesive hole may be enlarged to fit over the child's genital area. Then, peel back and cut away enough of the paper covered adhesive to make an oval frame about one inch wide. There are now sterile pediatric urine specimen collectors. These are convenient and available in newborn and infant sizes.

## Blood Tests

Several hemologic tests, as with the urinalysis, are done routinely in most offices and hospitals on a new patient or for a possible new diagnosis. Designating the test "routine" does not minimize its importance. On the contrary, a physician can obtain valuable information from these tests. They are performed more frequently than others and are therefore part of a complete physical examination. Tests performed on the blood are so numerous that they fill volumes of books. Only a few basic and routine tests will be mentioned here.

Generally there are two sources of blood for laboratory testing, *capillary* (also called *peripheral*) blood and *venous* blood. Capillary blood is usually obtained from the finger or ear lobe. The quantity of blood from this source is limited to a few drops but is sufficient for such tests as a complete blood count (C.B.C.), hematocrit, some bleeding and coagulating times, and many chemical tests. If several tests are to be done, then venous blood must be drawn by the intravenous method. This is called *I.V. blood*.

Persons in the medical profession must keep in mind that the average person is apprehensive, if not frightened, at having blood drawn by any method. Because medical personnel often appear heartless to a frightened patient, they must remember to be calm and sympathetic, and give a brief explanation of the procedure. If these procedures are done correctly there is little discomfort. To a patient, 10 cc. of blood withdrawn appears to be a great deal of "blood loss." This can be related to the patient as a "little more than a tablespoonful" and that it is replenished in the body almost immediately. It may also be advisable to use the term "blood test" very carefully, since most people associate this with a test for syphilis. A brief, friendly explanation of other kinds of blood tests will nullify this misunderstanding. Be careful about telling a patient what test is being done for him, since the physician may prefer the patient not be informed.

Capillary blood is usually obtained from the ring or great finger of the adult or older child. If the fingers are extremely rough and thick skinned, then the ear lobe is used. Actually the ear lobe prick is practically painless but patients are apprehensive about this. It is also advisable to use the ear lobe if the patient will be handling any materials that are highly contaminated. In infants the great toe or the heel of the foot is pricked. Venous blood is obtained from the veins found in the anterior cubitus (inner bend of the elbow) area of the arm. This blood is called *venous blood*. The new disposable vacuum needle and syringe units, such as the Vacutainer, make this procedure practically painless if correct technique is employed. The term *venipuncture* is used when the vein is punctured for any purpose, whether to withdraw blood or to administer a medication into the vein and circulatory system (Fig. 27–2).

Because there are so many different tests other than the ones termed hemologic done on blood, it is necessary to handle these specimens, especially venous blood, in different ways. Basically, venous blood is sent to the laboratory in one of two ways, either the blood is prevented from coagulating, or it is allowed to coagulate and form a clot, thus leaving a clot of blood and blood serum. Speaking very generally, the majority of blood chemistry tests and blood cell counts are done on whole blood that has had an anticoagulant added to prevent a clot from forming or on blood that has been physically prevented from clotting by chilling or shaking. Never add an anticoagulant agent unless so instructed. There are several different agents used, and it is very important that the correct one be used. Vacuum-type venous blood collecting containers are color coded for the various tests. These may be supplied by the laboratory, and they will give directions on which to use for the different tests. Blood that has had an anticoagulant added is sometimes called *oxalated blood*. If this oxalated blood were centrifuged, the cells would be spun to the bottom of the tube leaving "*plasma*" at the top. Plasma is the fluid portion of the blood from which the cells have been suspended, or forced to the bottom, by centrifuging.

The other method of handling blood is withdrawing the blood and allowing a clot to form. Nothing is added to the blood, nor is it shaken. In a moderately short time normal blood will form a clot, leaving a fluid called *blood serum*. Blood serum does not contain any cells or fibrin. This fluid is used for blood *serological* tests such as the tests for syphilis and tests for antigen-antibody reactions.

## how to assemble

**1**

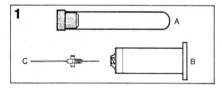

**Description of parts:**
A. Evacuated Glass Tube with Rubber Stopper
B. Plastic Holder with Guide Line
C. Double-Pointed Needle

**A**

**2**

**Thread needle into holder...tighten firmly!**
Place tube in holder with needle touching stopper.

**3**

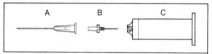

**Push tube forward until top of stopper meets guide line. Let go.** Tube stopper will retract below guide line—leave it in that position.
At this stage, the full point of the needle is embedded in the stopper (see cross section) thus avoiding blood leakage upon venipuncture and preventing premature loss of vacuum.

### Alternate Method
If needle and adapter are used, follow these instructions in place of steps 1 and 2.

| A | B | C |
|---|---|---|

**Description of parts:**
A. Luer Hub Needle
B. VACUTAINER Adapter
C. Plastic Holder
**Thread adapter into holder...tighten firmly!**
Attach Luer Needle to Adapter slip as you would needle to a syringe. Place tube in holder with needle touching stopper, then proceed to step 3, above.

## how to use

**1**

**With rear point embedded in stopper, enter tissue**—and immediately on tissue entry complete puncture of diaphragm.

**B**

**2**

**If in vein**—blood flows immediately. Note: Technologist with small hands, proceed as you would with a hypodermic syringe. Holder provides finger grip and tube acts as plunger (see inset).

**3**

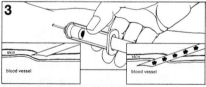

**If in tissue instead of vein**—blood will not be drawn. Proceed until venipuncture is signaled by intake of blood into VACUTAINER Tube, as shown.

**4**

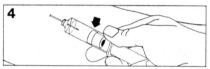

**Where vein cannot be located**—to conserve vacuum—remove tube from rear cannula (see arrow) before withdrawing needle from tissue.

**5**

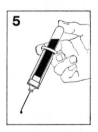

**How to obtain blood drops for red and white cell counts, blood smears, etc. After tube is filled**—grasp holder as illustrated and press firmly on bottom of tube. After each drop, release pressure and repeat for successive drops.

### Additional Information
**Incomplete Venipuncture,** which may cause the tube to fill slowly or partially, may be corrected by deeper vein entry.
**Transfixing of the vein** may be corrected by pulling back slowly with needle until flow of blood indicates vein re-entry.
**Multiple Specimens** (2, 3 or more) may be taken with one venipuncture and without loss of blood by releasing tourniquet while first tube is filling, and switching tubes while needle remains in vein.
**Vein occlusion** can be minimized by using VACUTAINER Adapter and smaller gauge needles (23, 24 or 25 gauge), thus slowing up flow of blood.
**Proper degree of vacuum** in each VACUTAINER Tube is doubly assured by the B-D Can Pack.

**Figure 27–2** B-D Vacutainer method of making a venipuncture. A. How to assemble B-D Vacutainer. B. How to use B-D Vacutainer. (Courtesy of Becton-Dickinson and Company.)

There is considerable difference between these two methods of handling venous blood, and they should not be confused. They are not interchangeable.

**Complete Blood Count (C.B.C.).**    This is the most frequently done blood test. It usually consists of a *white blood cell count (w.b.c.)*, also called *leukocyte* count; a *red blood cell count (r.b.c.)*, also called *erythrocyte* count; a *hemoglobin determination (h.g.b.)*; and a *white cell differential count (diff.)*. Frequently a *hematocrit (Hct.)* is also done with the complete blood count, or the physician may request a white blood cell count, a differential, and a hematocrit. There is some variance in the so-called routine complete blood count, depending on the physician's wishes. These tests are usually done on capillary blood but can be done on venous blood. There is no special patient preparation for these tests.

The *red cell count* is the number of red blood cells in one cubic millimeter of blood. The *normal range is 4.8 to 5.5 million/cu. mm. for men and 4.4 to 5.0 million/cu. mm. for women.* These may be written out in full, such as 4,400,000 to 5,000,000. An increase in erythrocytes is referred to as *polycythemia* and a decrease is called *anemia.* Technically, an anemia is a laboratory finding and not a diagnosis. For example, a normocytic normochromic anemia is a *finding* in malnutrition; mal-

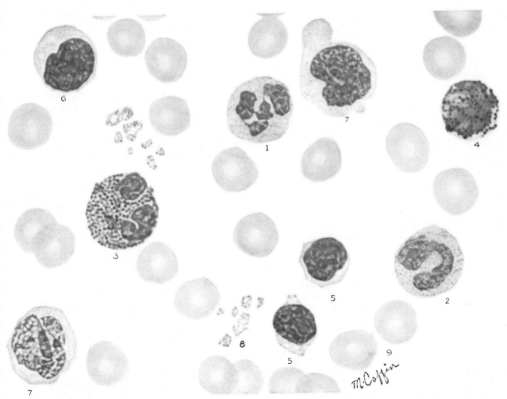

**Figure 27–3**   Normal cellular constituents of adult human blood. 1, Segmented (polymorphonuclear) neutrophil; 2, Band (stab) neutrophil; 3, Segmented eosinophil; 4, Basophil; 5, Small lymphocytes; 6, Large lymphocyte; 7, Monocytes; 8, Thrombocytes; and 9, Erythrocytes. (From Custer: *An Atlas of the Blood and Bone Marrow.*) In Leavell and Thorup: *Fundamentals of Clinical Hematology,* 3rd Ed., Philadelphia, 1971, W. B. Saunders Co.

nutrition is the *diagnosis*. There are many different types and causes for an anemia.

The *white cell count* is the number of white blood cells in one cubic millimeter of blood. The normal range varies with hematologists, but the *average is 5,000 to 10,000/cu. mm.* The white blood cell count is very diagnostic and can fluctuate fairly rapidly. In some diseases the count rises, and in other diseases the count falls. The rise and fall has been compared to a barometer that indicates the course of a disease or the progress of an infection. Leukocytes also play some role in the repair of injured tissue, but their chief function is to protect the body against microorganisms causing disease.

HEMOGLOBIN DETERMINATION. Hemoglobin is contained within the red blood cells. It is composed of heme (an organic compound of iron) and globin (a simple protein). The normal ranges are 14.5 to 16.0 gm./100 ml. blood for men and 13.0 to 15.5 gm./100 ml. blood for women. Hemoglobin is the essential carrier of oxygen in the body. The hemoglobin and red cell counts do not always rise and fall together, but there is generally some correlation between the two. In hemorrhage, the red cells and the hemoglobin both fall, but in an iron deficiency anemia the hemoglobin is reduced more than the red cells are. In pernicious anemia or in a polychromasia the red cells are reduced more than the hemoglobins.

DIFFERENTIAL WHITE CELL COUNT. There are several different white blood cells which can be identified microscopically when the blood is smeared on a microscopic slide and stained. It is very helpful to the physician to know whether the normal percentage range of these cells has changed. This change may indicate the progress or direction of a disease or infection. Because this change is so important, it should always be a part of a complete blood count. The number of white blood cells in the complete blood count does not tell which one of the various white cells has increased or decreased. These leukocytes are divided into five types, lymphocytes, monocytes, neutrophiles, eosinophiles, and basophiles. The last three are often referred to as granulocytes. A change in these cells is extremely important and especially so when considered with the white blood count and the patient's condition or diagnosis. An example of this is an increase in eosinophiles often seen in some parasitic diseases and some allergic conditions. A marked increase of younger, immature neutrophiles is called a "left shift" and can be prognostic to the physician. Frequently the progress of a disease will appear in the blood "picture" before the patient shows any clinical signs or symptoms.

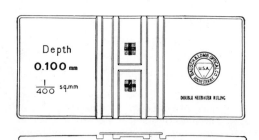

**Figure 27-4** Open counting chamber. The lower figure shows the chamber in cross section with coverglass in place.

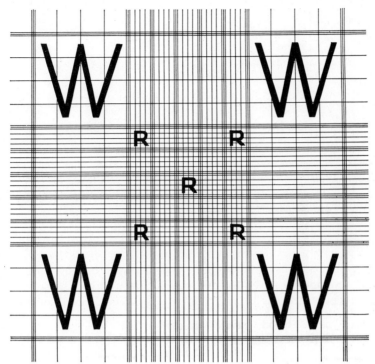

**Figure 27–5**   The area and depth of the counting chamber. (From Seiverd, C. E.: *Hematology for Medical Technologists*, 4th Ed., Philadelphia, 1972, Lea and Febiger.)

Normal ranges for these leukocytes are:

| | |
|---|---|
| Neutrophiles | 54 to 62 per cent |
| Eosinophiles | 1 to  3 per cent |
| Basophiles | 0 to  1 per cent |
| Lymphocytes | 25 to 33 per cent |
| Monocytes | 0 to  9 per cent |

While the hematologist is counting and studying the white blood cells, she is also examining the red blood cells seen on the slide. These erythrocytes, as they are correctly called, are examined for size and shape, for how they have taken the stain, or for any abnormality that may be seen.

HEMATOCRIT (HCT.).   This test measures the relative volume of cells and plasma in the blood. It is often done in combination with the red cell count and the hemoglobin, or in place of the hemoglobin. In anemias and after a hemorrhage the hematocrit reading is lower than normal, while in dehydration and polycythemia the reading is higher. Both capillary and venous blood are used. If the test is done with capillary blood it is then called "microhematocrit. ' There is no special preparation for the patient. The blood must be prevented from coagulating. If venous blood is used an anticoagulant is added to the blood. Special capillary tubes containing an anticoagulant are used for the micro method.

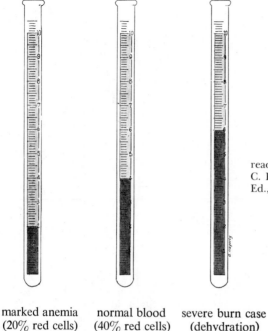

**Figure 27–6** High and low hematocrit readings. (Wintrobe tubes.) (From Seiverd, C. E.: *Hematology for Medical Technologists*, 4th Ed., Philadelphia, 1972, Lea and Febiger.)

marked anemia    normal blood    severe burn case
(20% red cells)    (40% red cells)    (dehydration)
                                                           (60% red cells)

The results are expressed in cubic millimeters per 100 ml. of blood, or in volumes/100 ml. Normal ranges are 45 to 50 vol./100 ml. for men and 40 to 45 vol./100 ml. for women.

ERYTHROCYTE SEDIMENTATION RATE (S.R., E.S.R., OR SED. RATE). When red blood cells are allowed to settle out of their plasma, the speed of their fall in a given length of time is known as the *sedimentation rate*. This rate has been found to depend, to some degree, on changes in the blood proteins. There are several different methods for running this test, and the normal ranges vary with each method. The laboratory will usually list the normal range for the method used. There are also differences of opinion as to the reliability of the test. It was once said that it "doesn't tell where the fire is, but does tell how hot it is." It is used as a rough index of the progress or presence of an inflammatory disease such as rheumatoid arthritis, rheumatic fever, or respiratory disease. Both capillary and venous blood are used. It is prevented from coagulating so that the cells can settle. There is no patient preparation for a sedimentation rate. Women tend to have a higher reading than men, especially during menstruation. Some samples of normal ranges are:

| | | | |
|---|---|---|---|
| Cutler Method | Men: 0–8 | Women: | 0–10 |
| Wintrope Method | 0–6.5 | | 0–15 |
| Westergren Method | 0–15 | | 0–20 |

PROTHROMBIN TIME (PRO. TIME OR P.T.). This is a test to measure the clotting ability of the blood. It is an essential test in establishing and maintaining an-

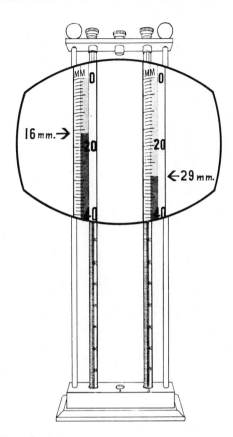

**Figure 27-7** Reading the sedimentation rate in a Westergren tube. In the circled inset, the upper very light portion of each tube is plasma. The lower darker portion is red cells. (From Seiverd, C. E.: *Hematology for Medical Technologists,* 4th Ed., Philadelphia, 1972, Lea and Febiger.)

ticoagulation therapy, such as the administration of Dicumarol and other similar drugs. This test may also be done daily during acute stages of myocardial infarction. Prothrombin content of the blood is often low in liver diseases, vitamin K deficiency, and thrombinemia of infants. Venous blood is used and mixed with a special solution. Certain medications such as barbiturates may interfere with accurate results; otherwise there is no special patient preparation. Normal ranges depend on the specific type of test done, but the usual range is from 11 to 18 seconds.

HETEROPHILE. Basically, this is a test used to confirm a clinical diagnosis of infectious mononucleosis, but it is also used in the diagnosis of serum sickness. It is an agglutination reaction between the patient's blood serum and washed sheep cells. A series of dilutions is made in test tubes, then incubated. The greatest dilution which agglutinates the erythrocytes is noted. There are no special restrictions or instructions for the patient. Venous blood is drawn and allowed to coagulate to obtain the blood serum. Normal range is near 1:28. A reading of 1:56 is considered diagnostic.

TESTS FOR THE PRESENCE OF BILE (BILIRUBIN) IN THE BLOOD

*Bilirubin (van den Bergh method).* This is to determine the presence of free bilirubin that is broken down from hemoglobin. It is an important liver function test and is also done on newborn infants to determine the possibility of performing an exchange transfusion. There are several drugs and some foods that, if

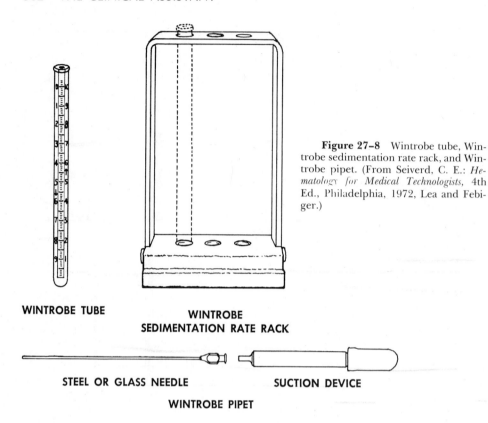

WINTROBE TUBE

WINTROBE
SEDIMENTATION RATE RACK

STEEL OR GLASS NEEDLE          SUCTION DEVICE

WINTROBE PIPET

**Figure 27–8** Wintrobe tube, Wintrobe sedimentation rate rack, and Wintrobe pipet. (From Seiverd, C. E.: *Hematology for Medical Technologists*, 4th Ed., Philadelphia, 1972, Lea and Febiger.)

taken in excess, can interfere with an accurate reading. It may be best to check with the laboratory if there is a question. It is preferred that fasting venous blood be used, but this is not absolutely necessary. The blood is allowed to coagulate and the serum is used. Normal range from 0.1 to 1.0 mg./100 ml. serum.

*Icterus Index.* This is a simple test to determine the amount of bilirubin in blood serum, but it does not differentiate between bilirubin due to hemolysis or due to a biliary obstruction, so this test does have limitations. It is useful in discovering an early jaundice condition before it is visible to the physician. The patient's serum is drawn the same as in the above bilirubin test. Normal range is 4 to 6 units.

MEAN CORPUSCULAR VOLUME (M.C.V.). This is a measurement calculated from the hematocrit reading and the red blood cell count. The M.C.V. in normal adults is between 80 and 90 microns. In some microcytic anemias it may go as high as 150 microns. This index is not valid unless the red blood cell count is absolutely accurate.

SERUM CALCIUM (CA). Calcium is essential in the formation of bone tissue, in muscular activity, and in blood coagulation. When there is a deficiency of calcium, tetany will occur. This condition is a twitching of muscle fibers and tetanic convulsions. An increase of blood calcium is found in hyperparathyroidism, multiple myeloma and some respiratory diseases. There is no preparation of the patient, nor any patient restrictions. Venous blood is drawn and allowed to clot, since this is a serum test. Normal range is 8 to 11 mg./100 ml. serum.

COOMBS' TEST, DIRECT.    This test is done basically on newborn infants for the diagnosis of erythroblastosis fetalis. In many hospitals it is done routinely in all umbilical cord blocks. Only about 2 cc. of blood is needed and is taken directly from the cord, or venous blood may be drawn. Normally the results are negative. The indirect Coombs' Test is used in the detection of various minor blood type factors, including Rh, and is used in cross-matching blood for blood transfusions. Normal reading is negative.

BLOOD UREA NITROGEN (BUN).    This is a kidney function test. Normally the kidneys excrete urea, a major product of the kidneys, the end product of protein metabolism. In some kidney diseases this may be impaired and the kidneys do not excrete urea sufficiently, so the urea nitrogen in the blood increases. This test gives essentially the same information as the Non-protein Nitrogen (N.P.N.) but is more accurate. There is no preparation of the patient nor any food restrictions. Venous blood is drawn, and an anticoagulant is added. Normal range is 8 to 28 mg./100 ml. blood.

URIC ACID.    This test is used basically to aid in the diagnosis of gout, a metabolic disease marked by acute arthritis and inflammation of the joints. Uric acid is the end product of purine (a protein) metabolism. An increase of uric acid is also seen in severe kidney damage and toxemias of pregnancy. There is no preparation of the patient or dietary restriction. Venous blood is used and an anticoagulant added. Normal range is 3.0 to 5.0 mg./100 ml. blood.

PROTEIN-BOUND IODINE (P.B.I.).    Since iodine is used by the thyroid gland to manufacture thyroxin, and since iodine is also stored in the thyroid gland, this test is basically a thyroid function test. Iodine in the blood serum is bound, or attached, to the protein molecule and is not free iodine in the blood, thus the name protein-bound iodine. Hypothyroidism will give a low reading, while hyperthyroidism produces an increased reading. There is no preparation of the patient, but this test is affected by many medications and by any radiographic contrast media. Some radiopaque iodine-containing injectable media can produce a falsely high P.B.I. reading for several months, or even years. The patient's history must be carefully checked. Venous blood is used and allowed to clot, since this is a serum test. Normal range is 5 to 8 micrograms per 100 ml. serum.

THYROXINE IODINE OR BUTANOL-EXTRACTABLE IODINE (B.E.I.).    These tests are for thyroid function and have a distinct advantage over the P.B.I. because radiographic contrast media do not interfere. It is generally preferred that the patient's diet be iodine-free for three days before the test. Venous blood is drawn and allowed to clot, since the test is done on blood serum. Normal range is 3.5 to 6.5 micrograms per 100 ml.

BLOOD GLUCOSE OR BLOOD SUGAR (BL. S.).    This is one of the most frequently performed blood chemistry tests. It is used in the diagnosis of diabetes and as an aid in the control of diabetic patients. This test is requested by a wide range of specialists in the medical profession. The ophthalmologist sees patients with blurred vision and the podiatrist sees patients with foot ulcers that are not healing normally. Each of these conditions is seen in a diabetic patient not receiving medical care.

An increase in the blood sugar is called *hyperglycemia* and a decrease is called *hypoglycemia*. Because "fasting blood" is used, patients are instructed to eat or drink nothing, except water, for 12 hours before the test is done. Diabetic patients should not take their dose of insulin until after the blood has been drawn.

Occasionally a physician will want to know a patient's response to food intake, and he will order a blood sugar test at a specific time after a meal. In this case the time of the meal and the time the blood is drawn must be noted. It is usually done two hours after the meal. The laboratory will usually ask the patient for a urine specimen at the time the blood is drawn. Venous blood is used and an anticoagulant is added. Normal range for fasting blood is 80 to 120 mg./100 ml.

GLUCOSE TOLERANCE OR SUGAR TOLERANCE. These tests are done to determine a patient's response to a standard amount of glucose. The patient reports to the laboratory in a fasting state the same as for a regular blood glucose. Fasting blood is drawn and a urine specimen requested. The patient is then given a rather large dose of glucose, usually in one of various flavors of a soda pop-type mixture that the patient drinks. At regular intervals thereafter, blood is drawn and a urine sample requested. These tests determine how the patient's body handles the added glucose. These tests are valuable in ruling out diabetes mellitus and in diagnosing a possible hyperinsulinism. The patient should be told that it will be necessary to stay at the laboratory for three to five hours, depending on the physician's request. Blood is drawn and an anticoagulant is added for each interval test. The normal response to the oral glucose intake is that the blood sugar peaks not more than 150 mg./100 ml. and returns to the fasting state within two hours. Very elderly patients may reach a slightly higher peak.

CHOLESTEROL (CHOL.). Cholesterol is normally found in the blood, but some disease states will raise or decrease the cholesterol concentration. An elevated reading may aid in the diagnosis of liver function, hypothyroidism, and a possibility of atherosclerosis, although this last condition is still in the research state. A decrease is found in hyperthyroidism, anemias, cachexia, and acute infections. The patient is often asked to avoid high cholesterol foods for a period of time before the test, or some physicians and laboratories want fasting blood used for the test. It is advisable to check with the physician and/or the laboratory before instructing the patient. The blood is drawn and allowed to coagulate. The normal range is 150 to 250 mg./100 ml.

SEROLOGICAL TEST FOR SYPHILIS (S.T.S.). It may also be referred to as a test for Venereal Disease, Syphilis (V.D.S.) or Venereal Disease Research Laboratory test (V.D.R.L.). There are several varieties of test for this disease, and there are too many to list here. Often the medical office is not concerned with the specific type of test run but with the results of the test. There are several factors that interfere with the results of various tests. The interpretation requires skill and experience, as well as correlation with the clinical findings and patient's medical history. All the questions on the laboratory request form must be answered, such as, whether it is a new case or treated case. Solomon Garb, M.D., in *Laboratory Tests in Common Use* has written: "In early primary syphilis the serology is negative. In late, adequately treated syphilis, the serology may be fixed at a high positive titer although the patient is, in effect, cured. In late, improperly treated syphilis, the serology may be negative even though the patient is not cured and is developing central nervous system involvement."

Many physicians' offices and most hospitals now require a routine S.T.S. on all patients. Most states have legal requirements for syphilitic testing before marriage and before the birth of a baby. These are the required "premarital" and "prenatal" tests.

There is no special patient preparation or restriction. Since the test is a serological test, the blood is drawn and allowed to coagulate. Normally the reaction is negative. A faintly positive reaction usually warrants further testing and study, because it may indicate some other disorder.

*Sputum* is the secretion from the lungs, bronchi, and trachea which is ejected through the mouth and is usually obtained by deep coughing. Sputum must not be confused with saliva and postnasal secretions. Saliva and postnasal secretions are considered contaminants in a sputum specimen and complicate or interfere with accurate sputum examination. Sputum is examined primarily for agents causing infectious diseases such as tuberculosis, pneumonia, and candidiasis (one of the many fungal infections found in the lungs). The Papanicolaou stain is also done on cells found in sputum to determine cancer.

Special containers should be provided to the patient. These are about two ounce wide-mouthed sterile jars or waxed paper cardboard containers. The caps should fit snugly. Instruct the patient to give only sputum and not saliva. Many patients have their most productive cough the first thing in the morning. Tell the patient to be very careful, not to contaminate the outside of the container, and not to fill it more than half full. If the specimen cannot be taken to the laboratory within the next few hours, or a 24 hour or three days' specimen is requested, then the container should be refrigerated. Most laboratories and public health department laboratories will furnish these containers.

## Examination of Feces (Stool) Specimens

If you compare feces to blood or urine, there are relatively few tests done on feces. However, these few tests are important to both the patient's health and as an aid to the physician's diagnosis. Maybe the infrequency with which the tests are performed is the reason for considerable mishandling of these specimens. It is very important that the medical assistant instruct the patient correctly, and that the specimen be taken to the laboratory as instructed. The laboratory technicians will appreciate this. Technicians say that of all the specimens brought into the laboratory, the feces specimen is the most mishandled, thus making it difficult for them to examine or causing them to instruct the patient and request another specimen. No one would appreciate repeating this procedure unless necessary for further testing and certainly not because of mishandling or poor instructions.

Because defecation does not take place at will, as urination does, the patient cannot be sent to the lavatory to get a specimen at any time. When a patient is told to bring a specimen to the laboratory he is usually embarrassed and somewhat confused as to how this procedure will have to take place. The medical assistant can ease the patient by simple matter-of-fact instructions. Remember to remind the patient that time is very often important, and that the feces must NOT be contaminated with urine. This is especially important when instructing the female patient. The patient must NOT take a laxative unless specifically instructed to do so, and then it is to be only a mild saline laxative and never one containing oil or a harsh chemical. These interfere with the tests.

Furnish the patient with a wide-mouthed container; the same type as used for a sputum test may be used. The patient may void into a plastic bag or onto a paper plate, then transfer a small amount, about the size of a walnut, into the container provided. Give the patient a few wooden tongue depressors to use for this transfer. This small amount is sufficient for most tests, unless otherwise specified.

**Some Specific Tests and Their Collection.** Specimens for *viral culture* must be taken to the laboratory immediately. It would be best to have the patient void while at the laboratory. If there is a delay between collecting the specimen and culturing it, then it must be kept very cold, even frozen, if necessary. *Bacterial culturing* also requires immediate examination. If the feces is diarrheal a sterile cotton swab dipped into the specimen and placed in a sterile test tube is sufficient. The swab is best dipped into an area of the specimen that appears purulent. If *dysentery bacilli* are suspected, the physician will probably take a swab from the rectal or lower bowel area by holding the anus open with an anoscope. Place the swab in a sterile test tube and deliver to the laboratory immediately.

**Specimens to Be Examined for Parasites.** Loose, fluid stools to be examined for *intestinal amebae* and other *flagellates* are to be kept at body temperature and examined within 30 minutes. Well-formed stools to be examined for *ova* or *cystic forms of parasites* do not have to be kept warm and can be taken to the laboratory within a few hours. A small amount is sufficient for both examinations. If there is a possibility of a *tapeworm* the specimen may first be examined for diagnosis by the examination of a small amount to find the ova of the tapeworm, but if a purgative medication was given, the patient must then bring in the *entire* feces so the laboratory can search for the head (scolex) of the tapeworm. This is important, since the patient must be given another purgative unless the head is found. A plastic bag or large jar is used.

*Pinworms* inhabit the lower intestinal tract and are diagnosed by the presence of the ova. The female pinworm migrates to the anus during periods of rest, particularly at night, and deposits her eggs (ova). The most satisfactory means of confirming this diagnosis is to use a piece of Scotch tape. The sticky side of the tape is pressed gently into the anal folds and then with the sticky side down the tape is placed on a microscopic glass slide and sent to the laboratory. This specimen should be taken immediately upon awakening, before any excess movement or going to the bathroom.

**Occult Blood.** The patient is instructed to eat no meat, including fish and poultry, for three days before a specimen is examined. Otherwise, false positive results may occur from the meat residue. Only a small amount of feces is needed.

**Chemical Analysis.** This requires the entire specimen defecated, since the amounts of the substances tested are reported and calculated on the basis of daily output. It would be advisable to keep the specimen cool to prevent excess bacterial growth.

Large amounts of undigested food in the stool may indicate abnormalities in digestion. Since this may be both a microscopic and macroscopic examination the amount needed may vary. It is best to check with the physician and the laboratory. A clay-colored stool may indicate a lack of the normal amounts of bile and assist the physician in diagnosing a biliary obstruction. A small amount of specimen would be needed for testing for urobilin, also called stercobilin.

# MYCOLOGY

Mycology is the study of fungus diseases. These vegetable cellular organisms are very numerous in the air, water and soil, but a very few of them are capable of causing disease. Fungus diseases are often slow to appear and are difficult to diagnose and sometimes treat. Although many are resistant to treatment only a very few are fatal. Among some fungus infections are histoplasmosis, coccidioidomycosis, ringworm, athlete's foot, and thrush.

*Histoplasmosis* is a disease caused by the inhalation of dust or decayed fowl and bird droppings containing the offending fungi. It begins in the lungs and then becomes systemic. It is not contagious between men. It first appears as an influenza and resembles tuberculosis when x-rayed. A sputum specimen is collected and tested to aid in this diagnosis.

*Coccidioidomycosis* is also a fungus affecting the respiratory tract, but it can be superficial as well as systemic. It is found in the dust in dry, hot southwestern areas of the United States and Mexico. It is called *desert fever* or *San Joaquin Valley fever*. It first appears as a respiratory, influenza-type disease. It is diagnosed by sputum examination, gastric washings, and skin scrapings, if the infection is superficial.

*Ringworm* (microsporum) causes some of the various dermatomycoses — diseases of the skin and hair. These are included in the large group of collagen diseases, and are diagnosed by scrapings of the skin, hair, and nails, and by ultraviolet light. *Athlete's foot* is also a dermatomycosis and may be caused by several different fungi.

*Thrush* is caused by *Candida albicans*. It involves mucous membranes of the mouth, anus, and vagina (see Chapter 32, Assisting in the Surgical Specialties: Obstetrics and Gynecology). Heavy antibiotic therapy may decrease the normal bacterial flora of these areas and thus allow *Candida* to flourish. It is found more frequently in babies, obese persons, and those who sweat profusely. It is diagnosed by direct examination and skin scrapings for microscopic slides and cultures. The student is referred to Chapter 22 for techniques of preparing and mounting slides for microscopic examination.

# ECTOPARASITES

These are parasites attached to, or living on, the outer surface of the body or immediately beneath the skin.

The most common of these is the well-known *itch mite* that causes *scabies*. It is highly contagious and holds no respect for its victim's pedigree or socioeconomic position. It usually infects the entire family. Schools will send a child home in haste if the mite is found. Patients are frequently shocked by this diagnosis. Examination of the skin is made with the aid of a magnifying lens to obtain skin scrapings for the mite and its eggs, also called *nits*.

The three lice that are found on man are identified by the area of the body they inhabit. They are: (1) *Pediculus humanus capitis* that is found in the hairs of the head by examining the hair for the eggs and the adult insect. (2) *Pediculus humanus corporis* is the so-called body louse that lives in the clothing but migrates to the body to feed. Its eggs are found in the seams and folds of clothing. (3) *Phthirus pubis (Pediculus pubis)* is the pubic louse and is found in the hairs of the pubic region. It is also diagnosed by examining the pubic hairs for the presence of eggs.

## BODY FLUIDS

*Transudates* are fluids that accumulate in body cavities, such as the abdominal or pericardial spaces. These fluids are not the result of an inflammation but are the result of edema and congestion. They are clear and light yellow in appearance. They are low in protein, contain very few white cells, and have no bacteria. Laboratory examinations include appearance, specific gravity, cell count, and protein determination. A Papanicolaou stain is done on the sediment for the possibility of malignancy. These fluids are taken from the body cavity by sterile puncture and draining technique.

*Exudates* are the product of an inflammatory condition. They may be found in a body cavity or in the tissues. They are usually cloudy, deeper yellow, and much thicker in appearance. They contain many blood cells, red and white, and usually bacteria are present. This fluid is also drained by sterile technique, but it frequently is obtained by a draining abscess or open wound. Bacterial cultures and stained smears are made from exudates; a "Pap" stain may also be done, but not as frequently as with a transudate.

*Synovial fluids* are obtained from a bursa, joint, or tendon sheath. A cell count is done, or it may be cultured or smeared for bacteria. The fluid is usually obtained by sterile puncture technique.

See Chapter 31, Assisting in Minor Surgery, for collection of these body fluid specimens.

## CYTOLOGICAL EXAMINATIONS

Exfoliated cells are cells that have sloughed off from both normal and malignant epithelial tissue. These exfoliated cells that lend themselves well to the Papanicolaou method of staining may be obtained from vaginal and cervical scrapings and secretions, bronchial secretions and washings, urinary sediment, pleural and peritoneal fluid sediments, and discharges from the mammary glands.

To insure accuracy of the "Pap smear," it should be fixed immediately after smearing on the microscopic slide in a solution of 50 per cent ether and 50 per cent ethyl alcohol. The slide should remain in this fixing solution for at least 30 minutes and then be removed and placed on end to air dry. Label with the patient's name and send to the laboratory for the cytotechnician or the pathologist to examine.

Papanicolaou smears are reported on a 5-point scale as follows:

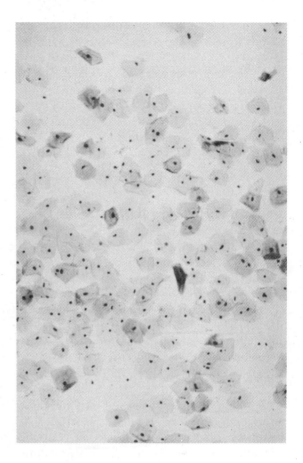

**Figure 27–9** Vaginal smear showing estrogen effect. Almost all the cells are mature superficial cells with pyknotic nuclei. Note the clean background. Papanicolaou stain × 115. (From Lynch, M. J., et al.: *Medical Laboratory Technology and Clinical Pathology*, 2nd Ed., Philadelphia, 1967, W. B. Saunders Co.)

| | |
|---|---|
| Grade I | Absence of atypical or abnormal cells |
| Grade II | Atypical cytology but no evidence of malignancy |
| Grade III | Cytology suggestive but not conclusive for malignancy |
| Grade IV | Strongly suggestive of malignancy |
| Grade V | Conclusive for malignancy |

See Chapter 32, Assisting in the Surgical Specialties: Obstetrics and Gynecology, for the procedure to obtain a cervical and vaginal cytological smear.

## HISTOLOGIC EXAMINATION

Histology is the microscopic study of the form and structure of the various tissues of the body. This differs from cytology, which is the study of the exfoliated cells themselves, not in relation to other cells. Specimens for histological study must be *fixed* as soon as possible. Fixation refers to arresting the life processes of the tissue cells. It also stops any dehydration, bacterial growth, or enzymatic activity. Tissue specimens are obtained by biopsy. The usual recommended fixative solution is 80 per cent alcohol and 10 per cent formalin with the ratio of the solution to specimen being ten to one. The specimen must be completely immersed and free from any side pressure. It is best to have it floating free.

The laboratory will then specially treat the tissue, so that it can be sliced microscopically thin and mounted on slides to be passed through a series of stains. It is then studied by the pathologist. The container must be properly labeled with the patient's full name, physician's name, the date, and the nature of the specimen. The possible diagnosis is sometimes included.

See Chapter 31, Assisting in Minor Surgery, for obtaining a specimen by biopsy.

## CEREBROSPINAL FLUID (C.S.F.)

The procedure to obtain cerebrospinal fluid, sometimes called spinal fluid, is usually done in a hospital on an out-patient basis, but occasionally, a physician will do a spinal puncture in the office. It is considered a minor surgical procedure.

Normally it is a clear, colorless fluid found in the ventricles of the brain and the central canal of the spinal cord. Approximately 100 cc. of fluid is present normally, and usually that amount is produced and reabsorbed daily. This fluid is obtained by a lumbar puncture, and about 2 to 3 cc. is allowed to drip into a series of small sterile vials. Three vials are usually taken; these vials are to be numbered 1, 2, and 3 in the sequence taken. A lumbar puncture is not too painful for the patient, but because of the reduced volume of fluid in the spine and ventricles, the patient is advised to remain flat for a few hours in order to prevent a severe headache. There is no special diet restriction or patient preparation for this procedure. It is also required in some institutions that the patient sign a permission form for a lumbar puncture to be performed.

Some tests done on this cerebrospinal fluid are the following. A *cell count* often indicates the presence of an infection. This should be done immediately after the fluid has been obtained. A high cell count is found in most cases of meningitis. A *serological test* is done to discover the presence of neurosyphilis and the involvement of this disease in the central nervous system. A *Colloidal-Gold* test aids in the diagnosis of multiple sclerosis. The *total protein* is increased in several diseases of the central nervous system, especially in meningitis, subarachnoid hemorrhage, or a spinal block due to a tumor.

## RADIOLOGICAL EXAMINATIONS

Ever since Wilhelm Konrad Roentgen discovered the x-ray in 1895, medicine has known the value of this almost miraculous discovery as an aid to diagnoses and a treatment of diseases. Great advances have been made since this discovery and, no doubt, the future holds even greater knowledge and use of it. The more knowledge gained, the safer the rays are to use. Early workers did not fully appreciate the dangers of this force, but nowadays great efforts are made to ensure more precise handling of this form of radiation equipment.

The term *x-ray* will, no doubt, be used for many years, but these rays have now been named *roentgen rays* in honor of their discoverer. The symbol "x" was used to represent the unknown. Very frequently the two terms used in the radiation world are confused. They are *roentgenology* and *radiology*. The term roentgenology is limited to the study and science of the roentgen ray, while radiology is the study and science of all forms of radiation including the x-ray, radioactive substances, and other forms of radiant energy. The films used as diagnostic aids are referred to as roentgenograms or radiographs. Films of specific areas of the body may be named, for example cholecystograms for gallbladder visualization or pyelograms for the pelvis of the kidney.

There are basically three methods of examination with the use of the roentgen ray. The radiogram (roentgenogram) is the picture taken that appears as a film negative (Fig. 27–11). The next is by the use of the ray to view a part of the body on a fluorescent screen. Examination by this method is called *fluoroscopy*. The advantage of this method is to view the action of the part exposed and the use of a radiopaque medium aids in this process. An example of this is to have the patient swallow a barium mixture while under the fluoroscope, and the radiologist or roentgenologist watches the barium pass through the esophagus as it passes into the stomach. The last method is a combination of these two methods, which records the results on a photographic film. These small films are called *photofluorograms*.

*Cineradiography* is a form of radiography that makes it possible to make a motion picture record of an examination. This enables the radiologist to study the events seen on the fluoroscope. This is of particular advantage in diagnosing pathology in the urinary tract.

*Contrast media* are materials used to alter the radiopacity of an area or part by forming a comparison with the surrounding parts. Contrast media are used essentially in body cavities, such as the digestive tract, urinary tract, ventricles, and meningeal spaces of the brain, bronchial tree, uterus, and fallopian tubes. Contrast media consist of gases (air, oxygen, $CO_2$), heavy metals (barium sulfate, bismuth carbonate), organic soluble and insoluble iodides, and others. Some of these are spoken of as radiopaque dyes that concentrate in a particular body organ such as the gallbladder. These dyes are administered orally, intravenously, or directly into the area, as in a retrograde pyelogram where the dye is introduced into the renal pelvis via cystoscopy.

Since individual radiologists have their own particular methods and preferences of patient preparation for the various procedures, it is advisable to check with them before instructing a patient on a procedure. The instructions given here will be standard generalities for each.

Patient preparation for diagnostic x-rays depends on the body region to be filmed and the purposes of the examination. In some instances, such as bone or lung studies, there is no special preparation necessary. In others, especially when a contrast medium is used to fill a hollow organ in the abdominal cavity, preparation of the patient is absolutely essential. Since gas in the intestinal tract has a degree of density and will not allow the x-rays to fully penetrate, it is essential that this gas be completely eliminated or a successful diagnostic film cannot be taken. It is equally important to have the intestinal tract free of gas and fecal material if a clear film of the ureters and kidneys is to be made, since these organs are posterior to the intestines.

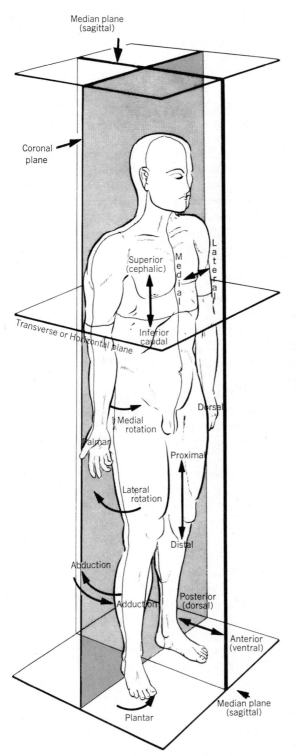

**Figure 27–10** A diagram illustrating the use of some anatomic terms referring to position and movement. (From *Radiography: A Tool of Medical Science,* GAF Corporation, 1970, p. 5.)

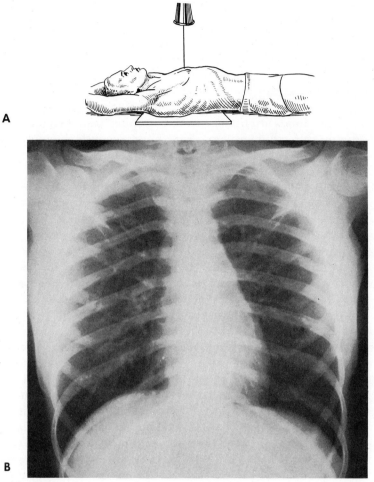

**Figure 27–11**   Antero-posterior recumbent study of chest: A. Positioning of patient. B. (From Meschan, I.: Radiographic Positioning and Related Anatomy. Philadelphia, 1968, W. B. Saunders Co.)

Because this cleansing of the intestines is so important, many radiological secretaries will supply the physician's office with printed instructions to be given to the patient. Success or failure of an x-ray examination depends greatly on how conscientiously a patient is given instructions and how carefully he follows these instructions. Most preparation instructions for the patient include dietary and/or fluid restrictions or eliminations and bowel cleansing procedures.

**Cleansing Enema Instructions.**   Many people do not know the proper technique for taking an enema and consequently get poor results. The patient should be instructed to take one quart of plain warm water, about 100° F. or a little warmer than body temperature. The patient should lie down, with the enema can or bag about three feet above head level. The first third of the enema should be taken lying on the left side, the middle third lying flat on the back, and the final third lying on the right side. The liquid should be held for several minutes before evacuating.

## Specific Roentgenography Tests

**Intravenous Pyelogram.**   This is the study of the ureters and kidneys after a contrast medium has been introduced intravenously. As mentioned above, gas and fecal material must be removed from the intestinal tract. This may be done by the administration of castor oil and a cleansing enema. The evening meal the night before the test should be light, consisting of toast, tea, and fruit. There must be no food or fluids after 9:00 P.M. that evening or in the morning before the test. The contrast medium is then injected intravenously the morning of the test at designated intervals, and the x-ray films are taken at given intervals to observe the rate of excretion, the concentration of the contrast medium in the kidney calices and pelves, the outline of the ureters, and the urinary bladder. The patient should be told there will probably be two venipunctures, and that the test will take about one hour. He may have breakfast after the test.

**Retrograde Pyelogram.**   This test is the same as the intravenous pyelogram except the contrast medium is introduced into the kidneys by means of a ureteral catheter through a cystoscope. The excretory procedure is not viewed adequately because the catheter is obstructing the ureters. This method is done when special studies of certain parts of the urinary tract are indicated or when adequate concentration of the contrast medium cannot be achieved by the intravenous method.

**Cholecystogram.**   This is an examination of the gallbladder, showing function, the presence of any gallstones, or anomalies. The intestinal tract must be cleared as instructed. The patient should eat a fat-free light meal the night before examination; he may usually have lean meat, vegetables, fruit, dry toast, tea, or coffee. Dye tablets (usually six or nine) are swallowed with the meal at regular intervals; specific instructions are issued with the tablets. Small amounts of water may be taken during the evening until bedtime. Patients should be warned that they may have some diarrhea and nausea after taking the tablets, but not to be alarmed. Many times after the first films are taken the patient may be instructed to eat a fatty meal, to stimulate functioning of the gallbladder, and then return for more films to be taken. This examination usually takes about one hour, including the fatty meal.

**Cholangiogram.**   This is done to view the cystic, hepatic and common bile ducts by using a radiopaque dye. In the intravenous method the dye is excreted by the liver into the bile ducts. X-ray films are taken at ten minute intervals. The procedure takes about four hours. The patient is instructed to restrict fluid intake in order to concentrate the dye. The evening meal the night before the test is fat free, and the intestines must be cleared by castor oil and an enema.

A postoperative cholangiogram utilizes the drainage tube left in place at surgery. The dye is injected through the drain tube and the series of films is started immediately.

**Barium Enema.**   This is valuable in viewing the colon. Obviously, the colon must be cleared of fecal material and gas. The day before the examination the patient is instructed to take castor oil and an enema. A light supper is eaten. Some radiologists prefer that the patient be placed on a low-residue diet for 24 hours before the examination. Nothing is taken by mouth after 9 P.M. the evening before, nor the morning of, the test. Tell the patient he will be given an enema of an opaque substance (barium sulfate) while on the table. He will be

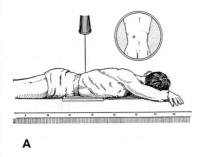

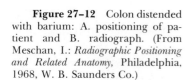

**A**

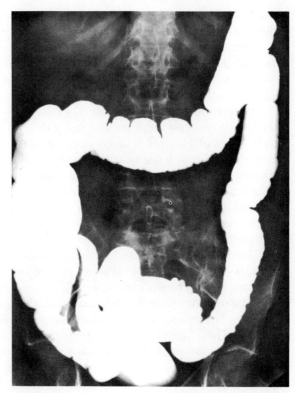

**Figure 27–12**   Colon distended with barium: A. positioning of patient and B. radiograph. (From Meschan, I.: *Radiographic Positioning and Related Anatomy*, Philadelphia, 1968, W. B. Saunders Co.)

**B**

moved from the left side, to the back, and to the right side to completely fill the colon. He is then fluoroscoped, and films are taken before he may evacuate the barium. The barium is then evacuated in the lavatory. If the physician requests, air is injected into the colon after the barium has been evacuated. The air is a contrast medium that gives a contrast to the barium which is coating the mucosa of the colon. This technique is done to better visualize polypoid masses. A barium enema will take from 15 to 30 minutes.

**Gastrointestinal Series.**   This is also sometimes called a Barium Meal, G.I. Series, or an Upper G.I. This is an x-ray series of the stomach and small intestine, depending on the physician's request. The radiologist observes by fluoroscope the filling of the stomach as the patient drinks a suspension of barium sulfate. Films are made during the filling or immediately after the fluoroscopic examination. This takes about 30 minutes. A physician may request more pictures be taken at a six hour period and/or at a 24 hour period. Patients are instructed to eat a light supper and take nothing by mouth after midnight the evening before the test. A patient may eat breakfast after the first series of films is taken. The patient may be requested to prepare the bowel with castor oil and/or an enema, if the barium is to be followed through more than the upper gastrointestinal area. The patient should be told that his stool may be light in color after the examination because of the barium passing. Some patients may need a cathartic or enema after all the films are taken if they have had difficulty with normal bowel movements.

**Pneumoencephalogram.**   This is a film study of the ventricles and meningeal spaces of the brain after the injection of air into the subarachnoid space, usually by spinal puncture. It is sometimes done to localize an abnormality that is filling a ventricle or meningeal space. A headache is a common after effect.

**Myelogram.** A myelogram is a film study of the spinal cord. Air is the contrast medium used and is injected into the subarachnoid space. The patient is instructed to lie flat for some time after this examination to minimize the headache.

**Intravenous Angiocardiogram.** This is a series of x-ray pictures taken of the heart. The contrast medium, organic iodide, is injected into the vein and a very rapid series of pictures is taken as the medium passes through the heart, to the lungs, back through the heart, and out through the aorta. The medium must be injected rapidly so a large gauge (12 gauge) needle is used. A vein "cutdown" is usually necessary. The entire series of pictures is taken while the patient holds an inspired breath. The complete series is taken during one complete circulation of the medium through the entire body. After the one circulation the opaque medium is too diluted for further filming.

This x-ray study is used to detect cardiac defects. As each chamber of the heart is visualized, pathways for the blood stream are demonstrated, and chamber enlargements can be seen.

The opaque medium may cause a flushing or hot flash as it passes through the body. Sometimes this procedure is done while the patient is under a mild anesthetic. There are no special patient preparations unless an anesthetic is to be given. Then the patient is instructed to take nothing by mouth for a few hours before the test.

**Aortogram.** An aortogram is a film study of the aorta and its branches after the injection of a contrast medium directly into the aorta. A *retrograde aortogram* means the study is done against the direction of the flow of blood. There is no special preparation of the patient for these studies.

**Bronchograms.** These are x-ray pictures of the bronchial tree. Small amounts of iodized oil are introduced by atomizer in order to visualize the outlines of the tubes and their branches. The films are taken immediately after the contrast medium has been introduced. A topical anesthetic is sprayed into the nose and throat to prevent coughing and gagging when the instrument is inserted to introduce the medium.

The patient is given nothing by mouth following this procedure until the anesthetic has worn off. The contrast medium is drained off by means of postural drainage. This is done by placing the patient in a prone position with the head and trunk of the body lower than the buttocks and legs.

**Hysterosalpingogram.** This procedure is also known as *uterosalpingogram.* A contrast medium is injected slowly through the cervical canal into the endometrium of the uterus and fallopian tubes. This is done to aid in the diagnosis of endometrial polyps, submucous fibroids, and tubal and uterine anomalies. Tubal patency (openness) and obstructions are also demonstrated. The patient may be instructed to clear the lower intestines and bowel by taking castor oil and an enema, but this is not always indicated. Otherwise, there are no special instructions to the patient.

**Mammography.** These are x-ray pictures taken of the breast tissue with or without an opaque medium introduced into the mammary ducts. A *simple mammography* is without the use of an opaque medium.

New films and exposure techniques, as well as the skill of the x-ray technician, now make it possible to view this soft tissue. This is an important aid to diagnosis but is not considered to be a substitute for biopsy. It is used to differentiate fibrocystic diseases and can help in the early detection of lesions too small to produce symptoms. It is used as a follow-up procedure in patients who have had a mastectomy. Periodic examinations can help detect early lesions in the remaining breast.

**Radioactive Isotopes (Radioisotopes).** These are used diagnostically and therapeutically. For diagnostic purposes the radioisotopes are administered intravenously and orally. The oral solution is a clear, colorless liquid.

Audrey L. Sutton, R.N., in *Bedside Nursing Techniques* has explained these radioisotopes very well by writing: "Radioactive isotopes emit both beta and gamma rays. An advantage in the use of these artificially made radioactive isotopes is that they emit mostly beta rays and very few gamma rays. Obviously this is a distinct advantage over the use of radium, which emits gamma rays. (Remember, gamma rays penetrate deeply, affecting the entire body; whereas beta rays can penetrate no more than a few millimeters of tissue.) For instance, the beta rays from iodine-131 are able to destroy thyroid tissue without harming the parathyroids.

"Another characteristic of the radioactive isotopes is the rapid rate of disintegration, ranging from several minutes to several years. The length of time required for 50 per cent of the radioactivity to disintegrate from an isotope is called *half-life*. In other words, if it takes two days for one half of gold-198 to disintegrate, the half life of gold is considered to be two days. Each particular radioactive isotope will always disintegrate at the same rate of speed."*

SOME DIAGNOSTIC TESTS WITH RADIOACTIVE ISOTOPES. Tests done with iodine-131 (half-life 8 days, beta and gamma radiation) include several different tests done on the thyroid gland. A good deal of information can be obtained about the status of this gland by the use of what is called *radioiodine*. A tracer dose is given to the patient and the fate of the iodine is followed by measuring its concentration in three areas—the thyroid gland, the urine, and the iodine bound to protein in the blood. These tests are called I-131 Uptake, Urinary excretion of I-131, and so forth. The tests are done with a counter, scintiscanner, or gamma camera. Other radioactive isotopes, such as phosphorus-32, gold-198, cobalt-60, and others, are used for diagnostic tests. These tests are used to locate brain tumors, intraocular tumors, pernicious anemia, to perform kidney scans, and many other procedures.

---

*From Sutton, A. L.: *Bedside Nursing Techniques in Medicine and Surgery*, 2nd Ed., Philadelphia, 1969, W. B. Saunders Co.

## BIBLIOGRAPHY

French, R. M.: *The Nurse's Guide to Diagnostic Procedures*, 3rd Ed., New York, McGraw-Hill Book Co.

Garb, S.: *Laboratory Tests in Common Use*, 5th Ed., New York, 1971, Springer Publishing Co., Inc.

Garnet, T., and Barbata, J.: *Laboratory Specimens*, Totowa, N.J., 1964, Littlefield.

Kark, R. M. et al.: *Primer of Urinalysis*, 2nd Ed., New York, 1963, Harper & Row.

Lynch, M. J., et al.: *Medical Laboratory Technology and Clinical Pathology*, 2nd Ed., Philadelphia, 1969, W. B. Saunders Co.

# Chapter 28

## BEHAVIORAL OBJECTIVES

*The medical office assistant should be able to:*

Identify the four vital signs and their normal limits.

Measure the cardinal signs using the instruments and techniques outlined in this chapter.

Prepare the patient for history taking and physical examination.

Record the patient's history based upon interrogation and examination of the patient.

Drape and position the patient appropriately preparatory to various forms of physical examination, including pelvic, abdominal, and proctoscopic.

Define the principal methodologies of the physical examination, including palpation, percussion, auscultation, mensuration, and manipulation.

Assist the physician in conducting the complete physical examination.

Set up the examination room with the materials discussed in this chapter to facilitate the physician's handling of the examination.

# Assisting with the Physical Examination

The clinical responsibilities of medical assistants vary widely, depending upon the physician's specialty and the extent of his reliance upon auxiliary personnel. Some physicians are reluctant to delegate clinical duties. However, the physician who does utilize competent help appreciates how his own time is saved and his professional skills amplified by the use of a well trained medical assistant. The clinical assistant can ease the role of both the physician and the patient in many office procedures.

The assistant must have the ability to (1) communicate with the patients and the physician, (2) evaluate their needs, and (3) follow instructions quickly and accurately. She must also be able to relay the physician's instructions to the patient accurately and clearly. There is much the assistant can do to save the physician's time in physical examinations. She has to maintain continuity between physician and patient as well as with the other office personnel and services. A good medical assistant follows an organized routine but is flexible enough to adjust to each individual problem.

Almost every patient has some degree of apprehension when called into the examining room. The clinical assistant can do much to ease the patient at this time. The tone of her voice, her ease, and her confidence in caring for the patient are very important. Remember, the medical assistant is present to aid the physician and the patient, not to impress them with her medical knowledge.

## VITAL SIGNS

Since an important part of every physical examination is the determination and recording of the patient's *cardinal signs*, often called *vital signs*, it is necessary for the medical assistant to have an understanding of these signs as well as the ability to determine and record them properly. These signs include the patient's *temperature, pulse, respiration,* and *blood pressure.*

## Temperature

A patient's temperature is an important part of the physical diagnosis. The Fahrenheit scale has been used most frequently in the United States, but many are now using the centigrade scale. Since most temperatures are taken orally, the quotes are assumed to be the oral temperature unless otherwise specified. If the patient is unable to cooperate the temperature is taken rectally and registers one degree higher than the oral temperature. Rectal temperature is generally considered more accurate than oral temperature but is not as convenient to obtain. Occasionally it may be necessary to place the thermometer under the arm. This reading is called the axillary temperature and will record one degree lower than the oral temperature. A patient's oral temperature should not be taken within thirty minutes after his having taken anything by mouth, even smoking.

The body temperature will vary during a 24-hour period. It is influenced by many things, especially the body metabolism and the presence of infection. Lower temperatures are found in the early morning hours. Shock, congestive heart failure, and exposure to extreme cold will lower the body temperature.

The so-called normal temperature is 98.6° F (37.0° C). When the body's temperature is elevated, it is frequently said that the person "has a temperature," but this figurative expression should be avoided since the person has a temperature, whether normal, subnormal, or elevated. The 98.6° F temperature is called the *normal* temperature, but it should be called the *average* temperature. There are some individuals with a normal temperature of 97° F, while others have a normal of 99.6° F. A persistently elevated temperature, called a *fever*, warrants a thorough investigation. There are several types of fevers.

In a *continuous* fever the temperature is elevated and remains consistently elevated with no, or very little, fluctuation during a 24-hour period. In an *intermittent* fever the temperature is elevated at times during the 24-hour period but falls to normal or even subnormal during this time. A *remittent* fever shows a con-

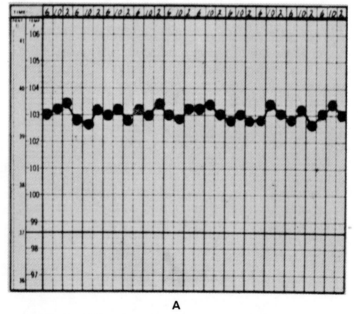

**A**

**Figure 28–1**   Temperature charts demonstrating A continuous fever.

*(Illustration continued on opposite page.)*

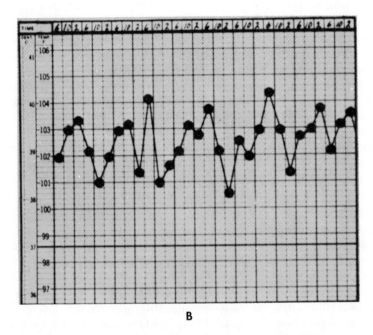

B

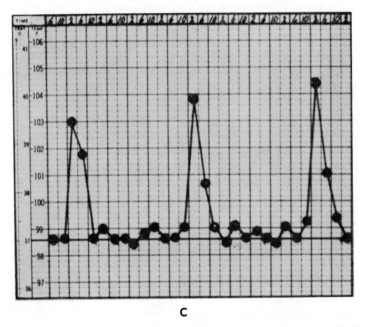

C

**Figure 28–1** *Continued.*  B remittent or septic fever, and C intermittent fever. In the latter case, the patient had benign tertian malaria, with chill and fever at 48-hour intervals. (From Hopkins, H. A.: *Leopold's Physical Diagnosis*, Philadelphia, 1965, W. B. Saunders Co.)

tinuous temperature elevation with a rise and fall but never a drop to the normal level. A remittent fever differs from the continuous fever in that there is a greater variance in the rise and fall of the remittent fever.

A fever is said to be *relapsing* when it recurs after one or more days of normal temperature. Fevers resolve or disappear by lysis or crisis. *Lysis* occurs when a fever gradually falls over a period of several days. If a fever abruptly falls within a 36-hour period it does so by *crisis*. Frequently a fever crisis is accompanied by profuse sweating *(diaphoresis)*. Diaphoresis also occurs in night sweats, extreme weakness and nervousness. Chills and rigor (shivering) are frequently found in patients who are having a fever crisis.

**Thermometers.** There are three types of fever thermometers used in a physician's office: oral, rectal, and security tips. Each thermometer should be stored in its individual container. *Do not* keep several thermometers in the same container. Label the container as to thermometer type, e.g., oral or rectal. Patients are very alert and apprehensive as to the type of thermometer, where it was used, and its cleanliness.

**How to Take a Temperature.** Rinse the thermometer well with cool water before using it. It is a good habit to hold your finger under the water tap before rinsing the thermometer. Someone may have just finished washing in hot water, and the warm water in the tap could cause difficulties. After rinsing the thermometer with cool water, check to see that the mercury is below 95° F. If not, shake the mercury down. To shake down, hold the top end between the thumb and first finger and swing the wrist down with a snap, as though shaking water off the fingers. Do not attempt to shake it down by grasping in the fingers and striking the hand against a solid object, as this will injure the thermometer. Place the thermometer in the patient's mouth under the tongue to one side. The patient should keep the mouth closed and the tongue down, breathing through the nose. An oral tip thermometer is kept in place for three minutes. Remove the thermometer from the patient's mouth and wipe the saliva and lipstick off with a rotary stroke over the bulb. Never touch the mercury bulb end. Hold the thermometer at eye level with the right hand so the calibrated scale is toward you. Rotate it slightly back and forth with the thumb and finger until the mercury column is clearly seen between the scale lines and the numbers. Read and record. Wash the thermometer with soap and cool water. Disinfect it with an antiseptic solution and rinse again with cool water before returning it to the container.

RECTAL TEMPERATURE. Rectal temperatures are taken on the very young

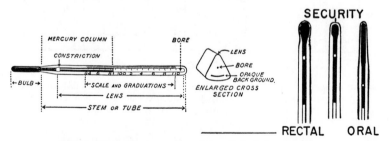

**Figure 28–2** Construction of the clinical thermometer.

patient, the patient with breathing difficulty, the uncooperative patient, and the unconscious patient. The rectal thermometer has a stubby bulb for safety purposes. NEVER use an oral thermometer in the rectum. Rectal thermometers should be carefully labeled and stored in a separate container. The procedure is the same as for the oral temperature, except the tip of the rectal thermometer is lubricated with vasoline or lubricating jelly and then gently inserted into the rectum past the constricting muscle of the anus, about one and one-half inches. The rectal thermometer is held in place for five minutes. Do not leave a patient alone while the thermometer is in the rectum. Remove, wipe and read. Record. The normal rectal temperature is usually one degree higher than the oral temperature.

The rectal temperature is most frequently done on the infant. The infant is placed on his back with the buttocks exposed. With the index finger between the ankles, grasp the legs and flex the knees over the infant's abdomen, exposing the anus; with the other hand insert the lubricated rectal thermometer into the anus about one inch. Keep a gentle but firm hold on the legs. Hold the thermometer in place between your index and great finger while the palm of the hand and thumb grasps the infant's buttocks. This hold will steady the infant and will also hold the thermometer secure. Be very careful not to let go of your holds on the legs and the buttocks while the thermometer is in place. After five minutes, remove, wipe and read. Record.

AXILLARY OR GROIN TEMPERATURE.   Use a rectal or security tip thermometer. Rinse thermometer and shake down. Wipe the area dry before putting the thermometer in place. Allow it to remain in place ten minutes. Instruct the patient to remain quiet during this time. Remove and record. The normal temperature reading taken by these methods will be 97.6° F, or one degree lower than a temperature reading obtained orally.

**Using the Electronic Thermometer.**   The electronic thermometers are very rapid, within five seconds, and claim an accuracy of within ± 0.2° F. They have disposable tips for both oral and rectal, which are color coded. The temperature reading on the dial remains in position until released, permitting an accurate recording on the patient's chart (Fig. 28–3).

These electronic thermometers require adjustment, and care must be taken to have the dial directly in front of you at eye level while adjusting it; otherwise, it will be inaccurately adjusted if you are viewing it from an oblique angle.

## Pulse Rate

This is such a routine part of the physical examination that it is often taken in a mechanical way, and some of the finer aspects are neglected. It is a method of counting the heartbeat through the walls of an artery. What is felt is a shock wave that travels along the fibers of the arteries as the heart contracts, similar to the sound of hammering as it travels through a pipe. The pulse rate varies from person to person. It is affected by the individual's activities and illnesses. The average adult pulse rate is from 60 to 90 beats per minute. During resting periods the rate is usually 60 to 70 beats per minute while during normal activity it may be from 70 to 90. The pulse rate of a young athlete may be as slow as 50

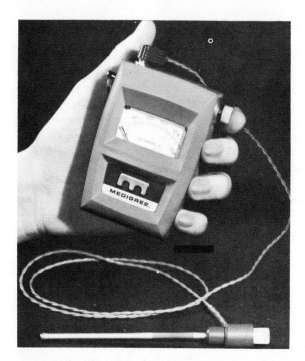

**Figure 28–3** Electronic thermometer. (Courtesy of Chesebrough-Pond's Inc.)

beats per minute. Infants and children usually have a slightly faster pulse rate of 90 to 120.

The radial artery at the wrist is the place most frequently used to take a pulse rate, but it may be taken any place where there is an artery near the body surface: the carotid artery at the neck, the temporal artery at the temporal area of the head, the brachial artery at the elbow, the popliteal artery at the back of the knee, and the dorsal pedis on the instep of the foot.

**How to Count the Pulse Rate.** The patient should be in a comfortable position with the wrist preferably near the same level as the heart. The arm should be well supported and relaxed. The patient may be sitting or lying down. With your first three fingers, locate the radial artery or another selected site and apply gentle pressure slightly above the wrist bone and the cords on the thumb side of the arm. Count the pulse for one minute. Make note of any irregularity or variations of the normal quality of the beat such as an arrhythmia (irregularity), strong or weak, jerky, unequal, and the like. Record the number of beats per minute.

## Respiration

The normal respiration rate is 16 to 20 per minute, somewhat slower in older persons and faster in infants and small children. The respiration rate gen-

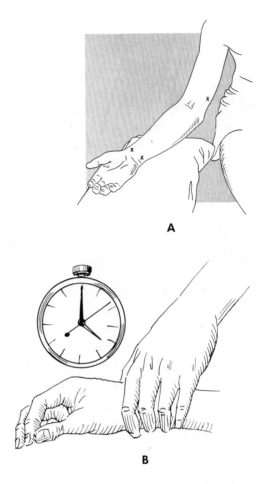

**Figure 28–4** A. Sites of palpation of the radial, ulnar, and brachial pulses. (From Dunphy, J. E., and Botsford, J. W.: *Physical Examination of the Surgical Patient*, 3rd Ed., Philadelphia, 1964, W. B. Saunders Co.) B. Counting pulsations. (From Wood, L. A.: *Nursing Skills for Allied Health Services*, Vol. II, Philadelphia, 1972, W. B. Saunders Co.)

erally increases as the body's temperature rises. An example of the respiration, pulse and temperature ratio is:

| Respiration | Pulse | Temperature |
|:-----------:|:-----:|:-----------:|
| 18 | 80 | 99°F |
| 21 | 96 | 101°F |
| 23 | 104 | 102°F |
| 28 | 126 | 105°F |

Variations occur in the respiratory rate (fast or slow), volume (deep or shallow), and rhythm (regular or irregular). There are specific medical terms used in describing the alterations that are found in breathing. *Dyspnea*, meaning difficult breathing, occurs in patients with pneumonia or asthma; it also occurs after physical exertion or at very high altitudes. Other alterations in breathing are *bradypnea* (abnormally slow respiration), *apnea* (temporary cessation of respiration), *tachypnea* (excessively rapid breathing), and *hyperpnea* (increased depth of breathing). Hyperpnea is usually accompanied by *hyperventilation* and is frequently found in emotional conditions. *Orthopnea* means a patient has dif-

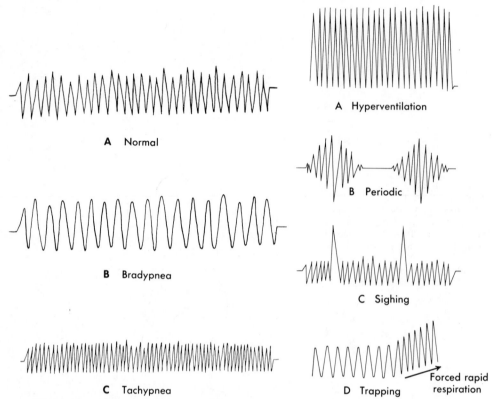

**Figure 28-5**  Spirograms demonstrating various respiratory patterns. (From Prior, J. A., and Silberstein, J. S.: *Physical Diagnosis*, 3rd Ed., St. Louis, 1973, The C. V. Mosby Co.)

ficulty breathing while in a supine position, as found in patients with congestive heart failure.

**How to Take the Respiration Rate.**    Because the respiration rate is easily controlled, and since a patient who is conscious of his breathing's being watched will control it to some extent, it is advisable to count the rate while appearing to be interested in something else, such as the pulse rate.

The medical assistant may keep her eyes alternately on the patient's chest and her watch while she is counting the pulse rate, and then, without taking her fingers from the pulse, she can count the respiration rate. If the patient is lying down, his arm can be crossed over his chest so the respirations can be felt with the rise and fall of the chest. Count the respirations for a minute and record. Also note any variations or irregularities in the rate.

## Blood Pressure

Arterial blood pressure is an important part of the physical examination and is recorded with the other vital signs – temperature, pulse, and respiration.

Blood pressure is the pressure of the blood against the walls of the arteries.

This pressure is determined by the pumping action of the heart, the resistance of the blood's flow through the arteries, the elasticity of the arterial walls, the amount of blood in the vessels, and the blood's viscosity (thickness). Because of these influencing factors, there are actually two blood pressures within the blood vessels. The *systolic* pressure is the highest pressure when the heart is contracting and when the pulse beat is felt. The *diastolic* pressure is the lowest pressure when the heart is relaxed and there is no pulse beat felt. The difference between the systolic and the diastolic is called the *pulse pressure.*

The normal average blood pressure of an adult is between 90 and 140 mm Hg (millimeters of mercury) systolic reading, and 60 to 90 mm Hg for the diastolic reading, with an average of 120/80 mm Hg. Blood pressure is recorded as a fraction, with the systolic reading on top and the diastolic reading on the bottom. The male adult has a slightly higher reading than the female. A child's reading is usually lower than an adult's. Older persons may have a slightly higher reading. A person of 60 years of age may have a normal reading of 140/90 mm. Hg. For routine frequent blood pressure checks the readings should be taken at about the same time of day and by the same person.

A person is said to have *hypertension* if his blood pressure is consistently above the normal pressure. It is not diagnostic of any one disease but can be found in various renal diseases, during pregnancy, in certain endocrine disturbances and in obesity. Blood pressure is increased in arteriosclerosis, atherosclerosis and brain injury. It is also influenced by pain, fear and exercise.

Low blood pressure is referred to as *hypotension* and is found in a wide variety of conditions such as hemorrhage, chronic wasting diseases and shock, both emotional and traumatic. *Orthostatic hypotension* is a form of low blood pressure that occurs when a person changes from a supine position to an upright position rather rapidly or when standing for a long period of time.

The instrument used to take blood pressure is called the *sphygmomanometer* and is aided by the *stethoscope.* A manometer is an instrument used to measure pressure of a liquid or gas. By adding *sphygmo-* (pulse) it means an instrument

**Figure 28–6**   Sphygmomanometer, (From Wood, L. A.: *Nursing Skills for Allied Health Services.* Vol. II, Philadelphia, 1972. W. B. Saunders Co.)

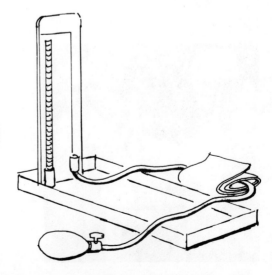

used to measure the arterial blood pressure; that is, the pulse pressure. There are two types of sphygmomanometers used, the mercury and the aneroid manometers. Both should be handled carefully; they are delicate and expensive instruments. The aneroid is easy to transport but should be frequently calibrated by the manufacturer. The mercury column is considered to be more accurate.

**How to Take a Blood Pressure.** The patient may be lying down with his arm resting beside him and the palm turned upward, or he may be sitting with the arm resting on a firm surface, palm upward and on the same level as his heart. Explain to the patient that the arm must be relaxed. Roll his sleeve about five inches above the bend of the elbow. Be careful the sleeve does not constrict the arm. Apply the completely deflated cuff around the arm about two inches above the bend. The cuff should be high enough to place the stethoscope without touching the cuff. The cuff is applied evenly and should be slightly snug. Place the stethoscope in your ears (the earpieces of the stethoscope should be pointing away from the face). Palpate the brachial artery and place the stethoscope over this point. Listen for the pulse. Hold the stethoscope over this point gently but firmly. Gently tighten the screw on the rubber bulb to close the air escape valve. By pumping the bulb, inflate the cuff until the pulse ceases, then inflate to 20 mm. higher. Now open the valve on the bulb slightly and listen for the return of the pulse beat, watching the mercury column or the aneroid dial. Slowly let the air escape from the bulb while watching the column and listening for the pulse beat. The first beat you hear is the systolic pressure. Continue to let the air escape slowly. The beat will become clearer and louder. Then suddenly the sound of the heart beat will be very dull and soft. This change in the beat is the diastolic pressure. Some physicians record the last sound heard as the diastolic pressure. It is advisable to check with your physician as to his preference (Fig. 28–7).

Clear all the air from the cuff and wait a few minutes; then repeat the procedure. Do not take one reading immediately after another and never take more than three successive readings on the same arm. Change arms. Record immediately. If others are using the stethoscope be sure to wipe the earpieces off with alcohol.

PALPATORY METHOD. The systolic pressure may be checked by feeling the

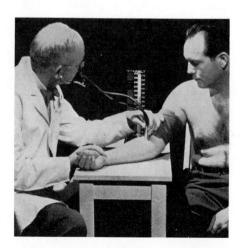

**Figure 28–7** Taking the blood pressure, employing both palpatory and auscultatory methods. (From Delp, L. H., and Manning, R. T.: *Major's Physical Diagnosis*, 7th Ed., Philadelphia, 1968, W. B. Saunders Co.)

radial pulse rather than using the stethoscope to hear the brachial pulse. Place the cuff in the usual position and palpate the radial pulse, noting the rate and rhythm. Now inflate the cuff until the pulse disappears and then go about 30 mm above this point. Do not remove your fingers from the pulse or change the pressure of your fingers. Now slowly let the pressure in the cuff down until the radial pulse is felt again. Note the mercury reading and record as the systolic pressure. The diastolic pressure is difficult to measure by this method and is not determined by the palpatory method.

COMMON CAUSES OF ERROR

1. The patient's arm is not at the same level as the heart. (It is not necessary for the manometer to be at the level of the heart.)
2. The rubber bladder in the cuff has not been deflated before starting or retaking a reading.
3. The mercury column is allowed to drop too rapidly, resulting in inaccurate readings.
4. The patient is nervous, uncomfortable or too anxious. This may cause a higher reading than the patient's actual blood pressure.
5. The cuff is improperly applied:
   a. Rubber bladder bulging out from the cover.
   b. Cuff not around arm smoothly.
   c. Cuff too tight or too loose.
6. Failing to wait a few minutes between retakes and not deflating the cuff completely between readings.
7. Defective apparatus:
   a. Air leak in a valve, especially the release valve.
   b. Leak in the rubber bladder.
   c. Mercury column is dirty.
   d. Mercury column is not at zero, although a zero reading on the aneroid manometer does not guarantee accuracy. It should be checked by the manufacturer.
8. On extremely obese patients it may be necessary to apply the cuff on the forearm and place the stethoscope over the radial artery.

# HISTORY TAKING

In order to understand the patient's needs it is necessary for the physician first to interview the patient and obtain a medical history. This permits the physician to correlate later the physical findings with information acquired in the history. Interrogation (history taking) and examination cannot be separated. They are the two basic skills of the medical profession.

The office assistant should assist the physician during this interview by making sure that the office surroundings are pleasant and by seeing that the physician is not interrupted. Good office and patient rapport, with respect for the patient, will enhance both the history taking and the physical examination.

Here are some terms used in writing a patient's medical history:

*Chief Complaint (C.C.).* This is usually the reason for the patient's seeking medical care. Often it is recorded in the patient's own words.

*Present Illness (P.I.).* This is an amplification of the chief complaint. It is usually written in chronological sequence with dates of onset.

*Systems Review (S.R.)* or *Review of Systems (R.O.S.).* This serves as a guide to general health and tends to detect conditions other than those covered in the present illness. It is obtained by logical sequence of questions beginning with the head and proceeding downward.

*Past History (P.H.)* or *Past Medical History (P.M.H.).* Questions regarding the patient's *Usual Childhood Diseases (U.C.H.D.)* are asked—major illnesses and operations, allergies, accidents, and immunizations.

*Family History (F.H.).* Details regarding the patient's mother and father are obtained—their health and, if deceased, the cause and age of death. Hereditary tendencies are recorded here.

The physician may wish to inquire about the patient's *Occupational History (O.H.)* and *Social History (S.H.).* Social history includes his eating and drinking habits, hobbies, and interests.

Many times you will hear that certain findings and conclusions in a medical history are either *subjective* or *objective.* These two terms are sometimes confused as are the terms *symptoms* and *signs* which are often used interchangeably with subjective and objective.

*Subjective* findings are the *symptoms* that are perceptible to only the patient; they pertain to the individual only. They are the subjective conclusions or symptoms that often bring the patient to the physician. An ache, pain, or vertigo is felt only by the patient. The patient tells the physician about these symptoms and the physician records them as subjective findings. *Cardinal symptoms* are the most significant of the patient's complaints, the ones that are used to establish a diagnosis.

*Objective* findings are perceptible to a person other than the patient. They are the *signs* that a physician detects when he examines a patient. A physician feels, sees or hears the signs that are often associated with a certain disease or abnormal condition. These objective findings are dependent on another's senses. A mass that a physician feels in the patient's abdomen is an *objective* finding. It is a *sign* of an abnormal condition.

Other terms used that require understanding are the words *functional* and *physical.* When a physician says a condition or disease is functional he means the disease is without discoverable lesion or organic cause. That is, the organ may appear "normal" but its function is not normal. A functional disease is any disease that alters the body functions but is not associated with any apparent organic or physical lesion. A physical disease or condition is one in which the abnormality or lesion can be seen or felt.

Some physicians may, at this time, make a summary of the history. Others may prefer to dictate it after the physical examination has been completed.

## PHYSICAL EXAMINATION

After the physician has talked with the patient he will request the medical assistant to prepare the patient for the physical examination. Frequently at this time the assistant will take the patient's weight and height. If the patient is to be weighed at each subsequent office visit, then it may be advisable to take the weight before the patient disrobes so the gain or loss will be consistent with the usual amount of clothing the patient will wear to the office. Place a paper towel on the scale and ask the patient to remove his shoes. For accurate height reading, have the patient face forward on the scale and record the height in inches. (For safety, remember to lower the head height bar the moment the patient steps off the scale.)

## Draping the Patient

Give the patient a gown or drape and ask him to disrobe sufficiently. Do not ask a patient to undress in an area that does not afford privacy or a place to leave personal belongings. If a patient appears to object to disrobing, then you must tactfully explain the necessity in order to have a complete examination of the area involved. It must be emphasized that failure to expose adequately will often lead to unnecessary delays and difficulties for the physician. Rapport is often accomplished by conversation, but as soon as the physician enters the room to start the examination the medical assistant should keep her conversation at a minimum.

If so directed by the physician, the medical assistant may take the patient's vital signs before informing the physician that the patient is ready.

## Positions and Draping of Patient for Physical Examinations

Here are instructions for placing patients in position and draping them for the various types of examinations (Fig. 28–8).

**Sims' Position.**   This position is sometimes called the "lateral" position, but since lateral only means "side" this does not clearly state the complete position. The patient is placed on the left side with a small towel under the left cheek. The left arm and shoulder are drawn back so the weight of the body is on the chest. The right arm is forward for support. The left leg is fairly straight, and the right leg is flexed upward sharply. The body is covered with a sheet that is raised over the rectal area. A towel is placed between the thighs near the rectum. This position is used for rectal examinations, and sometimes is used for pelvic examinations when the lithotomy position is not advisable.

**Lithotomy Position.**   Since this name is taken from history rather than describing the position, it is sometimes called *dorsosacral* position or *dorsal recumbent with knees flexed.* The patient is placed on the back with the knees flexed high, the arms at the side or folded over the chest, and the buttocks at the extreme edge of the table. The feet are supported in the examining table stirrups. The stirrups should be placed as far out as possible to swing the thighs well apart and not have the patient's heels too close to the thighs. The patient is less likely to have leg cramps with the stirrups far out. A towel is placed under the buttocks and a sheet draped over the abdomen and knees to the ankles. The physician will push the sheet back over the pubic area when he is ready to do the examination.

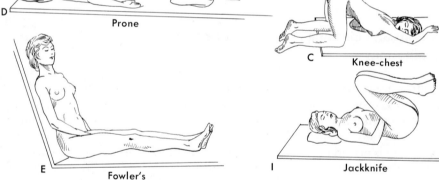

**Figure 28–8** Positioning during the physical examination.

When the patient is assisted down to the edge of the table it is not necessary to look but a quick movement of the assistant's hand can tell if the patient is at the table's edge.

**Knee-Chest Position.** As the term implies, the patient rests on the knees and chest. The head is turned to one side with one arm flexed under the abdomen and the other arm over the side of the table or above the head for support. The thighs are perpendicular to the table and slightly separated. This is a difficult position to maintain, but with assistance and support some patients can achieve a true knee-chest position. If not, it may be necessary to place the patient in a modified form of the knee-chest known as the *knee-elbow* or *genupectoral* position. A small pillow may be placed under the chest to aid in relaxation. The patient should be fully draped with only the anal and vaginal areas exposed. A fenestrated drape offers the best protection. This position is used for rectal examinations and some vaginal and prostatic examinations. It is also used for postpartum exercise.

**Proctological Position.**    This position necessitates an examining table that can be elevated in the center, lowering the head and foot, or a Procto-Rest (Fig. 28–9) may be used on the standard examining table. The patient's head and legs are lower than the buttocks. This position is used for proctological examinations, especially sigmoidoscopic examinations, because the sigmoid bowel is displaced into the abdominal cavity. A fenestrated sheet or two sheets are necessary for proper draping. Do not bind the legs together with the drape because it is often necessary for the legs to be separated for adequate examination. This position is sometimes incorrectly called the jackknife position. The true *jackknife* has the patient placed on his back with the shoulders slightly elevated and the legs flexed sharply with the thighs at right angles to the abdomen. This position is sometimes used to pass a urethral sound.

**Dorsal Position.**    The patient is lying on his back. In the *dorsal-recumbent* position the patient is on his back with the knees slightly flexed so as to have the soles of the feet flat on the table. In the *dorsal-elevated* position the patient is on his back with the head and shoulders slightly elevated, somewhat like the *Fowler's* position. The *supine* or *horizontal* position has the patient on his back. These two terms are frequently used in x-ray positioning. The *Walcher's* position has the patient on his back with the hips at the edge of the table and the legs hanging down.

The *prone* position has the patient lying face down or on the *ventral* surface of the body.

**Trendelenburg Position.**    This position is not used routinely for office examinations but is often used in the operating room. It displaces the intestines into the upper abdomen. The patient is placed on his back with the body on an incline, the head slightly lower, and the knees flexed over the lower end of the table. The patient should be supported to prevent slipping.

## Methods of Examination

A physician will employ several different methods to examine a patient. They are as follows.

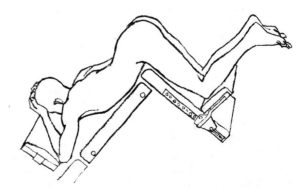

**Figure 28–9**   Inverted position on proctoscopic table. (See Figure 28–8F for proctological position.)

**Inspection.**  The visual study of that which can be seen, usually by the naked eye, such as the color of the skin, injuries, deformities, tremors, and rashes.

**Palpation.**  The feeling and manipulation of a part with the hand for the purpose of ascertaining its condition or that of the underlying organs. This method is used in feeling the skin and in feeling the abdomen for masses. Palpation may be done with both hands (bimanually) as in a pelvic examination or by one finger (digitally) as in an anal examination. (DO NOT CONFUSE with palpi-*t*ation which is a throbbing pulsation.)

**Percussion.**  The tapping of the surface of the body with a finger or a small hammer to elicit sounds or vibratory sensations. This method is often used in the examination of the chest and abdomen.

**Auscultation.**  The listening to sounds arising from within the body and from the various organs. This method is used chiefly to check the heart and lungs. Immediate auscultation is the direct application of the examiner's ear to the patient's body. Mediate auscultation is done with the aid of a stethoscope.

**Mensuration.**  The process of measuring as done in chest expansion. This method is often employed by orthopedists.

**Manipulation.**  The forceful passive movement of a joint to determine its range of extension or flexion. Manipulation may or may not be grouped with palpation. This is an important part of an orthopedic or neurological examination.

Because a complete physical examination varies with the physician's specialty and the patient's needs, this section will outline the general step-by-step sequence. Specialty examinations will be covered in a later chapter.

The patient's general appearance is an essential part of an examination. The body movements, both voluntary and involuntary, and posture are observed. Nutritional appearance, skin color and texture, voice, and speech pattern are also noted. The patient may be asked to walk, in order for the physician to observe any abnormalities in gait, such as limping or feet wide apart. Fat distribution is noted. Excessive perspiration and edema are diagnostic. Body hair distribution and the texture of the hair are observed.

With the patient seated on the examining table, the physician usually starts his examination with the head. The ears are examined with an otoscope for excessive wax and irritations of the external ear canal. Hearing acuity may be checked with a tuning fork. The nasal cavity is next examined with a nasal speculum. The physician may observe a deviated nasal septum or nasal polyps. The nasal mucosa is viewed for color and signs of irritation. The sinuses may be transilluminated. The oral cavity reveals many diagnostic signs, such as odor of breath, color and appearance of the mucosa, condition of the teeth and gums. The nasopharynx and larynx are examined. The floor of the mouth is palpated. The patient's oral hygiene and condition of the teeth are important health factors.

The eyes are examined for irritation of the conjunctiva, size and reaction of the pupils, intraocular pressure, ptosis of the eyelids, and ocular movements. The retina will be viewed with the ophthalmoscope. The distance visual acuity is checked, usually by the medical assistant, with the aid of the visual acuity chart.

Voluntary and involuntary movements of the head are examined. The neck is palpated for adenopathy, and the patient may be asked to swallow several times. The medical assistant may give the patient a small amount of water in a disposable cup to aid in swallowing. The back is viewed for mobility, kyphosis, scoliosis, and lordosis.

Auscultation of the lungs for breath sounds and rales is done and the sounds over the entire cardiac area are carefully checked. The patient's breast and axilla are palpated for adenopathy. The female breast is very carefully checked for consistency in texture, symmetry, tenderness, and palpable masses. The nipples are checked for possible discharge.

While the patient is still in the sitting position the reflexes are checked: biceps, quadriceps (knee jerk) and Achilles ankle jerk. Other reflexes may be tested with the patient in a supine position.

The patient is now lowered into a dorsal recumbent position (supine) and the abdomen exposed. If the female patient does not have a gown, then place a towel over the breasts. Here the physician is somewhat dependent on the patient's cooperation in telling him where the discomfort is located. It is necessary for the patient to be completely relaxed; this can only be obtained if the patient is comfortable and warm, without fear or apprehension. Sometimes abdominal relaxation is aided by having the patient's knees flexed. The internal organs are located by topographic anatomy, both by quadrants and regions (Fig. 28-10). Although palpation is the important method of abdominal examination, the physician will look for asymmetry, visible masses, and general appearance. The stethoscope may be used to locate bowel sounds or a bruit in the abdomen. Often abdominal pain is not experienced over the organ involved. Abdominal hernias may be checked in the dorsal position as well as in a standing position. To aid in further examination of the abdomen, the patient may be placed in other positions, such as knee-chest or Sims'.

After the abdominal examination the female patient will be given a pelvic examination (see Chapter 32). The external male genitalia are examined in the standing as well as in the dorsal position. The examination is basically inspection

**Figure 28-10**  A. Regions of the abdomen. B. Abdominal incisions.

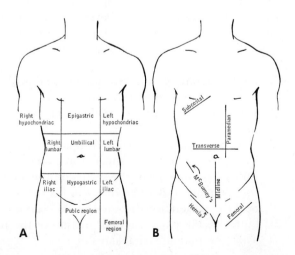

and palpation. Inspection of the foreskin and glans penis of the penis and palpation of the scrotum, as well as inspection for urethral anomalies are done. The prostate gland is usually palpated by having the patient bend at the waist over the examining table. The knee-chest position may be used to examine the obese male patient. The rectum of the female patient is palpated at the time of the pelvic examination. In the male, it is examined at the time of the prostatic examination. The rectum is palpated for sphincter tone, external and internal hemorrhoids, and palpable masses. (See Chapter 32 for proctoscopic examination.)

The sequence of a pediatric examination is essentially the same as that for the adult patient. The physician will be concerned with the child's sleeping, eating, and toilet habits. It is important that the physician and the office staff have good rapport with these little patients. Learn to listen to them and talk with them. For the routine well-baby examination the mother is usually asked to undress the baby. The baby's weight, height, and immunizations are carefully checked and recorded in the mother's record of the child as well as in the office record. Provide a drape or gown for older children.

## OUTLINE OF PROCEDURE AND SETUPS FOR PHYSICAL EXAMINATION

### Complete Physical Examination (Pelvic and Rectal not Included)

If a medical assistant is assisting the physician during this examination, it may not be necessary to have the needed items placed out on a tray. They may be handed to the physician from drawers or the side counter as they are needed.

Materials needed:

| | | |
|---|---|---|
| Otoscope | Sphygmomanometer | Disposable gloves |
| Tongue depressor | Percussion hammer | Tuning fork |
| Cleansing tissue | Ophthalmoscope | Stethoscope |
| Tape measure | Flashlight or headlight | |

1. After you have greeted the patient and made him feel at ease, explain briefly what examination is to be done.
2. Have the patient empty his bladder. Save the specimen for laboratory testing.
3. Ask the patient to disrobe completely and put on a gown. If a gown is not used give the patient a sheet. Some offices have the female patient leave her underslip on and slip the straps off the shoulders. Sometimes it is sufficient for the male to disrobe down to his trousers.
4. Seat the patient on the edge of the examining table with a towel under the buttocks. Place a sheet over the lap of the female patient.
5. Take the patient's vital signs.

6. Call the physician when the patient is ready. Remain in the room if a female patient is being examined, or if the physician requests your assistance.
7. After the patient has been examined in the sitting position, he is then placed in a dorsal-recumbent position. If the patient is ill or has had recent abdominal surgery, assist him down by giving him your arm as a support in order to prevent abdominal strain. Some physicians prefer the patient's hand placed over the chest; others prefer the arms at the sides. The patient may need to flex the knees slightly to obtain better abdominal relaxation. If the patient is extremely nervous and the knees are shaking, the assistant should support them, giving better relaxation.
8. After the examination is completed do not raise the patient too rapidly because dizziness may occur and the patient can easily fall forward or sideways. Also remember to raise and lower the footrest and leg support at the same time the patient is lying down or sitting up; otherwise, there is considerable strain on the back and abdominal muscles.
9. When the physician has finished his examination, assist the patient off the table and ask him to dress. If necessary, assist the patient in dressing; otherwise, respect his privacy.
10. Remember to give the patient any instructions before leaving the room. Too often patients are left in a room without knowing what they should do after they are dressed, or even if they *may* dress. Without instructions, they may leave the office without another appointment, a prescription, or treatment instructions.
11. Clean the room immediately. Put fresh paper on the table. A fresh towel should be placed on the pillow. Disinfect any surfaces that may need it. Remove all used instruments to be sanitized or sterilized. Return medications to their proper places. Check the room carefully and have it ready for the next patient.

# Chapter 29

**BEHAVIORAL OBJECTIVES**

*The medical office assistant should be able to:*

Identify the major apparatus used in office physical therapy and their applications.

Identify indications and contraindications for use of short-wave diathermy, radiation therapy, ultrasonic therapy, and other therapies introduced in this chapter.

Prepare the patient for physical therapy.

Assist the physician in administration of the physical therapies introduced in this chapter.

# Assisting in Physical
# Therapy

The duties of the medical assistant in physical therapy may be limited, and the authors recognize that it would be preferable if all medical offices employed graduate physical therapists to administer therapeutic treatment according to their employer's prescription. Since, however, there are a limited number of trained therapists, most of them being employed in hospitals and clinics, the medical assistant in the physician's office is almost universally required to learn to administer the various types of physical therapy treatments. Usually the physician himself administers the first treatment to the patient, directing and supervising subsequent treatments given by the medical assistant. This chapter is devoted simply to briefing the reader on the types of equipment employed and some suggestions on the use of these modalities.

Manufacturers of the various modalities provide materials that may be studied by the medical assistant to gain a better understanding of their nature and use. Manufacturers will frequently, on request, train the individual assistant in the proper handling of a given instrument so that the physician's orders may be carried out efficiently.

Mechanical and electrical modalities used in the office to treat the variety of conditions are considered *adjuncts.* Adjunctive therapy is an aid to another remedy or to the normal body functions in promoting a faster healing effect. This term is frequently applied to the various methods of physical therapy.

## SHORT WAVE DIATHERMY

The use of short wave diathermy has been popular for over forty years and is used in many physician's offices. The short wave diathermy machine is designed to produce energy very similar to that emitted by a radio station. Applied to human tissue, this energy penetrates deep within the body tissues and is expended in the form of heat. It is simply called "heat within," or diathermy (dia = through, thermy = heat). The temperature rise is the "yardstick" of the rate of energy expended in the tissues. This radio frequency energy produces heat within the tissues that dilates the blood capillaries, veins, and arteries, and a temperature rise of a few degrees above normal will greatly increase the rate of blood flow through the heated area. Diathermy is therefore prescribed in cases

**539**

in which the physician believes a materially increased blood supply is indicated. As a general rule, diathermy (heat) is indicated in all inflammatory processes, acute, subacute, or chronic, except where there is encapsulated pus without drainage or where there is danger of hemorrhage. Diathermy treatments over the abdominal area are contraindicated in the prepartum patient. The diabetic patient will be given special care, too. Diathermy heat will also concentrate in any conductive materials such as surgical implants and prostheses. A patient should be carefully questioned if there is a scar in the area to be treated to make certain there is no such implant beneath the area. Since scar tissue does not have the normal supply of blood vessels or nerves, precautions should be taken in applying the electrode pads over these areas. Areas that are suspected or known to be near a malignancy are also avoided. Be very cautious in cases where there is absence of or the possibility of impaired sensation. Infants and psychotic patients cannot always report excessive heat sensations. Erythema of the skin may be a possible indication of an underlying obstruction such as a blood clot in the vascular system. Other contraindications are cases of possible impairment in the cardiovascular and renal systems, respiratory diseases, and osteoporosis. Careful observation of the skin should be made for the possibility of blisters that may be the result of hot water bottles, heating pads, or skin ointments and salves that have been applied previously by the patient.

**Patient Preparation.** The patient should be disrobed and the area to be treated exposed and examined for scars, color changes of the skin, and any metals. Hearing aids and metal objects, such as rings, bra or underslip metal snaps, should be removed, because heat can concentrate in these objects. Do not place the patient on a metal table or permit him to come in contact with metal objects. Make certain the patient is comfortable before applying the electrodes (pads or drums). Possibly, this will prevent the patient from changing his position later to be more comfortable, resulting in the electrode's being moved to an incorrect position. For sanitary reasons and to collect perspiration place a towel over the patient between the skin and the electrode. Excessive perspiration may cause a steam blister if it is allowed to pool on the skin.

After the diathermy applicator has been applied to the desired area to be treated, the dosage power should be adjusted so only a mild sensation of warmth is felt by the patient. Ask the patient to tell you when he feels the first sensation of warmth. At this point deep tissue heating will be at maximum, and the surface heating will be at minimum. Many patients feel that if a little warmth will produce results more heat will produce greater results. This theory does not follow with short wave diathermy. DO NOT PERMIT THE PATIENT TO ASK FOR OR DEMAND MORE HEAT. NEVER INCREASE THE VOLUME OF ENERGY (HEAT) ABOVE THE INITIAL COMFORTABLE TOLERANCE OF THE PATIENT. The patient's receptor cells have become adjusted to the warmth; power has not been reduced. When the energy has been increased, it increases the temperature and the dose of treatment is increased. Remember that the patient cannot give you a true answer about what he feels because he does not know. DO NOT position the machine so the patient can reach it himself and turn up the energy. If the treatment temperature has been correct the patient should receive benefit within 36 to 48 hours after the treatment has been administered. If the patient has been overtreated (too much heat) he may not receive these benefits but may have pain or discomfort afterwards from the excessive energy expended in the tissues. The correct amount of heat in the underlying tissues results in dilation of the blood vessels in the area, which promotes a favorable amount of blood supply to the area not only during the treatment time but lasting for an additional period during the cooling off time. The average underlying muscular tissue temperature will reach around 105° F.

Diathermy treatments may be administered on a daily basis or three times a week depending on the physician's instructions. The average duration of the treatment is 20 to 30 minutes. Do not let the patient demand more time beyond the prescribed treatment.

Read the manufacturer's instructions carefully. The machine must be kept clean. Do not permit the electrical cords to kink or have any pull on the connections. The cords or cables leading to the patient electrodes should not be permitted to cross each other or to touch the patient in any way. Electricity follows the path of least resistance and will flow from one cord to another or to the places it touches and the patient will not receive any energy, since the current will be flowing from cord to cord. Almost all machines will have spacers on these cords to prevent this. Some machines may require a "warm up" period for the machine.

## RADIATION THERAPY

This is treatment by use of therapeutic rays. The two most used rays in the physician's office are the invisible infrared ray and the ultraviolet ray. The roentgen ray (x-ray) and radium emanations are akin to these but, because their use requires highly specialized training, they are not discussed in this book.

### Infrared Therapy

This type of therapy is produced by the infrared lamp which gives heat much the same as the diathermy machine. This heat, however, is generated by a metal coil element or a special heat-producing lamp. The beam from the infrared lamp is directed to the area of the patient's body needing treatment. The energy hits the skin surface, and since very shallow penetration occurs (the penetration is about 3 to 5 mm. (0.1 to 0.2 inch) (Fig. 29–1) and is dependent on conduction to the lower tissues) this results in about one degree of temperature elevation in those tissues. While not as effective as diathermy in producing a deep heat, the infrared lamp is very simple and fast.

**Patient Preparation.** The area to be treated by this modality should be exposed and examined for scars, redness, or any condition that contraindicates applying heat to the area. The patient should be placed in a comfortable position, either lying on a treatment table or sitting in a chair. Do not let the patient contact any metal surface that may also be heated by the lamp. Remove any metal from the treatment area. The lamp is positioned about 24 to 36 inches from the patient; an average of 30 inches is frequently used. Radiation is usually of 20 to 45 minutes' duration, according to the physician's instructions.

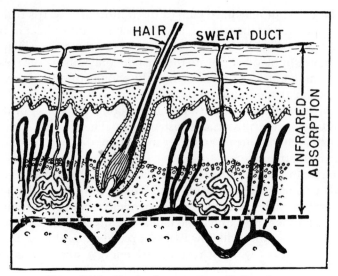

**Figure 29–1**   Depth of penetration of infrared rays.

During the course of the treatment the patient's skin will become flushed and pink, but a sunburn does not occur. DO NOT PERMIT THE PATIENT TO "GRIT HIS TEETH" AND TOLERATE EXCESSIVE HEAT. A gentle mild heat is sufficient. Remember, the infrared lamp can bring about a surface burn in exactly the same manner as any other source of heat, such as a hot stove or iron.

Infrared rays are used to promote muscular relaxation, speed circulation, and aid in the localization of an inflammatory process. They are also helpful in maintaining heat in a moist dressing. The infrared rays have no germicidal power any more than other forms of similar heat.

Maintenance of the infrared lamp is simple. The heating element is best kept in a down position when not in use to prevent dust from accumulating on the element. The electrical connections should be checked and kept in good working condition.

## Ultraviolet Radiation

This modality produces light energy in the same form as the rays from the sun that bring on the common sunburn. The portion of the sun's rays which we see is known as visible light; that portion we feel is heat, or infrared energy. Ultraviolet rays are themselves completely invisible, yet they bring about such a potent chemical reaction in the skin that in a few hours there follows the condition known as sunburn or erythema. Most of the sun's ultraviolet rays are absorbed or filtered out by the earth's dust and smoke. Ultraviolet rays are lethal to many microorganisms and when applied in intense amounts to a localized area are germicidal and effectively used in many skin diseases.

These rays are generated by different types of lamps. One way is to employ a high voltage, low current discharge through certain gases in a quartz tube which produces intense ultraviolet rays with very little generation of heat; this is known as the cold quartz method and is the one most frequently used in the physician's office. Another method is by electrically heating a quantity of mercury within a quartz tube. This is known as the hot quartz method. Still another method is to burn the chemical contents of carbon rods; this is the carbon arc method.

*Regardless of the method of generating the ultraviolet rays, great care must be employed in exposing the patient to this radiation.* There are two types of cold quartz ultraviolet lamps used in the medical office. One type produces the long waves in the ultraviolet spectrum and is used for general body radiation. This energy is very potent and care must be taken to avoid tissue damage by overexposure. The physician personally should direct the assistant as to the exact number of seconds or minutes for the duration of the treatment in order to avoid an excessive burn. The distance from the burner unit to the patient is exceedingly important, and this, too, should be carried out exactly as the physician directs. At a distance of 36 inches from the burner unit to the patient, a first degree burn can be produced in 30 seconds to one minute, a second degree burn in one to two minutes, and a third degree burn in two to four minutes. (See Figure 33–4).

The patient should be disrobed and the area to be treated sufficiently exposed. Extra care should be taken in treating areas that have impaired circulation or areas that have not been exposed during previous treatments. Portions of the patient's body that are not to be treated, such as the genital area, should be protected with a clean towel. Both the operator's and the patient's eyes should be protected with dark sun glasses to prevent the energy from entering the eyes.

For general body radiation it was previously said that the lamp should be held 36 inches from the patient. There are two important facts to keep in mind when administering this treatment. First, if the distance from the patient to the lamp is decreased by one half, then strength of the radiation is increased four times (Inverse square law). Second, the intensity of radiation striking the skin at right angles is greatest; at an angle of 30 degrees the intensity decreases to 80 per cent (Lambert's cosine law). Thus, it is important that the distance and the angle of the ultraviolet rays are the same for each treatment.

The size of the dose is usually governed by the erythematous response of the patient's skin. Treatments are generally given every other day, since 24 hours may not disclose the maximum erythematous response of the skin. The penetration of the rays is less than 0.1 mm. There is some tanning of the skin. The rays are considered to be carcinogenic if their use is prolonged for a considerable amount of time. Primary uses are for bactericidal and antirachitic therapy.

For small area therapy the hand-held portable cold quartz lamp can be very useful. This instrument, called the Spot-Quartz, is placed near to, or in contact with, the area to be treated. Since there is practically no heat generated in the lamp's coils, it will not burn the skin. The treatment time is from a few seconds to minutes, depending on the skin condition and the distance between patient and lamp (Fig. 29–2). A masking adapter for small areas attaches to the face of the lamp, and a filter to eliminate the visible light (Wood's Filter) for diagnostic use is available. The Spot-Quartz, when not in use, may be hung on the wall bracket supplied and is available for use after about one minute's warm-up of the quartz grid.

The glass coils of both the hand model and the larger lamp must be protected from breakage and kept free of dust and oil. They may be cleaned by carefully wiping with alcohol to remove oil.

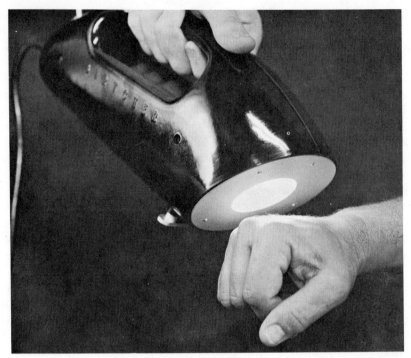

**Figure 29–2**   The Spot-Quartz, a portable cold quartz lamp. (Courtesy of the Birtcher Corporation.)

## ULTRASONIC ENERGY

This is the science of dealing with mechanical radiant energy. Since 1948 the use of ultrasonic energy as a therapeutic measure has been increasing. Early studies were first made in Europe, but the use of ultrasonic energy has advanced throughout the United States as well as other parts of the civilized world. Ultrasonic energy is simply sound energy, the same sort of energy that comes from a radio speaker or from the human voice. The customary sound with which we are familiar and which we hear is produced by sound waves vibrating at a rate of 100 to 12,000 cycles per second (frequency). A few exceptional people can hear sound waves vibrating at 15,000 cycles. Birds and dogs can hear frequencies of 25,000 cycles and more.

What is known as ultrasonics, as employed in therapeutic machines, is similar vibrating energy but at the rate of a million times per second. The mechanical energy at this frequency is created by an electronic machine which carries an electrical current up into an applicator or transducer. This electrical energy is fed to an element called a piezoelectric transducer. This material may be pure quartz or barium titanate. It is similar in size and shape to a half dollar coin. When activated by an electrical current it oscillates (vibrates) at a rate of one million times per second. This quartz crystal actually expands and contracts the same number of times per second as the frequency of the electrical current. When this crystal transducer is brought in contact with human tissue, the vibrating goes through the tissue. Though the frequency of this vibration is high, the total amount of energy is low. As measured by acoustical watts by engineers, the total energy administration to a patient is very small and is normally indicated on the output meter of the ultrasonic generator in total watts or watts per square centimeter of transducer element area. Acute ailments may be treated with the power as low as 0.5 to 1.0 watt per square centimeter as registered on the output meter on the generator. Chronic cases may be treated at a power output of 1.5 to 2.5 watts per square centimeter. The duration of a treatment will vary from 5 to 15 minutes, depending on the physician's instructions.

These ultrahigh frequency sound waves do not travel through air. The transducer (sound wave head or applicator) must be held snugly in contact with the body surface and aided in this contact by a coupling agent such as mineral oil. These sound waves do travel very well through water. Because of this, treatments are administered under water whenever it is convenient and that portion of the patient's anatomy needing treatment can be immersed. In deep body tissues that have a high water content, such as muscles, the ultrasonic waves penetrate better than the waves from the diathermy microwave; thus, absorption and heating are less. Ultrasound has less penetration and greater heating in tissues of low water content, such as bone. These minute sound waves bombard the tissues and cause the tissue to vibrate at the frequency rate. There is a small amount of heat generated in the tissue, but this is of limited importance. It is the extremely rapid vibrations that stimulate the circulation. One could say they cause the tissues to "flap" extremely rapidly. Results have been attributed to the vibrations causing the increase of blood flow, and this, in turn, creates a chemical action in the tissues that has a favorable effect in the body. All this takes place with little or no heat as experienced in the diathermy short wave and other heat modalities. The patient feels no sensation of pain and very little heat.

Ultrasonic therapy is used by orthopedic surgeons and neurosurgeons and is usually administered by a physical therapist on a physician's orders or prescription. Read the manufacturer's instructions carefully.

## ELECTROMUSCLE STIMULATORS

These low voltage machines provide an electrical current similar to that coming from an ordinary wall outlet, except the machine controls the wave form, the frequency, and the intensity. These low voltage currents are useful for stimulation of motor and sensory nerves. It is said to be a passive way to exercise a muscle when a patient cannot activate the muscle himself. It is used to revitalize a muscle or to keep a muscle from atrophying.

There are various types of waves, or sine currents, used. These are basically: (1) pulsating; (2) spasmodic or twitching; (3) surging, that is, a slow steady tightening; and (4) tetanizing, which contracts rapidly and holds tight. The type of current is prescribed by the physician.

Small electrode pads are saturated with tap water to moisten them in order to increase the contact with the patient's skin. These pads are held by the technician or strapped in place. The electrical current and vibrations of the muscle or muscles, depending on the placement of the pad, are varied in frequency as prescribed. An interrupted current will stimulate denervated muscles and is used by physicians to help maintain a nearly normal state of the muscle by frequent application, while awaiting reinnervation. Stimulation is also beneficial in retraining a patient to use a muscle or muscles. Various currents are used in electrodiagnosis.

Acute ailments are treated with a tetanizing effect which contracts the muscle and holds it in contraction for a period of 15 to 20 minutes. This causes the muscle to fatigue and allows the blood to flow through the area again with resulting pain. Chronic ailments are treated with a slow alternating muscle vibration for a period of 15 to 20 minutes, which promotes blood flow and encourages relief of pain. Proper use of this modality produces spectacular results and will often demonstrate to a patient that a muscle is not "dead" but can be revitalized.

## GALVANIC OR DIRECT CURRENT

The current found in some offices requires a machine to change the quality of the current supply from the wall outlet to one that flows continuously in the same direction, known as a direct or galvanic current. Sometimes the physician may have a machine which simply employs batteries for the electrical supply source. The direct or galvanic current has a chemical action. Exactly like the process of nickel-plating or silver-plating electrically in industry, certain drugs can be conducted into the human tissue by the use of direct or galvanic current. In some types of disorders this method is considered extremely effective. This process is sometimes referred to as "iontophoresis" or medical ionization. This treatment is usually employed by the physician himself. The assistant need only prepare the equipment for her employer's use.

Other modalities that may be used in a physician's office are as follows:

*Hydrotherapy* is the use of water in a tank. It provides buoyancy and gives a gentle support that favors body movements. The mild heat from the warm water also offers advantages.

A *paraffin bath* is especially useful in chronic joint diseases. A mixture of seven parts paraffin and one part mineral oil is heated to melting at about 126° F. The patient's hand or foot is dipped into the warm paraffin mixture, removed, and dipped again until a thick coat is formed on the part. This is left on for about 30 minutes and is then peeled off. It leaves the skin soft, warm, and pliable, with a slight erythema. Patients are usually very fond of this form of treatment.

*Psammotherapy* is similar to paraffin baths except that hot sand is used instead of paraffin. This is useful for treatment of the hands, although the entire body may be treated by this method.

A *contrast bath* utilizes two tanks. The patient's appendages are alternately immersed in hot and then cold water to enhance the flow of blood and stimulate the body's circulation.

## ELECTROSURGERY*

The use of electrosurgical modalities is an important part of the average physician's practice. They are therapeutic modalities with great versatility and are considered an important part of the medical care given to patients by dermatologists, gynecologists, otolaryngologists, urologists, proctologists, and oral surgeons. Although considerable major surgery is accomplished in the hospital by the use of the electrosurgical machines, in the physician's office only relatively

---

*Although electrosurgery is not a part of physical medicine, minor techniques are introduced here because the assistant's role in handling the equipment is very similar to her supportive function in electrotherapy.

minor surgery is done by this means. Such surgery is limited to the removal of unwanted tissue such as small growths, warts, moles, papillomas, skin tags, and small tumors, all on the surface of the body or within accessible orifices.

The chief reasons this modality is used in the medical office are the great versatility of the units themselves and the range of electrode tips that may be employed. It can be used for incision, excision, tissue destruction, or a combination of these. The cutting current may be used instead of a scalpel or curet; the coagulation current is used for effects similar, but often superior to, thermal cautery, carbon dioxide snow, or sclerosing injections. Some basic explanations of these currents will be helpful to the medical assistant, although she will never be applying these techniques; this is done only by the physician. The medical assistant will assist as she does in other forms of minor surgery; she will prepare the equipment and the patient for these procedures.

## Types of Currents Used

The types of currents used differ with the needs. They are basically classed as coagulation, desiccation, fulguration, and epilation (Fig. 29–3).

**Electrocoagulation.**   This means to clot by means of an electrical current, sometimes referred to as "to cook." This is accomplished by the biterminal method; that is, an indifferent plate is used, or a bipolar electrode tip is used so the current will flow between the two needle tips (Fig. 29–3). Coagulation tends to produce more necrosis than desiccation, but this current is often advantageous in the treatment of larger or deeper growths. The amount of destruction depends on the size of the current and the length of time applied. Coag-

A
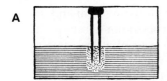 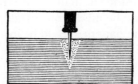 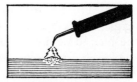

Biactive coagulation; no indifferent electrode. Current flows from one needle to other.

Desiccation current dehydrates tissue about needle, patient acting as indifferent electrode.

Fulguration current jumps across gap from needle to tissue. Sparks carbonize the tissue.

B
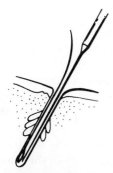

Epilation: insertion of electrode needle into hair follicle.

**Figure 29–3**   Hyfrecator electrodes. (Courtesy of the Birtcher Corporation.)

ulation takes place only between and immediately around the two tips. The destruction will cause the tissue to turn a greyish white and will slough in a few days, usually between five and fifteen, depending on the depth and size of the area treated. When the slough has completely separated, healthy granulation tissue appears beneath. Disinfectants are not necessary because the current itself creates a sterile area. To create this cell destruction, the electrode tip is placed within the tissue and then the current is turned on.

**Desiccation.** This is always done by means of a monoterminal electrode; that is, no indifferent plate is used. This of course, somewhat limits the effectiveness in elevated or deep growths. To desiccate means to *dry out.* Monoterminal desiccation, like fulguration, may be used for relatively superficial effects, such as on the nasal septum. It may also be used in destroying granulations or small polypoid recurrences. It is sometimes used to destroy the stem of a pedunculated growth after the growth has been removed by a cold snare, in order to provide hemostasis and minimize growth.

**Fulguration.** This term is taken from the Latin "fulgurare," meaning lighten or spark. It is the destruction of tissue by means of an electric spark. It is usually monoterminal, using the same electrode tip as desiccation BUT the needle-electrode tip is not inserted into the tissue. It is held about one or two millimeters away from the surface, allowing the current to spark to the tissue being treated. The power is cut in half if biterminal fulguration is employed. A greyish white coagulum is formed on the surface and will slough in a few hours to a few days, depending on the mass. Some small superficial growths will dehydrate and carbonize immediately.

**Epilation.** This procedure is not frequently done in a physician's office because of the length of time involved. The word is taken from epi = upon and pilus = hair. It is the art of extraction and destruction of the hair follicle. A biterminal technique is usually employed. A very fine steel noninsulated needle is inserted into the hair follicle beside the hair. These needles are very fragile and bend easily. The patient should be made comfortable. A strong light and a magnifying glass are essential. The patient should be instructed not to remove in any way the hair to be destroyed. It is necessary for a growth of at least two weeks to take place before it can be grasped sufficiently for removal. The hair must be held while the needle is inserted about one-fourth of an inch into the follicle.

## Preoperative Preparation of the Skin

This preparation will vary greatly with the procedure to be done, but a few general suggestions may be made to guide the medical assistant in assisting the physician.

The area of skin to be treated is usually cleansed with a surgical soap and water. It is then painted with a skin disinfectant. If an alcohol base disinfectant is used, be careful that it has been removed completely before using any type of treatment that may form a spark. This is especially important when working on the scalp or other hairy regions. Local anesthetics are not usually used, but this depends on the method of treatment and the age and sensitivity of the patient. If a local anesthesia is used, the physician may elect to use a small amount of 1 or 2 per cent procaine or xylocaine solution. Freezing with ethyl chloride is sometimes done, but care should be taken when using this substance near an electric spark.

## Postoperative Care

The after-care is simply to prevent trauma and infection. The crust remaining after desiccation is sterile, and the postoperative application of any antiseptic solution is not necessary. Nor is a dressing required when the treatment area is small and superficial. A small gauze dressing or Band-Aid may be applied to protect the area from trauma. Dressings are not usually advisable, since the crust in situ should be kept dry, and a dressing may become moist or hold the natural skin moisture in. The patient should be told to return in a few days so the area can be examined and any further treatment done.

## Care of Electrosurgical Equipment

As with all electrical appliances the electric cords must not be allowed to kink or become loose in their attachments. The wires inside the attachments are frag-

## Types of Electrodes

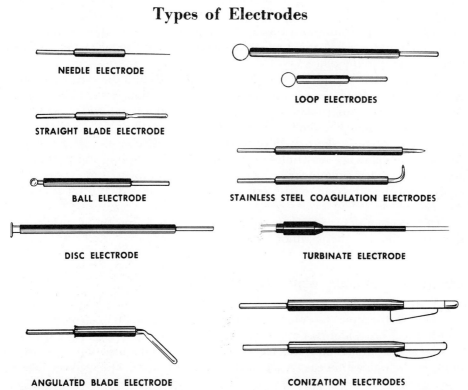

**Figure 29–4**   Types of electrodes used for electrosurgery. (From Otto, John F. Jr., M.D. (ed.): *Principles of Minor Electrosurgery,* Liebel-Flarsheim Co., 1957.)

ile and are easily broken if they are mistreated. The medical assistant should become familiar with the various electrodes used in electrosurgery (Fig. 29–4). The electrodes do not need to be sterilized because they sterilize themselves by means of the electric current, but they must be kept clean and polished. A piece of fine steel wool or emery paper can be used for this purpose. The handles and cords may be wiped with alcohol. Do not boil or autoclave these attachments unless the instructions state that they may be so sterilized.

## Cervical Conization

This procedure is frequently done in a gynecologist's office. It is relatively fast to do and with good hemostasis healing is usually quite fast.

The patient is instructed to take daily douches for a period of time before the procedure. The conization is usually done about a week after menstruation in order to permit the cervix to heal before the onset of the next period.

An indifferent electrode plate is used. It may be placed on the patient's abdomen and held in place by a sandbag or the patient's hands. Frequently it is placed under the sacral area of the patient's back. A coupling gel is generously applied to the plate and the patient's bare skin is contacted with the plate.

After the vaginal speculum is inserted the physician will cleanse the vagina and cervical area with a mild disinfectant. The cervical os must be free of any discharge or mucus. A topical or local anesthetic is sometimes applied. A cocaine solution is the most commonly used. This solution is applied to the cervical area by soaking an applicator with the cocaine and leaving it in the cervical os for about ten minutes. The patient may have been instructed to take a mild sedative before coming to the office.

Postoperative care varies with the patient's needs and the physician. Some physicians use a vaginal pack with or without medication. Sometimes an iodoform gauze wick is inserted into the cervical area and is removed from 24 hours to a few days later. The medical assistant should ask the physician before the procedure is done so she may have the correct items ready on the sterile tray. Antiseptic douches are sometimes prescribed after the packing and the tampons are removed. The patient may be given a later appointment after a week or two in order for the physician to pass a small uterine sound or dilator for patency of the cervical canal.

Cervical biopsies may be done in much the same way as the cervical conization. (See Chapter 31 for Minor Surgery.)

## Electrosurgical Equipment—The Hyfrecator

The Hyfrecator,* a coined name derived from "high frequency" and "eradicator," is a widely used instrument for simple electrosurgical techniques such as electrodesiccation and electrocoagulation. This instrument is usually hung on the wall within easy reach of the treatment table. The medical assistant

---

*Trade name for high frequency eradicator of The Birtcher Corporation, Los Angeles, California.

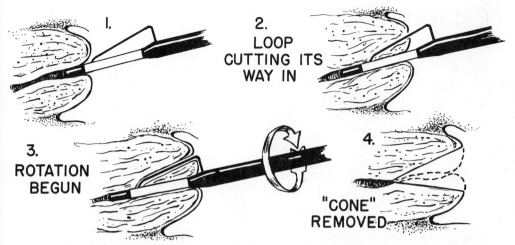

1.

2.
LOOP
CUTTING ITS
WAY IN

3.
ROTATION
BEGUN

4.

"CONE"
REMOVED

**Figure 29–5**  Cervical conization. Drawn by Patric Claiborne, Courtesy Medical Art Section, Medical Center of Washington, D.C. (From Otto, J. F. Jr., M.D. (ed.): *Principles of Minor Electrosurgery,* Liebel-Flarsheim Co., 1957).

never uses this instrument, but she will prepare the patient and attach the electrodes the physician has requested. Care of the equipment is very important, as with all the modalities. Metal attachments that do *not* have any insulation material may be sterilized by heat, but it is always safer to use a form of chemical disinfectant as suggested in the manufacturer's instructions. If the electrode tips have come in contact with any oily substance they should be cleaned with ether or alcohol. Never sterilize any plastic parts with heat unless the manufacturer advises this form of sterilization.

When preparing a patient for electrosurgery make certain that no portion of the metallic part of the electrode is in contact with the metal of the table. Protect the patient with a pad and towels.

Certain types of high frequency electrical current will actually cut tissue when guided through it by an ordinary wire or the point of a needle. A certain quality of high frequency current known as *undamped current* will cause the individual cells to explode in front of the guiding wire loop, blade, or needle point. The cutting is faster than with a sharp surgical blade. This current is used because, as it cuts, capillaries and smaller veins are sealed to reduce bleeding. The field is sterilized by the heat generated, and the shape of the wire loop or blade defines the shape of the cut. In the medical office only the physician uses the electrosurgical cutting machine, but the assistant is required to keep the equipment in order and to prepare the instrument setup properly for the physician's use.

## BIBLIOGRAPHY

Long, C. B.: *The Simple Story of Short-wave Therapy,* Los Angeles, California, The Birtcher Corporation, 1957.

Mennell, J. M.: The use and abuse of physical therapy in rehabilitation, *Clin. Orthop. 12*:131, 1958.

Otto, J. F., Jr. (ed.): *Principles of Minor Surgery: A Manual of Office Electrosurgical Practice,* 1957, The Liebel-Flarsheim Co.

# Chapter 30

**BEHAVIORAL OBJECTIVES**

*The medical office assistant should be able to:*

Identify the major medical specialties, their peculiar language, and particular problems treated by the specialist in allergy, dermatology, endocrinology, and so forth.

Prepare and maintain appropriate supplies and equipment in the clinical examination and treatment room for the medical specialist.

Assist the medical specialist in the routine testing and examination procedures and treatment modalities administered in his day-to-day practice.

# Assisting in the Medical Specialties

General aspects of assisting with the physical examination and the role of the assistant in measuring and recording the vital signs, positioning, and draping the patient were set forth in Chapter 28, Assisting with the Physical Examination.

In the specialist's office, emphasis is given to special areas of the body, or to special kinds of complaints. This chapter will outline the assistant's role in assisting in the most common medical specialties. Subsequent chapters will cover assisting in minor surgery and in the surgical specialties.

## ALLERGY

This is the specialty of diagnosing and treating allergic conditions. In normal immune reaction an antigen unites with an antibody and results in the elimination of the harmful antigen. An allergic reaction is the same, BUT the interaction of the antigen and the antibody is accompanied by a harmful effect on the body tissue and a substance called histamine is released in excess. This turn of events from the normal immune response is referred to as "hypersensitive reaction," and the diseases arising from it are called "diseases of hypersensitivity." Among such diseases are those of allergy, hay fever, serum sickness, and transfusion reactions. In short, the immune reaction can take two turns, a good turn or a bad turn.

Symptoms of an allergy can occur for the first time at any age. The substances that produce an allergic response can be eaten, inhaled, injected, or applied topically to the skin. The response of these antigens, or allergens, as the allergists prefer to call them, bears no relationship to the type of material involved. For example, foods may cause eczema, rhinitis, or asthma. Pollens may also cause any of these conditions. When rhinitis is caused by a pollen, it is given a very special name, hay fever, although "hay" is not necessarily the causative agent.

An allergic reaction does not occur on the first contact with the allergen because the antibodies have not yet been produced by the body. It *may* occur on the second contact, when the antibodies have been released and are in reserve in the body tissues, but not necessarily. The reaction may not occur until later in

**553**

life, when contact with the allergen suddenly develops into a sensitivity. An allergy is said to be a reaction to a substance that ordinarily is harmless to the majority of persons. There are almost as many allergens, such as pollens, foods, plants, animal fur, insect bites, chemicals, etc., as there are substances. The reactions range from a mild sneezing to a more severe serum sickness or anaphylactic shock that is serious and can be fatal unless immediate emergency measures are taken.

The diagnosis of an allergy is made by taking a very careful history from the patient, performing a careful and complete physical examination, and following this up with selected laboratory tests, which may include x-ray studies, blood and urine examination, and finally skin tests. This history and physical examination are always made by the physician, but the skin tests and laboratory tests are usually the responsibilities of a medical assistant or laboratory technician. Since skin tests are potentially very hazardous to perform, they should always be conducted under direct supervision of a physician. It should be emphasized that skin tests by themselves are not strictly diagnostic of an allergy, but, when combined with a careful history and other factors, they are helpful in establishing the diagnosis. Skin tests are ordinarily performed by one or more of several methods: scratch, intradermal, ophthalmic, or patch.

**Scratch Test.** The most common and possibly the least satisfactory is the scratch and puncture test. It is most popular because it is rapid and simple to perform. The tests may be performed on any smooth surface of the skin, but the forearm and back are most popular. Of the two, the forearm is safer, since a serious reaction may be limited by the application of a tourniquet above the elbow. However, the back is favored in infants and in young children because of the large area of skin available and the possibility of immobilizing such a patient if necessary.

Scrub the skin well with alcohol or acetone and allow to dry. If several tests are to be given, use a definite pattern in order to facilitate accurate reading of reactions. Make a scratch on the skin with a needle or scarifier. It is not necessary to draw blood; in fact, it is inadvisable. Scratch only deep enough to permit the extract to enter into the skin. The length of the scratch should be about one-eighth inch or less. If a scarifier is used, it should be placed on the skin and twirled with slight pressure. Then place one small drop of the extract over this scratch area.

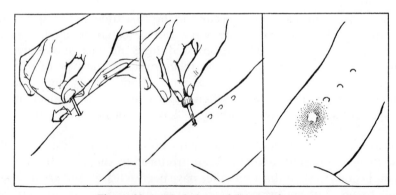

**Figure 30–1**   Technique of the scratch test.

Do not use too much because the fluid may run into an adjoining scratch and the test will be of no value.

A reaction will occur within 10 to 30 minutes. If the reaction is positive, a wheal (hive) will be formed at the site of the scratch. The interpretation of the test should always be compared with the control, which is a scratch with a plain base fluid free from any allergy-producing extract.

The interpretation or reading of the skin tests is performed by the physician. However, a few doctors delegate this step to the trained skin tester. Reactions are commonly graded from a 2 to a 4. No precise definition of a reaction can be given, and indeed the intensity may vary among individuals. However, as a general rule, a 2 reaction implies a wheal which is definitely larger than that of the control. A larger wheal is interpreted as a 3, whereas the presence of pseudopods — fingerlike extensions around the periphery of the wheal — should be read as 4. Erythema or reddening around the wheal is usually disregarded in the interpretations. Frequently the large or significant reactions are accompanied by local itching.

**Intradermal (Intracutaneous) Test.**   This method can be used if a patient has shown a questionable or negative reaction to the scratch method. This test is more sensitive than the scratch test. Extracts are injected into the skin, with usual sterile technique, in a dose of 0.01 cc. to 0.02 cc. The reaction time is identical with that of the scratch test. The antigen, however, is more dilute.

**Patch Test.**   This method of testing is of some value in tracking down the cause of contact dermatitis. In the patch test the suspected material is placed on the skin — near the original lesion, if possible — covered with a small square of cellophane, and held down with strips of adhesive or transparent tape or even collodion. The reaction is read within one to four days.

The tuberculin patch test is commonly used because of the ease in administering it. The tuberculin is incorporated into a small square of gauze which is held in place on the skin for two days. A red spot on the skin at the place of application is read as a positive reaction.

**Ophthalmic Test.**   This test is less common. The testing extract is dropped into the conjunctiva of the eye. This procedure is rarely done and is mentioned only for the sake of completeness.

Considerable controversy exists as to the best way of performing skin tests. But the one item which seems to be overlooked by even professional allergists is the nature of the materials that are used for skin testing. In the hands of the finest skin tester, poor testing materials are without value. Unfortunately there is no standardization of testing materials, and the potency and specificity will vary from one supplier to another. Furthermore, the number of materials that are available for skin testing are frequently ludicrous. Under active investigation are methods that use the patient's blood directly. However, such methods are still experimental.

# DERMATOLOGY

The human skin, also called the integument or integumentary system, is the largest organ of the body. It has many different functions; aids in controlling body temperature; is a barrier to most bacteria; furnishes a sensory system; and

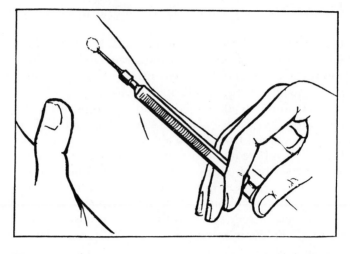

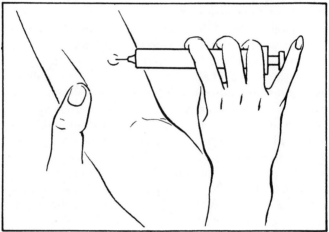

**Figure 30–2**   Methods of intradermal (intracutaneous) testing.

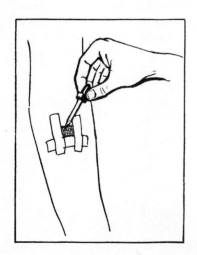

**Figure 30–3**   Patch test.

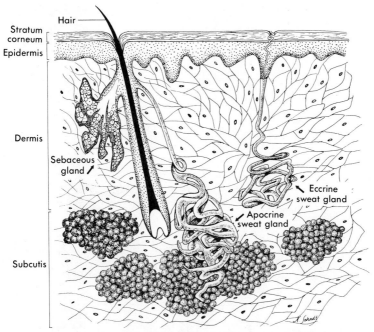

**Figure 30-4**  The histological anatomy of the skin and its appendages. (From Prior, J. A., and Silberstein, J. S.: *Physical Diagnosis*, 4th Ed. St. Louis, The C. V. Mosby Co., 1973.)

is an insulator against outside elements. Both the term "dermis" (Greek) and "cutis" (Latin) are used when referring to the skin. Dermatitis and cutitis are both inflammations of the skin and are synonymous, but dermatitis is by far the preferred term.

The skin has an outer layer, the epidermis, and an under layer, the dermis or corium. Blood vessels and nerves are located in the dermis as well as the sweat glands, hair roots, and the nail beds. Normality of the skin depends on the person's age, sex, physical, and emotional health. The skin reflects both internal systemic conditions and external contact reactions.

Examination of the skin is basically inspection, followed with detailed examination by palpation, diascopy, and special tests. The diascope is a glass plate pressed against the skin to permit observation of changes produced in the underlying areas by the pressure. The impairments that most frequently bring a patient to the dermatologist's office are (1) the cosmetic disfigurements a skin disease causes, (2) pain and pruritus, and (3) interference with sensations or movements. Fear that a skin lesion is the result of a systemic condition is sometimes a major concern.

Inspection of the skin may show color changes such as erythema, leukoderma, jaundice, or vitiligo. Localized red or purple changes may be the result of vascular neoplasms, birthmarks, or subcutaneous hemorrhages (petechiae and ecchymoses). Palpation is used to confirm and amplify findings seen by inspection. Inspection and palpation are interrelated in confirming diagnoses. Palpatory findings may be texture, elasticity, or edema.

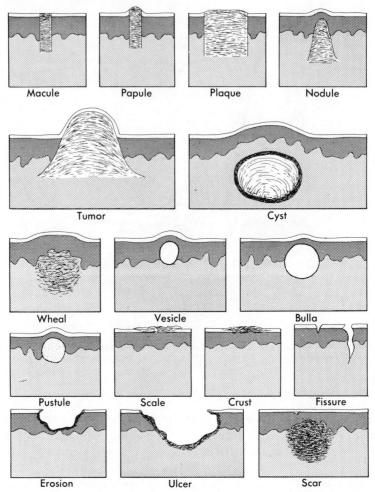

**Figure 30–5** Lesions of the skin. (Modified from Becker and Obermayer *Modern Dermatology and Syphilology* 2nd Ed. J. B. Lippincott Co. In Prior, J. A., and Silberstein, J. S.: *Physical Diagnosis,* 3rd Ed., St. Louis, The C. V. Mosby Co.)

Disorders of the skin may be divided into primary and secondary lesions. Primary lesions are those that appear immediately. Macules, papules, plaques, nodules, comedones, cysts, wheals, and pustules are all primary lesions. Secondary lesions never appear originally but are the result of alterations in a primary lesion. Examples of secondary lesions are scales, crusts, fissures, erosions, ulcerations, and scars. A burn gives a blister. The blister is the primary lesion; the blister breaks and an ulceration forms; then healing ends in a scar. The ulceration and the scar are secondary lesions.

Materials needed:

Good light                    Comedo extractor

Microscopic slides
Ultraviolet light with
Wood's Filter
#15 knife blade

Diascope
Dropper bottle of 10
per cent KOH (10 per
cent potassium hydroxide)

Draping a patient for a skin examination depends on the area to be examined. Remember to expose the area adequately but protect the patient's privacy. Try to make the patient as comfortable as possible and offer support when it is needed.

### Some Special Tests

*Potassium hydroxide examination* of the cornified surface of the skin, such as the palms and soles, is done by scraping a small amount off, placing it on a microscopic slide, mixing with the slightly warmed 10 per cent KOH solution, and placing it under the microscope. This is done in conjunction with a culture for fungi.

*Wood's light examination* is a visual examination of the skin made in a darkened room with the ultraviolet lamp. Differences in the ultraviolet light absorption and fluorescence bring out characteristics of some skin diseases, such as *tinea capitis* (ringworm).

## ENDOCRINOLOGY

Endocrinology is the study of the function and dysfunction of the glands of internal secretion. Changes due to an endocrine disease may cause alterations in body contour, size, fat distribution, skin texture and pigmentation, circulation, and may have considerable effect on the nervous system. The endocrinologist must be able to distinguish between the patient's hereditary pattern and endocrine dysfunction. This dysfunction falls into two categories—deficiency (hypo-) of a hormone and overproduction (hyper-) of a hormone.

Inspection and palpation are the most common methods employed in examining the patient, with inspection being the more prevalent. Of the six endocrine glands in the body, the thyroid and the male gonads (testes) are the most accessible to palpation. The female gonads (ovaries) are palpable to a degree.

Eponyms are used more frequently in endocrinology than in other specialties, but they are slowly being replaced with the true anatomical or pathologic name. A considerable amount of endocrine dysfunction is included in the therapy in other specialties. The gynecologist sees the patient with the ovarian changes of amenorrhea and menopause. The internist may examine an enlarged thyroid gland that has resulted from an iodine deficiency, or a myxedema from severe hypothyroidism. The ophthalmologist may examine the patient with exophthalmic goiter that gives the appearance of bulging eyes.

Besides the complete physical examination, the physician is aided in his diagnosis by a great variety of tests. Some of these tests are x-rays, radioisotopes and blood chemistry.

The medical assistant in an endocrinologist's office will be called upon to participate in the routine physical examination as outlined in Chapter 28.

## INTERNAL MEDICINE

The internist is often called the "diagnostician of medicine." There are several subspecialties of internal medicine, such as cardiology and gastroenterology. It is a nonsurgical specialty—one concerned with diseases not treated surgically.

## Abdominal Examination

Although an abdominal examination is a part of the routine physical examination, it is usually more comprehensive if the patient has complained of visceral discomfort. Considerable time is needed for a thorough abdominal investigation.

The abdomen is conveniently divided into topographic segments (Fig. 30–6). This permits precise location of physical signs and symptoms, and makes it possible to relate these to the underlying organs.

The abdomen must be adequately exposed. A small pillow is placed under the patient's head and the hands are crossed over the chest or the arms are at the patient's side, depending on the physician's preference. The knees may be slightly flexed to increase abdominal relaxation. The drape is lowered to the pubic hair line and the gown is raised to the xiphoid process. If the patient does not have a gown on, then a towel is placed over the female breast before the drape is lowered. The patient must be warm and comfortable in order to relax properly.

The abdominal examination is done by inspection, palpation, percussion and auscultation. The main purpose of inspection is to note the color and texture of the skin, as well as to look for striae, hair distribution, surgical scars, and

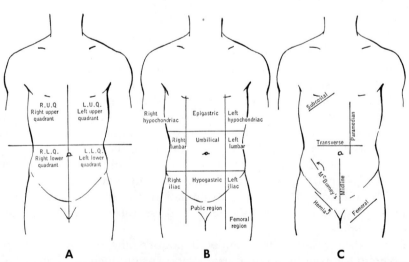

**A**        **B**        **C**

**Figure 30–6** *A.* Quadrants of the abdomen. *B.* Regions of the abdomen. *C.* Abdominal incisions.

**TABLE 30–1** STRUCTURES UNDERLYING THE ABDOMINAL QUADRANTS

| *Right Upper Quadrant* | *Left Upper Quadrant* |
|---|---|
| Liver | Stomach |
| Gallbladder | Spleen |
| Pylorus | Body of pancreas |
| Duodenum | Left kidney |
| Head of pancreas | Splenic flexure of colon |
| Right kidney | |
| Hepatic flexure of colon | |
| | |
| *Right Lower Quadrant* | *Left Lower Quadrant* |
| Cecum | Sigmoid colon |
| Appendix | Left ovary and tube |
| Right ovary and tube | |
| Portion of ascending colon | |

*Midline*
Bladder
Uterus

visible bulging or peristalsis. The physician will listen with the stethoscope for bowel sounds, which are varied and numerous, and bruit sounds. Percussion is used to determine the presence of gaseous distentions and free abdominal fluids. The medical assistant may be asked to place the ulnar edge of her hand parallel over the midline of the abdomen to prevent fluid wave sounds from transmitting through the abdominal wall. Palpation is the major part of the abdominal examination. The physician will usually stand on the patient's right side and the medical assistant stands opposite the physician. If the patient complains of being ticklish, it is best to ignore this and not make an issue of it. The medical assistant should keep her conversation at a minimum during the examination.

After the examination the patient may dress. Remember to give the patient any special instructions. Frequently gastrointestinal or gallbladder x-rays are ordered. It is important the patient be properly instructed in the preparation for these tests.

## Chest Examination

Although the thoracic cavity contains both the lungs and the heart, when one speaks of a chest examination it is assumed the lungs will be examined, not the heart. The chest, like the abdomen, is given topographical landmarks for the three views; anterior, posterior and lateral (Fig. 30–7). Although the lungs are basically examined by auscultation, inspection, percussion, and palpation are also employed. Inspection is concerned with symmetry, condition of the skin and the patient's nutrition. The posterior is viewed for scoliosis and kyphosis. Mensuration (measurement) is done on the chest expansion. Percussion is valuable in determining the relative amount of air or solid material in the underlying lung. Vibrations from the spoken voice are transmitted through the chest wall and felt by the physician's hand.

Auscultation is most useful in a chest examination. The room must be quiet

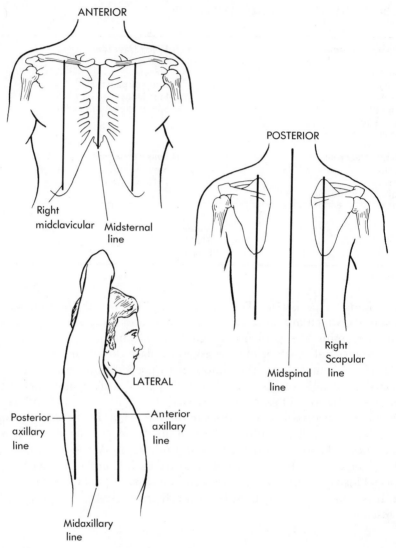

ANTERIOR

Right
midclavicular    Midsternal
line

POSTERIOR

Midspinal     Right
line          Scapular
              line

LATERAL

Posterior                    Anterior
axillary                     axillary
line                         line

Midaxillary
line

**Figure 30-7**  Topography of the chest. (Adopted from Prior. J. A., and Silberstein, J. S.: *Physical Diagnosis*, 4th Ed. St. Louis, The C. V. Mosby Co., 1972.)

and the medical assistant should assist the patient in remaining quiet. The assistant will soon learn whether the physician prefers the bell, diaphragm, or combination type of stethoscope.

Pulmonary Function Tests are often done in the specialist's office. An example of these tests is the Vital Capacity Test. This measures the volume of air a patient can forcibly expire from the lungs after a maximal inspiration. Chest x-rays are also a routine part of the chest examination. Frequently a physician will prefer the x-rays be taken before the physical examination so they are available for study at the time of the examination.

Materials needed:

| | |
|---|---|
| X-ray in view box | Stethoscopes |
| Cleansing tissues | Tongue depressor |
| Light | Otoscope |

## Heart Examination

Heart disease is the major cause of death in the United States, as well as being the cause of many chronic illnesses. People are concerned and apprehensive about their hearts. No physician would consider examining a patient without checking the patient's heart. Patients seem to derive some therapeutic value from just having a physician "listen to their heart." A heart attack or diagnosis of heart disease does not condemn a patient; in fact, if the physician's instructions are followed, the patient's life is often prolonged.

The topographical landmarks of the chest are helpful in localizing and describing the heart's location and borders. The heart is primarily examined by auscultation, but the other methods may also be employed. These methods of examination are aided by x-rays and the electrocardiogram. The cardiologist will also use such tests as heart catheterization and angiocardiogram. *Heart catheterization* is accomplished by introducing a small flexible catheter into the vein of the right arm and gently passing it into the vena cava, right atrium, right ventricle, and on to the pulmonary artery. The pressure of the blood is measured in these vessels and heart chambers. Samples of the blood are also withdrawn from these areas to determine their oxygen content. The *angiocardiogram* is a special x-ray procedure using an opaque dye to show the heart and its major blood vessels.

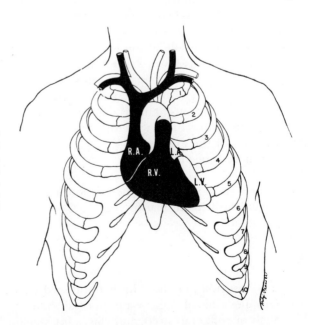

**Figure 30-8** Topographic anatomy of the heart. R.A. Right atrium, R.V. Right ventricle, L.A. Left atrium, L.V. Left ventricle. (From Prior, J. A., and Silberstein, J. S.: *Physical Diagnosis*, 4th Ed., St. Louis, The C. V. Mosby Co., 1973.)

Occasionally the physician will mark the patient's chest where he wishes the electrocardiogram electrodes to be placed.

The patient is disrobed to the waist and placed in a sitting position. To assist in attaining complete relaxation, ask the patient to void first. The room must be warm and the patient relaxed. Silence is a must while the physician is listening to the heart.


## NEUROLOGY

As in other physical examinations, a careful history provides valuable clues in diagnosing neurological malfunctions. These may be seizures, syncope, diplopia, incontinence, and subjective sensations. The patient's general health often complicates a neurological diagnosis. The purposes of a neurological examination are to (a) determine whether a nervous system malfunction is present, (b) discover its location, and (c) identify its type and extent. During the history taking the physician may determine the patient's emotional status, intellectual performance, and general behavior which may be evident in the patient's grooming and mannerisms. The patient's ability to communicate is also observed at this time.

Each cranial nerve is checked. For example, the first cranial nerve, the olfactory nerve, is examined by the patient's ability to identify familiar odors, such as coffee, tobacco, or cloves. The fifth cranial nerve, the trigeminal nerve, is checked by differentiating between warm or cold objects held on the patient's right and left cheeks.

The motor system is examined by the patient's muscular strength and movements. The diameters of the upper arms and the calves of the legs are measured for muscular atrophy. The sensory system notes the patient's ability to perceive superficial sensations, such as a wisp of cotton brushed on the skin, a light pinprick, or hot and cold touching on certain areas. Several reflexes, such as the patellar and Achilles, are examined. A stroke with a dull instrument on the lateral aspect of the sole of the foot may show the Babinski sign.

The patient is given a gown and disposable slippers, and asked to disrobe completely, except perhaps for brassiere and underpants. The patient is then seated on the edge of the examining table. The medical assistant will hand the physician the various items as they are needed. After she has gone through this examination a few times with the physician, she will know which item he needs at each point of the examination.

Materials needed:

| | |
|---|---|
| Neurological hammer or percussion hammer | Cotton |
| Small brush (paint brush type) | Tongue depressor |
| Large pin | Measuring tape |
| | Finger cot |
| | Applicator stick |

Two test tubes for holding hot and cold water.
Dropper vials of sugar water and salt water for tasting.
Vials of coffee, tobacco, and cloves for smelling.

# PEDIATRICS

A large percentage of the patients in the pediatric office are "well-baby" or "well-child" care patients. The role of the physician and the medical office staff is to supervise and help maintain the health of the patients. An increasing number of auxiliary health personnel are being involved in the health services given to young patients.

The frequency of the well-child visits will vary with the physician and the community. It may follow this pattern: 2 weeks, 7 weeks, 4 months, 1 year, 2 years, 5 years, 10 years and 15 years. Immunizations and illnesses will significantly increase the frequency of these visits.

As with any other physical examination, the medical history is an essential guide to the examination. With the infant, the physician is dependent on the parent for the history, but as the child gets older some history may be obtained from him, clarified or amplified by the parent. Generally a child is extremely honest in the facts of his illness. Close observation will also give the physician considerable information. A wince may indicate tenderness, the facial expression associated with nausea should alert the physician and his staff.

Explaining what is to be done and showing the child the instruments to be used will often contribute to his cooperation. The instruments and the examiner's hands should be warm. Quick "behind the back" moves will startle a child and make him suspicious. Small infants are usually undressed by the mother and examined while being held on the mother's lap. The duties of the medical assistant will be to (1) weigh and measure the infant, (2) record this information on the mother's records and on the office record, and (3) check whether immunizations are due.

The sequence of the examination will vary with the needs and cooperation of the patient. Sometimes a tongue depressor in each little hand will keep an infant from grabbing the stethoscope.

## Restraints for Children

For routine examinations it is usually not advisable to use strong restraints. A small child may be held on an adult's lap, with the child's right arm tucked under the adult's left arm. The child's left arm may be held in place by the adult's right hand. The adult's left hand is then free to support the child's head, as shown in Figure 30–9. For eyes, ears, nose, and throat examination and treatment, the child is placed on the examining table with the medical assistant at the child's head as shown in Figure 30–10. When picking up an infant's legs to expose the buttocks, make certain you have your index finger between the ankles to prevent the infant's two ankle bones from being pressed together. Frequently a child is crying from pain resulting from the restraining hold and not from the examination. If more extensive restraints are necessary you may place a child on a large sheet that has been folded lengthwise, the top of the sheet being even with the shoulders and the bottom of the sheet just below the feet. Leave a greater portion of the sheet on the left side of the child. Now bring this longer

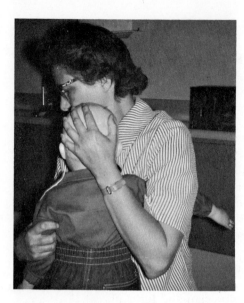

**Figure 30–9**

side back *over* the left arm and *under* the body *and* right arm. Next, bring the sheet back *over* the right arm and *under* the body again. The two arms will be completely restrained, leaving the abdomen exposed. If you wish to restrain the entire body, bring the right portion of the sheet over the abdomen and tuck it securely under the entire back and out again on the right side.

Another method of restraint is the mummy style. This is done by folding the sheet into a triangle and placing it on the examining table. The distance from the fold to the lower corner of the sheet should be twice the length of the child. Now place the child on the sheet with the fold slightly above the shoulders. Loosen any tight clothing and straighten the arms and legs of the child. Next, bring the lower corner of the sheet up over the child's body. Now the left corner is brought over the body and tucked under the body snugly, leaving the arm exposed. Next, bring the opposite corner over the exposed arm and under the child's body. This restraint is quick and easy to make and can be used to leave either arm exposed while securing the opposite arm and also the legs and body. It may be pinned if necessary. Elbow restraints may be made by using a blood pressure cuff or a towel wrapped around the elbow several times.

To prevent a small child or infant from rolling his head from side to side, the assistant should stand at the head of the table and support the child's head between her hands, making certain not to press on the ears, or the anterior or posterior fontanel. The reverse of this may be the assistant's restraining a child with her body by taking the place of the physician as shown in Figure 30–10B, and the physician's working from above the child's head. This may be used for an examination of the child's eyes. A small infant may be placed crosswise on the examining table which has both the head and base raised slightly, forming a large V in the table. This will prevent the infant from rolling as he might on a flat surface.

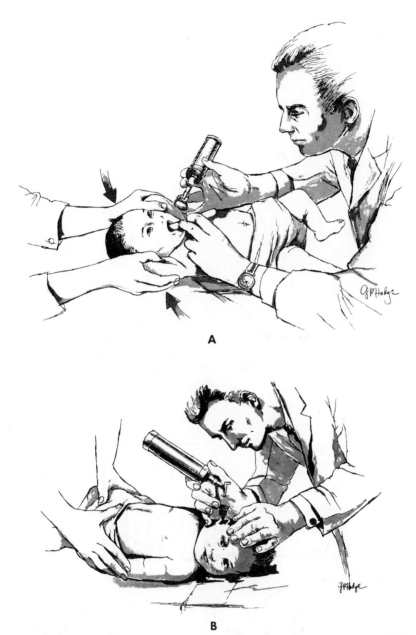

**Figure 30–10** A. Examination of the throat in the young patient. Note that the child's head is held still by exerting pressure on his arms against the sides of the head. In this manner one person can immobilize the head and arms. B. Technique of ear examination in the young child. Note that the examiner's hand holding the otoscope rests on the patient's head, so that any sudden movement will be transferred to both the hand and instrument and prevent trauma to the ear canal. (From Judge, R. D., and Zuidema, G. D.: *Physical Diagnosis: A Physiological Approach to the Clinical Examination,* 2nd Ed., Boston, Little, Brown & Co., 1968.)

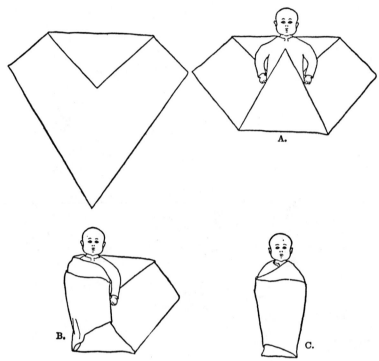

**Figure 30–11** Mummy restraint for infant. (From Standard Nursing Procedures of the Department of Hospitals, City of New York, published by The Macmillan Company.)

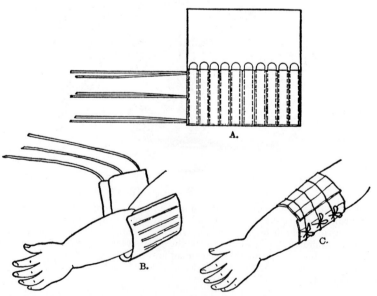

**Figure 30–12** Elbow restraint for infants. (From Standard Nursing Procedures of the Department of Hospitals, City of New York, published by The Macmillan Company.)

It is not necessary to drape an infant, but the older child's modesty should be respected. A friendly, rather nonchalant manner will help, but never be condescending or "talk down" to a child. Sincere respect and conversation at the child's level will accomplish a great deal. Be patient and wait for the child to understand what is expected of him.

## Other Examinations

The eyes are examined the same as in the adult, but more patience is required. The "E" Game Eye Chart or the Picture Visual Acuity Chart may be used. Ocular movements and pupillary responses may be checked on the infant. The ear, nose, and throat examination may be delayed until the end of the examination, because it may require restraints. The medical assistant can assist the physician by offering the child a distraction while the physician is examining the chest and abdomen. A rectal examination is important and may require a moderate restraint.

The neurological examination is usually accomplished by game playing, such as grasping a toy or putting blocks together. How a baby sits and how it moves its legs are important. The gait of a child tells a physician a considerable amount.

Materials needed:

Flashlight  
Illuminated diagnostic set  
Tongue depressor  
Scales  

Stethoscope  
Finger cots  
Tape measure

## PHYSIATRY

This specialty is practiced by a physician specializing in the use of physical agents such as heat, cold, light, water, electricity, and various mechanical apparatuses in the diagnosis and treatment of body disorders. These agents are employed in order to relieve pain and to rehabilitate and restore normal bodily functions. As with some other specialties, most of the patients entering the physiatrist's office have been referred by other physicians. Physical therapy is applied to the patient following an injury, after surgery, or when therapeutic exercise is prescribed. Exercise is the most widely used means of treatment in physical therapy. Methods vary widely, in gradations from passive to actively resistive exercise, depending on the physician's prescription. These exercises are aided by various physical modalities. The term "modalities" refers to all physical treatment measures which are applied to the patient and includes heat, massage, electricity, and various pieces of mechano-therapy equipment, such as ultrasound, muscle stimulation, diathermy, and others.

Most of the assisting and the administration of treatments as prescribed in the physiatrist's office is done by a physical therapist. For further information see Chapter 29, Assisting in Physical Therapy.

# Chapter 31

**BEHAVIORAL OBJECTIVES**

*The medical office assistant should be able to:*

Instruct the surgical outpatient in preoperative and postoperative care and procedures.

Prepare the patient both physically and emotionally for surgery.

Practice aseptic technique around the operating field and in handling sterile supplies.

Prepare the basic surgical setups for suturing, needle biopsy,

gynecologic procedures, and so forth.

Assist the surgeon in outpatient procedures for cyst removal, special irrigations, fracture casting and so on.

Apply and change dressings for incisions and wounds.

Identify apparatus and materials routinely used in minor surgery.

# Assisting in Minor Surgery

The amount of minor surgery done in a physician s office often depends upon the location of the office. In an urban area where hospitals are more accessible it is easy to use the hospital facilities on an outpatient basis, but many rural physicians find themselves doing more office surgery because of greater distances to hospitals. As a rule a physician will prefer to use hospital facilities if the patient is diabetic or has a heart condition or any blood dyscrasia. The removal of lesions and growths that may need immediate histological study presents a problem for office surgery. Performing office surgery is also difficult if the patient will be immobile after the procedure.

## GENERAL INSTRUCTIONS

When planning office surgery, the medical assistant should complete the following procedures before the time of the appointment.
1. Have all necessary consent forms signed.
2. Give the patient all the necessary preoperative instructions, such as medications to be used and special skin cleansing.
3. Ask the patient to arrange to have someone bring him to the office and take him home.
4. When appropriate, instruct the patient to wear special clothing that is easily removed and can be worn home over bulky dressings.
5. Always call the patient the day before the appointment to confirm special instructions.

Consideration should also be given to postoperative care.
1. Give the patient time to rest after the surgery. If sedation was given, make certain he is sufficiently recovered to avoid injury to himself.
2. If the patient was given a local anesthetic that will be wearing off, he should have this explained. Check with the physician to determine whether he wishes to prescribe some pain medication.
3. Do not allow the patient to leave the office without the physician's knowledge.
4. Make certain the patient has any necessary postoperative instructions, preferably in writing.

### Advice to Patients

Postoperative instructions may include (a) how to apply a compress, (b) elevation of a limb, (c) possibility of drainage if there is a drain or wick in the wound, (d) the necessity for and method of changing the dressing when there is drainage, (e) the date and time of the return appointment, and (f) the importance of calling the office if there are any changes or any questions. If the patient does not report in by telephone as requested, then the assistant should call the patient.

## Observing Sterile Technique

Although the procedures outlined in this chapter are called *minor surgery*, all the sterile techniques of major surgery must be observed. The medical assistant must have a sound knowledge of sterility and sterile technique. She should remember that air currents carry bacteria, so any body motions, coughing or talking over the area should be kept at a minimum. Hands are the greatest source of contamination and must be washed very carefully. Learn what can be touched with the hands and what must be handled with sterile forceps. Use sterile transfer forceps for handling only sterile items. Instruments are arranged on the field in the order in which they are used. Consider that the area within an inch around the edge of a field is contaminated.

If the medical assistant has an infection on her hands or if she is handling an infected area, she should wear gloves. Have a conveniently placed container to receive contaminated materials for both disposable and reusable items. These containers should be nonabsorptive, such as a plastic bag or a wax-lined paper bag. Instruments should be placed in a disinfectant solution in a receiving basin. Do not pass contaminated materials over the sterile field.

## Positioning the Patient

Always remember to have the patient disrobe sufficiently to completely expose the involved area. There is too much risk of contamination in doing a procedure while either the patient or the medical assistant is holding back clothing that may slide over the area where the physician is working. Clothing that is held back may also act as a tourniquet or make it extremely difficult to apply a dressing or bandage properly.

It is equally important to position the patient as comfortably as possible. An uncomfortable position can be held for a limited time, and then the patient will have to move, often in the middle of a procedure. If bandaging is applied to an area with the patient in an awkward position, the bandage will bind or fit improperly when the patient assumes a normal position.

## Handwashing

Washing the hands is the most effective means of preventing the spread of infection. The hands should be washed, using correct technique, before and after each patient. It is not necessary to do an extended scrub each time; only the first scrub in the morning is extensive. If a good surgical soap is used, it will leave a film of antiseptic that lasts several hours on the skin, and a normal wash is sufficient during the remainder of the day. It is not advisable to rinse the hands with alcohol because it will remove the antiseptic soap film, and alcohol is extremely drying to the skin. Buy a good soap that is gentle to the hands; the purchase of inexpensive surgical soap is a false economy. Each sink should be equipped with two dispensers, one with a liquid surgical soap and the other with a good grade of hospital hand lotion. Dry cracked skin is a source of infection.

Running water and friction are the two main factors in proper hand washing; surgical soap is of no value without these two. The water should be tepid, not hot. Water that is too hot or too cold is harmful to the skin and will cause chapping. Friction means the firm rubbing of all surfaces of the hands and forearms. The fingers should be interlaced and rubbed thoroughly. All jewelry except for a plain wedding band and engagement ring should be removed. Bracelets are never worn in the medical office.

**Procedure.** Wet the hands well and apply ample soap. Rub the soap around well with plenty of friction. Interlace the fingers and rub the finger sides well. Now start up the forearm by rubbing the wrists and on to the lower forearm. Rinse well under running water by starting at the fingertips and working up to the arms. Keep the hands held above the wrist level. If necessary, clean the fingernails with the blunt end of a toothpick. Repeat the soaping, scrubbing, and rinsing. For general office procedures it is not necessary to scrub the hands with a brush — good manual friction is sufficient. After the hands and arms have been rinsed well the second time, blot them dry by starting at the hands and working toward the elbow. Do not return down the arm. Use a fresh towel for each arm. Turn off the faucets with the used paper towel. It is advisable to use a good grade of paper towels that are gentle to the skin.

## Skin Preparation

The patient may have been instructed to cleanse the affected area with a surgical soap daily for a few days and again just before coming to the office. After the patient has been disrobed and positioned, the area is cleansed again with antiseptic soap. Be sure to have ample toweling around or under the area that is cleansed. If the area is to be shaved, this is done now. A wet shave is preferred because there is less danger of skin nicks and the moisture prevents the minute hairs from blowing around. Rinse the area again and blot dry with sterile sponges. Paint the skin with the selected skin antiseptic by starting in the center over the immediate site of the incision and working outward by a circular motion. Since you cannot sterilize the skin you do not want to rub over an area once cleansed. Wait a few moments and, with a fresh sterile sponge, repeat the disinfection of the skin by starting in the center again. Paint a wide area surrounding the operative site and go far under the sterile drapes that you or the physician are ready to put in place. Drapes may be four sterile towels held together at the corners by towel clamps or you may have a fenestrated fabric drape. Many offices are now using the presterilized disposable fenestrated Steri-Drapes. When opening a pack the first flap is opened away from you. Be careful

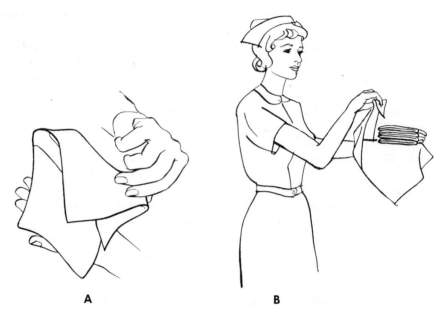

A                                    B

**Figure 31–1**   (From Sutton, A. L.: *Bedside Nursing Techniques in Medicine and Surgery,* 2nd Ed., Philadelphia, 1969, W. B. Saunders Co.)

not to lift a flap by reaching inside a pack but pinch up the flap as shown in Figure 31–1. Arrange articles in the order used so they may be picked up without touching the other items on the tray. Place items with the handles on the outside. Pick up instruments with sterile forceps so they may be handed to the physician correctly (Fig. 31–2).

*Handling sterile supplies* consists basically of knowledge and honesty. It requires constant vigilance and a degree of graceful dexterity. If you visualize and remember that everything that is sterile is white, everything that is nonsterile is black, and there is no gray, then you will have eliminated considerable difficulty in remembering sterile technique. Here are some basic rules to remember. Use only sterile forceps to handle sterile items. Keep wet forceps in a vertical position so the fluid does not run back over the nonsterile area (Fig. 31–3). Never touch the edge of a container. When removing a lid, keep the inside surface facing down and don't move it too far away (Fig. 31–4). If the lid MUST be placed on the table top then place it upside down. Don't talk over an open container.

When opening a solution container, lift off the top cover and be very careful not to touch the neck of the container. When pouring from a bottle, place your hand over the label and pour away from the label. Pour a small amount of the contents of the bottle into the sink or waste container to disinfect the lip of the bottle. Never rest the neck of a bottle on the rim of the container into which you are pouring the solution. Pour from directly above at a distance of at least 8 inches (Fig. 31–5). Prepackaged sterile disposable items, such as syringe and needle and suture material and needle, should be opened by touching the pull-

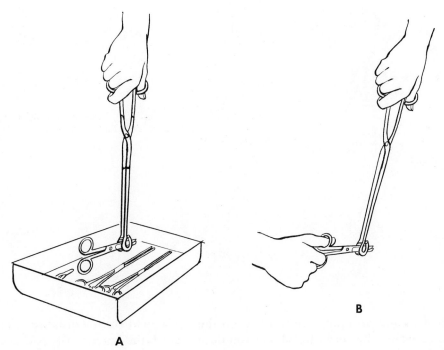

**A**

**B**

**Figure 31–2** (From Sutton, A. L.: *Bedside Nursing Techniques in Medicine and Surgery,* 2nd Ed., Philadelphia, 1969, W. B. Saunders Co.)

**Figure 31–3** (From Sutton, A. L.: *Bedside Nursing Techniques in Medicine and Surgery,* 2nd Ed., Philadelphia, 1969, W. B. Saunders Co.)

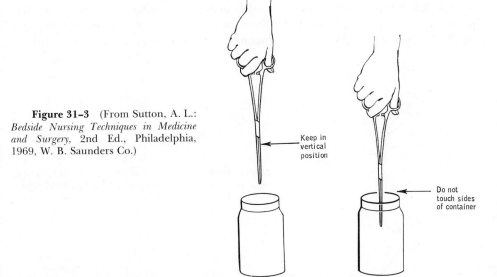

Keep in vertical position

Do not touch sides of container

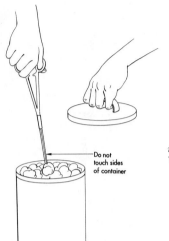

Do not
touch sides
of container

**Figure 31–4** (After Sutton, A. L.: *Bedside Nursing Techniques in Medicine and Surgery,* 2nd Ed., Philadelphia, 1969, W. B. Saunders Co.)

away flaps and dropping the contents on the sterile field from a distance of at least 12 inches. Be very careful that you do not touch the inner sterile package (Fig. 31–6).

## Dressings and Bandages

Dressings and bandages frequently appear easy and simple to apply, but a special skill is required to apply a good functional dressing that serves the purpose for which it was intended. To the patient, a neat, comfortable dressing is a mark of competence. Care must be taken to apply the bandage properly so it will

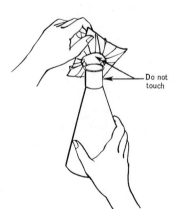

Do not
touch

**Figure 31–5** (From Sutton, A. L.: *Bedside Nursing Techniques in Medicine and Surgery.* 2nd Ed., Philadelphia, 1969, W. B. Saunders Co.)

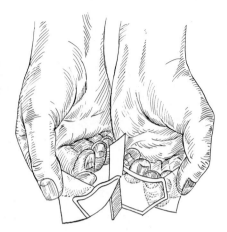

**Figure 31–6** Dropping sterile suture from outer package onto the sterile field. Do not touch inner package.

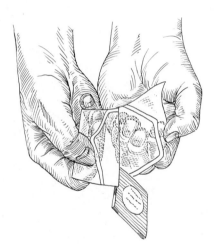

remain in place. It is distressing to the patient to have a dressing fall off before he reaches home.

Roller bandages are not applied directly over a wound. Gauze squares are placed over the wound, making sure the gauze completely covers the wound; then they are anchored in place with tape. Plain roller gauze is almost a thing of the past. It is difficult to apply because it must be put on with reverse spiral turns if the area is uneven. It also has no elasticity and tends to bind. Elastic bandages or wrinkled-crepe types lend themselves to various shapes and do not slide as easily. An elastic bandage with adhesive backing makes a secure but flexible cover (Fig. 31–7). When applying elastic bandage as a pressure dressing, especially to the lower limbs, it is absolutely essential to keep the bandage consistent in spacing and tension with even overall pressure over a large area. Gentle pressure stimulates circulation, but any unevenness will cause a constricture point and possibly create an ulcer.

Liquid adhesive dressings are useful for small areas that are difficult to ban-

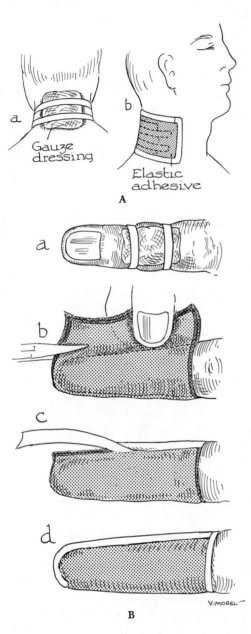

**Figure 31–7**  (From Ochsner, A., and DeBakey, M. E.: *Christopher's Minor Surgery,* 8th Ed., Philadelphia, 1959, W. B. Saunders Co.)

dage. Figure 31–8 illustrates the application. There are commercially made elastic adhesive bandages in various shapes that lend themselves to difficult spots (Fig. 31–9).

Seamless tubular gauze bandages, with or without elastic, are superior material for covering any round surface, such as arms, legs, fingers, and toes. These tubular bandages are applied with a cage-type applicator. With a little practice they save considerable time and are secure. Figures 31–10 through 31–14 illustrate various applications of a tubular gauze bandage.

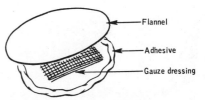

**Figure 31-8** (From Sutton, A. L.: *Bedside Nursing Techniques in Medicine and Surgery*, 2nd Ed., Philadelphia, 1969, W. B. Saunders Co.)

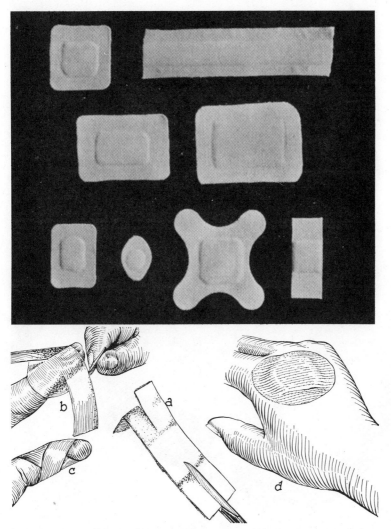

**Figure 31-9** (From Ochsner, A., and DeBakey, M. E.: *Christopher's Minor Surgery*, 8th Ed., Philadelphia, 1959, W. B. Saunders Co.)

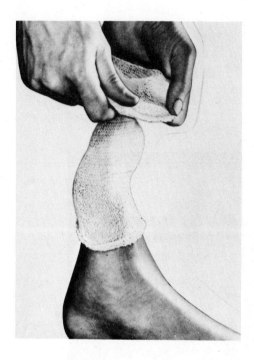

**Figure 31–10** (Courtesy Scholl, Inc., Hospital Products Division.)

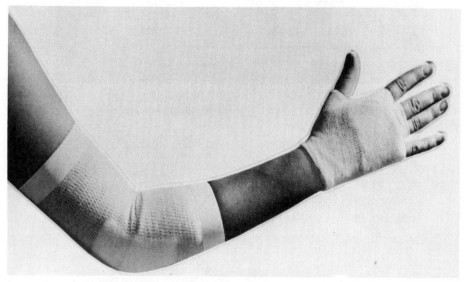

**Figure 31–11** (Courtesy Scholl, Inc., Hospital Products Division.)

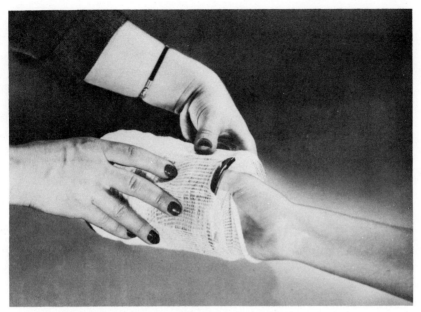

**Figure 31–12**   (Courtesy Scholl, Inc., Hospital Products Division.)

## BASIC SURGICAL SETUPS

Since there are so many different minor surgery setups, and since each physician has his own preferences, this book will not attempt to list all the specific items used for each technique. It is recommended that the medical assistant

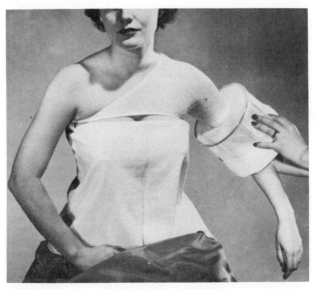

**Figure 31–13**   (Courtesy Scholl, Inc., Hospital Products Division.)

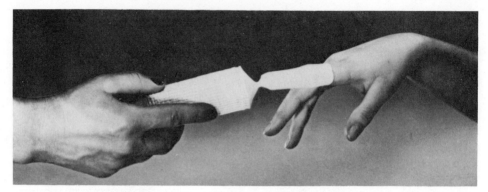

**Figure 31–14**   (Courtesy Scholl, Inc., Hospital Products Division.)

make a card file with the name of each procedure, the instruments used, medications needed, and any special wishes the physician may have for that particular procedure. With this handy file she will not forget seldom-done techniques, and she will not have to ask the physician each time.

The following setups will not include the general instructions for preparation of the patient, such as disrobing, emptying the bladder, positioning, and skin preparation, unless there is something particular to that procedure. Nor will bandaging and dressings be explained unless there are unique needs.

## Removal of Sutures

Instruments necessary for the removal of sutures are a 6-inch pair of dressing forceps and a cutting blade. This blade may be a Bard-Parker Disposable Blade, a pair of Littauer stitch scissors, or general operating scissors, sharp-sharp. The cutting blade or scissors should be sterile.

First, remove the dressing carefully. If the dressing is stuck to the incision, it must be soaked off with hydrogen peroxide. Do not oversoak. The area is then cleansed with alcohol or a skin antiseptic and sponged dry with a sterile sponge. Next, grasp the knot of the suture with the dressing forceps and cut the suture as nearly as possible at skin level and extract the suture by pulling toward the incision line very gently. Butterflies or Steri-Strip closures may be placed over the incision area to give support and strength. When removing these tape closures later, always pull each end of the closure strip toward the incision line.

Materials needed:

6-inch dressing forceps
Sterile cutting blade or stitch scissors
Skin antiseptic
Sterile sponges

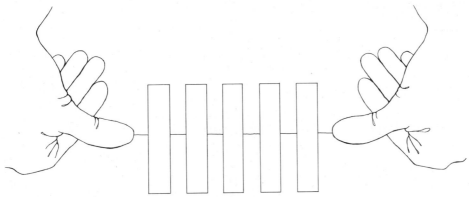

(Steri-Strip skin closures. Courtesy Minnesota Mining and Manufacturing Company. Medical Products Division, Erie, Pa.)

## Dressing Change

Materials Needed:

| | |
|---|---|
| Sterile dressing forceps (2) | Bandages |
| Bandage scissors (2) | Dressings |
| Gloves | Tape |
| Towels | Medication |

Check the patient's medical record and follow the physician's instructions carefully. Have the patient disrobe sufficiently to expose the area to be dressed and place the patient in a comfortable position with the area to be dressed well supported. Arrange sufficient toweling under the area. If the wound is infectious, you should wear gloves to handle the contaminated dressings; otherwise, use the "no-touch technique." Do not ask the patient to look at the wound. Be careful not to reveal any unpleasant reactions, either by your own comments or facial expressions.

Cut off the bandage with bandage scissors; do not unwind. Cut tape next to the dressing. Always remember to remove tape by pulling *toward* the wound. If old dressings adhere to a wound they may be soaked off with hydrogen peroxide. Do not pull off stuck dressings. Sometimes it is advisable to leave the old tape on, if it is adhering well, and place the new tape directly over the old. Frequent dressing changes and pulling off tape can make a patient's skin very tender.

Place the removed dressings directly in a container or covered receptacle. Do not leave them exposed on the dressing tray or counter top, within view of the patient. Cleanse the area and the wound and gently blot with a sterile sponge. It may be necessary to use hydrogen peroxide or a sterile saline solution for cleansing. Surgical soap may also be used. Avoid using cotton because it will adhere to granulation tissue.

If there is any question as to the type of fresh dressing to be used, consult

**TABLE 31-1** CONTAMINATION WHILE DRESSING A WOUND

| *Sources* | *Prevention* |
|---|---|
| *Mechanical* | |
| Hands and instruments | Dress one wound at a time |
| | Use instruments whenever possible to handle items |
| | Keep sterile items separate from contaminated items |
| *Environmental* | |
| Air currents from windows, moving drapes, and leaning over field | Keep moisture to a minimum |
| | Move drapes slowly and keep low over area |
| | Avoid passing over wound area; work from the side |
| | Avoid leaning over sterile field |
| *Personal* | |
| Talking, coughing, hair falling forward | Keep hair under control |
| | Avoid talking and coughing, or wear surgical mask |

the physician. Also, if the wound appears not to be healing properly or if there is any abnormal change, consult the physician and follow his instructions carefully.

Work from a dressing tray or counter where fresh supplies have been assembled. Apply any necessary medication. Sprays and powders do not present a problem, but ointments are more difficult to apply. Do not spread an ointment directly over the wound. Using a sterile tongue depressor, spread the ointment on the sterile dressing, being careful not to contaminate the dressing or medication. Make certain that you have covered an area larger than the wound, using large enough dressings. Secure the dressing with tape and do not let the tape touch the wound in any way. Apply an outer dressing or bandage if needed. Take great care that the dressing and bandages are even in pressure and that any splint or support does not cause needless pressure on one given area. An improper bandage can do considerable harm.

Be certain that you have recorded the dressing change accurately in the patient's medical record. Beside the date, the entry should include how much discharge there was on the old dressing, the condition of the wound (purulent matter, granulation tissue, etc.), what medication was applied, and when the patient is to return.

## Suture Setup

If an emergency patient arrives in the office with a pressure dressing over a laceration, do not remove the pressure dressing until the physician is ready to suture. Ask the patient the possible length and depth of the wound. Usually there is very limited cleansing of the wound because of bleeding. If not, let the physician instruct you on what cleansing is necessary.
On the side you should have:

| | |
|---|---|
| Local anesthetic | Extra sterile sponges |
| Dressings | Tape |
| Bandages | Splints or guards |
| | Drape |

On the sterile field:

| | |
|---|---|
| Gloves | Sponges |
| Syringe and needle | Suture and needle |
| Hemostats (3) str. | Tissue forceps or skin hook |
| Scissors | Needle holder |

## Needle Biopsy

A biopsy is the examination of tissue removed from the living body. Biopsies are usually done to determine whether a growth or swelling is malignant or benign; however, it may be done as a diagnostic aid in other diseases or infections. A needle biopsy may be done by aspiration with a needle and syringe or by a special biopsy needle. The specimen is then sent to a pathologist for either a cytological or histological examination. (See Chapter 27 on Specimen Collection).

On the side:

Specimen bottle with sufficient fixative solution in it
Laboratory form and label
Local anesthetic

On the sterile field:

| | |
|---|---|
| Gloves | Syringe and needle |
| Biopsy needle | Sponges |

Usually there is no dressing required after a needle biopsy. A Band-Aid is often sufficient.

## Abdominal Paracentesis

This is the insertion of a trocar into the peritoneal cavity for the removal of excessive fluids. The patient is instructed to empty his bladder. With the lower abdomen exposed, the patient is placed in a well supported sitting position. The skin just below the umbilicus is cleansed, and a local anesthetic is injected. A small incision is made to aid in the insertion of the trocar. The amount and character of the fluid obtained is recorded and the fluid saved if the physician requests it. Use sufficient towels under the buttocks and catch-basin.

On the side:

| | |
|---|---|
| Measuring vessel | Skin antiseptic solution |
| Local anesthetic | Specimen bottle with label |
| Extra sponges | Laboratory form |

On the sterile field:

| | |
|---|---|
| Gloves | Syringe and needle |
| Trocar | Sponges |
| Drain tube for trocar | Knife with #11 or #15 blade |

After the paracentesis, a small sterile dressing or a large Band-Aid is placed over the puncture site.

## Sebaceous Cyst Removal

This is a benign retention cyst of a sebaceous gland containing fatty substance of the gland. It is also called a wen. They may occur any place on the body with the exception of the palms of the hands and the soles of the feet. They are

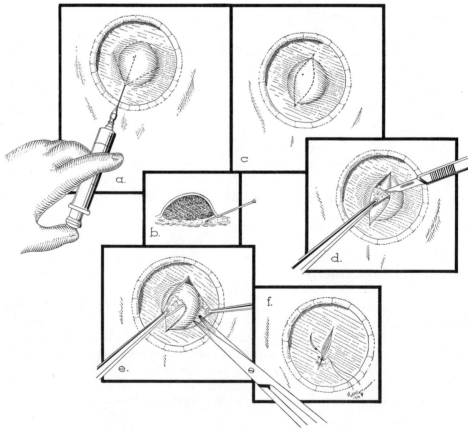

**Figure 31-15** Drawing showing technique of excision of sebaceous cysts or wens. *a* and *b*, Infiltration of the tissues surrounding the cyst is performed with procaine hydrochloride 0.5 per cent solution. *c* and *d*, An elliptical incision is made over the cyst to remove a small segment of skin including the puncta. *e*, Using the attached ellipse of skin for traction purposes the cyst is removed intact if possible. *f*, Bleeding points are controlled with fine catgut ligatures, and the skin incision is closed with nonabsorbable sutures. (From Ochsner, A., and DeBakey, M. E.: *Christopher's Minor Surgery*, 8th Ed., Philadelphia, 1959, W. B. Saunders Co.)

more common on the neck and shoulder and because they are frequently the source of irritation, they are removed. Ordinarily the cyst is attached only to the skin and moves freely over the underlying tissue. For cosmetic reasons the physician will make the incision on the natural skin crease lines. Figure 31–15 illustrates the procedure.

On the side:

Local anesthetic          Biopsy bottle with label
Disinfectant (skin prep)  Laboratory form

On the sterile field:

Gloves                      Syringe and needle
Drape and towel clamps      Knife handle with blade #15
Hemostats: 2 str. and 2 cvd. Tissue forceps (2)
Dressing forceps (2)        Allis forceps
Suture and needle           Needle holder
Scissors s/s or s/b         Sponges
*Dissector                  *Coagulant gel

## Draining an Abscess

An abscess is a localized collection of pus in a cavity formed by the disintegration of tissue. Abscesses may appear in any part of the body. "Furuncle," "boil," and "carbuncle" are names applied to different types of abscesses. In most abscesses pyogenic cocci, usually staphylococci, are found, but it is not uncommon to find secondary organisms. The treatment for abscesses, other than those on the face, is usually incision and drainage. Because of the infectious organisms, extreme caution should be taken in handling the contaminated materials and instruments.

On the side:

Wax or plastic bag for contaminants   Ethyl chloride spray
Extra sponges                         Extra applicators
Medications
Skin antiseptic
Bandages

On the sterile field:

Gloves          Gauze stripping, iodoform.
Hemostats (2)   Knife handle with blade #15

*Physician's choice

| | |
|---|---|
| Probe | Dressing forceps (2) |
| Scissors | Sponges |
| | Dressing |

The physician may choose to inject a local anesthetic if the abscess is deep rather than use the ethyl chloride to "freeze" the area. The medical assistant may cut the length of gauze stripping for packing at the physician's request. Several layers of gauze sponges should be placed over the abscess opening, especially if a drain has been inserted and the gauze anchored with bandage. Frequently a patient is instructed to apply warm moist packs for a couple of days. Daily dressing changes may also be indicated because of the copious drainage.

## Ear Irrigation

An ear irrigation is usually done to remove excessive or impacted cerumen from the auditory meatus. Occasionally a patient will have a foreign body in the ear canal, such as a bug, bean, or wad of paper. The physician will examine the ear and remove the foreign body, but occasionally the medical assistant will do the ear irrigation on the physician's orders. Usually the patient has been given pretreatment instructions to place drops of cerumen-removal medication in the ear before coming to the office in order to soften the cerumen. Have the patient lie on his side, place a few drops in his ear, remain in this position for 15 minutes, and then repeat on the other ear. Instruct the patient to make absolutely no attempt to "clean out the ear." Sometimes the patient is instructed to use 3 per cent hydrogen peroxide drops in the ear just before coming to the office. Have the patient assume a sitting position with the back well supported. The hair should be pinned up and away from the ear and a terry towel placed over the patient's shoulder. A large plastic drape over the patient's shoulder and lap will give good protection.
Have the following items ready:

| | |
|---|---|
| Medicine droppers (2) | Cotton |
| Metal applicator, str. | Cotton applicators |
| Medication | Ear basin |
| Illuminated otoscope | Irrigating syringe (Reiner or asepto) |

Prepare a quart of mild soapy or plain water at 98.6° F. It is important that the water be body temperature. Grasp the ear between the middle and index fingers, leaving the thumb free to act as a rest for the syringe. Gently place the syringe tip inside the meatus and very gently direct the flow of water up and back. Remember, do not force the water in and do not empty the syringe completely because the remaining bubbles will make a considerable roar in the ear that is quite annoying to the patient. It is necessary for the patient to hold the ear basin, but watch that it does not get too full and spill.

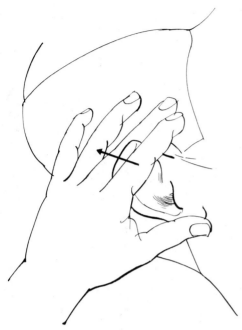

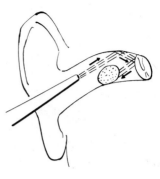

**Figure 31–16** (From Sutton, A. L.: *Bed-side Nursing Techniques in Medicine and Surgery*, 2nd Ed., Philadelphia, 1969, W. B. Saunders Co.)

## Nasal Pack

This dressing is inserted into the nasal cavity, usually for the purpose of stopping hemorrhage or for the application of medication. The patient is placed in a sitting position with the back well supported. Drape the front of the patient and give him some paper tissues.

On the side:

| | |
|---|---|
| Head mirror and light | Laryngeal mirror |
| Emesis basin | Tongue depressor (metal or wooden) |
| Medication | Topical anesthetic |

On the sterile field:

| | |
|---|---|
| Nasal speculum | Dressing forceps (bayonet) |
| Cotton applicators | Hemostatic forceps, str. |
| Scissors | Medicine glass |
| Metal applicator, str. and cvd. | Nasal pack, 1 inch, plain or iodoform |
| Nasal packing with string (4″) | |

This is not usually a painful procedure, but it is uncomfortable, and the patient may require moral support. If nose drops are to be administered, the patient is placed on his back with the head lower than the shoulders and turned to one side (Fig. 31–18). Draw sufficient medication into the dropper for both nostrils, turning the head for each side. Place the dropper about ⅓ of an inch inside the nos-

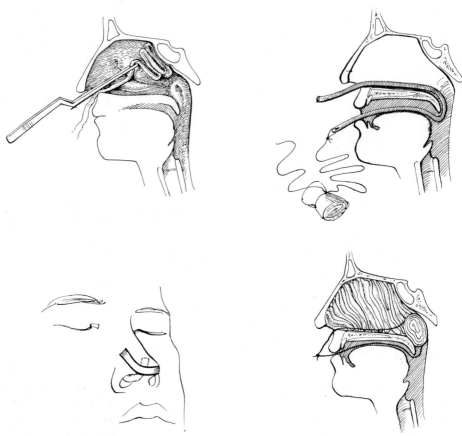

**Figure 31–17**   (From Sutton, A. L.: *Bedside Nursing Techniques in Medicine and Surgery*, 2nd Ed., Philadelphia, 1969, W. B. Saunders Co.)

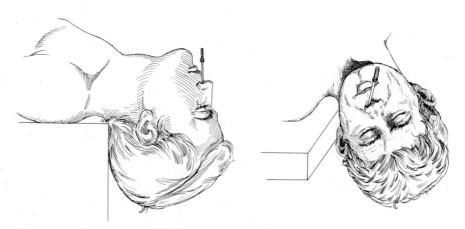

**Figure 31–18**   Instillation of nose drops.

tril. Instruct the patient to remain in this position for about 5 minutes. Provide the patient with a paper tissue. For infants and small children, it is best to use a rubber tipped dropper. Hold the child's head by cupping your hand under his chin.

## Eye Irrigation

Irrigation of the eye is done to cleanse it or apply a medication such as an irrigating solution. The sterile solution should be warmed to body temperature. The patient is placed on his side with the head turned to the side of the eye to be irrigated and the head held level by placing a pillow under the patient's neck as shown in Figure 31–19. A basin is placed under the temple. The patient may hold the basin, if necessary. Use a sterile syringe to moisten a cotton ball with solution to cleanse the eyelid and eyelashes of the affected eye. Be gentle. Instruct the patient to stare at a fixed spot during the irrigation. Place the sterile syringe filled with solution on the bridge of the nose parallel to the eye. The irrigating solution should move in a gentle, steady flow. Dry the eyelid with a sterile cotton ball or dressing.

On the side:

Curved basin and extra dressings

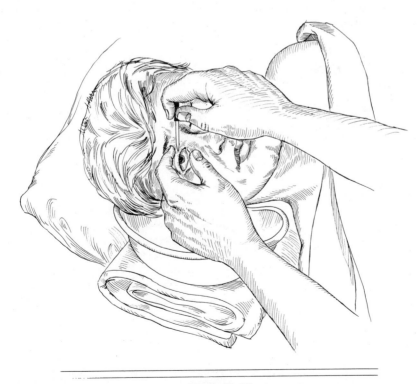

**Figure 31–19**

On the sterile field:

 Medicine droppers (one for each eye) or small asepto syringes.
 Cotton balls or gauze dressing squares
 Medication or irrigating solution

## Instillation of Eye Drops

This is done to introduce medication into the eye for examination or treatment of the eye. Always check an eye medication very carefully. Some medications are not stable, especially if exposed to the light. Improper use of the medicine dropper will cause contamination of the medication. DO NOT TILT THE MEDICINE DROPPER SO THE MEDICATION ENTERS THE RUBBER BULB. This is a major source of contamination and cross mixing of medications. Each medication must have its own sterile dropper. The patient is usually in a sitting position but may be supine with the head tilted backward. Draw the medication into the sterile dropper, don't tilt, and place the required drop(s) just inside the inner surface of the lower eyelid near the center. To pull the lower eyelid down place your finger on the patient's cheek bone and gently pull downward (Fig. 31–20). Pressure over the lacrimal sac will prevent the medication from draining into the nasal cavity if the physician so requests. Do not touch the eyelid or eyelashes with the medicine dropper but hold it about 1/2 inch above the eye. Instruct the patient to stare at a fixed spot on the ceiling. Then have the patient

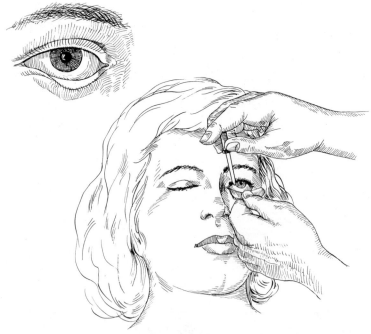

**Figure 31–20**

close the eye and roll the eyeball a few times, unless the motion of the eye is contraindicated. Gently blot the excess medication with a gauze or cotton ball.

The general physician does not do minor surgery of the eye in his office but will refer it to an ophthalmologist. With adequate facilities and a specially trained assistant the following two procedures may be done in the ophthalmic office.

Surgical technique and sterility must be maintained as with any other type of surgery.

## Chalazion

This is an obstruction of a sebaceous gland in the eyelid. It is removed from under the eyelid through a vertical conjunctival incision or through the external surface of the skin.
On the sterile field:

| | |
|---|---|
| Chalazion clamp | Knife (#11 blade and #7 handle) |
| Curette | Small scissors, s/s |
| Eye dressing forceps | Cotton applicators |
| Gauze dressings | Eye pad |

On the side:

| | |
|---|---|
| Topical anesthetic | Antibiotic ointment |
| | Ophthalmic antiseptic solution |

The patient is placed in the operating chair, and a drape is placed over the chest and lap. Hand the patient some tissues. Hemostasis is obtained by pressure directly over the site of the chalazion removal. After the ophthalmic antibiotic ointment has been applied, the eye patch is applied by folding the patch in half and fixing it firmly in place with tape. The tape should be placed in an overlapping fashion. Be careful not to have any of the patient's hair caught in the tape.

## Irrigation of the Naso-Lacrimal Duct

Occasionally the tear duct will become obstructed and cause watering of the eye, especially in the older patient. This is an office procedure if the patient is cooperative; otherwise, it may have to be done under general anesthetic in the hospital.
On the sterile field:

| | |
|---|---|
| Punctum dilator | Medicine glass |
| Syringe (2 cc) | Normal saline solution or |
| Lacrimal needle | Antibiotic solution |

It may be necessary for the medical assistant to assist the patient by supporting his head.

With an adult, the probing of a tear duct may be performed under local anesthetic and topical anesthetic.
On the sterile field:

Punctum dilator                     Medicine glass
Syringe (2 cc)                      Lacrimal needle
Probes, double ended sizes 00–2

On the side:

Local anesthetic        Topical anesthetic
Ophthalmic antiseptic

## Cervical Biopsy

This is the examination of the tissue removed from the cervical area of the uterus. Biopsies are usually done to determine whether there is a malignancy present. It is also a diagnostic aid in diagnosing other diseases. If the Papanicolaou Smear Test is positive, it is usually confirmed by a cervical biopsy. The patient is placed in the lithotomy position with a towel under the buttocks.
On the side:

Specimen bottle 10 per cent formalin        Skin antiseptic solution
Laboratory form

On the sterile field:

Gloves                              Coagulant foam or gel
Vaginal speculum                    Sponges
Uterine dressing forceps (2)        Uterine tenaculum
Cervical biopsy punch               Vaginal tampon or packing

Since the cervix is devoid of nerve endings that would respond to cutting and burning stimuli, there is very little discomfort. Postbiopsy bleeding may be controlled by the application of a coagulant gel or foam, or the physician may choose to lightly cauterize the area. The physician may also choose to remove a piece of tissue by means of electrical conization. (See the chapter on Assisting in Physical Therapy.)

Cervical polyps are frequently encountered, especially in women nearing menopause. They are asymptomatic and are usually removed in the medical office. The procedure is basically the same as for a cervical biopsy. The pedicle of the polyp is seized with a uterine sponge forceps and cut off with a blade or uterine polyp forcep. The removed polyp is then sent to the pathologist for a histological examination.

## Gynecological Pack

A pack is a dressing or similar material that is inserted into a body opening or cavity, usually to control bleeding and to hold medication in a given area. A cervical or gynecological pack may be inserted following cervical surgery. The patient is in the lithotomy position with a towel under the buttocks. The routine pelvic examination instruments are ready for use with the addition of a vaginal pack or tampon, uterine dressing forceps, medication glass, and medication. Explain to the patient that a pack has been inserted and relay any instruction from the physician. These instructions may advise her when to remove the pack, and whether she is to take a specific type of douche. Remember to give the patient a sanitary pad if there is an excess of medication on the pack.

## Rubin's Test

This is a test for the patency (openness) of the uterine tubes, made by the transuterine insufflation of carbon dioxide. If the tubes are patent (open) the gas will enter the peritoneal cavity and may be seen by x-ray or fluoroscope. The patient will feel some pain in the shoulders because of the subphrenic pneumoperitoneal pressure. Beside the regular pelvic examination setup you will have ready:
On the side:

Germicide solution      Carbon dioxide gas

On the sterile field:

Sterile towels        Tubal insufflator with cannula tip
Uterine tenaculum
Uterine sound

## Marshall-Marchetti Test

This is a urinary stress incontinence test. Incontinence is the inability to retain the urine under stress situations such as coughing and sneezing. It is involuntary escape of urine. The urinary bladder is filled with 200 to 300 cc. of sterile water or saline, and the patient is asked to cough or suddenly strain, "bear down." If the water escapes, then there is a weakness of the bladder sphincter. The patient is in the lithotomy position with a basin and ample toweling under the buttocks. A routine pelvic examination is usually done before the test.
On the side:

500 cc. sterile water or saline      Germicide solution
Lubricating jelly

On the sterile field:

   Catheter setup      Asepto syringe

## Huhner Test (hoon' er)

    The Huhner test involves the determination of the number and condition of spermatozoa in mucus aspirated from the vaginal canal within 2 hours after coitus and to what extent they have penetrated the cervical mucus. The patient is prepared as for a pelvic examination and with a pelvic examination setup. In addition, have ready a cervical aspirator and bulb and microscopic slides.

## Endometrial Lavage

    This is a diagnostic procedure for the detection of endometrial carcinoma. About 30 cc. sterile saline is washed through the uterine cavity in small amounts, dislodging cells and small particles of tissue and returning them to a reservoir. This is then sent to the pathologist for cytological or histological study. The patient is prepared the same as for a routine pelvic examination.
Materials needed:

   Routine pelvic setup
   Sterile disposable endometrial lavage set
   Sterile gloves

    Complete sterility must be maintained during this procedure. The physician will assemble the lavage set after he has put on the sterile gloves.

## Endometrial Curettage by Suction

    This is done for the purpose of obtaining a specimen of the lining of the uterus. There are differences of opinion as to the time during the menstrual cycle that this procedure should be done. The physician's orders should be given to the patient. Careful sterility must be maintained. Place patient in lithotomy position.
On the side:

   Specimen bottle with fixative     Antiseptic solution
   Laboratory form                  Lubricating gel

On the sterile field:

   Vaginal speculum         Gloves
   Uterine tenaculum       Sponges

Uterine dressing forceps        Cotton swabs
Uterine sponge forceps
Uterine suction curette

Have the patient remain in a dorsal position on the table for a few minutes after the procedure. Have a sanitary pad available. Send the specimen to the pathologist for examination.

## Insertion of an Intrauterine Device (IUD)

This is the insertion of a mechanical device into the uterine cavity for the purpose of contraception. These devices are made of various materials and come in various shapes. They are inserted by the physician, usually during the patient's menstrual period. The patient is prepared as for a pelvic examination with extra toweling under the buttocks.
On the side:

Germicide solution

On the sterile field:

IUD and inserter        Gloves
Uterine tenaculum       Uterine dressing forceps
Uterine sound           Sponges
Vaginal speculum

After insertion of the IUD the patient is generally instructed to examine herself to feel the transcervical appendage (if that type of device is used). The patient is instructed to return after one or two menstrual periods for a recheck.

## Thrombotic Hemorrhoid Incision

Hemorrhoids are varicosities, enlarged veins, within or just outside the rectum. They are usually caused by straining during stool evacuation or pressure from internal organs, such as the uterus during pregnancy. Ideally the patient should be placed in the proctological position and well supported by the table or a Procto Board. If this is not possible, then the lateral Sims' position or the knee-chest (or knee-elbow) position may be used. If the latter is used, the patient must have assistance in maintaining this uncomfortable position. The anal area is thoroughly, and gently, cleansed with soap, water, and cotton and then dried and painted with an antiseptic solution. The buttocks may be spread apart with 3 inch bands of adhesive tape.
On the side:

Local anesthetic, injectable and topical

On the sterile field:

| | |
|---|---|
| Gloves | Hemostat, mosquito (2) str. and (2) cvd. |
| Coagulant foam or gel | Surgical gut for possible ligation |
| Knife handle with blade | Scissors |
| Ample sponges | Padding material rolled or small roll of crepe roller bandage |

The physician may prefer to use electrosurgical cautery for the bleeding. After the blood clot is removed, the padding is placed against the anus and the buttocks are released and taped together.

## Urethral Dilation

This is done for the purpose of expanding or enlarging the urethral meatus. The female patient is placed in the lithotomy position. The male patient is in a dorsal recumbent position. Check the patient's record for the size dilators needed.
On the side:

| | |
|---|---|
| Basin | Antiseptic solution |
| Specimen bottle for urine | Laboratory form |
| Topical anesthetic jelly or solution | |

On the sterile field:

| | |
|---|---|
| Gloves | Sponges |
| Disposable catheter set | Urethral sounds |

## Toenail Resection

Ingrown toenails are usually the result of incorrect footwear or too short hosiery. Cutting the toenail corners back too far also contributes to this very painful condition. Severely ingrown nail must be removed surgically. This is usually done in the hospital but can be done in the office. The patient is placed in a semi-sitting position with the back and foot well supported. The toe is shaved and thoroughly cleansed.
On the side:

| | |
|---|---|
| Extra sponges | Local anesthetic, injectable |
| | Local anesthetic, topical |

On the sterile field:

| | |
|---|---|
| Knife handle with #10 blade | Sterile rubber bands |

Heavy hemostats (2) str.      Sture and needle
Needle holder                 Gloves
Scissors s/s                  Syringe and needle

A special nonadhesive dressing is used over the site. A silk or Teflon dressing is preferred along with petroleum gauze or topical anesthetic ointment. The patient may be instructed to keep the foot elevated for a couple of days.

## Plaster Cast Application

The application of a plaster cast to set a simple fracture is frequently done in the medical office. The comfort of the patient and the skill of the physician are greatly dependent on the help of a competent medical assistant. It is essential that she follow the physician's directions exactly, especially in holding the patient in the exact position he requests. She must also know the warning signs of a cast's becoming too tight so that proper care can be given before permanent damage is done.

Materials needed:

Stockinette                   Sheet wadding or cast padding
Plaster roller bandages       Cast cutter
Splint or guard               Cast knife
Adhesive tape                 Bandage scissors
Marking pencil                Felt or sponge padding

Pail of tepid water 95° F to 105° F      Patient's x-ray in viewer

The patient is placed in a comfortable position with the arm or leg completely exposed. Be very careful in moving the patient. If the clothing is cut off, try to cut on a seam so the garment can be repaired. Protect the patient with a sheet or plastic drape. Cleanse the area as the physician directs. This is important because a cast is usually on for some period of time, and skin rashes may occur. Measure the stockinette and allow at least two inches above AND below the needed length. If the physician instructs the medical assistant to dip the plaster rolls in water, they are dipped into the water vertically and then held horizontally. Bubbles will rise as the roll becomes saturated. (Instructions will be on the plaster roll package). The roll is then held horizontally between the palms of the two hands, and the excess water is expelled by a twist of the wrists.

Unroll the end of the bandage about two inches and hand it to the physician. Because plaster starts to set very rapidly, the medical assistant must pace herself with the physician.

Plaster warms slightly as it sets, so tell the patient to anticipate this, but it will not get hot. The physician will trim the cast and turn the stockinette down over the edges and secure it with tape. He may date it and draw where the fracture is located. As the cast is drying it should be supported with a pillow to prevent any strain and change in shape while it is drying. Instruct the patient to avoid any pressure on the cast for 24 hours. Do not hasten the drying by heat because the

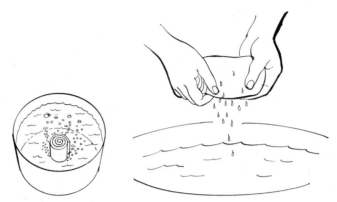

**Figure 31–21** (From Sutton, A. L.: *Bedside Nursing Techniques in Medicine and Surgery*, 2nd Ed., Philadelphia, 1969, W. B. Saunders Co.)

cast will dry from the outside inward with a resulting musty odor. When the cast is dry it will be white and shiny and will sound resonant when it is tapped.

The patient is instructed to watch for any signs of constricture such as numbness, tingling, heat or cold, and disturbances in the circulation such as undue swelling or change in color of the limb to white or bluish.

Some of the new porous honeycomb cast materials are much easier for the patient to care for. The patient may bathe and even go swimming with them because they dry quite readily but still give the same support as the plaster cast.

## TERMINOLOGY OF WOUNDS

The medical office assistant, whether she assists the doctor with minor surgery or is merely responsible for transcribing dictation or writing insurance reports, needs a clear understanding of the terminology used in the surgical areas. The clinical assistant especially will need to understand the types of wounds and the healing phases of the patient undergoing treatment. The assistant who is responsible for stocking the supplies must have a thorough knowledge of the materials needed. The remainder of this chapter will be directed toward these needs.

A *wound* is any interruption in the continuity of the internal or external body tissue. It may be *accidental* or *intentional, open* or *closed.* A surgical incision is an intentional wound. It is clean, neat, and made under controlled conditions; an accidental wound is none of these. An open wound is one with an outward opening where the skin is broken and underlying tissue exposed. A closed wound does not have an outward opening, but the underlying tissue is damaged, as in a hematoma or bruise. It is usually the result of a contusion.

An *abrasion* is a *superficial wound.* The depth is compared to that of a second degree burn. It is usually the result of friction, such as a skinned knee, and is usually accidental. An abrasion is painful and easily infected. A *puncture* or *penetrating wound* is intentional when made by a trocar for draining purposes or by a hypodermic needle. It is accidental when the patient has stepped on a nail. A *laceration* is usually thought of as being accidental and having the appearance of a tear, but a surgical incision may also be classed as a laceration. A "clean" laceration presents the same problems and management as a surgical incision would present.

All wounds go through a *healing* process, which is the restoration of the structure and function of the injured or diseased tissue. This healing process takes place in three phases. The *first phase* is the period when the blood serum and red cells form a network in the wound to act as "glue" and form a clot which plugs the wound, resulting in a scab. This first phase is also called the *lag phase*. The *second phase* is the mending process with the formation of granulation tissue. The same materials that arrest bleeding prepare the site for this mending. These fibrin threads contract and pull the edges of the wound together under the clot or scab. Epithelial cells start to form. This second phase is called *fibroplasia*, the development of fibrous tissue in the wound. These repair cells act as basting stitches and are disposed of when the permanent cells are joined. If the wound is a clean surgical cut there is practically no loss of the normal cells, and there is very little scarring. Scarring takes place in the *third phase*, also known as the *contraction phase*. In this third phase, if the edges are uneven or if there is considerable damage to the tissue, it is difficult for the repair cells to pull the edges together and they must build a bridge over the gap and form connective tissue. This is not true skin, nor can it change into true skin. It is scar tissue.

*Scar tissue* is usually very strong, but it cannot stand the tension of normal skin because of its loss of elasticity. It is also devoid of normal blood supply and nerves. There are several factors that influence the healing process. Healing is assisted by youth, adequate nutrition, and rest to the area. Destruction or reinjury during the second phase can increase the scarring and delay healing. Wounds are susceptible to infection because the normal skin barrier does not exist and this may result in *necrotic* tissue, which in turn acts as a culture for the infection. This necrotic tissue must be removed. This removal is called *debridement*. Pus is often seen with necrotic tissue. It is a combination of necrotic tissue, bacteria, dead leukocytes, exudates, and other tissue breakdown products.

## DRESSINGS

This term is used in the very broadest sense, since it can be applied to a bandage, a gauze pad, or a medication. But before discussing the many different uses of dressings, let us consider the other viewpoint, that of no dressing on the wound. This is the "open wound" method of healing. Some of the advantages of no dressings are (1) the wound will suffer no irritation or friction due to a dressing or bandage; (2) an open wound will stay drier and, therefore, will not be a medium for bacterial growth as is the moisture under a dressing; (3) sutures stay dry and hold tighter, and there is less danger of infection around the stitches; (4) if the patient has been closely shaved before surgery, small dry nicks will heal faster than the moist nicks; and (5) an existing infection may remain localized and

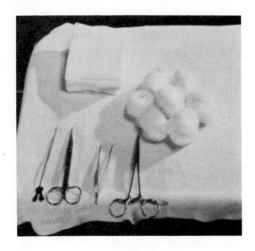

**Figure 31-22** (From Ochsner, A., and DeBakey, M. E.: *Christopher's Minor Surgery,* 8th Ed., Philadelphia, 1959, W. B. Saunders Co.)

not be spread by a dressing. These are all good points, but there are also many advantages to dressings.

A *wound dressing* will (1) prevent outside infection from entering a wound; (2) absorb secretions; (3) protect against trauma; and (4) restrict movement and act as a flexible splint. Dressings can also be used to (5) hold a medication in place; (6) close edges; and (7) cover a disfigurement. A dressing can act as a pressure area which is very important in the healing processes.

In addition to covering wounds, dressings immobilize and act as supports and provide great therapeutic value such as the pressure dressing just mentioned. They can also be used to apply cold packs and fomentations.

Dressings may be roller bandages, gauze squares of various sizes, and gauze in tube form such as a stockinette or Tubegauze and Surgifix. A good dressing must be effective, comfortable, and remain in place.

## OTHER MEDICAL SUPPLIES

Treatment room supplies include, in addition to the various types of dressings, some standard solutions and medications that are used in minor surgery and dressing changes. The solutions and medications listed here are basic and every physician will have his preferred items and methods of applying them. Many of these items will be used by the medical assistant as directed by the physician. Others are used by the physician only, but the assistant should be familiar with their usage.

*Sterile distilled water* is kept in two forms. Multiple-dose vials are used for the injectable distilled water and as a diluent for medications. Larger containers of sterile distilled water are used for rinsing instruments that have been in a chemical disinfectant solution. These containers of rinsing water may be prepared in the office. (See Chapter 26 for Sterilization of Solutions.)

*Sterile physiological saline* solution (0.85 per cent sodium chloride) is also stocked in two sizes. The smaller multiple-dose vials are used for injection (do not prepare these injectables in your office; purchase those commercially made).

Larger containers of physiological saline are used for rinsing and irrigating wounds.

*Alcohol* is usually 70 per cent isopropyl. It is used as a skin antiseptic, has moderate cidal power, is a fat solvent, and has wetting ability. Ethyl alcohol is also used and has the same properties as the isopropyl. It will not kill spores.

*Zephiran Chloride.* The tincture of Zephiran is colored and used as a skin antiseptic. The 1:1000 aqueous solution is used as an instrument disinfectant. Do not mix or confuse these two solutions. Each has a definite and different use.

*Tincture of Merthiolate* is also a skin antiseptic and is colored, as is *tincture of Mercresin.* Because they are alcoholic preparations they will evaporate if left in open containers.

*Bard-Parker germicide* is a popular instrument disinfectant and is used as is the aqueous Zephiran chloride. The instruments must be rinsed off before being used on tissue.

*Surgical soap* is an important item in the medical office. Examples are pHisohex, Septisol, and Gamophen. Surgical soaps are used for handwashing and for cleansing a patient's skin before the application of an antiseptic.

*Hydrogen peroxide* ($H_2O_2$) in a 3 per cent solution is used as a mild antiseptic. It kills by its oxidizing power. This oxidizing action creates minute bubbles when applied to a skin abrasion or wound and has cleansing action. It is used in irrigations and debridement, and is nonirritating.

*Local anesthetics* usually found in a physician's office are *Procaine, Xylocaine,* and many others. They may be plain or with epinephrine. These solutions are usually purchased in 30 to 50 cc. multiple-dose vials.

*Tincture of Benzoin* has many uses. It is used in inhalants and expectorants, but its main use in the office is as a protective coating over ulcers and abrasions. It is also used under adhesive tape to increase holding power and decrease skin sensitivity to tapes. It is supplied in spray cans as well as in solution for painting on the skin. Do not confuse tincture of Benzoin with benzene (benzol) that is used as a cleaning solvent. .

*Ethyl chloride* is a highly volatile liquid that is sprayed on the skin; it evaporates so quickly that the tissue is immediately cooled. It is used as a skin anesthetic. It is a topical anesthetic of very short duration, sometimes called "freezing."

*Epinephrine 1:1000* (Adrenalin) is a vasoconstrictor, used to check hemorrhages, asthmatic paroxysms, and shock. It prolongs the action of a local anesthetic. It is also used in allergic reactions. It is administered parenterally (injected), topically, and by inhalation.

*Aromatic spirits of ammonia* are usually found in small glass ampules covered with cotton and gauze that are easily crushed. Their most common use is for reviving persons who feel faint.

*Collodion,* sometimes called "new skin," is a flexible substance which acts as a local protector to the area when applied. It has a clear plastic appearance.

*Formalin,* 10 per cent solution, is used to preserve excised tissue, such as that taken in a biopsy, for histological study.

*Lubricating jelly* is used for the lubrication of instruments such as a vaginal speculum. It is packaged sterile in flexible tubes, like toothpaste. K-Y Jelly is a popular brand.

*Vaseline* (petroleum jelly or petrolatum) may be used plain as an ointment but is most frequently impregnated in gauze squares or strips.

*Iodoform gauze strips* are strips of gauze ¼ to ½ inch wide that are treated with iodoform, about 96 per cent iodine. They are used to pack into an abscess, acting as a wick to drain out the infection and also as a local antibacterial.

*Ether* is used in offices as an antiseptic and to cleanse the skin of skin oils.

*Silver nitrate* ($AgNO_3$) is found both in solution and on applicator sticks. It is a caustic and is applied topically. It must be kept in a lightproof brown container. The most commonly used solution is 20 per cent, but it also is used frequently in 10 and 50 per cent solutions. The applicator sticks are convenient for touching oral lesions.

## SUTURES AND NEEDLES

The word *suture* is used as both a noun and a verb. As a noun it refers to a surgical stitch or to the material used; as a verb it refers to the act of stitching. Sutures were used as long ago as 2000 B.C. History does not record the first surgical operations and the use of sutures, but ancient medical writings do make references to the use of sinews and strings to tie off bleeding blood vessels. Hippocrates wrote of his use of sutures and Aesculapius was said to have used sutures during the Trojan War. Before Joseph Lister, infection and pus were inevitable when a wound was closed by sutures. Modern surgery and the use of sutures began in 1865 when Dr. Lister developed antisepsis and the disinfection of suture materials. Many kinds of materials have been used over the centuries, including precious metals, horsehair, animal tendons, and cotton and linen cord. Most of the improvement in suture materials and techniques has occurred in the last fifty years.

A *suture* may also be used as a *ligature*. This is a strand of suture material used to tie off a blood vessel or to constrict tissue. To *ligate* means to apply a ligature.

**Types of Suture Materials.** Suture material may be classed as either absorbable or nonabsorbable. The absorbable suture is one that is digested and absorbed by the tissue enzymes during the process of wound healing. It is referred to as surgical gut, sometimes incorrectly called "catgut." The name came from the use of sheep intestines as fiddle strings by the Arabs. The Arabic word for fiddle is "kit" and these "kitgut" strings were used by surgeons for suturing. Surgical gut is still made from sheep intestines.

If the surgical gut is untreated it will be digested and absorbed by the body in a few days, usually about five days. Plain gut is used when healing is fairly fast and the need for the stitch does not exceed the usual five days. Treated gut is slower to absorb. It is coated with soluble chromium salts which delay absorption. The amount of coating controls the absorption from 20 to 40 days. This is somewhat dependent on the type of tissue it is in, the health of the patient, and the presence or absence of infection.

Nonabsorbable sutures are more frequently used in the medical office because a majority of suturing is superficial and in areas where sutures can be removed after healing has taken place. These removable sutures are made of

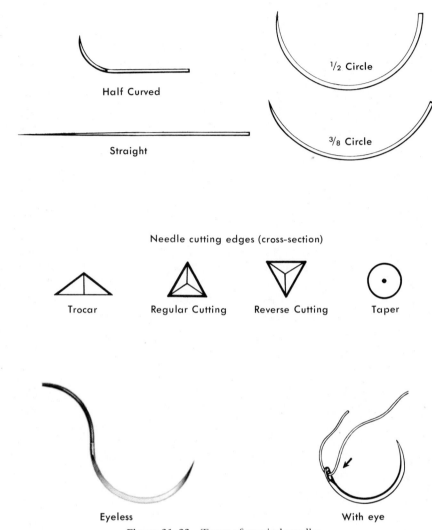

**Figure 31–23** Types of surgical needles.

many different materials. *Silk* is popular. It ties easily and can be autoclaved. It is twisted or braided and sometimes impregnated with wax or silicone coated. It is usually black. Dermal silk is a protein-coated silk that resists body action and is usually blue. Surgical *cotton* is very tough and resistant. It may be used internally when no absorption is desired, such as in a ligation. Cotton is white or may be dyed. *Stainless steel* is very strong and fine. It is noncorrosive and well tolerated. It may be a little more difficult to handle than other materials. *Nylon* and *polyethylene* are very strong and have a degree of elasticity. They are relatively nonirritating to the tissue. They are supplied in a single strand (monofilament) or in braided strands (multifilament). These synthetics have replaced the horsehair or silk-worm gut formerly used for very fine suturing needs. They are colorless, blue,

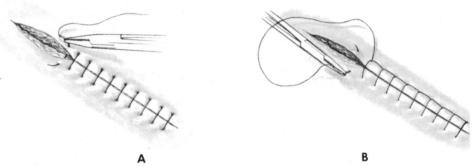

**Figure 31–24** Types of skin closures. A. Interrupted technique. B. Continuous technique. (Courtesy Ethicon, Inc.)

or green. The sizes of suture material are standard as set by the United States Pharmacopeia. They range from 7-0 to 3, with 7-0 being the smallest and 3 the largest. The 2-0 to 4-0 is used most frequently in the medical office. These may also be referred to as 000 or 0000 for the 3-0 and the 4-0.

**Needles.** These are chosen according to the area in which they are to be used and the depth and width of the desired stitch. They are classed according to their parts—eye or eyeless, straight or curved, cutting edge or noncutting (rounded) edge. The majority of suture materials used in the physician's office are presterilized and packaged ready for use. The needles are eyeless and much less traumatic because a single strand of suture is pulled through the tissue rather than the double strand of a threaded needle. Figure 31–23 illustrates the shape and edge of surgical needles as well as the eye and eyeless needles.

Techniques and types of skin closures vary greatly, and it would be impossible to describe or illustrate them. The majority of skin closures in an office are limited to superficial suturing by the interrupted and continuous (uninterrupted) techniques (Fig. 31–24).

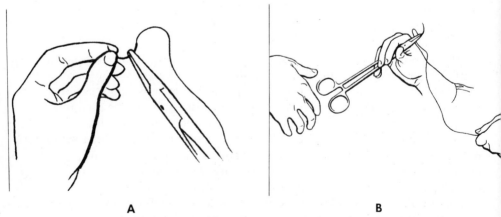

**Figure 31–25** A. Where to grip a needle. B. How to pass a needle holder. (Courtesy Ethicon, Inc.)

When handling suture materials, remember that sterility must be maintained. Do not attempt to straighten or remove a kink by jerking. If the suture is prepackaged in a fluid it should not be opened until ready for use because it will dry and become brittle.

If nonsterile suture is to be cut and threaded before autoclaving it should be loosely wrapped with care around a piece of gauze, and the needle tip should be stitched into the gauze. The needle holder may or may not be gripped onto the needle. A needle holder should not be placed too close to the tip, nor should it be placed over the eye of the needle and the suture strand. Remember, the needle is gripped in place for a right or left handed surgeon (Fig. 31–25).

## PREPARING STERILE PACKS

Before making up a pack to be sterilized, make absolutely certain you have checked and double-checked all items needed. Label the pack contents and date and initial the label. Prepackaged sterile drapes are convenient, and may be plain or fenestrated with tacky backs. Steri-Drapes are packaged in various sizes and save considerable time in drape preparation. If presterilized drapes are not used, then have two or four towels in fan fold in a separate pack. Clamps may be included with drapes or sterilized in separate packages. Packs for skin preparation may be prepared separately or disposable packs may be used. If the surgical procedure is not too complicated, skin preparation materials may be used directly from counter supplies or a side table.

## BIBLIOGRAPHY

International Association of Hospital Central Service Management: The Central Service Technician, 1969, Clissold Books, Inc., Chicago.
Keane, C. B.: Essentials of Nursing, 2nd Ed., Philadelphia, 1969, W. B. Saunders Co.
Ochsner, A., and DeBakey, M. E.: *Christopher's Minor Surgery*, 8th Ed., Philadelphia, 1959, W. B. Saunders Co.
Sutton, A. L.: Bedside Nursing Techniques in Medicine and Surgery, 2nd Ed., Philadelphia, 1969, W. B. Saunders Co.

# Chapter 32

**BEHAVIORAL OBJECTIVES**

*The medical office assistant should be able to:*

Identify the major surgical specialties, their language, and particular problems treated by the specialist in obstetrics and gynecology, ophthalmology, otorhinolaryngology, urology, and so forth.

Prepare and maintain appropriate supplies and equipment in the clinical examination and treatment room for the surgeon.

Assist the surgeon in the routine examination procedures and outpatient treatment administered in his office practice.

# Assisting in the Surgical Specialties

The assistant's role in assisting in the medical specialties was outlined in Chapter 30. This chapter will be directed toward the assistant in the most common surgical specialties. Much of the equipment peculiar to each specialty is described in Chapter 25.

## ANESTHESIOLOGY

Anesthesiology is the branch of medicine concerned with the administration of anesthetics and maintenance of the patient while under anesthesia. An *anesthesiologist* is a specialist in this branch of medicine, and the term is usually reserved for the physician administering the anesthetic. An *anesthetist* is one who administers anesthetics; this may be a nurse-anesthetist or a physician-anesthetist. The word "anesthetic" was given to medicine by Dr. Oliver Wendell Holmes (1809–1894).

Clinical assisting duties in an anesthesiologist's office are extremely limited and usually confined to the scheduling of appointments for the doctor to administer an anesthetic at a hospital and keeping the accounts. Many anesthesiologists do not maintain an office, as we think of a physician's office, but are hospital-based, using the services of a secretary. But medical assistants should be familiar with a few terms and definitions that are applicable to this specialty of medicine.

Anesthetics seem to fall into one of two groups, *general anesthetics* or *local anesthetics*. There is considerable controversy regarding these two terms, but for convenience they will be used here. A general anesthetic implies a state of unconsciousness, insusceptibility to pain, and a degree of muscle relaxation. General anesthetics are classed according to the route of administration. The *inhalants* are gases or highly volatile liquids; *intravenous* and *rectal* anesthetics are the nonvolatile drugs. The term local anesthetic is used when loss of sensation is confined to a limited area. Other terms used for local anesthetic are *conduction anesthesia* or *regional anesthesia*. Local anesthetics are also often referred to as *tissue infiltration anesthetics*. This is because the immediate surrounding tissue is injected or infiltrated with a local anesthetic so each individual nerve ending is blocked. This method may be used to induce spinal or caudal blocks. The names of local

**609**

anesthetics usually end with *-caine*. A *topical anesthetic* is a local anesthetic applied directly to the area involved, such as a spray on the nasal mucosa.

## GENERAL SURGERY

A surgeon's practice is what may be called a "referral specialty." That is, the patients are usually referred to the surgeon from other specialties or by the family physician. The procedure to be followed in the evaluation of the patient and the comprehensive preoperative examination requires teamwork between the surgeon and the referring physician. An effective working arrangement between these two physicians sometimes depends upon the cooperation of the medical assistant. The referring physician frequently takes care of the initial physical examination and basic preoperative laboratory tests. His knowledge of the patient's past medical and family history are shared with the surgeon. The surgeon will then have a clear understanding of the objectives of surgery and the patient's preoperative status. The surgeon may offer the patient a simple and understandable description of the operation, its rationale, and possible complications. (This is the basis of "informed consent.")

The psychological preparation of the patient is also shared by the referring physician and the surgeon. Anxieties of the patient are normal and inevitable and can be somewhat lessened by the attitude of a good medical assistant. The medical assistant in the surgeon's office can identify the patient with special needs. Families and relatives are anxious about the surgical patient. The medical assistant, with the surgeon's consent, can reduce some of these anxieties with simple explanations and reports.

Assisting the surgeon may include assisting with preoperative examinations and postoperative office visits. Physical examinations would follow the outline given in Chapter 28. The office postoperative care may include dressing changes and suture removal. These are described in Chapter 29, Assisting with Minor Surgery.

## OBSTETRICS AND GYNECOLOGY

Examination of the female reproductive system is done to assure normality of the reproductive organs, or to diagnose and/or treat abnormalities of these organs. Because of the intimate nature of the examination, every consideration must be given to the patient.

A gynecological history includes age at menarche; regularity of the menstrual cycle; amount and duration of the menstrual flow; menstrual disturbances such as dysmenorrhea; intermenstrual or postmenstrual bleeding; and vaginal discharges. Prenatal care is a major portion of the OB/Gyn office's appointments. The first prenatal visit is rather extensive with a complete history and physical examination and a pelvic examination that includes pelvic measurements, serological tests and routine laboratory tests. Follow-up prenatal visits include urinalysis, weight, blood pressure, and advice on diet and health habits. The patient's questions are answered, and she is given assurance.

The examining room must be adequately equipped and the surroundings pleasant. A dressing area with an adjacent toilet should be provided. The dressing area should assure privacy and be equipped with tissues and sanitary protection items. Some offices provide a little "goodie box" with safety pins and sanitary belts. Disposable examination gowns are also placed in this room. Check the supplies frequently throughout the day.

The patient should be instructed to empty her bladder and rectum, completely disrobe, and put on a gown. Unless contraindicated, the patient should have been advised at the time her appointment was made that she should NOT douche for 24 hours before the examination in order to properly evaluate vaginal discharges and to have a more satisfactory and accurate cytology study.

The medical assistant should remain in the examining room to provide reassurance to the patient, as well as offer legal protection to the physician. Furthermore, the patient should be given assistance in getting on and off the table. The lithotomy position is very awkward to get into unassisted and is embarrassing to the patient.

Dr. Allen C. Barnes, in *Physical Diagnosis: A Physiological Approach to Clinical Examination,* states: "For a woman in the lithotomy position on the examining table, this 'criterion of coverage,' interestingly enough, is most often the knee. There are said to be two principles of British Law: first, the trial must be fair; and secondly, the trial must give the illusion of being fair. The same might be said of draping the patient for gynecological examination; she should be decently covered, and she should have the illusion of being decently covered. As long as she does not look up to see her knee exposed, this illusion is largely maintained."

The physician will first inspect the external genitalia and palpate the perineal body, Bartholin and Skene's glands, and the urethral meatus. The patient may be asked to "bear down" in order to show any muscular weaknesses that may be the result of lacerations of the perineal body during childbirth. A third-degree laceration may have involved the rectal sphincter and cause rectal incontinence.

Next the vaginal speculum is inserted for examination of the cervix and vaginal canal. The normal cervix points posteriorly and is smooth, pink-colored squamous epithelium. Abnormalities most frequently seen are ulcerations (erosions), nabothian cysts, and cervical polyps. Since erosions cannot be palpated, inspection is the only method of knowing their presence. Healed lacerations resulting from childbirth are common in the multiparous patient. Pregnancy increases the size of the cervix, and hormone deficiency will cause it to atrophy. The vaginal wall is reddish-pink and has a corrugated appearance. Vaginal infections will change the appearance of the vaginal mucosa.

After the vaginal speculum has been removed the physician will do a bimanual examination; that is, the minor hand will be lubricated and inserted into the vaginal canal and the major hand will palpate the abdomen over the pelvic organs. The uterus is examined for shape, size and consistency. The position of the uterus is noted (see Fig. 32–1). The normal uterus is freely movable with limited discomfort. A laterally displaced uterus is usually the result of pelvic adhesions or displacement caused by a pelvic tumor.

The uterine adnexa (fallopian tubes and ovaries) are evaluated. The normal

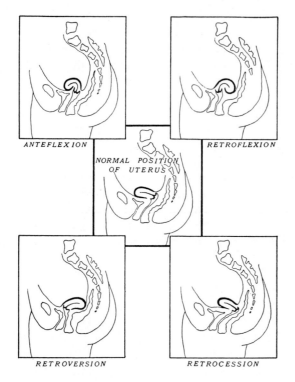

**Figure 32-1** Types of forward and backward uterine displacements. (From Miller, B. F., and Keane, C. B.: *Encyclopedia and Dictionary of Medicine and Nursing*, Philadelphia, W. B. Saunders Co., 1972.

tubes and ovaries are difficult to palpate. The physician may now complete the examination by rectovaginal abdominal examination. This is done when the middle finger of the minor hand is inserted into the rectum and the index finger is in the vaginal canal. The rectum is checked by the index finger inserted into the rectum.

Materials needed:

| | |
|---|---|
| Vaginal speculum | Uterine dressing forceps |
| Rubber gloves | Uterine sponge forceps |
| Lubricant | Gauze dressings or cotton balls |
| Cotton applicator sticks | Cleansing tissue |
| Spot light | |

1. Greet the patient and briefly explain what examination is to be done.
2. Have the patient empty her bladder and save the specimen.
3. Have the patient disrobe completely (except for her shoes if heel stirrups are used) and put on a gown.
4. Place a towel on the edge of the examining table and have the patient sit on the towel. Some offices put the patient directly into the lithotomy position from the sitting position but this should never be done unless the physician is ready to start the examination immediately. Never leave a patient waiting in the lithotomy position. Very common complaints from women regarding a pelvic examination are that they were (1) left waiting in the lithotomy posi-

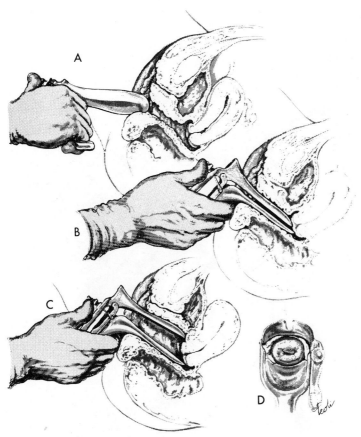

**Figure 32–2**  Insertion of vaginal speculum. A. Blades held obliquely on entering vagina. B. Blades rotated to the horizontal position as they pass introitus. C. Blades separated by depressing thumbpiece and elevating handle. D. Normal parous cervix. (From Judge, R. D., and Zuidema, G. D.: *Physical Diagnosis: A Physiological Approach to the Clinical Examination,* 2nd Ed., Boston, Little, Brown & Co., 1968.)

tion or (2) not assisted in sliding down to the edge of the table but were told to "scoot down" by themselves while the physician and the medical assistant stood and watched them struggle to the edge of the table. It is extremely awkward and embarrassing to "scoot down" by oneself, especially if the stirrups are not far enough out or the patient is nearing full term pregnancy. Please, medical assistants, assist the patient. This may be done simply by standing at the foot of the table and placing her heels in the stirrups. Next, lower or push in the foot board. Now reach up and grasp the patient under and just below the knees and easily slide her down so the buttocks rest on the edge of the table. This can be done without looking under the drape sheet while watching and talking to the patient. The physician will push the drape back when he starts the examination. Patients greatly appreciate this extra care and consideration.

There are several methods of draping for the lithotomy position. One method is to use a small square sheet. The patient holds one corner over her

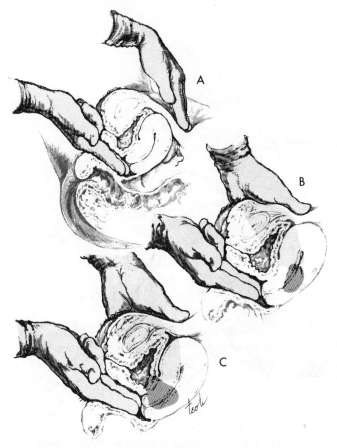

**Figure 32–3** Bimanual pelvic examination. The abdominal hand brings the pelvic contents to the intravaginal fingers. A. Palpation of the uterus. B. Palpation of right ovary. C. Palpation of right parametrial tissues. (From Judge, R. D., and Zuidema, G. D.: *Physical Diagnosis: A Physiological Approach to the Clinical Examination,* 2nd Ed., Boston, Little, Brown & Co., 1968.)

chest. The corners adjacent to this are draped over each knee and the far corner hangs between her legs, covering the perineum, and can be pushed back by the physician.

Some offices use a small sheet cut especially for the lithotomy position. This sheet is approximately 25 inches wide and 40 inches long. It is slit lengthwise about 24 inches. This drape does cover the knees but offers little protection from the side and, if made of disposable paper, tends to slide off easily.

Another method is to use a regular square sheet that has been folded into a triangle. The inside fold is placed over the patient's abdomen, the two adjacent corners go over the patient's knees, and the corner points are wrapped around the patient's ankles and tucked in place. The far corner from the fold hangs down over the perineum and can be pushed back by the physician.

Frequently a regular cot sheet is used and placed over the patient as a top sheet would be placed. Because there is ample sheet to drape over the entire area, there is no need for special placement of the sheet. The physician may then push back the sheet between the patient's legs and over her abdomen, thus exposing the perineum.

No matter what drape is preferred, its size must be ample to give the patient a feeling of security. If the patient is afraid a flimsy disposable sheet will slide off or too many areas are exposed, she will not relax, and relaxation is essential in a pelvic examination.

5. Direct the light source so the light is focused into the vaginal speculum.
6. Assisting the physician may consist of:
   A. Warming the speculum under warm running water.
   B. Assisting the physician with his gloves.
   C. Holding the microscopic slides or making the smear when he hands you the applicator. For easy identification of the source of the material to be smeared you can make a "V" for vaginal, "C" for cervical, and a "U" for urethral secretion.
   D. Handing the dressing forceps or sponge forceps with a sponge, handle first.
   E. Handing the sterile tenaculum for lifting the cervix.
   F. Applying the lubricant to the physician's fingers. Be careful not to touch the lubricant tube to his fingers. Apply about 1″ to 2″ of lubricant across the ends of his fingers.
   G. Placing the soiled instruments in a receiving basin.
7. Assist the patient to relax by having her breathe deeply and slowly. Instruct her to cross her hands over her chest. Sometimes a little conversation helps a patient to relax.
8. After the physician has completed the examination, *make certain the patient is pushed back on the table before sitting up.* Do not rush the patient. If there has been an extensive examination or treatment, it is best to slide the patient back on the table, raise the foot board and have the patient remain in a supine position for a few minutes. A patient may become dizzy when sitting up too rapidly after an examination, and there may be a tendency to fall forward. Records show some lawsuits resulting from this type of injury that probably could have been easily prevented.
9. In offices where vaginal specula are frequently used, they are kept warm by placing an electric pad in the drawer of the examining table and leaving it at the lowest temperature.
10. The patient may now dress. Remember to give her instructions.
11. Clean up the room immediately.

## Special Diagnostic Tests and Procedures

**Papanicolaou Smear ("Pap" Smear).**   Perhaps the single most important test done in a physician's office today is the obtaining of cells from the cervical area for a cytological study. This is done for the early detection of cancer of the cervix. These smears are best obtained when the patient has not douched for 24 hours prior to taking the specimen. It is done without the presence of any lubricating jelly or glove powder.

These cells are obtained by one of two methods: (1) the cells are scraped from the cervical os with a special cervical spatula or wooden tongue depressor and then spread on a glass microscopic slide, or (2) the cells may be obtained from secretions aspirated from the posterior fornix of the vagina by means of a glass cervical aspirator tube and bulb. The slide is immediately immersed in a fixing solution of 50 per cent alcohol and 50 per cent ether for at least 30 minutes, or it may be sprayed with a commercial fixative. Use whichever the pathologist prefers. Make certain the slide or slide container is correctly identified.

Materials needed: (other than the routine pelvic setup)

| | |
|---|---|
| Cervical spatula | Cervical aspirator |
| Microscopic slides (Make two slides for each area the specimen is taken from) | Labels and laboratory forms |
| | Fixative Solution |

**Maturation Index.**  This test is done to measure the patient's estrogen level—to determine whether the patient has an estrogen deficiency. The test results will aid in the diagnosis of endocrine disturbances such as are found in menopause or amenorrhea. The technique for obtaining the cells is the same as for other cytological studies, such as the "Pap" smear.

**Trichomoniasis.**  This vaginal discharge is caused by the protozoa *Trichomonas vaginalis*. The discharge is frothy pale yellow or white and has a distinct odor. The patient complains of burning and itching. It is a moderately common vaginal discharge, and the patient must be assured it is NOT a venereal disease. The vaginal trichomonad is an actively motile organism and the diagnosis is confirmed by a wet smear (hanging drop). This is usually done in the physician's office, since the organism is easily identified.

Materials needed:

| | |
|---|---|
| Microscope | Microscopic slide or |
| Normal saline | Hanging drop slide |
| Cervical aspirator | Cotton applicators |

**Candidiasis.**  This is an infection caused by the fungi of the genus *Candida*. It was formerly known as moniliasis, caused by the fungi of the genus *Monilia*. It is a yeast-like fungus. The vaginal discharge is clear with a curdlike substance in it. The patient complains of burning and itching. It is examined by a direct smear or by special culture media.

Materials needed:

| | |
|---|---|
| Microscopic slides | Culture media (especially for *Candida*) |
| Cotton applicators (sterile) | |

**Atrophic Vaginitis.**  Also called senile or adhaesiva vaginitis, this vaginitis occurring in older women is marked by the formation of raw patches on the vaginal walls. There is frequently a clear watery discharge. The patient complains of some burning and itching, as well as dyspareunia. A maturation index is usually done to confirm the diagnosis.

**Bacterial Vaginal Discharges.** Vaginal discharges due to bacterial origin are usually divided into two classes, *specific* and *nonspecific*. Those in the *specific* class are caused by a specific organism, usually *Neisseria gonorrhoeae*. Gonorrhea is a highly infectious venereal disease. Diagnosis is confirmed by a smear made from the discharge found in the vagina and urethral meatus. Occasionally a culture may be taken, but the majority of times two microscopic smears are taken and sent to the laboratory. If smears are taken from several places they are identified by smearing the exudate in the form of a "V" for the vaginal discharge, a "C" for cervical, and a "U" for the urethral smear. These smears are then air dried, labeled and sent to the laboratory. Take great care in handling the materials.

Materials needed:

Microscopic slides                    Cotton applicators (sterile)
Labels and laboratory forms

The *nonspecific* bacterial discharge may be caused by several different organisms. Because the organism(s) are unknown, the physician may do both bacterial smears and cultures. It is best to check with the laboratory for the type of culture media preferred.

**Cervical Cauterization.** The various electrosurgical currents are discussed in Chapter 29. Electrosurgical procedures are an important part of gynecological treatment of the cervix. Cervical erosions are usually treated in the physician's office with electrocautery without anesthesia unless they are unusually large. Chronic cervicitis is treated with electrocoagulation and conization by electrical current.

The patient is prepared in the same way as for a routine pelvic examination with the addition of the electrosurgical unit and its attachments. The electrosurgical unit should be carefully checked before using. Physicians will vary in the placement of the indifferent (dispersive) electrode. This electrode may be placed on the patient's abdomen and held in place by the patient's hands or by a sand bag. It is frequently placed under the sacral portion of the patient's buttocks. Be careful that the electrode does not touch any metal on the patient or on the examining table. The physician will select the electrode tip preferred. These tips do not need to be sterilized because they are self-sterilizing, but they must be kept polished and completely free of any residual material. When cleaning, be careful not to bend the wire on the conization tip.

Materials needed:

Vaginal speculum that is nonconductive may be preferred, such as disposable plastic
Routine pelvic setup
Sterile tenaculum
Sterile uterine sound
Electrosurgical unit and attachments
Contact paste or jelly

It should be explained to the patient, with the physician's permission, that there may be a slight sloughing off of the cauterized tissue within the next few days. She should also be given any postoperative instructions.

## BREAST EXAMINATION

Careful breast examination is part of the female examination, whether the patient is symptomatic or not. Breast cancer is the most common malignancy occurring in women. Early detection is the key to successful treatment. Women should also be instructed to examine their own breasts at regular intervals. The American Cancer Society has excellent pamphlets and films to supplement the physician's instructions.

The patient must disrobe to the waist. The breasts should remain covered until the actual examination. A small pillow or rolled towel may be needed to elevate the shoulder on the side being examined. This allows the breast to rest more evenly on the chest wall while the patient is in a supine position. The medical assistant should remain in the room during the examination.

The patient is examined in both sitting and supine positions. The examination is basically done by inspection and palpation of the breasts, axillae, and supraclavicular regions. In inspecting the breasts, the physician looks for asymmetry (which is not uncommon), skin conditions such as "orange peel" texture, and retractions and dimpling. Various gymnastics and positioning of the patient's arms are necessary to pull the suspensory ligaments of the breast and increase some retractions of the tissue or deviation of the nipples. The next portion of the examination is palpation. There is a wide variation in the consistency of the normal breast tissue depending on the patient's age, obesity, stage of the menstrual cycle, and pregnancy.

## OPHTHALMOLOGY

A complete examination of the eye is technical and requires expensive equipment, but the practitioner of general medicine does become involved with some examinations and treatments of the eye with the use of basic office equipment. The use of the ophthalmoscope to examine the retina of the eye is an essential part of every complete physical examination. The eye often reflects an individual's general health or may be involved in a systemic disease or injury. The eye may react to a systemic medication the patient is taking.

The most routine eye test, other than the use of the ophthalmoscope, is the distance acuity test, usually given with the *Snellen Chart*. This test may be administered by the medical assistant. She may also be trained to check the patient's near vision with the *Near Vision Acuity Chart*. This is especially done on the patient past 40 years of age for possible presbyopia. Testing a patient's color vision is important, especially if the patient is in certain occupations. All children by the age of five years should be checked by the color vision charts.

The eyelids are examined for edema, which may be the result of nephrosis, heart failure, allergy, or thyroid deficiency. Ptosis of the eyelid may be an involvement of the third cranial nerve. Infections of the eyelids are frequently a *sty* or *chalazion*. If the lacrimal ducts are obstructed, the patient will have constant tearing known as *epiphora*. The conjunctiva of the eye is the delicate membrane covering the eyeball and lining the eyelids. Inflammation of the conjunctiva may be bacterial or viral, and there is a highly contagious conjunctivitis commonly called *pinkeye*.

The *corneal reflex* or corneal sensitivity is tested by touching the cornea of the eye quickly with a wisp of cotton. The patient will blink. The pupils of the eye are normally round and equal in size. Normal pupils will constrict rapidly in response to light and during accommodation. This is seen by shining a bright pinpoint light into one eye from the side of the patient's head. The pupil of the illuminated eye will constrict, and the pupil of the other eye will also constrict equally. Each eye is checked this way. Then the patient is asked to look at the physician's finger as it is moved directly towards the patient's nose. This test is called *light and accommodation* (L&A). An older patient's eyes do not accommodate as well as a younger person's.

The *ophthalmoscope* is used for examining the interior of the eye. It projects a bright narrow beam of light which permits the physician to examine the interior parts of the eye and the retina through the lens of the eye. It is helpful in detecting possible disorders of the eyes as well as disorders of other organs, the conditions of which are reflected in the condition of the eyes.

*Intraocular pressure* has been checked by the ophthalmologist for many years, but nowadays many general practice physicians are also checking their patients (especially those past 35 years of age) for intraocular pressure. Elevated intraocular pressure, known as *glaucoma*, causes pressure on the nerve fibers and thus, may possibly result in blindness. The *tonometer* is used to measure this intraocular pressure. The patient is placed in a reclining position or sitting with the head resting back on a support. A topical anesthetic is instilled in each eye. After a minute the patient is instructed to fix his vision on a spot on the ceiling. The physician will then touch the sterile footplate of the tonometer to the cornea of the eye (Fig. 32–4).

*Strabismus*, crossed eye, is seen predominantly in a small percentage of small children because it is diagnosed early in life and treated as early as possible. There are several problems that cause eyes to turn, but more commonly it is due to weakness of an extraocular muscle. Evaluation of patients with strabismus includes a cover test, measurement of visual acuity, and a careful ophthalmoscopic examination.

Special techniques used in the ophthalmologist's office include the use of a *slit-lamp biomicroscope*. This is used to see the fine details in the anterior segment of the eye. It is used to view a corneal foreign body because it gives a well illuminated and highly magnified view of the area. The patient with *exophthalmia*, abnormal protrusion of the eye due possibly to overactive thyroid or a tumor behind the eye ball, is checked with the *exophthalmometer*. This instrument is designed to measure the forward protrusion of the eye. The *ophthalmodynamometer* is used to measure the pressure of the central retinal artery. It is helpful in patients with circulatory disease because it measures the blood pressure in the retinal artery.

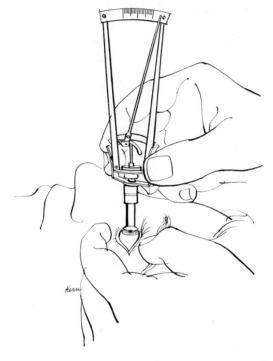

**Figure 32–4** Measurement of intraocular pressure by tonometry. (From Sutton, A. L.: *Bedside Nursing Techniques*, 2nd Ed., Philadelphia, W. B. Saunders Co., 1969.)

Materials needed:

Distance Acuity Chart
Near Vision Acuity
   Chart
Color-vision charts
Pencil flashlight

Ophthalmic topical anesthetic for
   corneal anesthesia
Cotton (sterile)
Tonometer (sterile)
Ophthalmoscope

The patient is placed in a sitting position. There is no special draping. Hand the patient some paper tissues.

**Distance Visual Acuity.** Distance visual acuity is frequently part of a complete physical examination. It is widely used in schools and industry. To date it is the best single test available for visual screening. Many cases of myopia, astigmatism or hyperopia have been detected by this routine test. The most common chart used is the Snellen Alphabetical or "E" chart (Fig. 32–5). This chart has various letters of the alphabet for general use. If the office has patients with an English language handicap, then the "E" chart may be used. This chart is also used for preschool patients, slow learners, or mentally retarded children who have not yet learned the English alphabet. The symbol on the top line of the chart can be read by persons of normal vision at 200 feet. In each of the succeeding rows, from the top down, the size of the symbols reduces to the point where a person with normal vision can see them at a distance of 100, 70, 50, 40, 30, and 20 feet.

The patient must not be allowed to study the chart before the test. The room or hall should be long enough so the 20 foot distance can be marked off accurately. The chart should be hung at eye level and with maximum light, without

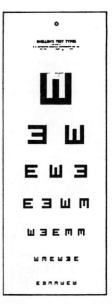

**Figure 32–5**   Snellen visual acuity chart. (From Harley, R. D. (Ed.) *Pediatric Ophthalmology*. Philadelphia, W. B. Saunders Co., 1975.)

glare on the chart. The patient may be standing or sitting with the chart at eye level.

Most adults do not need the chart explained, but you must have the patient's cooperation. If the "E" chart is used, explain how you want the patient to tell you which way the letter "E" is facing. The patient may point up or down or right or left. Or, he may hold his three fingers in the same direction the letter "E" is facing. Use the same routine each time the patient is tested by starting with the right eye. If the patient is wearing glasses the physician may want him tested first with

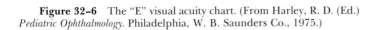

**Figure 32–6**   The "E" visual acuity chart. (From Harley, R. D. (Ed.) *Pediatric Ophthalmology*. Philadelphia, W. B. Saunders Co., 1975.)

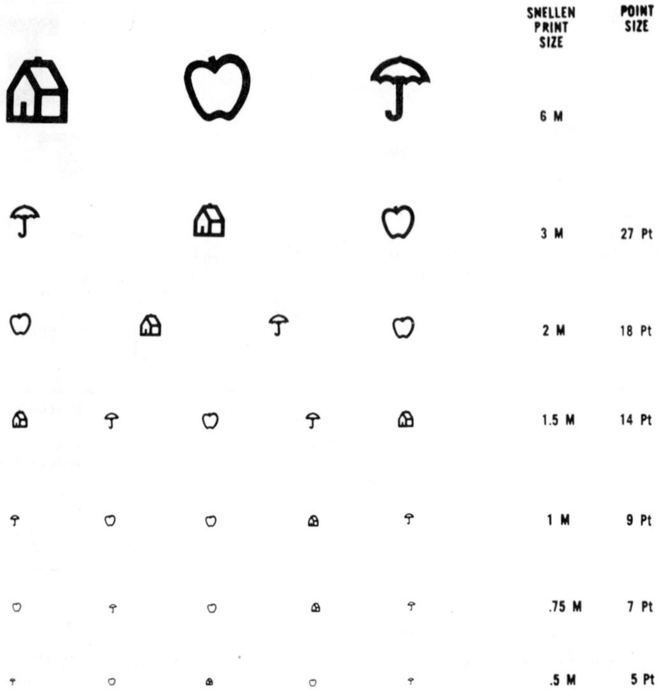

**Figure 32-7** Picture visual acuity chart. (From Harley, R. D. (Ed.) *Pediatric Ophthalmology*. Philadelphia, W. B. Saunders Co., 1975.)

the glasses on and then without the glasses. Make certain you record the "With" and "Without."

Test one eye at a time. Both eyes are to be kept open during the test, but the eye not being tested is to be covered with a paper cup or a piece of cardboard. The paper cup is best because a piece of paper should not touch the eye. Under no circumstances should the patient use his fingers to "hold the eye closed." Allow a moment between changing eyes. The medical assistant should stand beside the chart and point to the line to be read.

Start with the line having the larger symbols in order to help the patient develop confidence in himself; then proceed to the lower lines. If there is no apparent difficulty, skip to the 50 line. If the patient responds rapidly, then skip to the 20 line. Have the patient try to read another line after he says he cannot read one.

Observe the patient's behavior during the test to see if he squints, leans forward and appears to strain, or the eyes fill with tears. Record the reactions. Record the responses of each eye separately. The response is recorded in the form of a fraction. The numerator (top number) is the distance of the patient from the chart, the denominator (lower number) is the lowest line read satisfactorily by the patient tested. Allow one mistake per line. An example, if the patient reads the 20 line at 20 feet, the fraction 20/20 is recorded for that eye tested. If the 40 line is the lowest line the patient can read, the fraction 20/40 is recorded for that eye. Make certain the record reads "Right Eye" (O.D.) and "Left Eye" (O.S.), the record may show O.D. 20/20 and O.S. 20/40.

## OTORHINOLARYNGOLOGY

This is the medical specialty dealing with the ear, nose, and throat. It is frequently referred to as otolaryngology or even as a single specialty of otology or laryngology. Because the term otorhinolaryngology is difficult for the average person to understand, it is referred to simply as ear, nose, and throat (E.N.T.). Where the E.N.T. examination begins varies with the physician. Most of the involved area is visible to the physician, with the exception of the nasal accessory sinuses and the middle and inner ear. A large part of this examination consists of the inspection of the mucosa.

If the ears are examined first, the external auditory canal is viewed with an otoscope or light and ear speculum. The normal external canal has a small amount of cerumen (wax) in it. An excessive amount may be removed by the physician with an ear spoon or curette or by irrigation. (See Chapter 31, Ear Irrigation.) The patient may be given a hearing test with an audiometer to disclose any hearing loss. There are three types of hearing loss—conductive, perceptive, and mixed. *Conductive* hearing loss is a disturbance in the conduction of sound as it passes through the ear canal, tympanic membrane, and the ossicular chain to the oval window and to the inner ear. *Perceptive* deafness is a disturbance anywhere in the inner ear or in the hearing center of the brain. *Mixed* hearing loss is a combination of both conductive and perceptive. The anatomical differences between the adult's and the child's eustachian tube,* makes children far more susceptible to middle ear infections (*otitis media*). Occasionally it may be necessary to do a *myringotomy* to drain the exudate from the middle ear.

Examination of the nasal cavity is mainly inspection of the mucous membrane. The common cold and allergies are the main causes of changes in the mucosa. Because the physician cannot see into the nasal sinuses, these are examined by palpation and transillumination. If the mucosa is swollen, it may be necessary to spray the area with a vasoconstrictor. The throat is the area that includes the larynx and pharynx and is viewed with the aid of a mirror and tongue depressor. In the nasopharynx the physician will look for enlarged adenoids (pharyngeal tonsil) and the orifice of the eustachian tubes. It may be necessary to grasp the tongue with the aid of a piece of gauze in order to view the laryngopharynx. Spraying the throat with a topical anesthetic helps with the gagging patient.

In the oral cavity the patient's teeth and gums are carefully examined. The palatine (faucial) tonsils (if present) are checked for size and the presence of crypts. The lingual tonsils are also checked. The salivary glands are palpated.

Materials needed:

Laryngeal mirror                          Illuminated diagnostic set (optional)
Tongue depressor (wooden or metal)        Ear basin

*The tube from the middle ear to the pharynx.

| | |
|---|---|
| Nasal speculum | Gauze square (4 by 4) |
| Ear speculum | Cotton applicator sticks |
| Metal applicator | Cotton |
| Bayonet dressing forceps | Topical anesthetic spray |
| Ear curette or spoon | Vasoconstrictor medication spray |
| Head mirror and light | |

1. For a good E.N.T. examination the patient is in an upright position, sitting very erect with the head about 10 inches from the back of the chair. The correct E.N.T. position is not a restful position.
2. Place a drape around the patient's neck. If medications are to be used, drape the patient's lap.
3. Hand the patient several tissues.
4. Hold the ear basin, if necessary.
5. Most specialists prefer the head mirror rather than illuminated instruments. The light source is usually a 150 watt light globe placed directly behind and to the right of the patient.
6. If the laryngeal mirror fogs it may have to be warmed. This can be done with a small alcohol lamp flame, under warm water, or by holding it in your hand for a few moments.

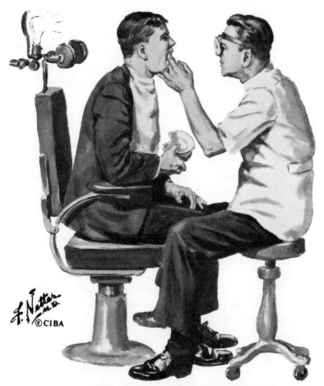

**Figure 32–8**  Position of physician and patient for an E.N.T. examination. © Copyright 1964 CIBA Pharmaceutical Company. Division of CIBA-GEIGY Corporation. Reproduced, with permission, from the CLINICAL SYMPOSIA, illustrated by Frank H. Netter, M.D. All rights reserved.

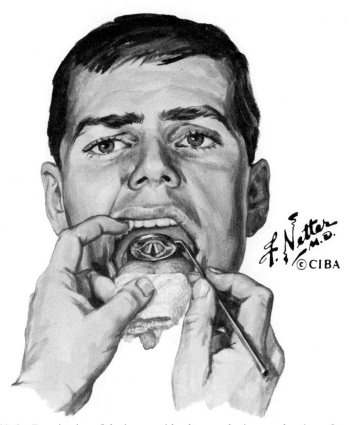

**Figure 32–9**   Examination of the larynx with a laryngeal mirror and a piece of gauze. © Copyright 1964 CIBA Pharmaceutical Company Division of CIBA-GEIGY Corporation. Reproduced, with permission, from the CLINICAL SYMPOSIA, illustrated by Frank H. Netter, M.D. All rights reserved.

7.  Specialists are also rather particular about the cotton applicator. They prefer a metal applicator with a wisp of cotton wrapped around the end of the applicator, leaving a small tuft of cotton at the tip. Be very careful that the metal tip is not at the very end but back about one-half inch.

## PROCTOLOGY

The proctosigmoidoscopic, or "procto" examination, as it is sometimes called, is the examination of the rectum and lower colon. It is an important part of a thorough physical examination. Since at least 70 per cent of cancers of the entire rectum and colon are anatomically within reach of the sigmoidoscope (25 cm. or 10 inches), it is obvious why a "procto" examination is important. About 13 per cent of the malignancies are found within digital reach (8 cm. or 3.2 inches). In past years the examination was done on the symptomatic patient, but because the examination is relatively simple and does not cause too much discomfort, it is fairly routine.

Some physicians feel there is no need for special bowel preparation if the patient is examined after normal defecation. They feel the use of laxatives or enemas does not preserve the normal appearance of the intestinal mucosa. If bowel preparation is desired the patient is instructed to use a laxative or one of the commercial saline enemas during the latter part of the day prior to the examination. The medical assistant should know the physician's desires and instruct the patient properly.

The anal area is first inspected for evidence of lesions, external hemorrhoids, fissures, or fistulas. Next, a small amount of lubricant is applied to the physician's index finger and the anal sphincter is dilated. The rectal sphincter muscle will relax after a few moments of pressure. Internal hemorrhoids cannot be felt unless they are thrombosed. Physicians will vary as to whether they use the sigmoidoscope, anoscope, or rectal speculum next. Besides inspecting for malignant lesions, the physician may observe polyps and/or abscesses.

Materials needed:

| | |
|---|---|
| Sigmoidoscope | Probe with bulb tip |
| Anoscope | Gloves |
| Rectal speculum | Finger cots |
| Insufflator | Long cotton applicators |
| Suction pump | Lubricating jelly |
| | Basin of water |

Before the examination starts be certain to check the illuminated instruments for light. See that the obturators are positioned correctly. Have a basin to receive the used instruments. The basin of water is to rinse out the suction pump immediately after each use. The pump tubing is very difficult to keep clean and free of odor.

1. Greet the patient and briefly explain the examination to be done. Patients are extremely apprehensive about this examination and will need extra assurance and consideration.
2. Have the patient empty his bladder and save the specimen.
3. It is best to have the patient disrobe completely and put on a gown.
4. Assist the patient into the correct position. Proper positioning is very important for the comfort of the patient and to insure accessibility of the rectum and sigmoid colon to the physician. An examining table that will adjust to the proctological position is far superior for both of the above reasons. With the proctological table, the patient assumes the position of kneeling on the knee board with the trunk of the body over the bend of the table and the forearms and elbows resting on the headboard. The patient may then rest his head on his arms. The table is next tilted forward, and his body trunk is then adjusted so the hips, NOT the waist, are bent over the bend of the table. If correctly positioned the abdomen will hang forward and downward freely. This allows the **S** curve of the sigmoid colon to straighten out somewhat. Since many offices do not have a procto table, other positions are used. The lift illustrated in Figure 32–10 gives the patient support, but remember, the trunk of the body must be forward with the patient bending at the hips

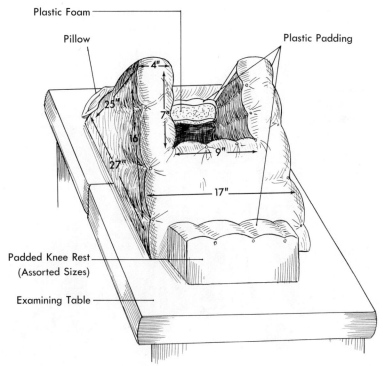

**Figure 32–10** The author's lift for positioning patients for proctosigmoidoscopic examination. Note the cut-out portion into which the abdominal contents fall, making the bowel examination much easier. Also note the knee lifts of different sizes to accommodate people of different heights. (From Conn, H. F., et al.: *Family Practice,* Philadelphia, W. B. Saunders Co., 1973.)

and not at the waist. The knee-chest or knee-elbow position is frequently used (Fig. 28–8). In the correct knee-chest position the patient's back is in a "swayback" position. This is difficult to maintain, and many patients cannot get into a true knee-chest position. It may help if the medical assistant stands beside the table and offers support to the patient. The Sims' position is used for rectal examinations or for patients who cannot be placed in the other more advantageous positions. However, the physician is somewhat limited in the depth of the bowel he can examine.

5. A fenestrated drape is superior for this examination, but two small sheets may be used and clipped together at the sides, or one larger sheet may be draped around and clipped over the patient's back. A small towel is placed directly under the anus and over the perineal body.

6. The medical assistant should watch the patient for any undue reactions and offer assurance.

7. Have tissues ready for the physician to wipe his gloved finger. Take the used instruments and applicators from the physician by the handle or with a tissue to protect yourself. Have the long applicators ready to hand the physician and remember to rinse out the suction tubing after each use.

8. The used instruments are placed in a basin of disinfectant solution and removed from the room to be sanitized and sterilized later.

CONDITIONS WHICH CAUSE ANAL PAIN
(Below the Pectinate Line)

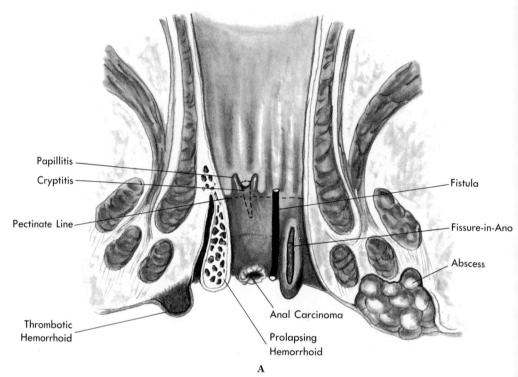

Papillitis

Cryptitis

Fistula

Pectinate Line

Fissure-in-Ano

Abscess

Thrombotic
Hemorrhoid

Anal Carcinoma

Prolapsing
Hemorrhoid

A

**Figure 32–11** **A.** Conditions occurring from the pectinate line to the perianal area which cause anal pain.

*Illustration continued on opposite page.*

9. When the physician has finished, assist the patient off the table or into a supine position. Do not let patients rise too rapidly because they are frequently dizzy after this examination. It is best to level the table and have the patient remain there for a few minutes.
10. The patient may then dress after the resting period. Be sure to have cleansing tissue in the dressing area and don't forget to give the patient any instructions the physician wanted him to have.

## ORTHOPEDIC SURGERY

An orthopedist is concerned with the body's mobility and diagnosing and treating diseases and abnormalities of the musculoskeletal system. A considerable part of this practice may be caring for fractures of the injured patient, especially in some resort areas. One orthopedist said the most common complaint to enter his office was the complaint of a "low back pain."

Besides a careful history, the examination covers basically the back and the

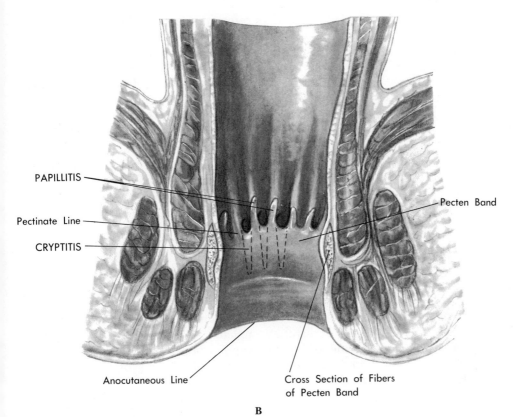

PAPILLITIS

Pectinate Line

CRYPTITIS

Pecten Band

Anocutaneous Line

Cross Section of Fibers
of Pecten Band

**B**

**Figure 32–11** *Continued.* **B.** The relationship of the pecten band to the pectinate line and its association with cryptitis and papillitis. (After Spiesman and Malow.) (From Conn, H. F., et al.: *Family Practice*, Philadelphia, W. B. Saunders Co., 1973.)

extremities. The physical examination of the musculo-skeletal system is performed largely by inspection, but palpation and mensuration are done. The orthopedic physician wants to determine the condition of the muscles, joints and bones. A considerable amount of the examination is done to determine the direction and range of active and passive motion in the joints.

The first step is usually inspection of the patient's posture in standing, sitting, and supine positions. A lateral view of the patient in a standing position shows the position of the head in relation to the trunk of the body. Normal or rigid curves of the cervical, thoracic, and lumbar spine may be seen. Abnormalities such as kyphosis or lordosis are seen in this lateral inspection. A scoliosis is seen from the posterior view. To determine the patient's gait, the physician will ask him to walk. The physician may observe a limp, possibly due to ankylosis, or a scissor gait as seen in spastic paraplegia.

Each major joint of the body is inspected for range of motion. A goniometer is used for precise measurement of a joint's flexion and extension. Muscles are examined for hypertrophy or atrophy. The measurement of the circumference of an extremity at a given point, such as the calf of the leg or the biceps of the arm, is compared with the opposite side. The tendon reflexes are checked.

The spine, or vertebral column, is referred to in divisions. The first seven vertebrae are the cervical spine, the next twelve are the thoracic spine, and the next five are the lumbar spine. These are the 24 movable vertebrae. Below the lumbar vertebrae are the sacrum and coccyx. When referring to the movable spine the physician will say C-5, meaning the fifth cervical vertebra or L-3, meaning the third lumbar vertebra.

A considerable part of an orthopedic examination looks like the patient is doing various gymnastics with the physician's help or guidance. Physicians specializing in industrial medicine and workmen's compensation cases have special terminology and methods for recording and measuring the musculoskeletal system. The American Academy of Orthopaedic Surgeons has published a guide called *Joint Motion: Method of Measuring and Recording.*

Materials needed:

| | |
|---|---|
| X-ray view box and x-rays | Goniometer |
| Tape measure | Dynamometer |
| Percussion hammer | |

In order for the physician to view the patient's entire back and the hip joints it is necessary for the patient to disrobe completely and be given a loin cloth-type garment. The female patient may also keep her brassiere on. Give the patient a gown and seat him on the edge of the examining table. Most physicians also prefer that the patient remove his shoes.

## UROLOGY

The urologist treats diseases of the genitourinary tract of the male and the urinary tract of the female. Frequently the urologist works with the gynecologist to treat the female patient.

The upper urinary system (kidneys and ureters) is assessed mainly by abdominal palpation. The urinary bladder is palpable when distended, but this is very discomforting to the patient. A considerable part of a urinary survey is dependent on the patient's history, such as frequency, urgency, dysuria, or incontinence. Cystitis is the most common disorder of the bladder, especially in the female. Renal calculi are the most painful. A major part of the examination is urinalysis. The medical assistant must be able to instruct the patient, especially the female, in the collection of a urine specimen, although a voided specimen is not always satisfactory, especially from the female. It is best to have the patient void in the physician's office so the specimen can be examined immediately. Most urologists prefer to examine a catheterized specimen.

Besides a careful urinalysis and urine culture, the physician may order an intravenous pyelogram, retrograde pyelogram, cystogram, or kidney function tests. Kidney function tests determine the kidneys' ability to concentrate and dilute urine, to excrete certain chemicals, and to excrete urea.

**Cystoscopy** is the examination of the bladder by means of a cystoscope which is passed through the urethra and into the bladder. The cystoscope illuminates the bladder interior. By means of special lenses and mirrors the bladder mucosa is examined for inflammation, tumors and calculi. A catheter can be passed through the cystoscope and on into the ureters and kidneys to obtain samples of urine or introduce an opaque substance for x-rays.

There is no special instrument setup for a routine urological examination unless a special procedure, such as obtaining a catheterized urine specimen, is done. Most offices are now using the prepackaged disposable units for catheterization and for bladder irrigations.

Both male and female patients are disrobed and given a gown. The female patient is placed in a lithotomy position, as for a pelvic examination. The male patient is seated on the examining table and the physician will instruct the patient to do what is needed.

# BIBLIOGRAPHY

Conn, H. F., Rakel, R. E., and Johnson, T. W. (eds.): *Family Practice,* Philadelphia, 1973, W. B. Saunders Co.

*Essentials of the Gynecological History and Examination,* 1965, Smith, Kline & French Laboratories.

*Essentials of the Neurological Examination,* 1968, Smith, Kline & French Laboratories.

*Proctosigmoidoscopy for the Detection of Asymptomatic Cancer,* 1962, American Cancer Society, Inc.

Judge, R. D., and Zuidema, G. D. (eds.): *Physical Diagnosis: A Physiological Approach to Clinical Examination,* 2nd Ed., Boston, 1968, Little, Brown and Co.

Prior, J. A., and Silberstein, J. S.: *Physical Diagnosis,* St. Louis, 1969, The C. V. Mosby Company.

Stein, H. A., and Slatt, B. J.: *The Ophthalmic Assistant: Fundamentals and Clinical Practice,* 2nd Ed., St. Louis, 1971, The C. V. Mosby Co.

Sutton, A. L.: *Bedside Nursing Techniques in Medicine and Surgery,* Philadelphia, 1969, W. B. Saunders Company.

# Chapter 33

**BEHAVIORAL OBJECTIVES**

*The medical office assistant should be able to:*

Accident-proof the physician's office to minimize risk of injury to visitors.

Familiarize herself with local emergency services so that the severely ill or injured can be transferred quickly for critical care.

Prepare and maintain a "crash tray" of essential drugs and equipment for emergency use.

Apply first aid in common presenting conditions such as poisoning, hemorrhaging, fractures, burns, and the like.

# First Aid and Medical Emergencies

There are many different approaches to the manner of emergency care, but this discussion will attempt to remain within general principles. Each medical assistant should consult with her physician-employer as to *his* desires and preferences for handling emergencies in his particular practice. Each medical assistant should enroll in an American Red Cross First Aid course and obtain an advanced certificate. A refresher course should be taken every few years. It is also strongly recommended that medical assistants encourage their local chapters of the A.A.M.A. to have workshops conducted by their local physicians and the emergency facilities in their community.

In a true emergency, the law permits anyone to do whatever is reasonably necessary, provided that the care given is within the scope and skill of the first aider's competence. The law holds persons giving emergency care to be responsible for any injury that they cause owing to their negligence or failure to exercise reasonable care.

Some medical emergencies may require the medical assistant to make an immediate decision that comes rather close to making a medical diagnosis. The obvious injury of spurting blood does not present this problem, but the ashen-faced patient gasping for breath and in obvious pain calls for medical knowledge in order to make a decision. The medical assistant must remember her limitations and never forget that her employer may be held liable for her mistakes.

## ACCIDENT-PROOF THE OFFICE

It is usually the medical assistant's responsibility to accident-proof the office as much as possible. Do not use scatter rugs, delicate chairs, or have slippery floors. Keep cupboard doors and drawers closed. Wipe up any spills immediately and pick up dropped objects. All medications should be kept out of sight; dangerous drugs should be kept in locked cupboards. If there are children in the office, keep all sharp objects out of reach. NEVER give a child a disposable syringe and needle for a toy or as a reward for being good. These items are not toys and should be destroyed and carefully discarded. Never leave a seriously ill patient or a restless, depressed, or unconscious patient unattended.

## PLAN AHEAD

The office staff should discuss possible emergencies that may occur in that office or area. Local industries, for instance, may present unique problems that call for very specialized care. Plan for these, and ask the doctor's advice on what procedure he wants you to follow. If there are several employees, each should be assigned specific duties. Organization and planning will make the difference between organized care for the patient and complete chaos. Some offices have set up the "buddy system." This system allows one person to take immediate charge of the patient while another obtains needed materials and calls for assistance. In this way the patient is not left unattended. They can also relieve each other in more strenuous work like resuscitation and external heart massage.

## COMMUNITY EMERGENCY SERVICES

In every area, the medical assistant should call the local fire department, police department, or rescue squad and know what is available to her and the patients. She should learn ahead what numbers to call and how these calls are handled. Usually one call will send all the help that is needed. These emergency services are extremely well coordinated in dispatching resuscitators, ambulances, and other emergency care.

Every office should have a list of emergency numbers posted. This list should include the Poison Control Center, the local rescue squad, or fire and police department numbers. The list should be in plain sight and known to all office personnel. When in doubt, dial "O" for operator. A fire department emergency rescue squad captain once told a group of medical assistants that the rescue squad made almost as many calls into physician's offices as they did to private homes. Remember, the fact that you are in a medical office does not mean you can handle all emergencies. Neither is the doctor always in the office when you are there.

## CRASH TRAY

The *emergency* or *crash tray* that is made up in your office should be kept in an easily accessible place known to all personnel in the office. A firm rule must be made that *no one* borrows *any* item from the tray. It should be checked periodically and all medications kept fresh and ready for use. The contents of the tray will vary to some degree according to the type of emergencies your office will possibly encounter. Listed below are some basic items found in crash trays.

Epinephrine (adrenalin), injectable
Apomorphine hydrochloride, injectable (This is a narcotic.)
Antihistamine, injectable and oral
Ipecac, oral
Isuprel, aerosol spray (isoproterenol hydrochloride)
Sterile dressings

Tourniquet (not often recommended)
Disposable syringe and needle units
Adhesive tape
Airways of various sizes
"Instant" type of hot and cold packs

The *epinephrine* should be in a ready-to-use cartridge syringe and needle unit. These are supplied in one cc cartridges. Then, in case of an insect sting, 0.5 cc may be given immediately at the site of the sting and 0.5 cc may be given in the opposite arm. Epinephrine is also used to check hemorrhage and relieve asthmatic paroxysm and shock. It is a vasoconstrictor, cardiac stimulant, and relaxes the bronchioles.

Other drugs that may be found in this section are *atropine, lanoxin,* and *xylocaine.* The *apomorphine hydrochloride* is a prompt and effective emetic and is used in cases of poisoning when a stomach pump cannot be employed. *Ipecac* is also an emetic and many physicians are recommending that mothers keep it on hand at home for use in cases of emergency. Antihistamine counteracts the effect of histamine and is used in the treatment of allergic reactions and anaphylaxis. *Isuprel* (isoproterenol hydrochloride) is an antispasmodic and is used in bronchial spasm; it is also a cardiac stimulant. Some trade names for this product are *Isuprel* (Winthrop), *Medihaler-Iso* (Riker) and *Norisodrine* (Abbott). Other medications found useful in a crash tray are *Aramine* for severe shock, *Amytal Sodium* and *Valium* for convulsions and as sedatives, dextrose and insulin to treat diabetics, and *Lasix* for congestive heart failure.

Many physicians and others involved in emergency care do not recommend the use of a tourniquet except in cases of insect or snake bites on the arms or legs because there is considerable danger from the *incorrect* use of a tourniquet. It should be used very cautiously. It is much better in cases of bleeding to apply pressure directly over the bleeding area. In cases of insect or snake bites, the tourniquet is applied just above the bite area, or just above the place where the offending medication was administered in the case of an error in injection of a medication.

If bottles of intravenous solutions are kept in the crash tray, then it has been suggested that a hammer and large nail also be kept in the tray. A nail quickly driven into the wall may relieve some person from having to hold the bottle above the patient. One can find oneself quite often without a place to hang a bottle or irrigation bag, and one small nail hole is well justified by the great convenience it affords.

Another good suggestion is to have cards in the tray that have the emergency numbers on them. By doing so, the person in charge can hand the correct number to a specific person with instructions to call that number. This may save a few moments searching for a number.

## GENERAL RULES

Make the patient as comfortable as possible. Do not leave an ill or emergency patient in the reception room. The first and most important rule is to

KEEP CALM. Stop for 30 seconds, survey the situation, and recognize what is the actual emergency. A decision must be made as to whether the need is immediate or nonimmediate. This decision may call for some medical knowledge and calm judgment. After you have surveyed the situation, calmly but firmly give specific instructions to the patient and the other office personnel. Never say, "Will someone call the doctor?" Say, "YOU call the doctor," "YOU get a blanket," and "YOU get the emergency tray." After the emergency is under control, make certain that all the events and medications used are recorded accurately. Be precise when recording. It is a good idea to have statements of how the accident happened or what events just preceded the emergency. If the patient is one of your employer's regular patients, make sure the patient's medical chart is flagged with this pertinent information. If the patient is not a regular patient in your office, he should be given any necessary information that he can take with him to prevent a possible recurrence of the emergency.

Whenever a patient is being sent to a hospital for an emergency that may require an anesthetic, it is advisable to instruct the patient not to take anything by mouth. Food in the stomach can present quite a problem when a patient is receiving a general anesthetic.

## SOME SPECIFIC PROBLEMS

### Poisoning

Each office should have the telephone number of the local poison control center. This center is often located in the largest local hospital or the county hospital. When a patient calls in to report a poisoning, ask him the name of the poison taken, how long ago it was taken, and how much was taken. Tell him to bring the poison with him to the office or to the hospital.

If the name of the poison is unknown, then ask what type it was; that is, was it a pill like aspirin or a fluid like kerosene. It is always best to send poison cases to the hospital, especially if it has a poison control center. You should know the location of the center well enough to instruct the patient on how to get there. Unless the antidote is written on the label of the poison, be cautious about advising the patient to take an emetic, although it is generally safe to try to dilute the poison with water or milk. Milk is frequently preferred. Then induce vomiting. Save the vomitus for analysis. Remember, DO NOT induce vomiting if the patient has ingested a strong alkaline, acid, kerosene, or gasoline. If ipecac is not available, large amounts of tepid water may be given. The universal antidote is one part strong tea, one part milk of magnesia and two slices of burnt toast, crumbled. Some first aiders recommend using lots of milk with egg white in it. It may be necessary to make the patient gag to start the vomiting. The gag reflex is started by touching the back of the tongue lightly.

### Fainting

One of the most common emergency problems to confront the medical assistant is a patient's fainting or feeling faint. Fainting is usually caused by a lack of oxygen in the blood with a consequent lack of oxygen to the brain. If a patient faints, or even says, "I feel faint," if his face becomes pale, or if perspiration becomes profuse, especially on the forehead, the patient should be positioned with the head lower than or on the same level as the heart. If the patient is placed on the treatment table, turn his head to one side and loosen all tight clothing. Give aromatic spirits of ammonia; be careful not to hold the ammonia directly under the patient's nostrils but pass it back and forth about six inches from the nose. Cold water lightly sprinkled on the face will help. Take the patient's pulse, respiration, and blood pressure; then report to the physician. Keep the patient in a supine position for at least ten minutes after he has regained consciousness.

If it is not possible to get the patient onto a bed, place him in a sitting position and lower his head between his knees. If the patient cannot sit or lie down, tell him to kneel on one knee as if tying a shoelace; this gets the head lower than the heart. Never try to hold up a patient who faints but ease him gently to the floor if he cannot be assisted to a bed. On the floor, he is placed in a level position. After the patient has regained consciousness he may be given some tea or coffee. Recovery usually occurs within five minutes. If it does not, a physician should be called.

## Head Injuries

Head injury may cause the patient to be dizzy, have a severe headache, or even be unconscious. The loss of consciousness may be brief or prolonged; it may appear immediately or be delayed for as long as a half hour. The pupils of the eyes may be unequal. If the patient is unconscious, do not attempt to arouse him. If the face is flushed, raise the head and shoulders slightly. If the face is gray and ashen, keep the patient flat. If there are signs of vomiting, place him on his abdomen. Do not give any stimulants. Use extreme caution in moving the patient. Watch the pupils of the eyes and record any changes. Also record the blood pressure. Report the time of any changes in the eyes and blood pressure. Check the ears for any bleeding in the canals. Keep the patient warm and quiet; do not allow him to move about. All head injuries must be considered serious and needing medical care. There may be bleeding around the brain even when there is no evidence of external bleeding or injury.

## Abdominal Pain

If a patient is vomiting, place him on his stomach with the head turned to one side or place him in a semi-sitting position. Have the emesis basin available. If possible, place the patient in a room near a toilet. Keep him warm and quiet. Give him nothing by mouth. You may allow him to rinse his mouth out after vomiting if he is fully conscious. DO NOT apply heat to the abdomen unless the physician instructs you to do so. If the patient is not vomiting, he may have a few sips of water occasionally, but give him nothing else by mouth. Abdominal pain may be due to the ingestion of a food or drug, heat exhaustion, gallstones, diarrhea, or many other causes. Severe and persistent abdominal pain should have medical attention as soon as possible. Gentle pressure over the abdomen will determine if the muscles are rigid. If they are "hard as a board," there may be a peritoneal irritation. Take the patient's temperature.

## Chest Pain

All patients with chest pain are treated as heart emergencies until a physician has ruled out this diagnosis. The patient is usually sweating and has a gray, ashen appearance. The lips and fingernails may be cyanotic. He is frequently clutching his chest in pain. This pain may radiate out to the left arm and up the left side of the neck. The pulse may be rapid and weak, and frequently there is

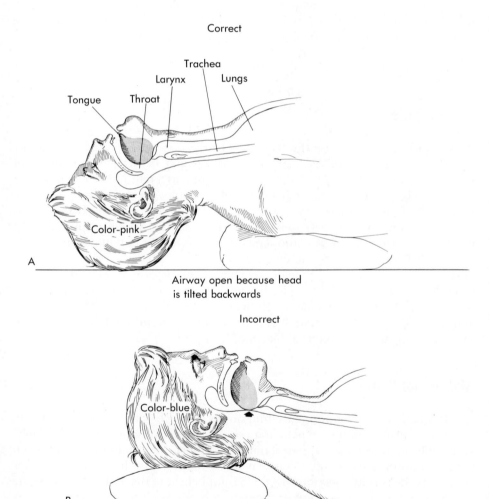

Figure 33–1   Position of head for mouth-to-mouth resuscitation.

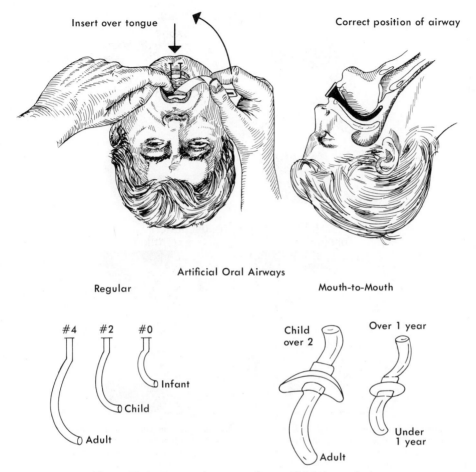

**Figure 33-2**   Proper placement of an artificial airway device.

nausea. DO NOT have the patient walk any distance. The secretary's chair with rollers is an excellent method of moving this patient to a quiet room where he can rest. The patient will probably prefer to have his head slightly elevated or even be in a semi-sitting position. Keep the patient quiet and warm but do not overheat him. Administer oxygen if the physician has previously given these instructions. Prepare the medication that the physician is most likely to use. This may be adrenalin (epinephrine), atropine, digitalis, or calcium gluconate.

If the physician cannot be reached, call the local emergency squad at the police or fire department. It may be necessary to start mouth-to-mouth resuscitation if the patient is unconscious and there is no evidence of breathing. Loosen all tight clothing. If necessary, insert an airway. Some physicians may give you permission to give the patient some aspirin if the patient is fully conscious. DO NOT give the patient anything such as alcohol, food, or water by mouth without the physician's permission. If the patient is conscious, ask him if he has any medication with him. This medication is usually nitroglycerine tablets that are ad-

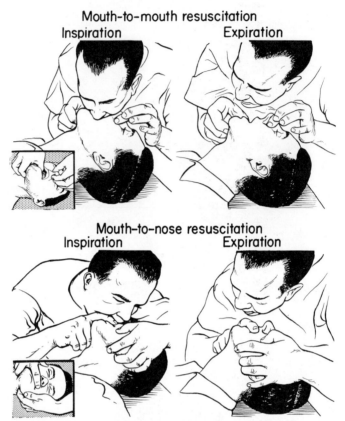

**Mouth-to-mouth resuscitation**
Inspiration          Expiration

**Mouth-to-nose resuscitation**
Inspiration          Expiration

**Figure 33–3**   *Mouth-to-Mouth.* 1. Remove any obstructions from the mouth. 2. Hyperextend the patient's neck. 3. With your thumb hold the jaw open. 4. Pinch patient's nostrils closed. 5. Take a deep breath then breathe directly between the patient's lips, forming an air-tight seal with your mouth. 6. Allow the patient to exhale. 7. Repeat every 4 or 5 seconds in the adult, slightly faster for a child. 8. For the small child the resuscitator's mouth may cover the patient's nose and mouth. *Mouth-to-nose.* Same procedure, except the patient's mouth is held closed and air is breathed into the nostrils. (From Gordon, A. S., et al.: J.A.M.A. *167*:320, 1958).

ministered sublingually. The patient will tell you what to do. DO NOT give any smelling salts.

If the physician is in the office or immediately on his way in, connect the patient to the electrocardiograph and make some tracings. Limb lead #2 is usually considered to be the monitoring lead. It is extremely important that the office staff remain calm, since all heart patients are extremely frightened persons and will need assurance.

Only a physician can tell the difference between a heart attack and a case of acute indigestion.

## Asthma

Since only a physician can treat asthma, the medical assistant should give the patient all the assurance she can. Have the respiratory medication ready for the physician's orders. Some asthmatic patients will carry a respiratory inhalator with them. In this case, you can assist them in using this inhalator. A bronchodilator such as epinephrine or aminophylline may be ordered by the physician.

Other medications are used to thin the mucus in the air passages so the patient may clear his lungs more easily. Emotions play a very important part in the severe asthmatic, and he must be assured and kept calm.

## Anaphylactic Reactions

This is an extremely broad range of reactions, ranging from mild itching to anaphylactic shock. It is the anaphylactic shock that presents a true emergency because it can occur very suddenly and without warning. The patient will have dyspnea, cyanosis, and may sometimes have convulsions. Epinephrine and oxygen should be immediately ready for administration on the physician's orders. The patient will appear flushed and have a rapid pulse as a result of the administration of the epinephrine, and he should be told that these are side effects of the medication and not to be alarmed.

## Shock

In this state, the patient's peripheral blood circulation is impaired. Shock is the result of a traumatic condition, such as hemorrhage, injury, pain, or fear. It may follow the changing of a surgical dressing or the administration of a medication by injection. It may be immediate or delayed, severe or mild. The patient is pale, clammy feeling, often has dilated pupils, weak and rapid pulse, low blood pressure, and complains of thirst and feels lethargic and faint. He may have labored breathing. Place the patient on his back with the legs elevated, loosen all tight clothing, and keep the patient warm. Do not give the patient any stimulants. If medical care will arrive within about twenty minutes, it is best not to give the patient anything by mouth. Tea or coffee may be given later if there is no evidence of internal hemorrhage or head injury. Because there are so many different causes of shock, it is advisable to administer only basic first aid care and get immediate medical help.

## Burns

Burns are extremely painful and dangerous. There is always the danger of infection from contamination because the burned tissue acts as a culture medium for bacteria. The most frequently recommended first aid for a burn is to immerse it immediately in cool water. This will give immediate relief from the pain. The other danger that a burned patient has is the possibility of shock. Shock can be very serious in burn cases. If immersion in water is not possible, then apply sterile wet compresses to the area. DO NOT apply any medications or ointments unless instructed to do so by a physician. If the burn is over a large area, wrap a clean towel (sterile, if possible) over the area and get the patient to the hospital as soon as possible. If clothing is to be removed, do not pull it off; cut it away carefully. DO NOT open blisters. Chemical burns should be thoroughly rinsed with plenty of water and covered with a sterile moist dressing.

Depth of Burn Injury

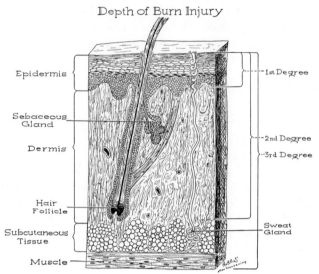

**Figure 33–4** (From Haynes, Jr., B. W., Ochsner, A., and DeBakey, M. E., Eds.: *Christopher's Minor Surgery*, 8th Ed., Philadelphia, 1959, W. B. Saunders Co.)

A *first degree burn* shows erythema of the epidermis only. The tissue destruction is superficial without blistering. There is little or no pain.

A *second degree burn* includes the entire epidermal layer and varying depths of the dermis. Blisters are usually formed, and there is some pain. There is also danger of infection in the blistered area. If the burn is deep enough there may be some destruction of the hair follicles and the sebaceous glands.

A *third degree burn* is the destruction of all the epithelial structure. The destroyed skin will slough off, leaving a raw area. It may be necessary to have skin grafts. There is great pain and danger of infection.

A *fourth degree burn* is sometimes known as a "charred burn." This burn reaches the underlying muscular tissue and is extremely painful. There is great danger of infection. Grafts and plastic surgery are usually necessary. Diagnosis of the depth or degree of a burn differs because skin varies in depth in different locations of the body. A burn is usually mixed in degrees in the different areas that are burned.

## Hemorrhages

Bleeding may be external or internal. First aiders can do little about internal bleeding, except keep the patient very quiet and warm to prevent shock. Get medical help immediately.

External bleeding is not as complex as internal bleeding. You can frequently see the source of the bleeding. There are three practical ways to control bleeding. First, use direct pressure over the area by applying a sterile pad. Do not press too hard, especially if there is the possibility of a fracture beneath the bleeding area. The second method is to apply pressure over the nearest pressure point between the bleeding area and the heart. The third method is to apply a tourniquet. A tourniquet is used only as a last resort. A broad flat tourniquet is best, and a pad should be used under the area of the tie. Gently tighten the tourniquet until the bleeding is stopped. Do not make it any tighter, since the tissues beyond the tourniquet can die without blood circulation. Do not release the tourniquet every twenty minutes, but get medical help within that period of time. Most physicians recommend the first method of direct pressure over the bleeding area. If a sterile dressing is available it, of course, is best to use; otherwise, use the cleanest material available. With the newer antibiotics the threat of infection is not as great as in the past.

## Nosebleeds

If the patient is cooperative, bleeding from the nose may be controlled by inserting a ball of cotton into the bleeding nostril and then applying external pressure to the side of the offending nostril. Sometimes a cotton ball placed between the upper lip and teeth, with outside pressure over this area, will help. Cold compresses to the face may also be of value. The patient's head should be elevated.

## Lacerations

Lacerations are a great part of general practice and pediatrics. Have the patient lie down and cover the injured area with a sterile dressing. Use enough thicknesses to absorb the bleeding. If the bleeding persists or is profuse, apply pressure to the dressing and also to the area just above the wound. For any type of hemorrhage, the patient should be kept quiet. Do not use any disinfectant unless the physician has given you previous instructions. If the laceration is extremely dirty, it may be irrigated with sterile normal saline solution. Hydrogen peroxide is frequently used to irrigate small areas. A butterfly closure strip may be used over small lacerations to hold the edges together.

Closure of a wound with microporous tape eliminates the discomfort of suturing and suture removal, as well as some of the risks of infection imposed by sutures. The figure on page 583 shows the steps in closure by the tape method. First the skin and the wound, if necessary, should be cleansed to assure a clean dry skin. The tape in 1/4 or 1/2 inch widths is placed at approximately 1/4 inch intervals until the wound is closed. Generally, closure is started near one end, but a longer wound could be brought together in quarters and then the intervening spaces closed next. A dry dressing may be placed over the area although it is usually not necessary.

## Fractures

When a patient with a fracture is brought into the office, there is little the medical assistant can do other than make the patient comfortable, support the

Simple (closed) fracture
— No open wound

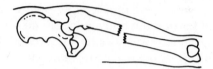

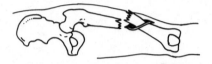

Compound (open) fracture—Wound in
skin communicates with fracture

Extracapsular fracture—Bone broken
outside joint

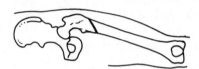

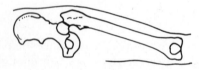

Intracapsular fracture—Bone broken
inside joint

Comminuted fracture—Bone
splintered into fragments

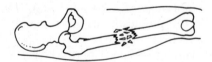

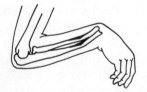

Greenstick fracture—Bone broken,
bent but still securely hinged at one
side

Longitudinal fracture—Break runs
parallel with bone

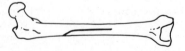

**Figure 33–5**   (From Ethicon, Inc.: *Nursing Care of the Patient in the O.R.*, 1973.)

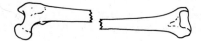

Transverse fracture—Break runs across bone

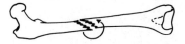

Oblique fracture—Break runs in slanting direction on bone

Spiral fracture—Break coils around bone

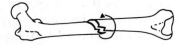

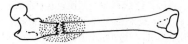

Pathologic fracture—Break is at site of bone disease

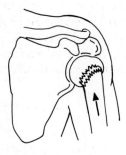

Impacted fracture—Bone broken and wedged into other break

Fracture dislocation—Break complicated by bone out of joint

Depressed fracture—Broken skull bone driven inward

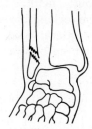

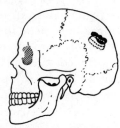

**Figure 33–6**    (From Ethicon, Inc.: *Nursing Care of the Patient in the O.R.*, 1973.)

fractured area, and keep the patient quiet. Have the patient lie down in a position that will not place a strain on the area and that will prevent any movement. If there is an abrasion or bleeding, place a sterile dressing over the area. Do not apply too much pressure on the bleeding area if there is a fracture beneath. Be gentle. DO NOT ATTEMPT TO STRAIGHTEN THE FRACTURE or move it in any way. If the patient must be moved, then give support to the fracture before moving. If it is possible, many physicians would appreciate having an x-ray of the area ready when they arrive.

## Obstetrical Emergencies

An obstetrical office presents problems that are unique to this specialty. Every medical assistant employed in this specialty or any office where the physician delivers babies should be trained to handle the emergencies. The majority of these problems will be presented to you over the telephone. Of course, if the physician is in the office the call should be transferred to him immediately.

If a pregnant patient calls in to report a vaginal bleeding, you must ask some specific questions. Is the bleeding like a menstrual flow or is it a gushing type of hemorrhage? Is it painful or without any pain? If the bleeding is gushing, then the patient must be told to lie down immediately while you send for an ambulance. It takes only a few minutes for both mother and baby to bleed to death from a ruptured uterus. If the bleeding is like a normal menstrual flow, have the patient go to bed with the foot of the bed elevated and tell her you will report this to the physician immediately.

If the tissue passed is liver-like, it may possibly be a blood clot; white tissue may be the fetus. No matter what the tissue appears to be, have the patient save it, if possible, and take it with her to the hospital.

## Seizures

Seizures are frightening to witness, but the patient is not usually suffering, nor is he in great danger. Tranquility is usually an essential component of such care. Loosen the clothing, but do not attempt to restrain the patient's movements except to protect him from injuring himself. Move anything that might be in the way and cause the patient injury. Give nothing by mouth, neither fluids nor medication. If the patient remains unconscious after the jerking has subsided, turn his face to one side because there is frequently considerable saliva. Many physicians do not recommend attempting to place anything between the patient's teeth during the convulsion, unless there is evidence that the patient is chewing his tongue. In this case, a piece of gauze wrapped around two tongue depressors may be placed in the mouth between the teeth. Do not use your fingers.

If the patient has not regained consciousness within 10 to 15 minutes, it may be advisable to call a physician. After the seizure is over, let the patient rest or sleep in a quiet room. If the seizure has occurred in an inconvenient place for the patient to rest, he may be moved to a quiet place after he has regained consciousness and can tell you his name and where he is. This way you will know he is sufficiently oriented.

## Choking

There is considerable controversy over the immediate care of a choking person. Many experts say not to slap a choking person on the back, while others say to strike the person sharply over the back to aid in dislodging the object. They all agree that it is best to hang the head *and* trunk of the body over the edge of a table, bed, or another person's lap. DO NOT give the victim soft bread or a drink of water—nothing by mouth. If the victim is a child, then simply turn the child upside down or across your lap with the trunk of the body hanging down. Firm taps on the back may help. If the upside down treatment does not help, it may be necessary to search for the object in the victim's throat. Do not probe without looking. Use a light. Be very careful in retrieving the object with an instrument. It is best to use your fingers. Usually air can pass around the object and the person can be given mouth-to-mouth resuscitation. If the object cannot be immediately removed then medical help must be gotten immediately. Time of the essence with a choking person.

## Foreign Body in the Eye

This kind of emergency is most uncomfortable, and it is often extremely difficult to keep the patient from rubbing the eye. However, he must be instructed not to touch the eye in any way. If the doctor has given you prior permission, you may put a few drops of ophthalmic topical anesthetic in the eye. The patient will greatly appreciate this and will experience almost immediate relief. Unless the foreign object is clearly visible, do not attempt to search for it or remove it. The patient should be placed in a darkened room to wait. Have plenty of tissues available. If there is a contusion and swelling, cold wet compresses will help. If you have been trained to turn an upper eyelid out, then do so gently and search for the foreign body. Be very careful not to place any pressure on the eye. If the foreign body cannot be found, then ask the patient to close his eye normally, place a pad over the eye, and hold it in place with a strip of Scotch tape. Get medical care.

## Animal Bites

Any animal bite that breaks the skin should be seen by a physician and reported to the authorities. The animal must be identified and confined for quarantine. The animal should not be killed because a positive rabies identification is almost impossible to make if the animal has been dead for a while. Many pet owners will not admit their pet has bitten a person because they fear the animal will be killed. Assure them the Health Department authorities only want to confine the animal for observation. The bite should be washed thoroughly with soap and water and treated as any other wound would be. The victim should be seen by a physician.

## Insect Stings

If the insect's stinger is still in the skin, it should be removed by brushing it off or by using a fine tweezer. Be very careful not to squeeze the stinger and inject more venom into the skin but place the tweezers close to the skin and not over the stinger sac. Apply an ice compress to the area. To relieve itching, a paste of baking soda may be applied or a compress of ammonia water used. If the patient gives a history of allergies, the physician should be consulted immediately. Do not delay. If the sting is on an arm or leg, a broad flat tourniquet may be applied above the site of the sting. Release the tourniquet every ten minutes for about a minute. Have the patient report to the nearest hospital or physician's office. Do not give the patient any alcohol or stimulants. Keep the patient's activities at a minimum in order to limit circulation.

*Appendix One*

# Suggested Readings and Reference Books for Medical Assistants

American Medical Association: The Business Side of Medical Practice, Chicago, American Medical Association, 1974

_____: Current Medical Terminology, 4th edition, Chicago, American Medical Association, 1971

_____: Judicial Council Opinions and Reports, Chicago, American Medical Association, latest edition

_____: Medicolegal Forms with Legal Analysis, Chicago, American Medical Association, 1973

_____: The Physician's Career, 2nd edition, Chicago, American Medical Association, 1967

_____: Principles of Medical Ethics, Chicago, American Medical Association

_____: The Wonderful Human Machine, Chicago, American Medical Association, latest edition

_____: X-ray Examinations, Guide to Good Practice, Chicago, American Medical Association, latest edition

American National Red Cross: Standard First Aid and Personal Safety, Garden City, Doubleday & Company, 1973

Anthony, Catherine Parker: Basic Concepts in Anatomy and Physiology, 2nd edition, St. Louis, C. V. Mosby Company, 1970

_____: Structure and Function of the Body, revised 4th edition, St. Louis, C. V. Mosby Company, 1972

Aurner, Robert and Paul S. Burtness: Effective English for Business Communication, 6th edition, Cincinnati, South-Western Publishing Company, 1970

Bredow, Miriam: Medical Office Procedures, 6th edition, New York, McGraw-Hill Book Company, 1973

Bredow, Miriam and Marian Cooper: The Medical Assistant, 3rd edition, New York, McGraw-Hill Book Company, 1970

Brunson, Evelyn V.: The Professional Secretary, Englewood Cliffs, Prentice-Hall, Inc., 1974

Bryan, Arthur H.: Bacteriology: Principles and Practice, 6th edition, College Outline Series, New York, Barnes & Noble, 1962

Burke, Shirley R.: The Composition and Functions of Body Fluids, St. Louis, C. V. Mosby Company, 1972

Burton, Genevieve: Personal, Impersonal and Interpersonal Relations, a Guide for Nurses, 3rd edition, New York, Springer Publishing Company, 1970

Carson, A. B., Arthur E. Carlson, and Mary E. Burnet: Accounting Essentials for Career Secretaries, 3rd edition, Cincinnati, South-Western Publishing Company, 1972

Carvel, Fred J.: Human Relations in Business, New York, The MacMillan Publishing Company, 1970

Creighton, Helen: Law Every Nurse Should Know, 2nd edition, Philadelphia, W. B. Saunders Company, 1970

Curran, William J.: Tracy's The Doctor as a Witness, 2nd edition, Philadelphia, W. B. Saunders Company, 1965

Cusumano, Charles L.: Malpractice Law Dissected for Quick Grasping, Philadelphia, J. B. Lippincott Company, 1969

Dennis, Robert Lee and Jean Monty Doyle: The Complete Handbook for Medical Secretaries and Assistants, Boston, Little, Brown & Company, 1971

Dennis, Lorraine: Psychology of Human Behavior for Nurses, 3rd edition, Philadelphia, W. B. Saunders Company, 1967

Dienhart, Charlotte M.: Basic Human Anatomy and Physiology, 2nd edition, Philadelphia, W. B. Saunders, 1973

Dorland's Pocket Medical Dictionary, 21st edition, Philadelphia, W. B. Saunders Company, 1968

Frenay, Sister Agnes Clare: Understanding Medical Terminology, 5th edition, St. Louis, Catholic Hospital Association, 1973

French, R. M.: The Nurse's Guide to Diagnostic Procedures, 3rd edition, New York, McGraw-Hill Book Company, 1971

Garb, Solomon: Laboratory Tests in Common Use, 5th edition, New York, Springer Publishing Company, 1971

Gavin, Ruth E. and W. A. Sabin: Reference Manual for Stenographers and Typists, 4th edition, New York, McGraw-Hill Book Company, 1970

Gross, Verlee E.: The Structure of Medical Terms, revised 2nd edition, North Hollywood, Halls of Ivy Press, 1973

———: Mastering Medical Terminology, 4th edition, North Hollywood, Halls of Ivy Press, 1969

———: Illustrated Programmed Gross Anatomy, North Hollywood, Halls of Ivy Press, 1973

Hadley, Anne: Forty-Five Lessons in Surgical Terminology, Philadelphia, J. B. Lippincott Company, 1972

———: Medical Secretary as a Word Technician, Philadelphia, J. B. Lippincott Company, 1968

Hanna, J. Marshall, Estelle L. Popham and Rita S. Tilton: Secretarial Procedures And Administration, 6th edition, Cincinnati, South-Western Publishing Company, 1973

Hill, George J. II: Outpatient Surgery, Philadelphia, W. B. Saunders Company, 1973

House, Clifford, R. and Apollonia M. Koebele: Reference Manual for Office Personnel, Cincinnati, South-Western Publishing Company, 1970

Hutchinson, Lois: Standard Handbook for Secretaries, 8th edition, New York, McGraw-Hill Book Company, 1971

Jacob, Stanley W. and Clarice A. Francone: Structure and Function in Man, Philadelphia, W. B. Saunders Company, 3rd edition, 1974

JeHarned, R. N.: Medical Terminology Made Easy, 2nd edition, Chicago, Physicians Record Company, 1968.

Johnson, Margaret A.: Developing the Art of Understanding, 2nd edition, New York, Springer Publishing Company, 1972

Kahn, Gilbert, Theodore Yerian and Jeffrey R. Stewart, Jr.: Filing Systems and Records Management, 2nd edition, New York, McGraw-Hill Book Company, 1971

Kalish, Richard A.: The Psychology of Human Behavior, 3rd edition, Brooks-Cole Publishing Company, 1973

Kimber, Diana C., Carolyn E. Gray, Caroline Stackpole, and Lutie C. Leavell: Anatomy and Physiology, 15th edition, New York, The MacMillan Publishing Company, 1966

Klein, A. E.: New World Concise Secretarial Handbook, Cleveland, World Publishing Company, 1973

Krueger, Elizabeth A.: The Hypodermic Injection, Philadelphia, J. B. Lippincott Company, 1965

Laird, Donald A. and Eleanor C. Laird: The Technique of Handling People, 2nd edition, New York, McGraw-Hill Book Company, 1954

――――: Psychology: Human Relations and Motivations, 4th edition, New York, McGraw-Hill Book Company, 1967

Langley, Leroy L., E. Cheraskin and Ruth Sleeper: Dynamic Anatomy and Physiology, 3rd edition, New York, McGraw-Hill Book Company, 1969

Levine, Myra E.: Introduction to Clinical Nursing, 2nd edition, Philadelphia, F. A. Davis Company, 1973

Maedke, Wilmer, Mary F. Robek and Gerald Brown: Information and Records Management, Beverly Hills, Glencoe Press, 1974

Mager, N. H. and S. K.: The Office Encyclopedia, 8th edition, New York, Pocket Books division of Simon & Schuster, 1966

Miller, B. F. and Claire Keane: Encyclopedia and Dictionary of Medicine and Nursing, Philadelphia, W. B. Saunders Company, 1972

Moellring, F. K.: Beginning with the Microscope, New York, Sterling Publishing Company, 1972

Morgan, James A.: The Art and Science of Medical Radiography, 3rd edition, St. Louis, Catholic Hospital Association, 1971

Moritz, Alan R. and R. Crawford Morris: Handbook of Legal Medicine, 3rd edition, St. Louis, C. V. Mosby Company, 1970

Morris, R. Crawford and Alan R. Moritz: Doctor and Patient and the Law, revised 5th edition, St. Louis, C. V. Mosby Company, 1971

Nursing Examination Review Book, Volumes 4 and 5, Flushing, New York, Medical Examination Publishing Company, Inc., 1967

Purtilo, Ruth: The Allied Health Professional and the Patient, Philadelphia, W. B. Saunders Company, 1973

Schnitzer, Kurt, M.D.: Electrocardiographic Technique, 2nd edition, New York, Grune & Stratton, 1960

Seedor, Marie M.: Introduction to Asepsis, Philadelphia, J. B. Lippincott Company, 1969

Sferra, Adam, et al.: Personality and Human Relations, 2nd edition, New York, McGraw-Hill Book Company, 1961

Sloane, Sheila B.: The Medical Word Book, Philadelphia, W. B. Saunders Company, 1972

Smith, Samuel: Atlas of Human Anatomy, 6th edition, New York, College Series, Barnes & Noble

Steen, Edwin: Medical Abbreviations, 3rd edition, Philadelphia, F. A. Davis Company, 1971

Stehli, George: Microscope and How to Use It, New York, Sterling Publishing Company, 1970

Strand, Helen R.: An Illustrated Guide to Medical Terminology, Baltimore, Williams & Wilkins Company, 1968

Strunk, William, Jr. and E. B. White: The Elements of Style, 2nd edition, New York, The Macmillan Publishing Company, 1972

Thomas, C. L.: Taber's Cyclopedic Medical Dictionary, 12th edition, Philadelphia, F. A. Davis Company, 1973

Tokay, Elbert: Fundamentals of Physiology: The Human Body and How it Works, New York, Barnes & Noble, 1967

Waltz, J. R. and F. E. Inbau: Medical Jurisprudence, New York, The Macmillan Publishing Company, 1971

Widmann, Frances K.: Goodale's Clinical Interpretation of Laboratory Tests, 7th edition, Philadelphia, F. A. Davis Company, 1973

Young, Clara G. and James D. Barger: Introduction to Medical Science, 2nd edition, St. Louis, C. V. Mosby Company, 1973

_____: Learning Medical Terminology Step by Step, 2nd edition, St. Louis, C. V. Mosby Company, 1971

# Appendix Two

# Combining Forms in Medical Terminology*

The following is a list of combining forms encountered frequently in the vocabulary of medicine. A dash or dashes are appended to indicate whether the form usually precedes (as *ante-*) or follows (as *-agra*) the other elements of the compound or usually appears between the other elements (as *-em-*). Following each combining form, the first item of information is the Greek or Latin word, or both a Greek and a Latin word, from which it is derived. Those words that are not printed in Greek characters are Latin. Information necessary to an understanding of the form appears next in parentheses. Then the meaning or meanings of the word are given, followed where appropriate by reference to a synonymous combining form. Finally, an example is given to illustrate the use of the combining form in a compound English derivative.

| | | | |
|---|---|---|---|
| a- | *a-* (*n* is added before words beginning with a vowel) negative prefix. Cf. in-³. a*metria* | -agogue | ἀγωγός leading, inducing. ga-lact*agogue* |
| ab- | *ab* away from. Cf. apo-. *ab*ducent | -agra | ἄγρα catching, seizure. pod*agra* |
| abdomin- | *abdomen, abdominis. abdomi*noscopy | alb- | *albus* white. Cf. leuk-. *albo*cinereous |
| ac- | See ad-. *ac*cretion | alg- | ἄλγος pain. neur*algia* |
| acet- | *acetum* vinegar. *acet*ometer | all- | ἄλλος other, different. *allergy* |
| acid- | *acidus* sour. *acid*uric | alve- | *alveus* trough, channel, cavity. *alve*olar |
| acou- | ἀκούω hear. *acou*esthesia. (Also spelled acu-) | amph- | See amphi-. *amph*eclexis |
| acr- | ἄκρον extremity, peak. *acro*megaly | amphi- | ἀμφί (*i* is dropped before words beginning with a vowel) both, doubly. *amphi*celous |
| act- | *ago, actus* do, drive, act. re*action* | amyl- | ἄμυλον starch. *amylo*synthesis |
| actin- | ἀκτίς, ἀκτῖνος ray, radius. Cf. radi-. *actino*genesis | an-¹ | See ana-. *an*agogic |
| | | an-² | See a-. *an*omalous |
| acu- | See acou-. osteo*acusis* | ana- | ἀνά (final *a* is dropped before words beginning with a vowel) up, positive. *ana*phoresis |
| ad- | *ad* (*d* changes to c, f, g, p, s, or *t* before words beginning with those consonants) to. *ad*renal | | |
| | | ancyl- | See ankyl-. *ancyl*ostomiasis |
| | | andr- | ἀνήρ, ἀνδρός man. gyn*andr*oid |
| aden- | ἀδήν gland. Cf. gland-. *ade*noma | angi- | ἀγγεῖον vessel. Cf. vas-. *angi*emphraxis |
| adip- | *adeps, adipis* fat. Cf. lip- and stear-. *adip*ocellular | ankyl- | ἀγκύλος crooked, looped. *anky*lodactylia. (Also spelled ancyl-) |
| aer- | ἀήρ air. *anaer*obiosis | ant- | See anti-. *ant*ophthalmic |
| aesthe- | See esthe-. *aesthe*sioneurosis | ante- | *ante* before. *ante*flexion |
| af- | See ad-. *af*ferent | anti- | ἀντί (*i* is dropped before words beginning with a vowel) |
| ag- | See ad-. *ag*glutinant | | |

*Compiled by Lloyd W. Daly, A. M., Ph.D., Litt. D., Allen Memorial Professor of Greek, University of Pennsylvania. *In* Dorland's Pocket Medical Dictionary, 21st Ed., Philadelphia, W. B. Saunders Co., 1968.

against, counter. Cf. contra-. *antipyogenic*

**antr-** ἄντρον cavern. *antrodynia*

**ap-[1]** See apo-. *apheter*

**ap-[2]** See ad-. *append*

**-aph-** ἅπτω, ἀφ- touch. *dysaphia*. (See also hapt-)

**apo-** ἀπό (*o* is dropped before words beginning with a vowel) away from, detached. Cf. ab-. *apophysis*

**arachn-** ἀράχνη spider. *arachnodactyly*

**arch-** ἀρχή beginning, origin. *archenteron*

**arter(i)-** ἀρτηρία elevator (?), artery. *arteriosclerosis, periarteritis*

**arthr-** ἄρθρον joint. Cf. articul-. *synarthrosis*

**articul-** *articulus* joint. Cf. arthr-. *disarticulation*

**as-** See ad-. *assimilation*

**at-** See ad-. *attrition*

**aur-** *auris* ear. Cf. ot-. *aurinasal*

**aux-** αὔξω increase. *enterauxe*

**ax-** ἄξων or *axis* axis. *axofugal*

**axon-** ἄξων axis. *axonometer*

**ba-** βαίνω, βα- go, walk, stand. *hypnobatia*

**bacill-** *bacillus* small staff, rod. Cf. bacter-. *actinobacillosis*

**bacter-** βακτήριον small staff, rod. Cf. bacill-. *bacteriophage*

**ball-** βάλλω, βολ- throw. *ballistics*. (See also bol-)

**bar-** βάρος weight. *pedobarometer*

**bi-[1]** βίος life. Cf. vit-. *aerobic*

**bi-[2]** bi- two (see also di-[1]). *bilobate*

**bil-** *bilis* bile. Cf. chol-. *biliary*

**blast-** βλαστός bud, child, a growing thing in its early stages. Cf. germ-. *blastoma, zygotoblast.*

**blep-** βλέπω look, see. *hemiablepsia*

**blephar-** βλέφαρον (from βλέπω; see blep-) eyelid. Cf. cili-. *blepharoncus*

**bol-** See ball-. *embolism*

**brachi-** βραχίων arm. *brachiocephalic*

**brachy-** βραχύς short. *brachycephalic*

**brady-** βραδύς slow. *bradycardia*

**brom-** βρῶμος stench. *podobromidrosis*

**bronch-** βρόγχος windpipe. *bronchoscopy*

**bry-** βρύω be full of life. *embryonic*

**bucc-** *bucca* cheek. *distobuccal*

**cac-** κακός bad, abnormal. Cf. mal-. *cacodontia, arthrocace.* (See also dys-)

**calc-[1]** *calx, calcis* stone (cf. lith-), limestone, lime. *calcipexy*

**calc-[2]** *calx, calcis* heel. *calcaneotibial*

**calor-** *calor* heat. Cf. therm-. *calorimeter*

**cancr-** *cancer, cancri* crab, cancer. Cf. carcin-. *cancrology.* (Also spelled chancr-)

**capit-** *caput, capitis* head. Cf. cephal-. *decapitator*

**caps-** *capsa* (from *capio;* see cept-) container. *encapsulation*

**carbo(n)-** *carbo, carbonis* coal, charcoal. *carbohydrate, carbonuria*

**carcin-** καρκίνος crab, cancer. Cf. cancr-. *carcinoma*

**cardi-** καρδία heart. *lipocardiac*

**cary-** See kary-. *caryokinesis*

**cat-** See cata-. *cathode*

**cata-** κατά (final *a* is dropped before words beginning with a vowel) down, negative. *catabatic*

**caud-** *cauda* tail. *caudad*

**cav-** *cavus* hollow. Cf. coel-. *concave*

**cec-** *caecus* blind. Cf. typhl-. *cecopexy*

**cel-[1]** See coel-. *amphicelous*

**cel-[2]** See -cele. *celectome*

**-cele** κήλη tumor, hernia. *gastrocele*

**cell-** *cella* room, cell. Cf. cyt-. *celliferous*

**cen-** κοινός common. *cenesthesia*

**cent-** *centum* hundred. Cf. hect-. Indicates fraction in metric system. [This exemplifies the custom in the metric system of identifying fractions of units by stems from the Latin, as centimeter, decimeter, millimeter, and multiples of units by the similar stems from the Greek, as hectometer, decameter, and kilometer.] *centimeter, centipede*

**cente-** κεντέω puncture. Cf. punct-. *enterocentesis*

**centr-** κέντρον or *centrum* point, center. *neurocentral*

**cephal-** κεφαλή head. Cf. capit-. *encephalitis*

**cept-** *capio, -cipientis, -ceptus* take, receive. *receptor*

**cer-** κηρός or *cera* wax. *ceroplasty, ceromel*

**cerat-** See kerat-. *aceratosis*

**cerebr-** *cerebrum. cerebrospinal*

**cervic-** *cervix, cervicis* neck. Cf. trachel-. *cervicitis*

**chancr-** See cancr-. *chancriform*

**cheil-** χεῖλος lip. Cf. labi-. *cheiloschisis*

**cheir-** χείρ hand. Cf. man-. *macrocheiria.* (Also spelled chir-)

**chir-** See cheir-. *chiromegaly*

**chlor-** χλωρός green. *achloropsia*

**chol-** χολή bile. Cf. bil-. *hepatocholangenia*

**chondr-** χόνδρος cartilage. *chondromalacia*

**chord-** χορδή string, cord. *perichordal*

**chori-** χόριον protective fetal membrane. *endochorion*

**chro-** χρώς color. *polychromatic*

**chron-** χρόνος time. *synchronous*

**chy-** χέω, χυ- pour. *ecchymosis*

**-cid(e)** *caedo, -cisus* cut, kill. *infanticide, germicidal*

**cili-** *cilium* eyelid. Cf. blephar-. *superciliary*

**cine-** See kine-. *autocinesis*

**-cipient** See cept-. *incipient*

**circum-** *circum* around. Cf. peri-. *circumferential*

**-cis-** *caedo, -cisus* cut, kill. *excision*

**clas-** κλάω, κλασ- break. *cranioclast*

**clin-** κλίνω bend, incline, make lie down. *clinometer*

**clus-** *claudo, -clusus* shut. *Malocclusion*

**co-** See con-. *cohesion*

**cocc-** κόκκος seed, pill. *gonococcus*

**coel-** κοῖλος hollow. Cf. cav-. *coelenteron.* (Also spelled cel-)

**col-[1]** See colon-. *colic*

**col-[2]** See con-. *collapse*

**colon-** κόλον lower intestine. *colonic*

**colp-** κόλπος hollow, vagina. Cf. sin-. *endocolpitis*

**com-** See con-. *commasculation*

**con-** con- (becomes co- before vowels or *h;* col- before *l;* com- before *b, m,* or *p;* cor- before *r*) with, together. Cf. syn-. *contraction*

**contra-** *contra* against, counter. Cf. anti-. *contraindication*

**copr-** κόπρος dung. Cf. sterco-. *coproma*

**cor-[1]** κόρη doll, little image, pupil. *isocoria*

cor-² — See con-. corrugator

corpor- — *corpus, corporis* body. Cf. somat-. intracorporal

cortic- — *cortex, corticis* bark, rind. corticosterone

cost- — *costa* rib. Cf. pleur-. intercostal

crani- — κρανίον or *cranium* skull. pericranium

creat- — κρέας, κρεατ- meat, flesh. creatorrhea

-crescent — *cresco, crescentis, cretus* grow. excrescent

cret-¹ — *cerno, cretus* distinguish, separate off. Cf. crin-. discrete

cret-² — See -crescent. accretion

crin- — κρίνω distinguish, separate off. Cf. cret-¹. endocrinology

crur- — *crus, cruris* shin, leg. brachiocrural

cry- — κρύος cold. cryesthesia

crypt- — κρύπτω hide, conceal. cryptorchism

cult- — *colo, cultus* tend, cultivate. culture

cune- — *cuneus* wedge Cf. sphen-. cuneiform

cut- — *cutis* skin. Cf. derm(at)-. subcutaneous

cyan- — κύανος blue. anthocyanin

cycl- — κύκλος circle, cycle. cyclophoria

cyst- — κύστις bladder. Cf. vesic-. nephrocystitis

cyt- — κύτος cell. Cf. cell-. plasmocytoma

dacry- — δάκρυ tear. dacryocyst

dactyl- — δάκτυλος finger, toe. Cf. digit-. hexadactylism

de- — *de* down from. decomposition

dec-¹ — δέκα ten. Indicates multiple in metric system. Cf. dec-². decagram

dec-² — *decem* ten. Indicates fraction in metric system. Cf. dec-¹. decipara, decimeter

dendr- — δένδρον tree. neurodendrite

dent- — *dens, dentis* tooth. Cf. odont-. interdental

derm(at)- — δέρμα, δέρματος skin. Cf. cut-. endoderm, dermatitis

desm- — δεσμός band, ligament. syndesmopexy

dextr- — *dexter, dextr-* right-hand. ambidextrous

di-¹ — di- two. dimorphic. (See also bi-²)

di-² — See dia-. diuresis.

di-³ — See dis-. divergent.

dia- — διά (*a* is dropped before words beginning with a vowel) through, apart. Cf. per-. diagnosis

didym- — δίδυμος twin. Cf. gemin-. epididymal

digit- — *digitus* finger, toe. Cf. dactyl-. digitigrade

diplo- — διπλόος double. diplomyelia

dis- — dis- (*s* may be dropped before a word beginning with a consonant) apart, away from. dislocation

disc- — δίσκος or *discus* disk. discoplacenta

dors- — *dorsum* back. ventrodorsal

drom- — δρόμος course. hemodromometer

-ducent — See duct-. adducent

duct- — *duco, ducentis, ductus* lead, conduct. oviduct

dur- — *durus* hard. Cf. scler-. induration

dynam(i)- — δύναμις power. dynamoneure, neurodynamic

dys- — δυσ- bad, improper. Cf. mal-. dystrophic. (See also cac-)

e- — *e* out from. Cf. ec- and ex-. emission

ec- — ἐκ out of. Cf. e- eccentric

-ech- — ἔχω have, hold, be. synechotomy

ect- — ἐκτός outside. Cf. extra-. ectoplasm

ede- — οἰδέω swell. edematous

ef- — See ex-. efflorescent

-elc- — ἕλκος sore, ulcer. enterelcosis. (See also helc-)

electr- — ἤλεκτρον amber. electrotherapy

em- — See en-. embolism, empathy, emphlysis

-em- — αἷμα blood. anemia. (See also hem(at)-)

en- — ἐν (*n* changes to *m* before *b, p,* or *ph*) in, on. Cf. in-². encelitis

end- — ἔνδον inside. Cf. intra-. endangium.

enter- — ἔντερον intestine. dysentery

ep- — See epi-. epaxial

epi- — ἐπί (*i* is dropped before words beginning with a vowel) upon, after, in addition. epiglottis

erg- — ἔργον work, deed. energy

erythr- — ἐρυθρός red. Cf. rub(r)-. erythrochromia

eso- — ἔσω inside. Cf. intra-. esophylactic

esthe- — αἰσθάνομαι, αἰσθη- perceive, feel. Cf. sens-. anesthesia

eu- — εὖ good, normal. eupepsia

ex- — ἐξ or *ex* out of. Cf. e-. excretion

exo- — ἔξω outside. Cf. extra-. exopathic

extra- — *extra* outside of, beyond. Cf. ect- and exo-. extracellular

faci- — *facies* face. Cf. prosop-. brachiofaciolingual

-facient — *facio, facientis, factus, -fectus* make. Cf. poie-. calefacient

-fact- — See facient-. artefact

fasci- — *fascia* band. fasciorrhaphy

febr- — *febris* fever. Cf. pyr-. febricide

-fect- — See -facient. defective

-ferent — *fero, ferentis, latus* bear, carry. Cf. phor-. efferent

ferr- — *ferrum* iron. ferroprotein

fibr- — *fibra* fibre. Cf. in-¹. chondrofibroma

fil- — *filum* thread. filiform

fiss- — *findo, fissus* split. Cf. schis-. fission

flagell- — *flagellum* whip. flagellation

flav- — *flavus* yellow. Cf. xanth-. riboflavin

-flect- — *flecto, flexus* bend, divert. deflection

-flex- — See -flect-. reflexometer

flu- — *fluo, fluxus* flow. Cf. rhe-. fluid

flux- — See flu-. affluxion

for- — *foris* door, opening. perforated

-form — *forma* shape. Cf. -oid. ossiform

fract- — *frango, fractus* break. refractive

front- — *frons, frontis* forehead, front. nasofrontal

-fug(e) — *fugio* flee, avoid. vermifuge, centrifugal

funct- — *fungor, functus* perform, serve, function. malfunction

fund- — *fundo, fusus* pour. infundibulum

fus- — See fund-. diffusible

galact- — γάλα, γάλακτος milk. Cf. lact-. dysgalactia

gam- — γάμος marriage, reproductive union. agamont

gangli- — γάγγλιον swelling, plexus. neurogangliitis

gastr- — γαστήρ, γαστρός stomach. cholangiogastrostomy

gelat- — *gelo, gelatus* freeze, congeal. gelatin

gemin- — *geminus* twin, double. Cf. didym-. quadrigeminal

gen- γίγνομαι, γεν-, γον- become, be produced, originate, or γεννάω produce, originate. cytogenic

germ- germen, germinis bud, a growing thing in its early stages. Cf. blast-. germinal, ovigerm

gest- gero, gerentis, gestus bear, carry. congestion

gland- glans, glandis acorn. Cf. aden-. intraglandular

-glia γλία glue. neuroglia

gloss- γλῶσσα tongue. Cf. lingu-. trichoglossia

glott- γλῶττα tongue, language. glottic

gluc- See glyc(y)-. glucophenetidin

glutin- gluten, glutinis glue. agglutination

glyc(y)- γλυκύς sweet. glycemia, glycyrrhizin. (Also spelled gluc-)

gnath- γνάθος jaw. orthognathous

gno- γιγνώσκω, γνω- know, discern. diagnosis

gon- See gen-. amphigony

grad- gradior walk, take steps. retrograde

-gram γράφω, γραφ- + -μα scratch, write, record. cardiogram

gran- granum grain, particle. lipogranuloma

graph- γράφω scratch, write, record. histography

grav- gravis heavy. multigravida

gyn(ec)- γυνή, γυναικός woman, wife. androgyny, gynecologic

gyr- γῦρος ring, circle. gyrospasm

haem(at)- See hem(at)-. haemorrhagia, haematoxylon

hapt- ἅπτω touch. haptometer

hect- ἑκτ- hundred. Cf. cent-. Indicates multiple in metric system. hectometer

helc- ἕλκος sore, ulcer. helcosis

hem(at)- αἷμα, αἵματος blood. Cf. sanguin-. hemangioma, hematocyturia. (See also -em-)

hemi- ἡμι- half. Cf. semi-. hemiageusia

hen- εἷς, ἑνός one. Cf. un-. henogenesis

hepat- ἧπαρ, ἥπατος liver. gastrohepatic

hept(a)- ἑπτά seven. Cf. sept-². heptatomic, heptavalent

hered- heres, heredis heir. heredoimmunity

hex-¹ ἕξ six. Cf. sex-. hexyl-. An a is added in some combinations.

hex-² ἔχω, ἑχ- (added to σ becomes ἑξ-) have, hold, be. cachexy

hexa- See hex-¹. hexachromic

hidr- ἱδρώς sweat. hyperhidrosis

hist- ἱστός web, tissue. histodialysis

hod- ὁδός road, path. hodoneuromere. (See also od- and -ode¹)

hom- ὁμός common, same. homomorphic

horm- ὁρμή impetus, impulse. hormone

hydat- ὕδωρ, ὕδατος water. hydatism

hydr- ὕδωρ, ὑδρ- water. Cf. lymph-. achlorhydria

hyp- See hypo-. hypaxial

hyper- ὑπέρ above, beyond, extreme. Cf. super-. hypertrophy

hypn- ὕπνος sleep. hypnotic

hypo- ὑπό (o is dropped before words beginning with a vowel) under, below. Cf. sub-. hypometabolism

hyster- ὑστέρα womb. colpohysteropexy

iatr- ἰατρός physician. pediatrics

idi- ἴδιος peculiar, separate, distinct. idiosyncrasy

il- See in-². ³. illinition (in, on), illegible (negative prefix)

ile- See ili- [ile- is commonly used to refer to the portion of the intestines known as the ileum]. ileostomy

ili- ilium (ileum) lower abdomen, intestines [ili- is commonly used to refer to the flaring part of the hip bone known as the ilium]. iliosacral

im- See in-². ³. immersion (in, on), imperforation (negative prefix)

in-¹ ἵς, ἰνός fiber. Cf. fibr-. inosteatoma

in-² in (n changes to l, m, or r before words beginning with those consonants) in, on. Cf. en-. insertion

in-³ in- (n changes to l, m, or r before words beginning with those consonants) negative prefix. Cf. a-. invalid

infra- infra beneath. infraorbital

insul- insula island. insulin

inter- inter among, between. intercarpal

intra- intra inside. Cf. end- and eso-. intravenous

ir- See in-². ³. irradiation (in, on), irreducible (negative prefix)

irid- ἴρις, ἴριδος rainbow, colored circle. keratoiridocyclitis

is- ἴσος equal. isotope

ischi- ἰσχίον hip, haunch. ischiopubic

jact- iacio, iactus throw. jactitation

ject- iacio, -iectus throw. injection

jejun- ieiunus hungry, not partaking of food. gastrojejunostomy

jug- iugum yoke. conjugation

junct- iungo, iunctus yoke, join. conjunctiva

kary- κάρυον nut, kernel, nucleus. Cf. nucle-. megakaryocyte. (Also spelled cary-)

kerat- κέρας, κέρατος horn. keratolysis. (Also spelled cerat-)

kil- χίλιοι one thousand. Cf. mill-. Indicates multiple in metric system. kilogram

kine- κινέω move. kinematograph. (Also spelled cine-)

labi- labium lip. Cf. cheil-. gingivolabial

lact- lac, lactis milk. Cf. galact-. glucolactone

lal- λαλέω talk, babble. glossolalia

lapar- λαπάρα flank. laparotomy

laryng- λάρυγξ, λάρυγγος windpipe. laryngendoscope

lat- fero, latus bear, carry. See -ferent. translation

later- latus, lateris side. ventrolateral

lent- lens, lentis lentil. Cf. phac-. lenticonus

lep- λαμβάνω, ληπ- take, seize. cataleptic

leuc- See leuk-. leucinuria

leuk- λευκός white. Cf. alb-. leukorrhea. (Also spelled leuc-)

lien- lien spleen. Cf. splen-. lienocele

lig- ligo tie, bind. ligate

lingu- lingua tongue. Cf. gloss-. sublingual

lip- λίπος fat. Cf. adip-. glycolipin

lith- λίθος stone. Cf. calc-¹. nephrolithotomy

loc- locus place. Cf. top-. locomotion

log- λέγω, λογ- speak, give an account. logorrhea, embryology

lumb- lumbus loin. dorsolumbar

lute- luteus yellow. Cf. xanth-. luteoma

ly- λύω loose, dissolve. Cf. solut-. keratolysis

lymph- lympha water. Cf. hydr-. lymphadenosis

macr- μακρός long, large. macromyeloblast

mal- malus bad, abnormal. Cf. cac- and dys-. malfunction

malac- μαλακός soft. osteomalacia

mamm-    *mamma* breast. Cf. mast-. sub*mamm*ary

man-    *manus* hand. Cf. cheir-. *man*iphalanx

mani-    μανία mental aberration. *ma*nigraphy, klepto*mania*

mast-    μαστός breast. Cf. mamm-. hyper*mast*ia

medi-    *medius* middle. Cf. mes-. *medi*frontal

mega-    μέγας great, large. Also indicates multiple (1,000,000) in metric system. *mega*colon, *mega*dyne. (See also megal-)

megal-    μέγας, μεγάλου great, large. acro*megaly*

mel-    μέλος limb, member. sym*melia*

melan-    μέλας, μέλανος black. hippo*melanin*

men-    μήν month. dys*men*orrhea

mening-    μῆνιγξ, μήνιγγος membrane. encephalo*mening*itis

ment-    *mens, mentis* mind. Cf. phren-, psych- and thym-. de*ment*ia

mer-    μέρος part. poly*mer*ic

mes-    μέσος middle. Cf. medi-. *mes*oderm

met-    See meta-. *met*allergy

meta-    μετά (*a* is dropped before words beginning with a vowel) after, beyond, accompanying. *meta*carpal

metr-¹    μέτρον measure. stere*ometry*

metr-²    μήτρα womb. endo*metr*itis

micr-    μικρός small. photo*micr*ograph

mill-    *mille* one thousand. Cf. kil-. Indicates fraction in metric system. *milli*gram, *milli*pede

miss-    See -mittent. intro*miss*ion

-mittent    *mitto, mittentis, missus* send. inter*mittent*

mne-    μιμνήσκω, μνη- remember. pseudo*mne*sia

mon-    μόνος only, sole. *mon*oplegia

morph-    μορφή form, shape. poly*morph*onuclear

mot-    *moveo, motus* move. vaso*mot*or

my-    μῦς, μυός muscle. ino*leiomy*oma

-myces    μύκης, μύκητος fungus. myelo*myces*

myc(et)-    See -myces. asco*myc*etes, strepto*myc*in

myel-    μυελός marrow. polio*myel*itis

myx-    μύξα mucus. *myx*edema

narc-    νάρκη numbness. topo*narc*osis

nas-    *nasus* nose. Cf. rhin-. palato*nas*al

ne-    νέος new, young. *ne*ocyte

necr-    νεκρός corpse. *necr*ocytosis

nephr-    νεφρός kidney. Cf. ren-. para*nephr*ic

neur-    νεῦρον nerve. esthesio*neur*e

nod-    *nodus* knot. *nod*osity

nom-    νόμος (from νέμω deal out, distribute) law, custom. tax*onomy*

non-    *nona* nine. *non*acosane

nos-    νόσος disease. *nos*ology

nucle-    *nucleus* (from *nux, nucis* nut) kernel. Cf. kary-. *nucle*ide

nutri-    *nutrio* nourish. mal*nutri*tion

ob-    *ob* (*b* changes to *c* before words beginning with that consonant) against, toward, etc. *ob*tuse

oc-    See ob-. *oc*clude.

ocul-    *oculus* eye. Cf. ophthalm-. *ocul*omotor

-od-    See -ode¹. peri*od*ic

-ode¹    ὁδός road, path. cath*ode*. (See also hod-)

-ode²    See -oid. nemat*ode*

odont-    ὀδούς, ὀδόντος tooth. Cf. dent-. orth*odont*ia

-odyn-    ὀδύνη pain, distress. gastr*odyn*ia

-oid    εἶδος form. Cf. -form. hy*oid*

-ol    See ole-. cholester*ol*

ole-    *oleum* oil. *ole*oresin

olig-    ὀλίγος few, small. *olig*ospermia

omphal-    ὀμφαλός navel. peri*omphal*ic

onc-    ὄγκος bulk, mass. hemat*onc*ometry

onych-    ὄνυξ, ὄνυχος claw, nail. an*onych*ia

oo-    ᾠόν egg. Cf. ov-. peri*oo*thecitis

op-    ὁράω, ὀπ- see. erythr*op*sia

ophthalm-    ὀφθαλμός eye. Cf. ocul-. ex*ophthalm*ic

or-    *os, oris* mouth. Cf. stom(at)-. intra*or*al

orb-    *orbis* circle. sub*orb*ital

orchi-    ὄρχις testicle. Cf. test-. *orchi*opathy

organ-    ὄργανον implement, instrument. *organ*oleptic

orth-    ὀρθός straight, right, normal. *orth*opedics

oss-    *os, ossis* bone. Cf. ost(e)-. *ossi*phone

ost(e)-    ὀστέον bone. Cf. oss-. en*ost*osis, *oste*anaphysis

ot-    οὖς, ὠτός ear. Cf. aur-. par*ot*id

ov-    *ovum* egg. Cf. oo-. syn*ov*ia

oxy-    ὀξύς sharp. *oxy*cephalic

pachy(n)-    παχύνω thicken. *pachy*derma, myo*pachyn*sis

pag-    πήγνυμι, παγ- fix, make fast. thoraco*pag*us

par-¹    *pario* bear, give birth to. primi*par*ous

par-²    See para-. *par*epigastric

para-    παρά (final *a* is dropped before words beginning with a vowel) beside, beyond. *para*mastoid

part-    *pario, partus* bear, give birth to. *part*urition

path-    πάθος that which one undergoes, sickness. psycho*path*ic

pec-    πήγνυμι, πηγ- (πηκ- before τ) fix, make fast. sym*pec*tothiene. (See also pex-)

ped-    παῖς, παιδός child. orth*oped*ic

pell-    *pellis* skin, hide. *pell*agra

-pellent    *pello, pellentis, pulsus* drive. re*pellent*

pen-    πένομαι need, lack. erythrocyto*pen*ia

pend-    *pendeo* hang down. ap*pend*ix

pent(a)-    πέντε five. Cf. quinque-. *pent*ose, *penta*ploid

peps-    πέπτω, πεψ- (before σ) digest brady*peps*ia

pept-    πέπτω digest. dys*pept*ic

per-    *per* through. Cf. dia-. *per*nasal

peri-    περί around. Cf. circum-. *peri*phery

pet-    *peto* seek, tend toward. centrip*et*al

pex-    πήγνυμι, πηγ- (added to σ becomes πηξ-) fix, make fast. hepato*pex*y

pha-    φημί, φα- say, speak. dys*pha*sia

phac-    φακός lentil, lens. Cf. lent-. *phac*osclerosis. (Also spelled phak-)

phag-    φαγεῖν eat. lipo*phag*ic

phak-    See phac-. *phak*itis

phan-    See phen-. dia*phan*oscopy

pharmac-    φάρμακον drug. *pharmac*ognosy

pharyng-    φάρυγξ, φαρυγγ- throat. glosso*pharyng*eal

phen-    φαίνω, φαν- show, be seen. phos*phen*e

pher-    φέρω, φορ- bear, support. peri*pher*y

phil-    φιλέω like, have affinity for. eosino*phil*ia

phleb-    φλέψ, φλεβός vein. peri*phleb*itis

phleg-    φλέγω, φλογ- burn, inflame. adeno*phleg*mon

phlog-    See phleg-. anti*phlog*istic

phob-    φόβος fear, dread. claustro*phob*ia

phon-    φωνή sound. echo*phon*y

phor- See pher-. Cf. -ferent. exo-*phoria*

phos- See phot-. *phosphorus*

phot- φῶς, φωτός light. *phot*erythrous

phrag- φράσσω, φραγ- fence, wall off, stop up. Cf. sept-[1]. dia*phragm*

phrax- φράσσω, φραγ- (added to σ becomes φραξ-) fence, wall off, stop up. em*phraxis*

phren- φρήν mind, midriff. Cf. ment-. meta*phrenia*, meta*phrenon*

phthi- φθίνω decay, waste away. ophthalmo*phthisis*

phy- φύω beget, bring forth, produce, be by nature. noso*phyte*

phyl- φῦλον tribe, kind. *phyl*ogeny

-phyll φύλλον leaf. xantho*phyll*

phylac- φύλαξ guard. pro*phylactic*

phys(a)- φυσάω blow, inflate. *phys*ocele, *phys*alis

physe- φυσάω, φυση- blow, inflate. em*physema*

pil- pilus hair. epi*lation*

pituit- *pituita* phlegm, rheum. *pitui-tous*

placent- *placenta* (from πλακοῦς) cake. extra*placental*

plas- πλάσσω mold, shape. cine*plasty*

platy- πλατύς broad, flat. *platy*rrhine

pleg- πλήσσω, πληγ- strike. di*plegia*

plet- *pleo, -pletus* fill. de*pletion*

pleur- πλευρά rib, side. Cf. cost-. peri*pleural*

plex- πλήσσω, πληγ- (added to σ becomes πληξ-) strike. apo*plexy*

plic- *plico* fold. com*plication*

pne- πνοιά breathing. traumato*pnea*

pneum(at)- πνεῦμα, πνεύματος breath, air. *pneumo*dynamics, *pneumato*thorax

pneumo(n)- πνεύμων lung. Cf. pulmo(n)-. *pneumo*centesis, *pneumonot*omy

pod- πούς, ποδός foot. *pod*iatry

poie- ποιέω make, produce. Cf. -facient. sarco*poietic*

pol- πόλος axis of a sphere. peri*polar*

poly- πολύς much, many. *poly*spermia

pont- *pons, pontis* bridge. *ponto*cerebellar

por-[1] πόρος passage. myelo*pore*

por-[2] πῶρος callus. *poro*cele

posit- *pono, positus* put, place. re*positor*

post- *post* after, behind in time or place. *post*natal, *post*oral

pre- *prae* before in time or place. *pre*natal, *pre*vesical

press- *premo, pressus* press. *pressore*ceptive

pro- πρό or *pro* before in time or place. *pro*gamous, *pro*cheilon, *pro*lapse

proct- πρωκτός anus. entero*proctia*

prosop- πρόσωπον face. Cf. faci-. di*prosopus*

pseud- ψευδής false. *pseudo*paraplegia

psych- ψυχή soul, mind. Cf. ment-. *psych*osomatic

pto- πίπτω, πτω- fall. nephro*ptosis*

pub- *pubes* & *puber, puberis* adult. ischio*pubic*. (See also puber-)

puber- *puber* adult. *puber*ty

pulmo(n)- *pulmo, pulmonis* lung. Cf. pneumo(n)-. *pulmo*lith, cardio*pulmonary*

puls- *pello, pellentis, pulsus* drive. *pro*pulsion

punct- *pungo, punctus* prick, pierce. Cf. cente-. *puncti*form

pur- *pus, puris* pus. Cf. py-. sup*puration*

py- πύον pus. Cf. pur-. nephro*pyosis*

pyel- πύελος trough, basin, pelvis. nephro*pyelitis*

pyl- πύλη door, orifice. *pyle*phlebitis

pyr- πῦρ fire. Cf. febr-. galacto*pyra*

quadr- *quadr-* four. Cf. tetra-. *quadri*geminal

quinque- *quinque* five. Cf. pent(a)-. *quinque*cuspid

rachi- ῥαχίς spine. Cf. spin-. enceph*alorachi*dian

radi- *radius* ray. Cf. actin-. ir*radia*tion

re- *re-* back, again. *re*traction

ren- *renes* kidneys. Cf. nephr-. ad*renal*

ret- *rete* net. *reto*thelium

retro- *retro* backwards. *retro*deviation

rhag- ῥήγνυμι, ῥαγ- break, burst. hemor*rhagic*

rhaph- ῥαφή suture. gastror*rhaphy*

rhe- ῥέω flow. Cf. flu-. diar*rheal*

rhex- ῥήγνυμι, ῥηγ- (added to σ becomes ῥηξ-) break, burst. metror*rhexis*

rhin- ῥίς, ῥινός nose. Cf. nas-. basi*rhinal*

rot- *rota* wheel. *rot*ator

rub(r)- *ruber, rubri* red. Cf. erythr-. bili*rubin*, *rubro*spinal

salping- σάλπιγξ, σάλπιγγος tube, trumpet. *salping*itis

sanguin- *sanguis, sanguinis* blood. Cf. hem(at)-. *sanguin*eous

sarc- σάρξ, σαρκός flesh. *sarc*oma

schis- σχίζω, σχιδ- (before τ or added to σ becomes σχισ-) split. Cf. fiss-. *schist*orachis, rachi*schisis*

scler- σκληρός hard. Cf. dur-. *sclero*sis

scop- σκοπέω look at, observe. endo*scope*

sect- *seco, sectus* cut. Cf. tom-. *sectile*

semi- *semi-* half. Cf. hemi-. *semi*flexion

sens- *sentio, sensus* perceive, feel. Cf. esthe-. *sens*ory

sep- σήπω rot, decay. *sep*sis

sept-[1] *saepio, saeptus* fence, wall off, stop up. Cf. phrag-. naso*septal*

sept-[2] *septem* seven. Cf. hept(a)-. *sept*an

ser- *serum* whey, watery substance. *sero*synovitis

sex- *sex* six. Cf. hex-[1]. *sex*digitate

sial- σίαλον saliva. poly*sialia*

sin- *sinus* hollow, fold. Cf. colp-. *sino*bronchitis

sit- σῖτος food. para*sitic*

solut- *solvo, solventis, solutus* loose, dissolve, set free. Cf. ly-. dis*solution*

-solvent See solut-. dis*solvent*

somat- σῶμα, σώματος body. Cf. corpor-. psycho*somatic*

-some See somat-. dictyo*some*

spas- σπάω, σπασ- draw, pull. *spas*m, *spas*tic

spectr- *spectrum* appearance, what is seen. micro*spectr*oscope

sperm(at)- σπέρμα, σπέρματος seed. *sperm*acrasia, *spermato*zoon

spers- *spargo, -spersus* scatter. di*spersion*

sphen- σφήν wedge. Cf. cune-. *sphen*oid

spher- σφαῖρα ball. hemi*sphere*

sphygm- σφυγμός pulsation. *sphygmo*manometer

spin- *spina* spine. Cf. rachi-. cerebro*spinal*

spirat- *spiro, spiratus* breathe. in*spirat*ory

splanchn- σπλάγχνα entrails, viscera. neuro*splanchn*ic

splen- σπλήν spleen. Cf. lien-. *splen*omegaly

spor- σπόρος seed. *sporo*phyte, zygo*spore*

squam-   *squama* scale. de*squam*ation
sta-   ἵστημι, στα- make stand, stop. genesi*stasis*
stal-   στέλλω, σταλ- send. peri*stal*sis. (See also stol-)
staphyl-   σταφυλή bunch of grapes, uvula. *staphyl*ococcus, *staphyl*ectomy
stear-   στέαρ, στέατος fat. Cf. adip-. *stear*odermia
steat-   See stear-. *steat*opygous
sten-   στενός narrow, compressed. *sten*ocardia
ster-   στερεός·solid. chole*ster*ol
sterc-   *stercus* dung. Cf. copr-. *sterco*porphyrin
sthen-   σθένος strength. a*sthen*ia
stol-   στέλλω, στολ- send. dia*stole*
stom(at)-   στόμα, στόματος mouth, orifice. Cf. or-. ana*stom*osis, *stom*atogastric
strep(h)-   στρέφω, στρεπ- (before τ) twist. Cf. tors-. *streph*osymbolia, *strep*tomycin. (See also stroph-)
strict-   *stringo, stringentis, strictus* draw tight, compress, cause pain. con*strict*ion
-stringent   See strict-. a*stringent*
stroph-   στρέφω, στροφ- twist. ana*stroph*ic. (See also strep(h)-)
struct-   *struo, structus* pile up (against). ob*struct*ion
sub-   *sub* (*b* changes to *f* or *p* before words beginning with those consonants) under, below. Cf. hypo-. *sub*lumbar
suf-   See sub-. *suf*fusion
sup-   See sub-. *sup*pository
super-   *super* above, beyond, extreme. Cf. hyper-. *super*motility
sy-   See syn-. *sy*stole
syl-   See syn-. *syl*lepsiology
sym-   See syn-. *sym*biosis, *sym*metry, *sym*pathetic, *sym*physis
syn-   σύν (*n* disappears before *s*, changes to *l* before *l*, and changes to *m* before *b, m, p,* and *ph*) with, together. Cf. con-. myo*syn*izesis
ta-   See ton-. ec*ta*sis
tac-   τάσσω, ταγ- (τακ- before τ) order, arrange. a*tac*tic
tact-   *tango, tactus* touch. con*tact*
tax-   τάσσω, ταγ- (added to σ becomes ταξ-) order, arrange. a*tax*ia
tect-   See teg-. pro*tect*ive
teg-   *tego, tectus* cover. in*teg*ument
tel-   τέλος end. *tel*osynapsis
tele-   τῆλε at a distance. *tele*ceptor
tempor-   *tempus, temporis* time, timely or fatal spot, temple. *tempo*romalar
ten(ont)-   τένων, τένοντος (from τείνω stretch) tight stretched band. *teno*dynia, *teno*nitis, *tenon*tagra
tens-   *tendo, tensus* stretch. Cf. ton-. ex*tens*or
test-   *testis* testicle. Cf. orchi-. *test*itis

tetra-   τετρα- four. Cf. quadr-. *tetrag*enous
the-   τίθημι, θη- put, place. syn*the*sis
thec-   θήκη repository, case. *theco*stegnosis
thel-   θηλή teat, nipple. *thel*erethism
therap-   θεραπεία treatment. hydro*therapy*
therm-   θέρμη heat. Cf. calor-. dia*therm*y
thi-   θεῖον sulfur. *thi*ogenic
thorac-   θώραξ, θώρακος chest. *thoraco*plasty
thromb-   θρόμβος lump, clot. *thrombo*penia
thym-   θυμός spirit. Cf. ment-. dys*thym*ia
thyr-   θυρεός shield (shaped like a door θύρα). *thyr*oid
tme-   τέμνω, τμη- cut. axono*tme*sis
toc-   τόκος childbirth. dys*toc*ia
tom-   τέμνω, τομ- cut. Cf. sect-. ap*pen*d*ectom*y
ton-   τείνω, τον- stretch, put under tension. Cf. tens-. peri*ton*eum
top-   τόπος place. Cf. loc-. *top*esthesia
tors-   *torqueo, torsus* twist. Cf. strep-. ex*tors*ion
tox-   τοξικόν (from τόξον bow) arrow poison, poison. *tox*emia
trache-   τραχεῖα windpipe. *trache*otomy
trachel-   τράχηλος neck. Cf. cervic-. *trachel*opexy
tract-   *traho, tractus* draw, drag. pro*tract*ion
traumat-   τραῦμα, τραύματος wound. *traumat*ic
tri-   τρεῖς, τρία or *tri-* three. *tri*gonid
trich-   θρίξ, τριχός hair. *trich*oid
trip-   τρίβω rub. en*trip*sis
trop-   τρέπω, τροπ- turn, react. sitot*rop*ism
troph-   τρέφω, τροφ- nurture. a*troph*y
tuber-   *tuber* swelling, node. *tuber*cle
typ-   τύπος (from τύπτω strike) type. a*typ*ical
typh-   τῦφος fog, stupor. adeno*typh*us
typhl-   τυφλός blind. Cf. cec-. *typhl*ectasis
un-   *unus* one. Cf. hen-. *un*ioval
ur-   οὖρον urine. poly*ur*ia
vacc-   *vacca* cow. *vacc*ine
vagin-   *vagina* sheath. in*vagin*ated
vas-   *vas* vessel. Cf. angi-. *vas*cular
vers-   See vert-. in*vers*ion
vert-   *verto, versus* turn. di*vert*iculum
vesic-   *vesica* bladder. Cf. cyst-. *vesico*vaginal
vit-   *vita* life. Cf. bi-¹. de*vit*alize
vuls-   *vello, vulsus* pull, twitch. con*vuls*ion
xanth-   ξανθός yellow, blond. Cf. flav- and lute-. *xanth*ophyll
-yl-   ὕλη substance. cacod*yl*
zo-   ζωή life, ζῷον animal. micro*zo*aria
zyg-   ζυγόν yoke, union. *zyg*odactyly
zym-   ζύμη ferment. en*zym*e

# Appendix Three

# Common Abbreviations

| | | | |
|---|---|---|---|
| Abdom. | Abdomen | E.D.C. | Expected date of confinement |
| Acc. | Accommodation | | |
| A.C.S. | American College of Surgeons | EEG | Electroencephalogram |
| | | E.E.N.T. | Eye, ear, nose, and throat |
| aet. | At the age of | | |
| AgNO₃ | Silver nitrate | EKG | Electrocardiogram |
| A.H.A. | American Hospital Association | E.N.T. | Ear, nose, and throat |
| | | Etiol. | Etiology |
| Alb. | Albumin | F. | Fahrenheit |
| A.M.A. | American Medical Association | F.A.C.P. | Fellow, American College of Physicians |
| Anes. | Anesthesia | F.A.C.S. | Fellow, American College of Surgeons |
| A.P. | Anteroposterior | | |
| A.P. & L. | Anterior, posterior, and lateral | F.H. | Family history |
| | | F.H.S. | Fetal heart sounds |
| Ast. | Astigmatism | Fluor. | Fluoroscopy |
| A.Z. | Aschheim-Zondek test | Fried. test | Friedman test |
| B.M. | Bowel movement | G.A. | Gastric analysis |
| B.M.R. | Basal metabolic rate | G.B. | Gallbladder |
| B.P. | Blood pressure | G.C. | Gonorrhea |
| C. | Centigrade | G.E. | Gastroenterology |
| Ca. | Carcinoma | G.G.E. | Generalized glandular enlargement |
| Cardio. | Cardiology | | |
| C.B.C. | Complete blood count | G.I. | Gastrointestinal |
| cc. | Cubic centimeter | G.P. | General practitioner |
| C.C. | Chief complaint | G.U. | Genitourinary |
| C.D.C. | Calculated date of confinement | Gyn. | Gynecology |
| | | Hb. | Hemoglobin |
| chr. | Chronic | HCl | Hydrochloric acid |
| C.I. | Color index | Hgb. | Hemoglobin |
| cm. | Centimeter | H₂O | Water |
| C.N.S. | Central nervous system | I & D | Incision and drainage |
| CO₂ | Carbon dioxide | I.M. | Intramuscular |
| C.V. | Cardiovascular | inf. | Infected |
| C.V.A. | Cerebrovascular accident | inj. | Injection |
| | | Int. Med. | Internal medicine |
| D. & C. | Dilatation and curettage | I.Q. | Intelligence quotient |
| Derm. | Dermatology | I.V. | Intravenous |
| Diff. | Differential blood count | K.U.B. | Kidney, ureter and bladder |
| D.M.F. | Decayed, missing, and filled | | |
| | | L & A (l/a) | Light and accommodation |
| D.O.A. | Dead on arrival | | |
| ECG | Electrocardiogram | L & W | Living and well |

**660**

| | | | |
|---|---|---|---|
| Lat. | Lateral | P. Surg. | Plastic surgery |
| L.L.Q. | Left lower quadrant | Psy. | Psychiatry |
| L.M.P. | Last menstrual period | Psych. | Psychology |
| L.U.Q. | Left upper quadrant | pt. | Patient |
| M.A. | Mental age | P.T. | Physical therapy |
| M.M. | Mucous membrane | P.X. | Physical examination |
| NaCl | Sodium chloride (common salt) | R.B.C. | Red blood cell (count) |
| | | R.L.Q. | Right lower quadrant |
| N.A.D. | No appreciable disease | R.O. | Rule out |
| Neg. | Negative | R.U.Q. | Right upper quadrant |
| Neuro. | Neurology | S.M.W.D. | Single, married, |
| N.P.N. | Nonprotein nitrogen | Sep | widowed, divorced, |
| N.Y.D. | Not yet diagnosed | | separated |
| O.B. (Ob.) | Obstetrics | Sp. gr. | Specific gravity |
| O.D. | Right eye | S.R. | Sedimentation rate |
| O.L. | Left eye | Stat | Immediately |
| ol. | Oil | Strab. | Strabismus |
| O.P.D. | Outpatient department | Subcu. | Subcutaneous |
| Ophth. | Ophthalmology | Surg. | Surgery, surgical, |
| O.R. | Operating room | | surgeon |
| Orth. | Orthopedics | T. | Temperature |
| O.S. | Left eye | T. & A. | Tonsils and adenoids |
| O.T. | Old tuberculin | T.B. (Tbc.) | Tuberculosis |
| O.T.C. | Over the counter | Temp. | Temperature |
| Oto. | Otology | T.P.R. | Temperature, pulse, |
| Ov. | Ovum, egg | | and respiration |
| P. | Pulse | TUR | Transurethral resection |
| Para I | Woman having borne one child | u. | Unit |
| | | U.C.H.D. | Usual childhood |
| Para II | Woman having borne two children | | diseases |
| | | Ur.(or urn.) | Urine |
| Path. | Pathology | U.R.I. | Upper respiratory |
| PBI | Protein-bound iodine | | infection |
| P.E. | Physical examination | Urol. | Urology |
| Ped. | Pediatrics | U.S.P. | United States |
| pH | Hydrogen ion concentration: 7 neutral, above 7 alkaline, and below 7 acid | | Pharmacopeia |
| | | U.S.P.H.S. | United States Public Health Service |
| | | V.D. | Venereal disease |
| P.H. | Past history | V.D.G. | Venereal disease— |
| P.I. | Present illness | | gonorrhea |
| P.I.D. | Pelvic inflammatory disease | V.D.S. | Venereal disease— syphilis |
| P.N.D. | Post-nasal drip | W.B.C. | White blood cell |
| P. Op. | Postoperative | | (count) |
| Pos. | Positive | W.F. | White female |
| Prog. | Prognosis | W.M. | White male |
| P.S.P. | Phenolsulfonphthalein (kidney) test | W.R. | Wassermann reaction |
| | | Wt. | Weight |

**Symbols**

| | | | |
|---|---|---|---|
| * | birth | ♀ | female |
| — | negative | c̄ | with |
| + | positive | s̄ | without |
| ± | negative or positive (indefinite) | μ | micron |
| ♂ | male | † | death |

*Appendix Four*

# Color Atlas of Anatomy

# THE HUMAN BODY
## HIGHLIGHTS of STRUCTURE and FUNCTION

# SKELETAL SYSTEM

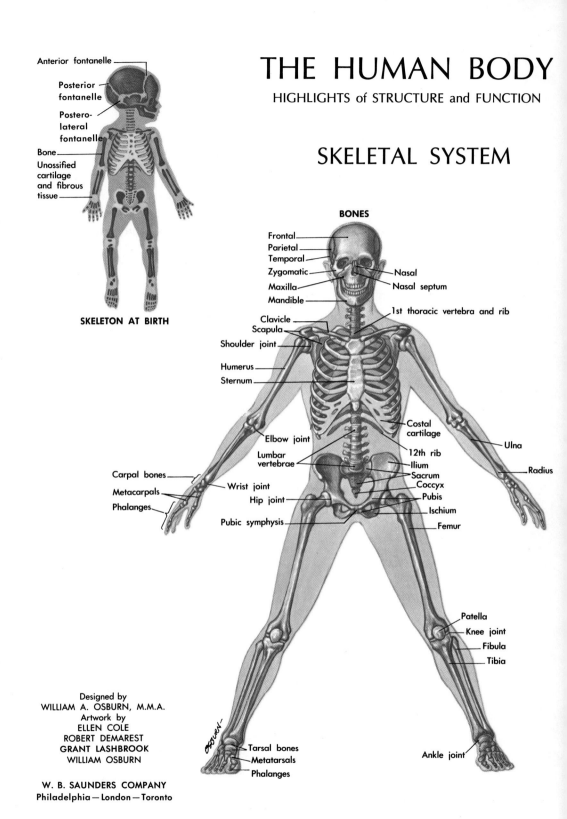

**SKELETON AT BIRTH**

Anterior fontanelle

Posterior fontanelle

Postero-lateral fontanelle

Bone

Unossified cartilage and fibrous tissue

**BONES**

Frontal

Parietal

Temporal

Zygomatic

Maxilla

Mandible

Nasal

Nasal septum

1st thoracic vertebra and rib

Clavicle

Scapula

Shoulder joint

Humerus

Sternum

Costal cartilage

Elbow joint

12th rib

Lumbar vertebrae

Ilium

Sacrum

Coccyx

Ulna

Radius

Carpal bones

Metacarpals

Phalanges

Wrist joint

Hip joint

Pubis

Ischium

Femur

Pubic symphysis

Patella

Knee joint

Fibula

Tibia

Tarsal bones

Metatarsals

Phalanges

Ankle joint

Designed by
WILLIAM A. OSBURN, M.M.A.
Artwork by
ELLEN COLE
ROBERT DEMAREST
GRANT LASHBROOK
WILLIAM OSBURN

W. B. SAUNDERS COMPANY
Philadelphia — London — Toronto

**Plate 1**

# SKELETAL SYSTEM—*Continued*

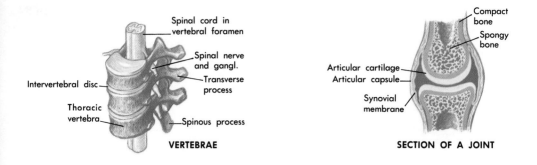

Spinal cord in vertebral foramen
Spinal nerve and gangl.
Transverse process
Intervertebral disc
Thoracic vertebra
Spinous process

**VERTEBRAE**

Compact bone
Spongy bone
Articular cartilage
Articular capsule
Synovial membrane

**SECTION OF A JOINT**

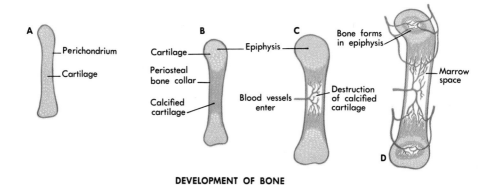

A
Perichondrium
Cartilage

B
Cartilage
Periosteal bone collar
Calcified cartilage
Epiphysis

C
Blood vessels enter
Destruction of calcified cartilage

Bone forms in epiphysis
Marrow space
D

**DEVELOPMENT OF BONE**

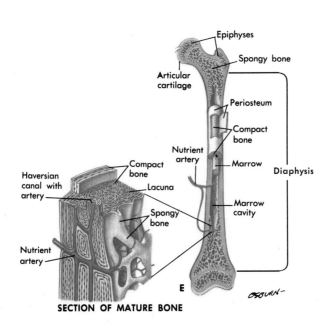

Epiphyses
Spongy bone
Articular cartilage
Periosteum
Compact bone
Nutrient artery
Marrow
Diaphysis
Marrow cavity

Haversian canal with artery
Compact bone
Lacuna
Spongy bone
Compact bone
Nutrient artery
E

**SECTION OF MATURE BONE**

**Plate 2**

# SKELETAL MUSCLES

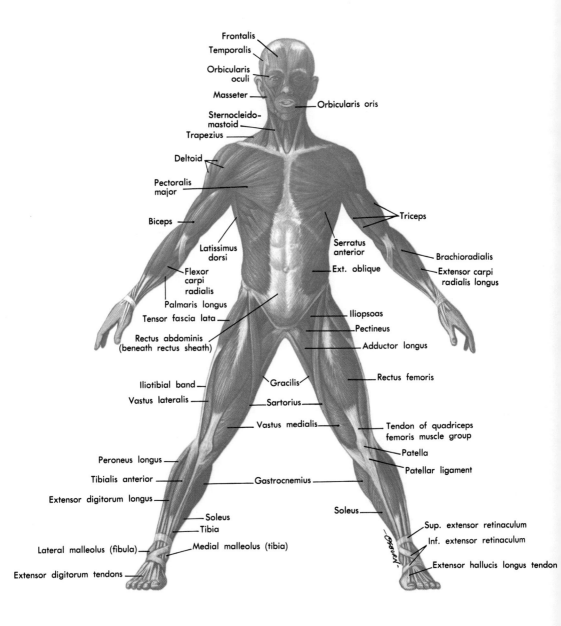

Frontalis
Temporalis
Orbicularis oculi
Masseter
Orbicularis oris
Sternocleido-mastoid
Trapezius
Deltoid
Pectoralis major
Biceps
Triceps
Latissimus dorsi
Serratus anterior
Brachioradialis
Flexor carpi radialis
Ext. oblique
Extensor carpi radialis longus
Palmaris longus
Tensor fascia lata
Iliopsoas
Pectineus
Rectus abdominis (beneath rectus sheath)
Adductor longus
Iliotibial band
Gracilis
Rectus femoris
Vastus lateralis
Sartorius
Vastus medialis
Tendon of quadriceps femoris muscle group
Peroneus longus
Patella
Patellar ligament
Tibialis anterior
Gastrocnemius
Extensor digitorum longus
Soleus
Soleus
Tibia
Sup. extensor retinaculum
Inf. extensor retinaculum
Lateral malleolus (fibula)
Medial malleolus (tibia)
Extensor digitorum tendons
Extensor hallucis longus tendon

**Plate 3**

## HOW A MUSCLE PRODUCES MOVEMENT

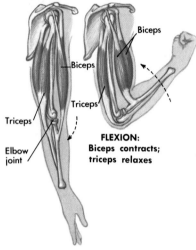

Biceps

Biceps

Triceps

Triceps

Elbow joint

**FLEXION:**
**Biceps contracts;**
**triceps relaxes**

**EXTENSION:**
**Triceps contracts;**
**biceps relaxes**

## HOW A MUSCLE ATTACHES TO BONE

Penetrating fibers          Periosteum

Muscle fiber
Int. perimysium

Ext. perimysium

Muscle fasciculus {

Tendon

The connective tissue which surrounds the muscle fibers and bundles may (1) form a tendon which fuses with the periosteum, or (2) may fuse directly with the periosteum without forming a tendon.

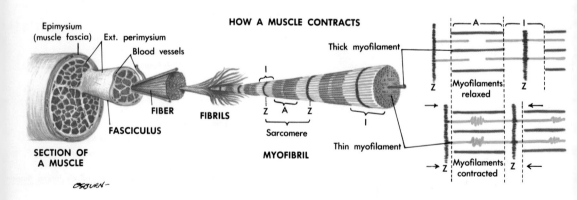

## HOW A MUSCLE CONTRACTS

Epimysium
(muscle fascia)

Ext. perimysium

Blood vessels

Thick myofilament

Z   A   Z

Sarcomere

Thin myofilament

FIBER

FIBRILS

FASCICULUS

**SECTION OF**
**A MUSCLE**

**MYOFIBRIL**

A — I

Z   Myofilaments
relaxed   Z

Z   Myofilaments
contracted   Z

OSBURN-

**Plate 4**

# RESPIRATION AND THE HEART

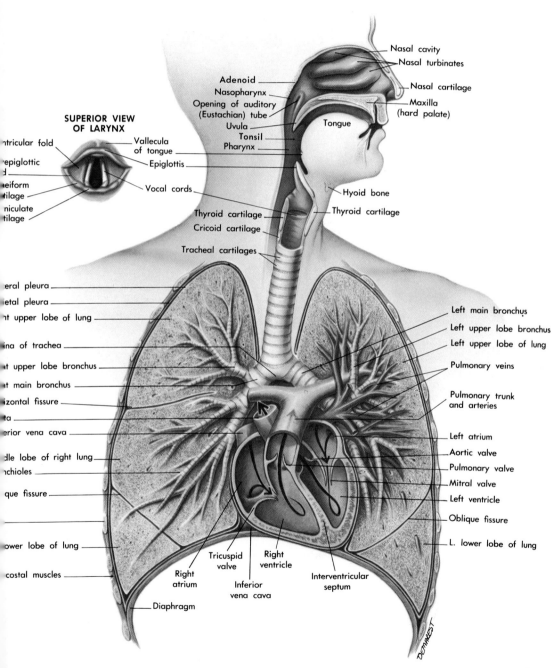

Nasal cavity

Nasal turbinates

Adenoid

Nasopharynx

Opening of auditory
(Eustachian) tube

Nasal cartilage

Maxilla
(hard palate)

Uvula

Tongue

Tonsil

Pharynx

## SUPERIOR VIEW
OF LARYNX

ntricular fold

Vallecula
of tongue

epiglottic
d

Epiglottis

Hyoid bone

eiform
tilage

Vocal cords

Thyroid cartilage

niculate
tilage

Thyroid cartilage

Cricoid cartilage

Tracheal cartilages

eral pleura

Left main bronchus

ietal pleura

Left upper lobe bronchus

nt upper lobe of lung

Left upper lobe of lung

ina of trachea

Pulmonary veins

nt upper lobe bronchus

nt main bronchus

Pulmonary trunk
and arteries

izontal fissure

ta

Left atrium

erior vena cava

Aortic valve

dle lobe of right lung

Pulmonary valve

nchioles

Mitral valve

que fissure

Left ventricle

ower lobe of lung

Oblique fissure

L. lower lobe of lung

costal muscles

Tricuspid
valve

Right
ventricle

Right
atrium

Inferior
vena cava

Interventricular
septum

Diaphragm

DEMAREST

**Plate 5**

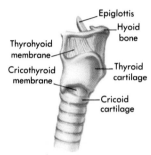

Epiglottis

Hyoid bone

Thyrohyoid membrane

Cricothyroid membrane

Thyroid cartilage

Cricoid cartilage

**LATERAL VIEW OF THE LARYNX**

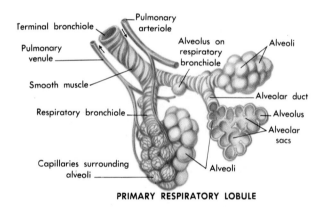

Terminal bronchiole

Pulmonary arteriole

Pulmonary venule

Alveolus on respiratory bronchiole

Alveoli

Smooth muscle

Respiratory bronchiole

Alveolar duct

Alveolus

Alveolar sacs

Capillaries surrounding alveoli

Alveoli

**PRIMARY RESPIRATORY LOBULE**

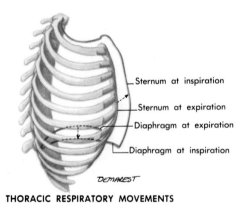

Sternum at inspiration

Sternum at expiration

Diaphragm at expiration

Diaphragm at inspiration

DEMAREST

**THORACIC RESPIRATORY MOVEMENTS**

**Plate 6**

# BLOOD VASCULAR SYSTEM

## VEINS

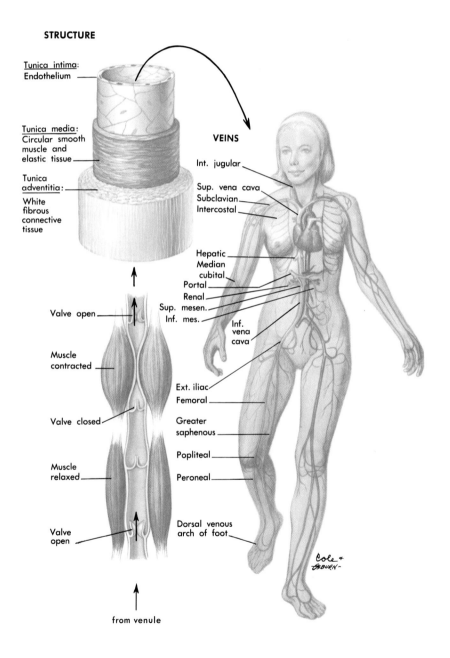

**STRUCTURE**

Tunica intima:
Endothelium

Tunica media:
Circular smooth
muscle and
elastic tissue

Tunica
adventitia:

White
fibrous
connective
tissue

Valve open

Muscle
contracted

Valve closed

Muscle
relaxed

Valve
open

from venule

**VEINS**

Int. jugular

Sup. vena cava
Subclavian
Intercostal

Hepatic
Median
cubital
Portal
Renal
Sup. mesen.
Inf. mes.
Inf.
vena
cava

Ext. iliac
Femoral

Greater
saphenous

Popliteal

Peroneal

Dorsal venous
arch of foot

Cole +
Coburn

**Plate 7**

# ARTERIES

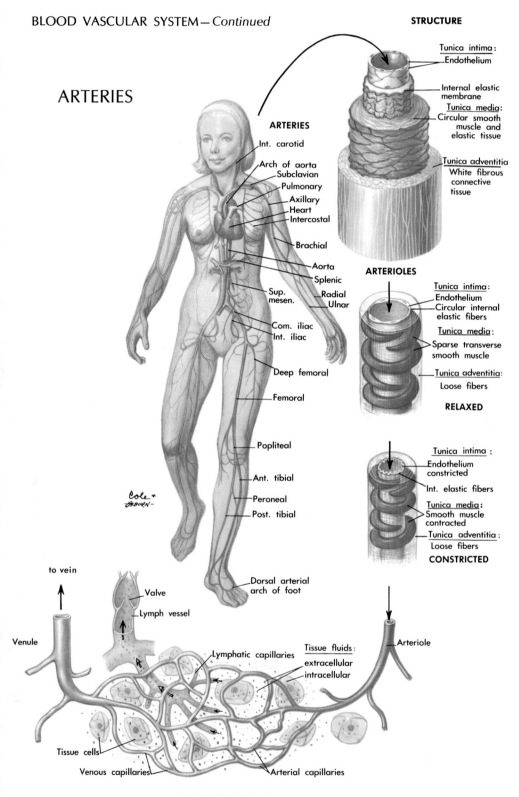

**STRUCTURE**

Tunica intima:
Endothelium

Internal elastic membrane

Tunica media:
Circular smooth muscle and elastic tissue

Tunica adventitia
White fibrous connective tissue

**ARTERIES**

Int. carotid
Arch of aorta
Subclavian
Pulmonary
Axillary
Heart
Intercostal
Brachial
Aorta
Splenic
Sup. mesen.
Radial
Ulnar
Com. iliac
Int. iliac
Deep femoral
Femoral
Popliteal
Ant. tibial
Peroneal
Post. tibial
Dorsal arterial arch of foot

Cole + OSBURN

**ARTERIOLES**

Tunica intima:
Endothelium
Circular internal elastic fibers

Tunica media:
Sparse transverse smooth muscle

Tunica adventitia:
Loose fibers

**RELAXED**

Tunica intima:
Endothelium constricted

Int. elastic fibers

Tunica media:
Smooth muscle contracted

Tunica adventitia:
Loose fibers

**CONSTRICTED**

to vein

Valve
Lymph vessel

Venule

Lymphatic capillaries

Tissue fluids:
extracellular
intracellular

Arteriole

Tissue cells

Venous capillaries

Arterial capillaries

**A CAPILLARY BED**

**Plate 8**

# DIGESTIVE SYSTEM

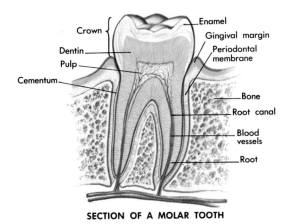

Crown
Enamel
Gingival margin
Dentin
Periodontal membrane
Pulp
Cementum
Bone
Root canal
Blood vessels
Root

**SECTION OF A MOLAR TOOTH**

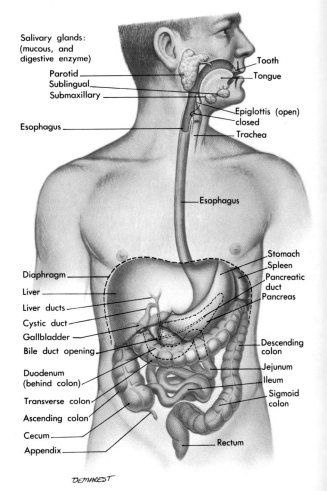

Salivary glands:
(mucous, and digestive enzyme)

Parotid
Sublingual
Submaxillary

Tooth
Tongue
Epiglottis (open)
closed
Trachea

Esophagus

Esophagus

Stomach
Spleen
Pancreatic duct
Pancreas

Diaphragm
Liver
Liver ducts
Cystic duct
Gallbladder
Bile duct opening
Duodenum (behind colon)
Transverse colon
Ascending colon
Cecum
Appendix

Descending colon
Jejunum
Ileum
Sigmoid colon

Rectum

DEMAREST

**Plate 9**

# DIGESTIVE SYSTEM—*Continued*

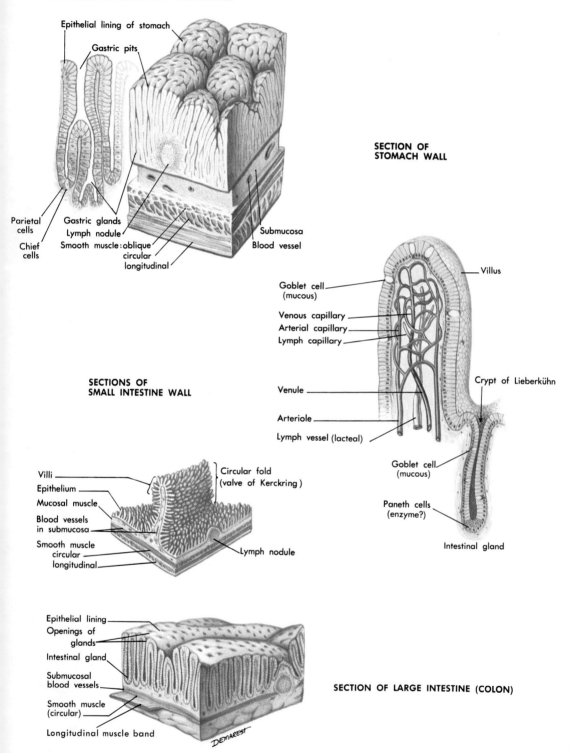

Epithelial lining of stomach

Gastric pits

Parietal cells

Chief cells

Gastric glands
Lymph nodule
Smooth muscle: oblique
circular
longitudinal

Submucosa
Blood vessel

**SECTION OF
STOMACH WALL**

Goblet cell
(mucous)

Venous capillary
Arterial capillary
Lymph capillary

Villus

Venule

Arteriole

Lymph vessel (lacteal)

Crypt of Lieberkühn

**SECTIONS OF
SMALL INTESTINE WALL**

Goblet cell
(mucous)

Paneth cells
(enzyme?)

Intestinal gland

Villi
Epithelium
Mucosal muscle
Blood vessels
in submucosa
Smooth muscle
circular
longitudinal

Circular fold
(valve of Kerckring)

Lymph nodule

Epithelial lining
Openings of
glands
Intestinal gland
Submucosal
blood vessels
Smooth muscle
(circular)
Longitudinal muscle band

**SECTION OF LARGE INTESTINE (COLON)**

DEMAREST

**Plate 10**

# GENITOURINARY SYSTEM

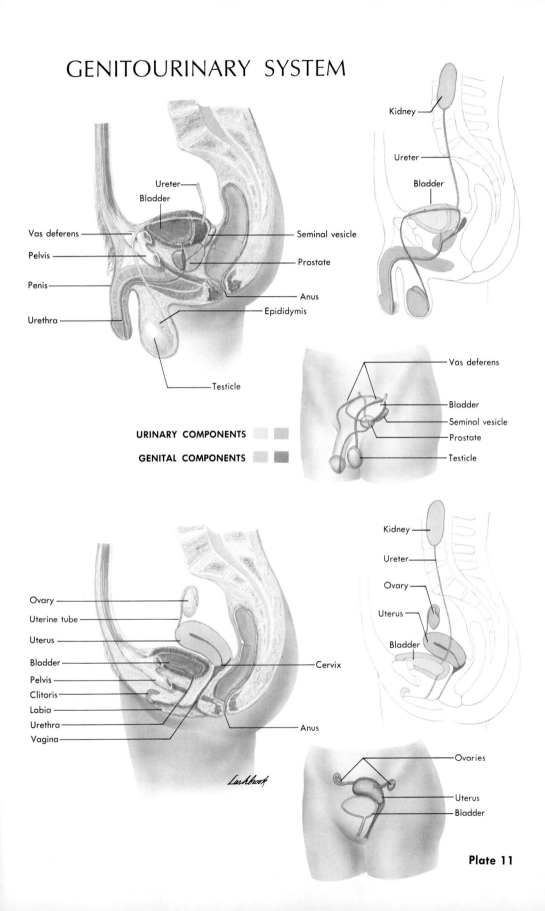

Ureter
Bladder
Vas deferens
Pelvis
Penis
Urethra
Seminal vesicle
Prostate
Anus
Epididymis
Testicle

Kidney
Ureter
Bladder

URINARY COMPONENTS
GENITAL COMPONENTS

Vas deferens
Bladder
Seminal vesicle
Prostate
Testicle

Ovary
Uterine tube
Uterus
Bladder
Pelvis
Clitoris
Labia
Urethra
Vagina
Cervix
Anus

Kidney
Ureter
Ovary
Uterus
Bladder

Ovaries
Uterus
Bladder

Lashbook

**Plate 11**

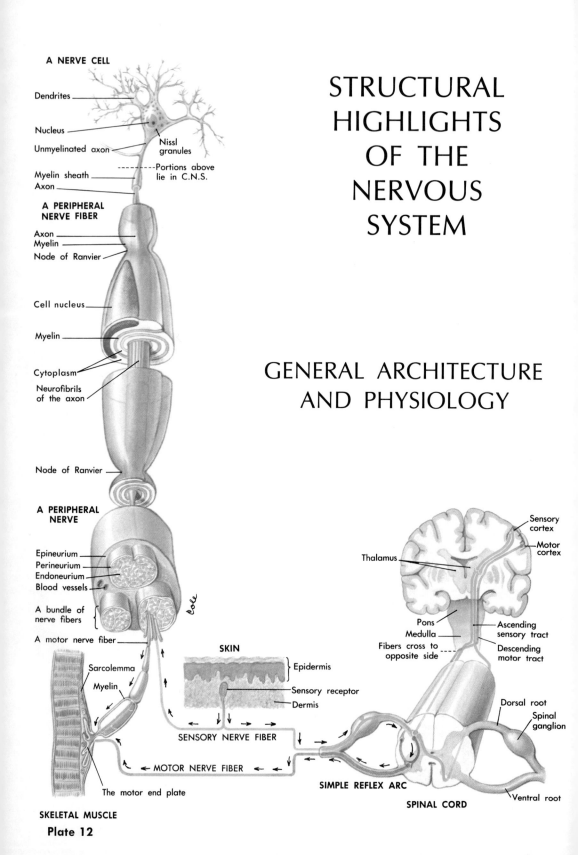

A NERVE CELL

Dendrites

Nucleus

Unmyelinated axon

Nissl granules

Portions above lie in C.N.S.

Myelin sheath

Axon

A PERIPHERAL NERVE FIBER

Axon

Myelin

Node of Ranvier

Cell nucleus

Myelin

Cytoplasm

Neurofibrils of the axon

Node of Ranvier

A PERIPHERAL NERVE

Epineurium

Perineurium

Endoneurium

Blood vessels

A bundle of nerve fibers

A motor nerve fiber

Sarcolemma

Myelin

The motor end plate

SKELETAL MUSCLE

Plate 12

STRUCTURAL HIGHLIGHTS OF THE NERVOUS SYSTEM

GENERAL ARCHITECTURE AND PHYSIOLOGY

Thalamus

Sensory cortex

Motor cortex

Pons

Medulla

Fibers cross to opposite side

Ascending sensory tract

Descending motor tract

Dorsal root

Spinal ganglion

Ventral root

SPINAL CORD

SKIN

Epidermis

Sensory receptor

Dermis

SENSORY NERVE FIBER

MOTOR NERVE FIBER

SIMPLE REFLEX ARC

# BRAIN AND SPINAL NERVES

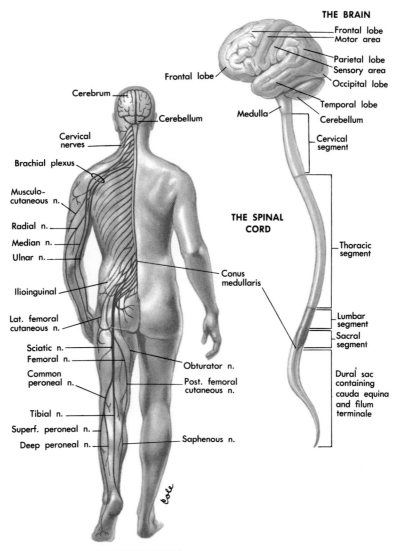

**THE BRAIN**

- Frontal lobe
- Motor area
- Parietal lobe
- Sensory area
- Occipital lobe
- Temporal lobe
- Cerebellum

Frontal lobe

Medulla

Cerebrum

Cerebellum

Cervical
nerves

Brachial plexus

Musculo-
cutaneous n.

Radial n.

Median n.

Ulnar n.

Ilioinguinal

Lat. femoral
cutaneous n.

Sciatic n.
Femoral n.
Common
peroneal n.

Tibial n.

Superf. peroneal n.

Deep peroneal n.

Conus
medullaris

Obturator n.

Post. femoral
cutaneous n.

Saphenous n.

**THE SPINAL
CORD**

Cervical
segment

Thoracic
segment

Lumbar
segment
Sacral
segment

Dural sac
containing
cauda equina
and filum
terminale

**THE MAJOR SPINAL NERVES**

**Plate 13**

# AUTONOMIC NERVES

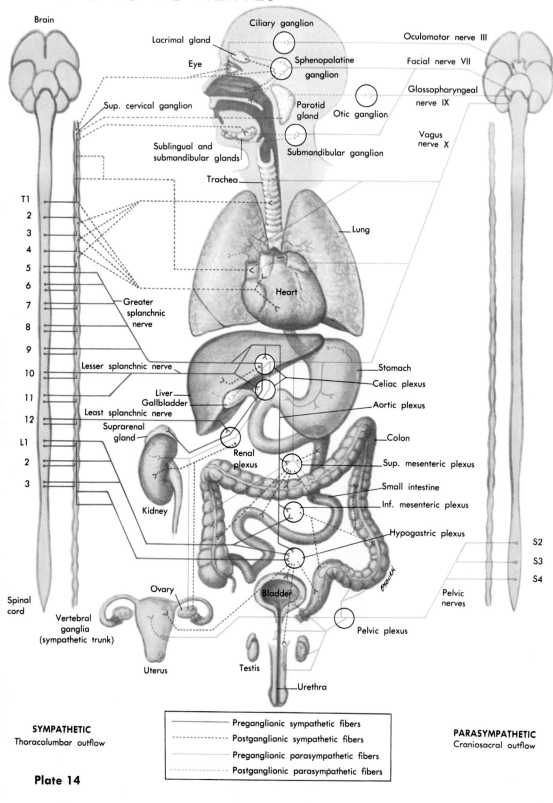

Brain

Ciliary ganglion

Lacrimal gland

Eye

Sphenopalatine ganglion

Sup. cervical ganglion

Parotid gland

Otic ganglion

Sublingual and submandibular glands

Submandibular ganglion

Oculomotor nerve III

Facial nerve VII

Glossopharyngeal nerve IX

Vagus nerve X

Trachea

T1
2
3
4
5
6
7
8
9
10
11
12
L1
2
3

Lung

Heart

Greater splanchnic nerve

Lesser splanchnic nerve

Liver
Gallbladder

Least splanchnic nerve

Suprarenal gland

Renal plexus

Kidney

Stomach

Celiac plexus

Aortic plexus

Colon

Sup. mesenteric plexus

Small intestine

Inf. mesenteric plexus

Hypogastric plexus

S2
S3
S4

Pelvic nerves

Spinal cord

Vertebral ganglia (sympathetic trunk)

Ovary

Uterus

Bladder

Testis

Urethra

Pelvic plexus

**SYMPATHETIC**
Thoracolumbar outflow

**PARASYMPATHETIC**
Craniosacral outflow

Preganglionic sympathetic fibers
Postganglionic sympathetic fibers
Preganglionic parasympathetic fibers
Postganglionic parasympathetic fibers

**Plate 14**

# ORGANS OF SPECIAL SENSE

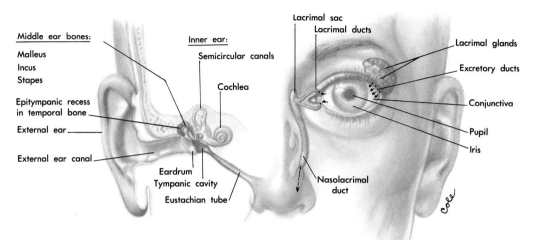

Middle ear bones:

Malleus
Incus
Stapes

Epitympanic recess
in temporal bone

External ear

External ear canal

Inner ear:

Semicircular canals

Cochlea

Eardrum
Tympanic cavity

Eustachian tube

**THE ORGAN OF HEARING**

Lacrimal sac
Lacrimal ducts

Lacrimal glands

Excretory ducts

Conjunctiva

Pupil

Iris

Nasolacrimal
duct

**THE LACRIMAL APPARATUS AND THE EYE**

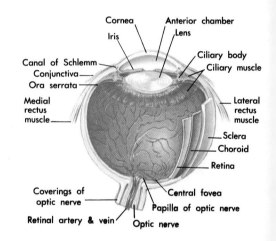

**HORIZONTAL SECTION OF THE EYE**

Cornea

Iris

Canal of Schlemm
Conjunctiva
Ora serrata

Medial
rectus
muscle

Anterior chamber
Lens

Ciliary body
Ciliary muscle

Lateral
rectus
muscle

Sclera
Choroid
Retina

Coverings of
optic nerve

Retinal artery & vein

Central fovea
Papilla of optic nerve

Optic nerve

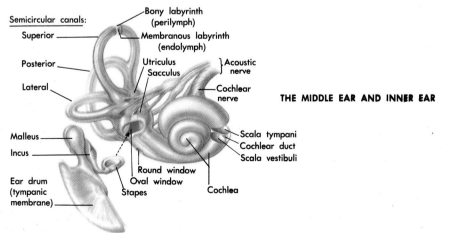

Semicircular canals:

Superior

Posterior

Lateral

Malleus

Incus

Ear drum
(tympanic
membrane)

Bony labyrinth
(perilymph)
Membranous labyrinth
(endolymph)

Utriculus
Sacculus

Acoustic
nerve

Cochlear
nerve

Round window
Oval window
Stapes

Scala tympani
Cochlear duct
Scala vestibuli

Cochlea

**THE MIDDLE EAR AND INNER EAR**

**Plate 15**

# PARANASAL
# SINUSES

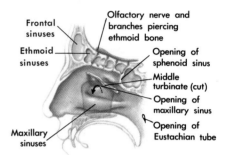

Frontal sinuses

Ethmoid sinuses

Olfactory nerve and branches piercing ethmoid bone

Opening of sphenoid sinus

Middle turbinate (cut)

Opening of maxillary sinus

Opening of Eustachian tube

Maxillary sinuses

**SAGITTAL SECTION OF THE NOSE**

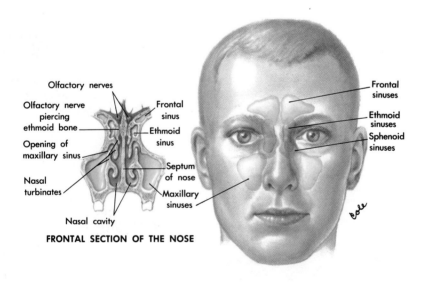

Olfactory nerves

Olfactory nerve piercing ethmoid bone

Opening of maxillary sinus

Nasal turbinates

Frontal sinus

Ethmoid sinus

Septum of nose

Maxillary sinuses

Nasal cavity

Frontal sinuses

Ethmoid sinuses

Sphenoid sinuses

**FRONTAL SECTION OF THE NOSE**

**Plate 16**

# *Appendix Five*

# Canadian Law and Health Insurance

The provisions of Canadian law governing medical practice and of provincial health insurance plans in Canada differ strikingly from those of the United States. Hence this supplement is provided to address these variations in practice between the two countries. In nearly all other respects the content of the book applies equally to the work of the medical office assistant in both countries.

# Canadian Law and Health Insurance for the Medical Secretary

Rhoda G. Finneron

## INTRODUCTION

There is no comprehensive textbook written expressly for the Canadian Medical Assistant-secretary. There is an excellent introduction to the administrative and clinical duties of the medical assistant to be found in the 33 chapters comprising the heart of this book, and although written by American authors, most of this information has universal application. In matters of medicine and the law, however, and in health and accident insurance, the Canadian situation varies quite markedly. The purpose of this Appendix, then, is to describe the peculiarities in the laws and in health insurance matters as they exist not only between the United States and Canada but from province to province in the Dominion as well. Full consideration could not be given to every provincial health insurance scheme; however, several are described, and the Ontario Hospital Insurance Plan is described in detail as being exemplary of other provincial plans. In addition, Workmen's Compensation is described in some detail.

This work was done with the help of those experts in their fields who were kind enough to aid me as I went along. I wish to thank particularly Dr. B. S. Borden, my own doctor, who proofread "Medicine and the Law in Canada" and answered my queries; and Mrs. Lorna Heer, B.A., B.L.S., and D. Turner, Esq., B.A., both of Osgoode Hall's Great Library, who researched the Canadian laws and statutes governing the practice of medicine in Canada. The Workmen's Compensation Board in Toronto and all the Canadian Provincial Health Insurance Organizations, sent me literature to work with. The former organization corrected what I wrote to bring it up to date where information had changed. My secretary, Ann Hurlburt, did the typing, and my daughter Penny gave me the time.

# MEDICINE AND THE LAW IN CANADA

Canadian law regarding medicine and its practice does not vary in any great extent from that of the United States. *Licencing** of physicians is strictly governed, and each province in Canada has its own Licencing Board. All students wishing to be doctors must attend a university which has a medical school. The examinations which entitle candidates to call themselves doctors are taken in the last year of medical school and are established by the Medical Council of Canada. These examinations are usually followed by one year of internship, after which the doctor applies to the Provincial Licencing Board for a licence to practice medicine in a particular province. For example, an intern wishing to practice in Ontario would apply to the College of Physicians and Surgeons of Ontario for a licence to practice in that province. If he wished to practice in any other province in Canada he would apply to a similar licencing body for that province.

There are two registers of doctors in Canada, the General Register for fully licenced doctors, and the Special Register, which is essentially for foreign doctors practicing in Canada. Doctors on the General Register must renew their licence every two years for as long as they practice. Doctors on the Special Register are, in general, those who have come to practice in Canada from other countries, such England, Pakistan, and India, or who are doing locum duty for another doctor. The latter must renew their registration every year.

Should a doctor, having been granted a licence to practice in, say, Manitoba, decide after a few years to move to British Columbia or Nova Scotia, he would have to apply to the appropriate licencing board of the chosen province, and might be required by that province to take formal examinations before its licencing body will allow him to practice. Once a province has licenced a doctor, that licence applies for the doctor's lifetime, so long as it is renewed as required or until retirement. Should he wish to change from one area to specialize in another, he would need further training in his new specialty and would be required to take the Medical Council of Canada and/or the provincial "board" examinations in that field.

Should a general practitioner decide that general practice was not for him and that he wanted to specialize in some field of medicine or surgery, the transition would be impossible without further training, examination, and relicencing or additional licencing, so that he might then be designated as M.D., followed by the new specialty designation e.g., Dorothy Johnson, M.D., F.R.C.S. (Otolaryngology).

As in the United States, anyone who practices medicine without the appropriate licence commits an offence against the federal laws. The practice of medicine in Canada is governed by Canadian law and Canadian statute, such as the following:

### Legislation with Respect to the Practice of Medicine in Canada

#### Federal
Canadian Medical Act, R.S.C. 1952, c. 27, as amended.
Established Programmes (Interim Arrangements) Act, R.S.C. 1970, c. E-8.

*LICENCE is the correct spelling in Canada; it is incorrect to spell it "license" in this particular instance.

Food and Drugs Act, R.S.C. 1970, c. F-27.
Health Resources Fund Act, R.S.C. 1970, c. H-4.
Hospital Insurance and Diagnostic Services Act, R.S.C., 1970, c. H-8.
Medical Care Act, R.S.C. 1970, c. M-8.
Medical Research Council Act, R.S.C. 1970, c. M-9.
Narcotic Control Act, R.S.C. 1970, c. N-1, as amended.
Department of National Health and Welfare Act, R.S.C. 1970, c. N-9, as amended.
Proprietary or Patent Medicine Act, R.S.C. 1970, c. P-25.
Public Works Health Act, R.S.C. 1970, c. P-39.
Quarantine Act, R.S.C. 1970, c. 33 (1st supp.).
Canada Temperance Act, R.S.C. 1970, c. T-5.

A licence may be revoked or suspended by the Canadian Medical Association (C.M.A.), whose headquarters are in Ottawa. Negligence, driving while intoxicated, imprisonment, and unprofessionalism represent grounds for suspension or revocation of a practitioner's licence.

## Professional Liability

A doctor practicing in Canada is responsible to do all in his power for anyone coming to him as a patient and whom he accepts for treatment. Further, he has a duty to refer the patient to a hospital or to a specialist if the problem is one he cannot deal with or one which he feels requires another doctor's opinion or surgical specialization.

## Malpractice

Malpractice is the word used, regrettably and all too often, as a blanket description for negligence on the part of a practitioner, nursing home, hospital, or mental institution.

Institutions and hospitals, as in any principal-agent relationship, are responsible for the behavior of their employees, and doctors are responsible for the actions of nurses and other health professionals employed in their offices or clinics. If the doctor is sued as a result of the negligence or carelessness of someone in his employ, his only resort in law is to sue the employee privately. Doctors and their nurses, secretaries, and medical assistants have an extremely delicate trust relationship with patients. Any harm done to this feeling of trust will damage the practice badly.

Doctors carry malpractice insurance (as do hospitals, clinics, institutions and nursing homes), to protect themselves against claims for negligence or incorrect treatment brought by patients or their estates. With today's wide coverage through the media of all that is happening in the medical and hospital world, patients too often expect miracles. If the doctors' and hospitals' best efforts fall short of expectation, patients may file suit for damage for malpractice or, to put it into contractual terms, for nonperformance of contract.

Canadian doctors are insured by the C.M.A. and, if there is any threat of or claim for damages, the doctor notifies the C.M.A. immediately. The C.M.A. then contests the claim with its *own* lawyers, and settles any claim for damages. The C.M.A. will *NOT* act on behalf of any doctor who uses his own lawyer. With such a strong organization behind him, it is in the doctor's best interest to let the C.M.A. handle the case. The practitioner may not discuss the case with anyone else at all, especially his own lawyer. The doctor will generally write or telephone the C.M.A. when a suit is begun against him. If his assistant should be asked to do this, she must realize the tremendous responsibility placed upon her to keep all she says and hears completely confidential, in the same way that she treats all other information about her employer's patients.

The C.M.A. sends its members a yearly report on all cases received and dealt with, so that every doctor will have the information. Most cases are dismissed as invalid; where validity is proved most cases are settled out of court. When this is not possible, cases proceed to court where judgment is handed down and a consideration for compensation stated. Whether a claim is settled in or out of court, the doctor can be penalized by the C.M.A. and his licence revoked or suspended. However, all human beings are fallible; doctors can make mistakes like everyone else. If, in spite of the best possible effort at correct diagnosis and treatment, a genuine mistake was made, or an incorrect conclusion drawn, neither negligence nor carelessness would likely be adjudged. No one would enter any field of endeavor, particularly law or medicine, if it was stipulated that should he make an error he faced revocation of his licence. Negligent behavior or carelessness must be proved to have existed and to have caused harm to the patient as a direct result.

Sometimes a patient will have cause to sue another party for damages for injuries he has received; he may be the victim of a careless driver, may have slipped and broken a leg in a department store because the floor was wet, or may have fallen on ice in front of someone's house. As a result, his insurance company may send the claimant to his own doctor for a prognosis, in order to confirm the opinion of the doctor employed by the company. Sometimes, however, in trying to deny a claim or lessen the amount, the patient is sent to an unfamiliar doctor so that (hopefully) a prognosis will be obtained which confirms that of the insurance company's doctor. In either case, if the amount of damages cannot be agreed upon, the insurance company will consult counsel (Queen's Counsel, Q.C., while Canada has a Queen; it is a King's Counsel, K.C., should Canada next have a king) and ask for "advice on quantum," which in lay terms means "will you advise us what is a fair settlement in this case." Counsel will take into consideration all that has happened to the plaintiff, or injured party; whether he has already lost money; if there is permanent disability; if his future earning capacity is affected; and so on.

After consideration of all factors, Counsel will suggest a sum of money the plaintiff might expect to receive as adequate compensation. The lawyers for both parties confer and try to reach an agreement. If no compromise can be reached, the case must go to court; there judgment will be handed down. Costs may be awarded the plaintiff along with damages; damages may be awarded with no costs (in which case both parties bear responsibility for their own costs); or the case may not be proved and neither party may win. There are many possibilities which may occur.

Please reply to the undersigned.                          ST. PETER'S HOSPITAL
Quoting HOSPITAL Ref. No: 4793                                Frederickton
                                                              New Brunswick

                                                          TEL. 506-1234-441
**CONFIDENTIAL**                                          29th July 1974

## MEDICAL REPORT

### MRS. RHODA GRACE FINNERON

This lady is a housewife and also a student at Brooklands Teacher's College. She was seen in the Accident Centre at St. Peter's on 3rd February, 1974 at 9:05 a.m., having been brought there by ambulance. She stated that she was standing behind her car, which was stationary, when another car ran into the back of her car, catching her legs between the two bumpers.

ON EXAMINATION: She had a large hematoma in the mid-tibia region of the right leg, with a small abrasion. An x-ray was taken of this leg but no bone injury was discovered. She was advised to rest the leg at home, where she was sent by ambulance, and to return to St. Peter's Hospital in one week's time. She was, however, followed-up by her own doctor while at home, where she stayed in bed for one week, after which time she got up and returned to her studies at the Teacher's College. She was seen about three times during the first week by her own doctor and had an x-ray of her left leg at Weybridge Hospital. This film showed an undisplaced, minor fracture of the upper end of the fibula. She was seen about every 10 to 12 days by her own doctor until two months ago. During this time she was having dressings to the abrasions on her right leg, which took some time to heal. She was unable to do her housework for one month and did not drive her car for two months. She was also unable to indulge in her hobbies of swimming, golf, sailing, and gardening.

*(Figure continued on opposite page.)*

It should be emphasized that everyone concerned will try to obtain a settlement out of court. In Ontario, for example, before pursuing a writ to court, and after lawyers for both sides have talked together, the case may be taken before a Master at Osgoode Hall, to see whether or not an amicable settlement can be reached. Only after every avenue has been explored does the case go to court. Settlement out of court is usually far less costly and far more advantageous to all concerned.

Doctors frequently prepare reports on the condition of an accident victim and give as fair a prognosis as possible. The reports should be stated clearly on stationery bearing the doctor's letterhead. If short, the reports may be double spaced. The two examples shown here are single spaced as they are rather long. If one report is to be prepared for the Workmen's Compensation Board, and the forms supplied (see page 710) are inadequate, the report should be similar in style to that submitted to a lawyer or court. This report will be sent to the lawyer for the Workmen's Compensation Board, as it employs its own lawyers

PRESENT POSITION: Left leg—no complaints or abnormality was reported for this leg.
Right leg—patient complains of prickling on the medial side of the right leg and numbness on the lateral side of that leg. There is some aching in the calf area of the leg, which is worse after any great amount of working. Patient is able to walk as far as she wants, however, despite the pain, but she cannot run as yet. She is able to do all her housework. She also complains of scars on her right leg and a depression on the lateral side of the mid-tibial region.

ON EXAMINATION: There is a 1½-inch tender scar on the lateral side of the right leg. This scar is noticeable because it is in a larger depressed area. There is also a small depressed scar on the medial side of the leg at the same level. There is some swelling around the scar and a small area of diminished sensation. There is also an area of hyperesthesia around the medial scar. The circumference of leg is ¼-inch less on the right than on the left side around the calf and there is an increase of ¼-inch in the circumference of the leg just above the ankle.

PROGNOSIS: Patient is unlikely to have any trouble in the future from her left leg. The scars on the right leg will fade for a further period of about six months but it is likely that patient will always have a scar on this leg that will be noticeable through all but the thickest stockings. The difference in circumference of the two legs and the depressed area should all improve during the course of the next six months, as should the sensory changes, but it is possible that she might always retain minimal difference in the circumference of the two legs.

B. S. Borden, M.D., F.R.C.S.(C)

BB/ab

for all such work. Either of the two report forms shown here are suitably designed for such work.

In Canada certain associations in business are called partnerships (Smyth and Soberman; Pollock; Underhill), and may not become incorporated. Among these associations are those of doctors and lawyers. A doctor may, of course, be the sole owner of his business or a sole practitioner, or he may choose to become one of several doctors who work under the umbrella of a partnership. A partnership agreement does not always have to be in writing but it should be to avoid problems which could arise. For instance, in the case of dissolution, when there is no specific partnership agreement which states otherwise, the *general* rule is that all partners share equally in both profits and losses. The argument *for* a written agreement is obvious. Such an agreement should be drawn by a lawyer and not by the doctors themselves.

Under Canadian law the word "partnership," in general, refers to a joint business enterprise carried on for profit. All the partners in the firm are jointly responsible for all debts and liabilities incurred while they are partners. The

TELEPHONE 922-451 (code 1-604)
W. BORDEN, M.D., F.R.C.S.(C) (ORTH)
1152 Skana Drive,
Tswassan, Delta,
British Columbia

November 21, 1974

**PRIVATE and CONFIDENTIAL**
**MEDICAL LEGAL ORTHOPAEDIC CONSULTATION NOTE**

Mr. H. Brodie,
Superintendent, Claims Department
Vancouver Region
Starlight Assurance Company
7 Right Street East, Sixth Floor
Vancouver, British Columbia
M2H 2C2

Dear Mr. Brodie:        Re: Peter R. Taylor
                        (Your Policy No. 9130770)

This 47-year-old insurance adjuster has been reviewed today with regard to residual disability following an accident which occurred on May 13th, 1974.

PRESENT COMPLAINTS: At the present time the patient's complaints are minimal. He complains of intermittent discomfort localized to the base of the neck. He also complains of occasional discomfort in the low back area, particularly if he has been sitting for a long time and also occasionally in the morning. The patient finds that his symptoms are gradually decreasing. They do not constitute a serious problem at the present time.

HISTORY OF ACCIDENT: At the time of the accident, the patient states that he was struck from the rear by another car. He had a seat belt fastened. He states that he was "stretched" over the back of the seat and at one point he was momentarily and fleetingly aware of looking at the ceiling. He felt pain and soreness in his neck and soreness in his legs, feet, and knees and also soreness in his arms.

The patient states that his severe symptoms subsided in about eight days and that he became quite better from a practical standpoint, in about three months. For three months after the accident he continued to have occasional discomfort as previously noted.

*(Figure continued on opposite page.)*

partnership's creditors' claims take precedence over the personal creditors of each doctor. All partnerships must be registered and must provide the names and addresses of all partners, the terms of the partnership, the name under which the partnership will operate, and how long the partnership has existed. All the members of the partnership must be named; no names may be omitted or added. Dissolution of the partnership must be registered.

It is not proposed here to go into the status of sleeping, dormant, silent, or any other kind of partners but active partners. A list of reference books at the end of this section indicates material one might read to find out more about partnerships and the laws applying to them in Canada.

**Good Samaritan Acts.**   In Canada a physician is responsible for any action

Peter R. Taylor, continued.

PERSONAL HISTORY: The patient is 47 years of age; in good general health. He had pneumonia and empyema in 1940, but aside from this, he has not had any serious illness.

Since the time of the accident, the patient has not received any specific therapy.

EXAMINATION: At the time of the present examination, the patient's disability appears to be quite slight. He moves about the examining room freely. There is no abnormality in gait.

Inspection of the neck does not reveal the presence of any deformity. There is a full range of motion with only slight discomfort at extremes. There is no spasm, no crepitus.

Upper extremity examination is negative for the presence of reflex, motor, sensory, or vascular abnormality.

The low back examination does not show the presence of any significant deformity. There is tenderness at the lumbosacral level. This is not severe. The range of motion of the lumbar spine is full with slight pain at extremes.

The lower extremity examination is negative for the presence of reflex, motor, sensory or vascular abnormality.

X-ray examination of this patient's cervical spine has been carried out today. The x-rays show the presence of degenerative changes. These degenerative changes are mainly localized to the C.5–6 level.

OPINION: This patient has sustained soft tissue sprain to the neck and low back as the result of a rear-end collision accident. At the present time, his disability is minimal and he is recovering. I think it is reasonable to expect that he will go on to full and complete recovery without any residual problem. I would not anticipate the need for future treatment as a result of this accident.

Yours sincerely,

WB/ab
Enclosure.

W. BORDEN, M.D., F.R.C.S.(C) (ORTH.)

he may take in administering aid. He is not required by law to stop at the scene of an accident, heart attack, or for any other incident. If he does administer aid to the victims of illness or accidents he is responsible for his action and its results. In an extreme case, the physician can be sued by the person treated or by his family, if the person should die, no matter how well-intentioned the physician's actions were and regardless of the fact that the victim may have died anyway. Again, this is an extreme example of what might happen.

Anyone working in the medical field, however, who is called upon for help, for instance to aid a heart attack victim, may instruct the person to lie down while someone calls an ambulance. It is unlikely that anyone, particularly a doctor or nurse, would hesitate to loosen clothing around the neck or, in severe attack, attempt mouth-to-mouth resuscitation, and it is also highly unlikely that a family would sue because of such well-intentioned acts. Nevertheless, the statement of the law mentioned previously does still apply in Canada throughout all its provinces.

**Controlled Substances.** In Canada, controlled substances, such as narcotics and all drugs, are subject to laws laid down by the Criminal Code of Canada (Narcotic Division) and particularly the Food and Drugs Act. The Narcotic Division of the Criminal code, and especially the Narcotic Control Act, oversees all distribution of narcotics, such as morphine and heroin, and phenobarbital and other barbiturates, while the Food and Drugs Act controls the manufacture and prescription of drugs like antibiotics, insulin, and so on. Obviously there is some overlap between the two control acts because prescriptions issued by doctors and filled by pharmacists may use barbiturates and other narcotics.

The manufacture of narcotics is also strictly controlled. First the manufacturer is screened, and then all his employees. He may manufacture only what he is permitted to do, and under controlled and supervised conditions. The manufacturer must have a licence before commencing business, and even before he may buy the necessary materials to do so. Pharmacists who use narcotics in prescriptions are very closely supervised by the Narcotic Division.

As far as drugstore owners are concerned, they keep a list of all drugs and narcotics, and must account for every milligram of drugs and narcotics used for prescriptions or in any other way, as must hospitals, nursing homes, clinics, and other pharmacists. Doctors keep a table of all drugs they use and/or prescribe. These lists or tables can be requested and examined by the agency at any time, so accuracy is all-important.

The drugs subject to the most stringent controls are those which come under the general heading of "narcotics." Other non-narcotic drugs must still be carefully accounted for; and some drugs, listed as still in the experimental stage, are placed on schedule "G," which means they are not available to all doctors, hospitals, or pharmacists. They are available only to a chosen few who work with them and report back on the results of the administration of the new drugs. These drugs would be issued by a pharmacist only upon presentation of a prescription calling for an experimental schedule "G" drug received from a doctor who had permission to use it, and under no other circumstances.

**Anatomical Gift Act.** A misconception held by many people is that unless a body is perfect—that is, it has not been opened or operated upon—it is not wanted or of use as a cadaver. This is incorrect. The 16 Canadian medical schools and research facilities need cadavers, and anyone wanting to promote the training of doctors can make no more welcome gift to a university than that of his body after death. If someone enters the hospital and dies within 24 hours, an autopsy is automatically performed. If a body is found under inexplicable circumstances, or if there is suspicion of foul play, an autopsy may be ordered. The cadaver is usually coffined afterward, as the work a training school would do has virtually been completed. Although this is usually the case, there are exceptions to the rule.

The use of all cadavers is subject to the wishes of the next-of-kin, regardless of what the person may have wanted when alive. For instance, a person may have wanted his eyes, kidneys, and heart to be donated after his death. Should the immediate next-of-kin object, he has a prior claim on the body and may refuse to carry out such wishes.

A person wishing to donate his eyes to the Eye Bank of Canada can write or telephone the Canadian National Institute for the Blind, with headquarters at 1929 Bayview Avenue, Toronto, for the proper forms. There are local branches of this institute throughout Canada that will supply the same information. (See the following donor cards and those on page 675.)

There is a National Kidney Foundation of Canada, which has its main office in Montreal, Quebec (P.O. 422, Montreal, Quebec), and it has branches in all the major cities of Canada. This foundation, too, gladly sends forms to anyone wishing to donate kidneys after death. Similarly, there is a Canadian Heart Foundation, which has its main office at 310 Davenport Avenue, Toronto, and, again, forms will be sent to anyone wishing to donate his heart after death. Examples of these forms are shown below. Since Canada is a bilingual country, the donor cards are printed in both English and French.

The donor should arrange through his doctor or lawyer to have all or part of his body assigned for use for teaching purposes, or in the case of heart,

---

**PLEASE PRINT IN BLOCK LETTERS**

NAME  Mr. / Mrs. / Miss   Rhoda Finneron

STREET  199 McNicoll Avenue

CITY  Willowdale, Ontario M2H 2C2

DATE  9 May, 1974

Please complete this card, detach and mail to the address on the reverse side. It shows that you have expressed the wish to leave your eyes for restoration of sight and will be kept on permanent file.

---

## CONSENT FORM

I, .................................................................. the (husband) (wife), (next-of-kin), or (person lawfully in charge of the body of the deceased), do hereby consent to the removal of the eyes of the deceased, according to his expressed wish.

Date _____  Signature _____

Witness _____

---

### EYE BANK OF CANADA
(Ontario Division)

Sponsored by
The Department of Ophthalmology, University of Toronto and The Canadian National Institute for the Blind

1929 Bayview Ave.   Toronto 17, Ont.   485-8644
Nights & Holidays   485-9476

At the time of death please notify above immediately.

---

## IN CASE OF ACCIDENT PLEASE NOTIFY

NAME  Miss P. Finneron

ADDRESS  199 McNicoll Avenue

CITY  Willowdale, M2H 2C2

PROVINCE  Ontario   PHONE  491-7357

RELATIONSHIP  Daughter

---

Please sign this card and show it to your next-of-kin, and doctor and keep it where it may be found quickly. Instructions to next-of-kin, nearest relative, guardian or person lawfully in charge of the body of the deceased: Immediately on my death, please sign the consent form on the reverse side and give it to my doctor or hospital authority.

Date _____  Signature of donor _____

---

Detach this portion when completed and mail to:

Eye Bank of Canada,  (Ontario Division)

The Canadian National Institute for the Blind

1929 Bayview Avenue,

Toronto 17, Ontario.

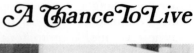

# *Une Chance de Vivre*     *A Chance To Live*

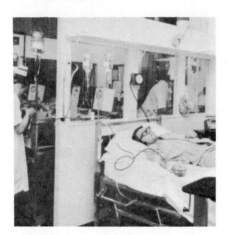 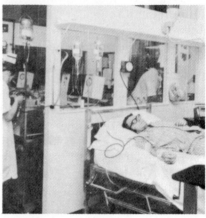

**NOUS AVONS BESOIN DE VOTRE AIDE.** Si vous voulez vous joindre à nous et accorder votre appui financier à la Fondation Canadienne des Maladies du Rein, veuillez bien compléter la formule ci-dessous et envoyer votre chèque à votre succursale locale

ou à

**LA FONDATION CANADIENNE DES MALADIES DU REIN**
5744, boul. Décarie, Montréal 252, Québec

Nom

Adresse

Ville          Zone     Province     Tél.

Veuillez ajouter:

Nom de la compagnie

Adresse

Ville          Zone     Province     Tél.

Occupation

Veuillez adresser le courrier au bureau ☐ à mon domicile ☐

Nom de l'époux ou épouse

☐ Souscripteur $ 3.00 ☐ Donateur $ 25.00
☐ Collaborateur $ 5.00 ☐ Patron $ 50.00
☐ Boursier $ 10.00 ☐ Gouverneur $100.00
☐ Bienfaiteur $100.00 et plus

**VOTRE DON EST DEDUCTIBLE POUR FINS D'IMPOT**

**YOUR HELP IS NEEDED** If you want to join or financially support the Kidney Foundation of Canada, please complete the form below and mail with your cheque to your local chapter.

or the

**KIDNEY FOUNDATION OF CANADA**
5744 Decarie Blvd., Montreal 252, Quebec

Name

Address

City          Zone     Province     Tel.

If you wish, please add:

Firm Name

Address

City          Zone     Province     Tel.

Occupation

Please send mail to Business ☐ Residence ☐

Husband or Wife's name

☐ Subscriber $ 3.00 ☐ Donor $ 25.00
☐ Contributor $ 5.00 ☐ Patron $ 50.00
☐ Fellow $ 10.00 ☐ Governor $100.00
☐ Benefactor over $ 100.00

**YOUR DONATION IS TAX DEDUCTIBLE**

cornea, liver, or kidney donations, for transplant. One thing the donor should *not* do is to put his request only in his will without also taking one of the steps mentioned previously. Usually disposal of the body takes place before the will is read, and it would be too late for the donations to be received if they were mentioned only in the will.

The survivors of the deceased, such as parents, sisters, or brothers, could agree to a donation of organs or of the entire cadaver in cases where a donation has never been mentioned, or they could consent to an autopsy at the request of the hospital or doctor in the interest of research. However, it is far better for anyone wishing to donate to do so before death so that his wishes are perfectly clear.

| ORGAN DONOR CARD | CARTE DE DONATION D'ORGANES |
|---|---|
| OF_____<br>Print or type name of donor<br>In the hope that I may help others, I hereby make this anatomical gift, if medically acceptable, to take effect upon my death. The words and marks below indicate my desires.<br><br>I give, direct, consent and request:<br>   ☐ (a) — any needed organs or parts<br>   ☐ (b) — only the following organs or parts<br>_____<br>Specify the organ(s) or part(s)<br>for the purposes of transplantation, therapy, medical research, or education.<br>Limitations or<br>Special wishes, if any:_____<br>FOLD                FOLD<br>FOLD Signed by the donor and the following witness in the presence of each other:<br><br>_____  _____<br>Signature of Donor    Date of Birth of Donor<br><br>_____  _____<br>Date Signed       Witness<br><br>_____<br>City   Zone   Province<br>This is a legal document under the Human Tissue Act or similar laws.<br>For further information contact your physician or the<br>KIDNEY FOUNDATION OF CANADA<br>Post Office Box 422, Montreal 379, Quebec. | M._____<br>Mme<br>Mlle_____<br>Ecrire en lettres moulées le nom du donneur.<br>Espérant que ce don servira à quelqu'un, je, soussigné, par la présente, consens au prélèvement lors de mon décès:<br>   ☐ (a) — de tous les organes ou parties de mon corps qui peuvent être utiles,<br>   ☐ (b) — uniquement des parties ou organes suivants:<br><br>à des fins de transplantation, traitement, recherche médicale et éducation.<br><br>Voeux particuliers: _____<br>PLIER            PLIER<br>PLIER            PLIER<br>Signé par le donneur en présence du témoin qui devra contresigner:<br><br>_____  _____<br>Signature du donneur    Date de naissance<br><br>_____  _____<br>Signé en date du     Signature du témoin<br><br>_____<br>Ville,   Zone,   Province<br>Ce document est valide en vertu de la loi de la donation des organes humains ou des lois similaires.<br>Pour de plus amples renseignements veuillez consulter votre médecin ou<br>LA FONDATION CANADIENNE DES MALADIES DU REIN,<br>Case Postale 422, Montréal 379, Québec. |

**Patients' Consent.**   If a minor (someone under 18 years of age in Canada), needs surgery, the consent of the parents, guardians, or guardian *ad litem* must be obtained or, when none of these persons can be traced and an emergency exists, a court order must be sought in order to proceed with treatment necessary to save the patient's life. The court which issues permission becomes guardian *ad litem* until the parents or the guardian can be traced. Anyone over 18 years of age signs his own consent forms for an operation and anesthetic, and accepts responsibility for undergoing surgery. The form on page 52, in Chapter 5, *Medicine and the Law,* is quite similar to·one which any Canadian hospital might use. Should an adult be unconscious or unable to sign, his next-of-kin would do so. In cases in which the patient's life is in immediate danger and no one can be found to sign the consent forms, the hospital or surgeon would, upon consultation, do whatever was necessary to save the patient's life.

**Voluntary Sterilization.**   Voluntary sterilization and vasectomy, but not abortion, will be performed on demand in Canada. The patient signs a request form similar to that shown on page 56, Figure 5–4, which is a consent to the operation for sterilization or vasectomy. It is essential, though, that the doctor have the appropriate signatures before commencing any such operation.

Abortion continues to be a very delicate matter in Canada, especially abortion on demand as a method of controlling family size. In general, a pregnant woman contracting a communicable disease or a disease which will probably adversely affect the fetus, such as rubella (and where the three-month stage of pregnancy has not been passed), or one whose own physical or mental health is threatened by the birth may be able to obtain a medical abortion. A woman wishing to abort an unwanted fetus must bring her case before a local committee of three, which will probably be comprised of a psychologist and two gynecologists. The committee will listen to the woman's doctor, and they may ask to see the woman too. Should they agree that she is a suitable case for abortion in that having the child will endanger her health or life, or that she is mentally incapable of accepting childbirth and caring for the child, the committee may consent to an abortion for her. The law states that each case is to be examined individually.

Obviously, there are enormous possibilities for discrepancies in the application of these abortion laws.

Above this committee of three is the hospital committee, which will be asked to give its consent to the operation. It, too, usually numbers three persons. Should they give their consent, the hospital committee will instruct the hospital to accept the woman and perform the abortion. It should be understood, however, that by no means do all hospitals in Canada perform abortions unless they are medically necessary to save the mother's life or for some equally valid reason. The difference in standards makes this whole situation intensely controversial.

## LEGAL RESPONSIBILITY OF THE MEDICAL ASSISTANT

The legal responsibility of the medical assistant has been well covered on pages 57 to 62 of Chapter 5. Even though this information specifically pertains to the United States, all that is said applies equally to Canada since all employees of doctors, hospitals, clinics, and other medical institutions act as agents of the employer. The employer-physician is responsible for any acts of the employee while on duty.

The forms shown on pages 57 and 58 are equally applicable in Canada, but the latter would be called a "self-discharge" form, and the first would not be used too frequently, except, possibly, by a doctor who has excluded himself from his provincial medical plan. Provincial plans are dealt with separately in this appendix.

It is unnecessary to repeat all that has been said in this book about responsibility for equipment and the behavior of both doctors and assistants; it cannot be emphasized too strongly that no medical assistant is licenced to practice medicine, to prescribe drugs, to instruct or to diagnose, or in any way to usurp the doctor's area of authority. These practices are called, whether in Canada or the United States, "the illegal practice of medicine," and are absolutely against Canadian law. The medical assistant or secretary must not attempt to treat a patient in the doctor's absence or to offer telephone advice. In an emergency she must act in as humane a manner as is conducive to saving the patient's life, while remembering that she is *not* covered by a "Good Samaritan Act" any more than is her employer. She must remember too that her employer is responsible for her actions if she is on duty at the time of the emergency. Whatever first-aid she administers, she must subsequently call a doctor or an ambulance and seek professional advice. The Medical Protective Association of each province establishes its own precise rules of behavior, and the medical assistant should be encouraged at the start of her career to seek advice there if she is in doubt as to what she should do in emergency situations.

The Canadian Medical Association Code of Ethics governs all behavior in the medical professions, and each year issues a list of "crimes" committed against this Code. These crimes could occur in advertising, overcharging, and the like; therefore, to avoid unfavorable consequences the Code must be adhered to by all doctors and their assistants.

# ACCIDENT AND HEALTH INSURANCE IN CANADA

Most provinces have a Federal Medical Care Program, though not all offer the same coverage. Not all provinces charge the same premium for membership, and the benefits offered are similar but not precisely the same across Canada. Not all doctors accept the fees the various programs offer and that are established by the Canadian Medical Association (C.M.A.). This may occur when the fees are not high enough to cover their services. In these cases, patients will see a notice to this effect on the doctor's waiting-room wall, usually coupled with an invitation to discuss fees with the doctor. Not all doctors are willing to collect their fees directly from the provincial authority, especially if this means a disparity between the fees paid by a medical program and those suggested by the Medical Association. In Ontario, for example, with O.H.I.P. (Ontario Health Insurance Plan) membership, 10 per cent less is paid than the scale established by the Ontario Medical Association (O.M.A.).

Each provincial medical association, under the guidance of the C.M.A., determines the amounts to be paid for the various types of services the doctor, hospital, or other medical service agency offers. The doctor may be paid directly by the provincial plan, or the patient may pay the doctor first and be reimbursed by the provincial plan. Where a doctor has opted out of his provincial plan, the patient will invariably pay the doctor and then be reimbursed by the provincial plan. Each provincial plan covers basic medical necessities, plus some extra benefits.

Extra health benefits, extra hospitalization, such as semiprivate accommodation, or payment for drugs may be covered under separate plans. Associated Medical Services Incorporated (A.M.S.), a Canada-wide organization with headquarters in Toronto, offers plans for drug coverage, as does Blue Cross. Blue Cross and Hospital Medical Care (H.M.C.) also offer coverage to immigrants entering Canada who must comply with the waiting period which some provinces have, and also to visitors staying for a short period of time, such as for a holiday. These situations apply throughout Canada. Coverage provided by organizations such as Blue Cross and Hospital Medical Care is usually offered to groups of eight or more people but this is not always so, since it is impossible to generalize about medical coverage from province to province.

## General Information

The most common procedure is that a company applies to the provincial plan for coverage for its employees, provides a list of employees, and indicates the marital status of each, along with his or her dependents, and the employee receives an identification card from the plan. Over 90 per cent of doctors bill the plan directly, accepting the provincial medical association fee, which is taken from the C.M.A. Fee Schedule (1971), as full payment, and the patient may never see a bill if his doctor has opted into the plan. When a doctor bills directly, he can use letterhead invoices or plan claim cards which can be forwarded either to the patient or the plan. If he bills the plan directly, he will usually receive payment directly; if the patient pays the doctor directly and claims the investment from the plan, only the subscriber will receive the claim settlement from the plan.

If the number of people employed by a company and insured as a group drops below six, the employer continues to remit monthly reports and remittances or premiums until his application to the board or the agent/carrier for an order terminating the group has been received. Thereafter the employer is relieved from further responsibility regarding the group and the members become pay-direct participants of the insurance plan. Generally, if a group has terminated for some reason, a member who does not join another group may send his certificate of payment to the insurance plan, along with his application to become a pay-direct member, 30 days prior to termination of the group, and thereby avoid waiting time for coverage.

The person who wishes to become a nongroup member of a plan, or who cannot become a member of a group for some reason, for example, because he is self-employed, may apply to the plan, and if eligible, pays the appropriate subscription rate. He is then enrolled in the plan as a nongroup, insured participant. As an example, in Ontario, under O.H.I.P., the new pay-direct participant is covered on the first day of the third month after enrollment, except when he has transferred from a terminated group. In that case, if he followed the instructions and notified the plan 30 days prior to the group's termination, he remains covered. Similarly, if he has transferred from another province's health care insurance plan, his coverage will commence on termination of that plan, providing an application for O.H.I.P. coverage was made within 30 days of the date of entitlement to payment under the other province's plan. Most provinces observe similar rules of eligibility. Generally speaking, to be eligible for any plan, a subscriber must

(1) be living in the province at the time of application;
(2) have resided in the province for at least 90 days, although there are exceptions to this;
(3) not be a tourist, transient, or a visitor to the province, or, by Federal Law, not be a member of the Canadian Forces, a member of the Royal Canadian Mounted Police Force, or a person serving a term of imprisonment in a penitentiary, although all their dependents are eligible.

However, if an applicant is only partially covered for medical care by, for example, the Department of Veterans' Affairs (D.V.A.), he is entitled to plan coverage for all benefits not covered by D.V.A. Further, dependents of persons not eligible for plan coverage are themselves considered eligible if they are residents of the province and are not covered for total medical care by the Federal Government Act.

Anyone entering the Canadian medical assistant-secretarial field would be wise to obtain all the material she can concerning the insurance plan for the province where she intends to work. Folders are available with samples of the cards used, and full instructions regarding eligibility, payment, and procedure. Everything covered by a plan is stated in clear terms so the medical assistant who reads the material can be informed and advise a patient what to do in case of doubt. The assistant-secretary should also know exactly what benefits are offered as extended health benefits by organizations such as H.M.C. and Blue Cross.

Probably only one common assumption can be made for every province across Canada, and that is that everyone carries Federal Medical Care Insurance under the provincial medical care insurance plan for the province in which he lives. It would be impossible to go into great detail for *every* provincial insurance plan, but *some* of the provinces should be examined as examples. It would be equally impossible to give examples of all the forms used by all the provinces in Canada; some forms for Ontario have been shown as examples, and those in other provinces would be similar. We will look at Alberta, British Columbia, Manitoba, Newfoundland, Ontario, Nova Scotia, and Saskatchewan as being representative of provincial plans established by the federal government.

## PROVINCE OF ALBERTA

*Name of Plan:* Alberta Health Care Insurance Plan.

*Provincial Legislation:* The Alberta Health Care Insurance Act & Regulations;* The Health Insurance Premium Act & Regulations.*

*Effective Date:* July 1, 1969.

*Administration and Method of Operation:* Administered and operated by the Alberta Health Care Insurance Commission.

*Method of Provincial Financing:* Annual premiums: $69 single; $138 family of two or more. A resident whose taxable income was not more than $500 for the preceding taxation year pays $36 annually, or $3 monthly. A family with a taxable income of not more than $1000 pays $72 annually; a single person with no taxable income pays $24 annually; a family with no taxable income pays $48 annually. A person over 65 years of age pays no premium for himself/herself or dependents. A resident in receipt of social assistance benefits from the Department of Social Development has his full premium paid.

*Utilization Fees:* None.

Every resident *must* register himself and his dependents with the Commission. A new resident must register by the first day of the month following his arrival.

*Date upon which Resident becomes a Beneficiary:* On registration.

*Insured Services:* The Alberta Plan provides coverage for "basic health services" in which are included the "insured services" under the federal act. Only the "insured services" are eligible for cost-sharing with the federal government.

"Basic health services" are
    insured services: all services rendered by physicians that are medically required; services rendered by a dental surgeon in the field of oral surgery that are specified in regulations;
    services rendered by a dental surgeon in the field of oral surgery that are specified in regulations but are not "insured services";

---

*Published by the Queen's Printer for the Province of Alberta.

*PROVINCE OF ALBERTA* (Continued)

optometric services limited to refraction of the eyes for the fitting of eye glasses not oftener than once every two benefit periods (the first benefit period was from July 1, 1969 to March 31, 1970; subsequent periods will be from April 1st of each year to March 31st of the next year) for adults and once each benefit period for children under 18 years of age. The benefit payable shall not exceed $12.50 for each refraction;

chiropractic services: benefits payable are actual charges not exceeding $6 per visit and not exceeding $10 for one x-ray for a particular disability, and benefit is subject to a total of $100 per benefit period for any resident and his dependents;

services rendered by and appliances provided by a podiatrist: benefits payable in accordance with the Alberta Podiatry Association schedule of fees approved by the Commission; and

services of an osteopath: benefits payable are actual charges but do not exceed $5 per visit.

(Benefits payable for podiatric and osteopathic services combined are limited to $100 per benefit period for any single resident and $150 for those with one or more dependents.)

*Exclusions:* Services that a person is eligible for and entitled to under various provincial and federal acts, such as the Workmen's Compensation Act; examinations required for the use of third parties; services not medically required; laboratory and x-ray procedures performed in facilities not approved by the Commission; and other similar services.

*Out-of-Province Benefits:* A resident continues to be entitled to benefits for insured services during *temporary* absence from Alberta.

*Extension of Coverage after Loss of Residence:* If a person becomes a resident of another participating province, traveling time and the minimum waiting period are imposed by that province's plan. If a person becomes a resident of a nonparticipating province, the waiting period shall not exceed three months. If a person is leaving Canada, coverage continues during traveling time within Canada and does not exceed a period of one month.

*Method and Scale of Payments to Physicians:* A practitioner may send accounts to the Commission on the form prescribed and receive payment. A beneficiary may submit the itemized receipt or the account of the practitioner to the Commission and receive payment. Practitioners sending an account to beneficiaries are required to provide information so that beneficiaries are able to submit claims to the Commission.

Rates of benefits paid for physicians' services are prescribed in Commission by-laws. Currently payment is 100 per cent of the 1968 Schedule of Fees of the Alberta College of Physicians and Surgeons. (This is 93½ per cent of the College's 1969 Schedule, introduced on July 1, 1969.)

*Provision for Extra Billing by Physicians:* Physicians and other practitioners have the right to make an agreement or arrangement with any person for remunera-

*PROVINCE OF ALBERTA* (Continued)

tion to be paid to them if the agreement or arrangement is made before services are rendered.

*Provision for Private Insurance Coverage:*

Act stipulates that an insurer shall not enter into, maintain in force, issue or renew a contract *which duplicates the benefits provided by the Plan.* However, insurers may issue contracts under which a resident is indemnified for the cost of any basic health service *rendered outside Alberta* that is over and above the benefits payable by the Commission and, to the extent prescribed by and specified in the regulations, for the cost of any basic health service, other than insured services, over and above the benefits payable by the Commission.

*Optional Health Services:*

For those persons wishing it, or companies buying it for their own group, Alberta Blue Cross membership provides coverage for hospital differential charges for semiprivate and private ward care; ambulance services; drugs; appliances; home nursing; naturopathic services; clinical psychological services, and dental care needed because of accidental injury. A special Blue Cross pamphlet, and the Alberta Commission's application for Optional Health Services are available from the Alberta Blue Cross Office. Claims are sent directly to the plan.
Premiums are: $24 single; $48 per family.
Subsidized rates are: $18 single, for an annual income not in excess of $500; $36 per family; for an annual income not in excess of $1000.
Groups pay by payroll deduction.
Individuals are billed quarterly.

*PROVINCE OF BRITISH COLUMBIA*

*Name of Plan:*
*Provincial Legislation:*

Overall Medical Services Plan of British Columbia.
Medical Grant Act and Regulations; Medical Services Act and Regulations.*

*Effective Date:*
July 1, 1968.

*Administration and Method of Operation:*

Administered by the Medical Services Commission of British Columbia through licenced, nonprofit carriers which may act only as agents of the Commission to enroll residents, collect premiums and pay accounts, and shall not assess or approve accounts or determine amounts to be paid for insured services. (Seven nonprofit societies are licenced carriers at this date.)

*Method of Provincial Financing:*

Monthly premiums: Single $5; family of two, $10; family of three or more, $12.50. Subsidies are available that reduce monthly premiums to $.50, $1, and $1.25 for residents with no taxable income, and to $2.50, $5, and $6.25 for residents whose taxable income does not exceed $1000 (Medical Grant Stabilization Fund.)

---

*See *The Medical Services Act and Regulations,* Chap. 24 (1967), The Queen's Printer, for the Province of British Columbia.

*PROVINCE OF BRITISH COLUMBIA* (Continued)

| | |
|---|---|
| *Utilization Fees:* | None. |
| *Insured Persons:* | It is the responsibility of every resident to become enrolled in and maintain coverage under the Plan for himself and his dependents, either personally or through arrangement with his employer or a person acting on his behalf. |
| *Date upon which Resident becomes a Beneficiary:* | Coverage effective on first day of second calendar month following the month in which application is accepted. |
| *Insured Services:* | Services rendered by a physician, surgeon or osteopathic physician that are medically required; <br> diagnostic x-ray and laboratory services; <br> anesthetic services; <br> x-ray, radium, cobalt, or isotope therapy, under supervision or order of attending physician; <br> psychiatric treatment limited to 15 hours of psychotherapy, after which psychiatrist must confirm that further treatment is necessary; <br> physiotherapy treatments not in excess of $50 per patient in any one year, and a maximum of $100 per family in any one year; <br> special nursing services by a registered nurse to a maximum of $40 per patient in any one year, where services deemed advisable by a physician or surgeon; <br> orthoptic treatment when on instructions of or referral by a physician but not to exceed $50 per patient in any one year, and a maximum of $100 per family in any one year; <br> administration of injections that follow accepted therapeutic practice for up to $50 per patient in any one year, when provided or administered by a physician; <br> services of chiropractors for up to $50 per patient in any one year, and up to a maximum of $100 per family in any one year; <br> services of a naturopathic physician for up to $50 per patient in any one year, and to a maximum of $100 in any one year per contract; <br> services of podiatrists, not to exceed $50 per patient in any one year, and a maximum of $100 per family in any one year, for services rendered otherwise than on instructions of or referral by a physician; <br> services of optometrists for tests of visual acuity but no more than one payment per patient per year; <br> medically required surgical procedures commonly performed only by a surgeon or a dental surgeon when done in a hospital. |
| *Exclusions:* | Services a person is eligible for and entitled to under various provincial and federal acts, such as Workman's Compensation Act, Hospital Insurance Act, Veterans' Rehabilitation Act, and so on. Medicolegal services: services for industrial or insurance purposes; advice by telephone; traveling; cosmetic services to a person over age 15; services which, on review of medical evidence, the Commission determines are not medically required. |
| *Out-of-Province Benefits:* | Payment for costs of insured services up to an amount not exceeding the amount otherwise payable under the plan. |

*PROVINCE OF BRITISH COLUMBIA* (Continued)

*Extension of Coverage*
*after Loss of Residence:*

Ninety days. If insured becomes a resident of another province participating under the federal Medical Care Act;
coverage extends 90 days plus traveling time. Students in
full-time attendance at recognized institutions outside the
province may continue to be insured persons under the
plan. Head of family receives coverage beyond 90 days absence if dependents continue to reside in the province and
are maintained by him.

*Method and Scale of*
*Payments to Physicians:*

A medical practitioner may elect to collect fees otherwise
than from the plan without loss of benefit to the insured.
Participating physicians submit claims to and receive payment from the Commission or licenced carrier. Payment
based on a tariff of fees agreed upon between the Commission and the British Columbia Medical Association. Nonparticipating physicians must complete claim form for or
furnish information to an insured person so that he may
obtain his benefit under the plan.

*Provision for Extra-*
*billing by Physicians:*

Participating physicians: only if reasonable notice given to
insured person, insured consents in writing and the amount
made known to the Commission. Nonparticipating physicians; may deal directly with patient for payment but insured entitled to reimbursement under the plan only when
physician has given notice in writing, there is written agreement between physician and insured on amount of extra-
billing, and the insured submits the claim to the Commission. If any insured person agrees to pay an amount in
excess of the fee prescribed by the Commission, neither the
Commission nor any carrier shall be liable for the excess.

*Provision for Private*
*Insurance Coverage:*

Regulations provide that a carrier which is not a licenced
carrier should not sell, provide, or offer to sell or provide
medical insurance or a plan for the prepayment of insured
services to residents of the province.

*Licenced Carriers:*

The British Columbia Medical Plan
1410 Government Street, Victoria, B.C.;
The Health Services Society
22 East 8th Avenue, Vancouver, B.C.; and
Medical Services Association
2045 West Broadway, Vancouver, B.C.,
There are seven offices in all for licenced carriers.

*PROVINCE OF MANITOBA*

*Name of Plan:* Manitoba Health Plan.
*Provincial Legislation:* The Manitoba Health Services Insurance Act and Regulations.*

*Effective Date:* April 1, 1969.
*Administration and*
*Method of Operation:* Administered by the Manitoba Health Services Commission
through Manitoba Medical Service.

---

*Published by the Queen's Printer for the Province of Manitoba.

*PROVINCE OF MANITOBA* (Continued)

*Method of Provincial*
*Financing:*

Monthly premiums: single $4.15, family $8.30, as of January, 1973. Tax revenue made available to the Commission through the Manitoba Health Services Insurance Fund.

*Utilization Fees:* None.

*Insured Persons:* Every resident of Manitoba must register himself and his dependents. Every resident liable to the Commission for payment of premium for himself and dependents. No waiting period for immigrants.

*Date upon which Resident*
*becomes a Beneficiary:* On becoming a resident and completing registration.

*Insured Services:* All personal health care services that are medically required and rendered by a medical practitioner, including specified surgical procedures performed by a registered oral surgeon or dental surgeon in a hospital.

optometric services: One eye examination, including refraction and prescription once a year. When the Commission is satisfied a need exists, an additional complete eye examination, including refraction, may be allowed.

chiropractic services: benefits payable up to $50 per single person, $100 for a family of up to three members, and $150 for larger families of four or more, each year.

hospital: immunization or examination for purposes of travel, employment or emigration; mileage, traveling time, advice by telephone; elective plastic surgery for cosmetic purposes except where Commission is satisfied on medical evidence that such surgery is not necessary; laboratory and x-ray procedures performed in facilities approved by the Commission; any service provided under the Hospital Services Insurance Act and Regulations.

*Out-of-Province*
*Benefits:*

Payment for the cost of issued services up to an amount not exceeding the amount that would otherwise be payable under the plan.

*Extension of Coverage*
*after loss of Residence:*

three months if insured person obtains an out-of-province certificate from the Commission. Traveling time not exceeding one month may be allowed.

*Method and Scale of*
*Payments to Physician:*

A medical practitioner may elect to collect his fees other than from the Commission.

Participating physician: reimbursed directly by the Commission. Payment at about 85 per cent of Manitoba Medical Association 1967 Schedule of Fees.

Nonparticipating physicians: must give reasonable notice that he proposes to collect payment from the insured.

*Provision for Extra-*
*billing by Physicians:*

Participating physician: not permitted to extra-bill.

Nonparticipating physician: may extra-bill if reasonable notice given and if insured person agrees to pay fee in excess of benefit.

*Provision for Private*
*Insurance Coverage:*

Act prohibits private insurance coverage for the cost of services that are benefits under the plan.

*Personal Care*
*Home Program:*

Personal care is assistance received by persons requiring

*PROVINCE OF MANITOBA* (Continued)

nursing care or personal attention or supervision with activities of daily living. It is given in personal care homes and hostels designated by the Manitoba Health Services Commission. All details as to which are approved homes, how one applies, who is eligible, what are the benefits, the choice of where to go, and charges for noninsured services above the residential charge of $4.50 per day may be obtained from the Commission.

## PROVINCE OF NEWFOUNDLAND

*Name of Plan:*     Newfoundland Medical Care Plan.

*Provincial Legislation:*     The Newfoundland Medical Care Insurance Act, 1968;* The Newfoundland Medical Care Insurance (Insured Services) Regulations, 1969; The Newfoundland Medical Care Insurance (Beneficiaries and Enquiries) Regulations, 1969; The Newfoundland Medical Services Insurance (Physicians and Fees) Regulations, 1969.

*Effective Date:*     April 1, 1969.

*Administration and Method of Operation:*     Administered and operated by the Newfoundland Medical Care Commission.

*Method of Provincial Financing:*     Tax revenue made available to the Commission through the Newfoundland Medical Care Insurance Fund. No direct payment or premium. Each person registered is issued a personal identity number of 12 digits; cost of replacement is $10.

*Utilization Fees:*     None.

*Insured Persons:*     Every resident *must* register himself and his dependents.

*Date upon which Resident becomes a Beneficiary:*     If individual enters Newfoundland from another province participating in a plan for which a contribution is payable under the Medical Care Act (Canada), coverage begins three months after arrival. Otherwise from date of arrival, including immigrants.

*Insured Services:*     All physicians' services medically required, including office, hospital or home visits; diagnosis and treatment of illness and injuries, and treatment of fractures and dislocations; care and treatment before, during and after operations; anesthetics; complete maternity care; services of specialists on referral; specific surgical procedures rendered in hospital by dentists.

*Physicians:*     Services to which a beneficiary is entitled under any federal or provincial act or any laws in force where services are provided; advice by telephone; cost of preparation by a physician of records, reports, or certificates for or on behalf of a beneficiary; any diagnostic, therapeutic, x-ray or laboratory services other than those listed in the diagnostic and therapeutic procedures section of the fee schedule; transportation charges for patient or doctor; examinations at request

---

*Published by the Queen's Printer for the Province of Newfoundland.

*PROVINCE OF NEWFOUNDLAND* (Continued)

of a third party; glasses, hearing aids, splints and appliances. No plastic or other surgery for cosmetic purposes unless medically indicated.

*Out-of-Province*
*Benefits:*

During temporary absence: same as those specified; if absence is *outside* of Canada, upon receipt of proof; at rate normally paid under the other province's medical care plan, if inside Canada.

*Extension of Coverage*
*after Loss of Residence:*

Three months if a person remains in Canada; if he becomes a resident of another participating province, traveling time also allowed.
A physician may elect to collect payments other than from the Commission.
    Participating physician: accepts payment from Commission as payment in full for services rendered.
    Nonparticipating physician: bills patients, who have right to receive amount of benefit from Commission.
    Payments by Commission are at 90 per cent of the 1967 Newfoundland Medical Association Schedule of Fees.

*Provision for Extra-*
*billing by Physicians:*

Participating physician: not permitted to extra-bill.
    Nonparticipating physician: may extra-bill provided he informs the beneficiary and provides the information required by the Commission to enable payment to be made under the Act to the beneficiary.

*Provision for Private*
*Insurance Coverage:*

No prohibition in legislation against private carriers providing coverage for cost of medical services that are insured services under the plan.

*PROVINCE OF NOVA SCOTIA*

*Name of Plan:*    Nova Scotia Medical Services Insurance.
*Provincial Legislation:*    Medical Care Insurance Act and Regulations.*
*Effective Date:*    April 1, 1969.
*Administration and*
*Method of Operation:*

Policy direction by Nova Scotia Medical Care Insurance Commission. Administered by Maritime Medical Care Incorporated on a nonprofit basis, in cooperation with Provincial Government's Division of Administrative Services.

*Method of*
*Provincial Financing:*    Taxation, as in Newfoundland.
*Utilization Fees:*    None.
*Insured Persons:*    All residents who are registered.
*Date upon which Resident*
*becomes a Beneficiary:*

After three months' residency, on registration; immigrants on the day they become a resident of the province. Transients, tourists, and visitors not eligible under M.S.I.

*Insured Services:*    All necessary medical and surgical services, including:
anesthetists' services;
complete obstetrical care;

---

*Published by The Queen's Printer for the Province of Nova Scotia.

*PROVINCE OF NOVA SCOTIA* (Continued)

treatment of fractures and dislocations;

all necessary referred specialist services;

all required diagnostic services, except those available under the Hospital Insurance Act;

eye examinations (including refraction);

well-baby care and physical examinations when deemed medically required by the physician;

specified surgical dental procedures (listed in Schedule "A" to Regulations) when performed in a hospital by a dental surgeon.

*Exclusions:*      Services available under Workmen's Compensation Act, N.S. Hospital Insurance Act, or other Government statute; ambulance; doctor's mileage or advice by telephone; routine physical examinations; cost of preparation of records, reports and certificates by a physician; eye glasses, hearing aids, surgical appliances, crutches, artificial limbs or other prosthetic appliances; dental services (other than those listed in Schedule "A"); services of optometrists, chiropractors, podiatrists, physiotherapists, nurses, or paramedical personnel; laboratory or diagnostic radiological services rendered in Nova Scotia.

*Out-of-Province*
*Benefits:*      All insured services; benefit entitlement not to exceed amount that would have been paid had the services been provided in Nova Scotia.

In hospitals elsewhere in the world, a payment of up to $40 per day for services provided from January 1, 1968 to December 31, 1970; $70 from January 1, 1971 to October 31, 1972, and $100 plus 75 per cent of the remainder from November 1, 1972 may be made for any adult or child, and up to $7 per day for an infant less than 15 days old, for services provided on and from May 1, 1966, and $11 from January 1, 1970.

*Extension of Coverage*
*after Loss of Residence:*      If a person becomes a resident of another province, he is covered for normal traveling time and any waiting period not exceeding three months that may be necessary in order to qualify for benefits under that province's plan. If the head of family moves to a new province, and leaves family behind, he will be considered as *temporarily* absent.

*Method and Scale of*
*Payments to Physicians:*      A physician may elect to collect his fees other than from the Corporation.

Participating physician: submits claims to and receives payment from the Corporation.

Nonparticipating physician: not entitled to charge for services to a resident unless he gives reasonable notice of his election to do so to the resident. If requested by the resident, must complete prescribed claim form or provide sufficient information to enable resident to complete form.

Benefits payments in accordance with tariff established by Commission, based on 1967 Schedule of Fees of Medical Society of Nova Scotia.

*PROVINCE OF NOVA SCOTIA* (Continued)

*Provision for Extra-*
*billing by Physicians:*     Physicians may charge a fee in excess of the tariff if they give reasonable notice of intention to charge a greater amount, the insured consents in writing to the extra charge, and the amount of the extra charge is made known to the Commission.

*Provision for Private*
*Insurance Coverage:*     No prohibition in legislation against private carriers providing coverage for cost of medical services that are insured services under the plan.

*PROVINCE OF SASKATCHEWAN*

*Name of Plan:*     Saskatchewan Medical Care Insurance Plan.
Saskatchewan Hospital Services Plan.

*Provincial Legislation:*     The Saskatchewan Medical Care Insurance Act and Regulations. The Medical Care Insurance Supplementary Provisions Act, 1968.*

*Effective Date:*     July 1, 1962.

*Administration and*
*Method of Operation:*     Administered by the Saskatchewan Medical Care Insurance Commission, and the Saskatchewan Hospital Services Plan. Approved nonprofit health agencies may provide services on receiving statements of accounts from medical members for insured services, receiving payments from the Commission and making payments to medical members.

*Method of Provincial*
*Financing:*     1973 Joint Tax Rates. *Swift Current:* single $24, family $48. Residents are liable for hospitalization only. *Other:* single $36; family head and spouse, plus dependents $72; single family head and dependents $36.

*Insured Persons:*     Every resident *must* register himself and his dependents.
*Date upon which Resident*
*becomes a Beneficiary:*     After three months' residency, on payment of tax. One month waiting period following payment of tax before eligibility for benefits.

*Insured Services:*     Medical services: diagnosis and treatment of all medical disabilities and conditions;
surgical services: diagnosis, preoperative care and treatment, surgical procedures, and postoperative care;
maternity services;
newborn care;
special services;
anesthesia;
x-ray laboratory and other diagnostic procedures;
preventive medical services: inoculations and vaccinations, routine physical examination but not for the purpose of marriage, insurance, or employment or at the request of a third party;
dental services when provided by a dentist in conjunction with maxillofacial surgery;
ocular examination by an optometrist to whom person

---

*Published by The Queen's Printer for the Province of Saskatchewan.

PROVINCE OF SASKATCHEWAN (Continued)

*Insured Services  Continued):*  has been referred by a physician. Does not include determination of refractive error;

refraction provided by a physician or an optometrist but limited to one per year where beneficiary has not reached seventeenth birthday; one every three years for persons aged 17 to 46 years, and one every two years for persons beyond age 46.

*Exclusions:*  Services received by beneficiaries under various provincial and federal acts, such as Workmen's Compensation Act, Saskatchewan Hospitalization Act, the Mental Health Act, and so forth.

Traveling by a physician; ambulance services and other forms of transportation of patients; services of special duty nurses; services for diagnosis or treatment of cancer; plastic or other surgery for cosmetic purposes; drugs and appliances; advice by telephone; examinations required for information of a third party; intermittent positive pressure breathing devices.

*Out-of-Province
Benefits:*  All insured services if provided by authorized persons, at rate payable in Saskatchewan, if in any province in Canada. Outside Canada, *up to* $50 per day (the latter rate would be emergency only), for a total of $2000 for one admission, when it reverts to $30 per day. Where required treatment is not available in Saskatchewan, payment will be made at 85 per cent of average daily charge to a maximum of $85 per day to a maximum of $4000.

*Extension of Coverage
after Loss of Residence:*  Three months.
*Method and Scale of
Payments to Physicians:*  Physicians may enter into agreement with Commission with respect to payment or may remain outside the plan.

Participating physicians submit claims to and receive payment from Commission. Payment is 85 per cent of schedule adopted by Commission after negotiation with doctor representatives.

Nonparticipating physicians must furnish information to patient to permit payment to be made by Commission to beneficiary.

*Provision for Extra-
billing by Physicians:*  Participating physician: accepts payment from Commission as payment in full for service. Nonparticipating physician: may deal directly with patient in respect to payment, in which event patient may receive the amount from Commission to which he is entitled under the plan.

*Provision for Private
Insurance Coverage:*  No prohibition in legislation against private carriers providing coverage for cost of medical services that are insured services under the plan.

The insurance organization of each province issues an annual report. This report contains information that is invaluable to a medical assistant-secretary and her employer. For example, Ontario issues a joint hospital/medical report; Saskatchewan issues two reports—one on medical care and one on hospitalization; Quebec and Manitoba each issue one report. The medical assistant should obtain the annual report for the province where she works, as it will bring her up-to-date on her province's plan.

At this point it will have become clear that not all provinces have only *one* type of coverage. Some have hospital care separated from medical care, although one payment may cover both. The Alberta Health Care Insurance Plan is a provincial plan with no private carriers, and excludes such items as Workmen's compensation payments, as is done in most provinces, while British Columbia has private carriers. No one in any province who is over 65 years of age pays a premium, but only some provinces extend immediate coverage to immigrants. Nova Scotia Medical Services Insurance combines with the Nova Scotia Hospital Insurance Commission to take care of residents. There are special arrangements for nursing homes and homes for the aged in some provinces, such as in Manitoba where they are considered under "personal care for residents," and, as well shall see, in Ontario. Other provinces have similar arrangements but few of the provinces are exactly the same as one another.

One may look at Ontario as a fairly typical example of what occurred in organizing a provincial insurance plan. The Plan was born when the Ontario Health Services Insurance Plan and the Ontario Hospital Services Commission were joined and all private carriers were abolished. The two organizations united to become the Ontario Health Insurance Plan. Similar occurrences brought about the same effect in other provinces across Canada.

## The Plan

OHIP = OHSIP + OHSC combined for:
(A) benefits
(B) premiums
A. Benefits are those currently being paid by one plan, i.e. doctors' bills formerly OHSIP), hospital bills (formerly OHSC), plus (as of April first) nursing homes and homes for the aged.
B. Premiums payable are reduced in that one lower premium covers both benefits.

Effective date was 1 April, 1972. (See Figure, *Introducing Your New Combined Government Plan*, from OHIP.)

Under OHIP, the new policy consisted of four major changes: abolition of premiums for all pensioners aged 65 and over; reduction in premium levels generally; improvement in premium assistance provisions; and replacement of the separate OHSIP and OHSC premiums with a single combined Health Insurance premium. All residents of Ontario kept their Ontario hospital insurance number as their new OHIP number. The new premiums were less than the old premiums, becoming $11 for an individual and $22 for a family, representing a savings of $4.80 for single people, $9.60 a year for couples, and $45 a year for families compared with the old system. Membership in OHIP is possible for groups through an employer and, of course, is also available as a pay-direct service for people who are, for instance, self-employed, or where an employer has too few employees to allow him to join OHIP as a group membership. In Ontario a group must consist of 15 or more people, and it is mandatory for an

## HEALTH INSURANCE FINANCING UNDER THE NEW POLICY AS COMPARED WITH THE PRESENT SYSTEM

### SOURCES AND APPLICATION OF FUNDS IN 1972-73

| | New Policy $ Millions | Present System $ Millions |
|---|---|---|
| Hospital and medical costs | 1585 | 1585 |
| Nursing home costs | 100 | 100 |
| TOTAL EXPENDITURE | 1685 | 1685 |
| Federal contributions | 695 = 41.2% | 695 = 41.2% |
| Premium Revenues | 498 = 29.6% | 625 = 37.1% |
| General provincial revenues | 492 = 29.2% | 365 = 21.7% |
| TOTAL FINANCING | 1685 | 1685 |

### WHO PAYS THE PREMIUMS

| | New Policy $ Million | Present System $ Million |
|---|---|---|
| Premiums paid by employers | 300 = 60.2% | 300 = 48.0% |
| Premiums paid by individuals | 198 = 39.8% | 325 = 52.0% |
| | 498 | 625 |
| Premium-free coverage | 1,534,000 persons | 458,000 persons |
| Half-premium coverage | 400,000 persons | 125,000 persons |

### PREMIUM PAYABLE BY A REPRESENTATIVE FAMILY

| Gross Income $ | Taxable Income $ | Full Premium Paid by Taxpayer — New Policy $ | Full Premium Paid by Taxpayer — Present System $ | Employer Pays $150 Towards Premium — New Policy $ | Employer Pays $150 Towards Premium — Present System $ |
|---|---|---|---|---|---|
| 2,000 | | nil | 132.00 | nil | nil |
| 3,000 | | nil | 132.00 | nil | nil |
| 3,000 | 330 | 132.00 | 202.80 | nil | 52.80 |
| 5,000 | 1,300 | 132.00 | 202.80 | nil | 52.80 |
| 7,000 | 3,300 | 264.00 | 309.00 | 159.00 | 159.00 |
| 10,000 | 6,300 | 264.00 | 309.00 | 159.00 | 159.00 |
| 15,000 | 11,300 | 264.00 | 309.00 | 159.00 | 159.00 |
| 20,000 | 16,300 | 264.00 | 309.00 | 159.00 | 159.00 |
| 30,000 | 26,300 | 264.00 | 309.00 | 159.00 | 159.00 |

Note:— Representative family consists of married taxpayer with two dependent children.
— Taxable income used in determining premium assistance is as calculated under the reformed income tax (i.e. 1972 rate structure, $3450 personal exemptions, 3% employment expense deduction and $100 standard deduction).

OHI-2

---

## HOW IT WILL WORK

### OHI Number and Billing System
Under the new plan combined coverage will be continued under the resident's present Ontario Hospital Insurance number and billing system. The OHSIP numbers and billing system will be discontinued.

### New Premiums
The first payment of premiums at the new combined rates of $11.00 for an individual and $22.00 for a family will be due in January, 1972, to cover benefit periods beginning April 1 and thereafter.

### Pensioners Who Now Remit Directly
All residents 65 or over who now remit Ontario Hospital Insurance premiums on a pay-direct basis will be sent a premium exemption application to complete and return to the plan. These will be mailed during the latter part of October, 1971. (See "Persons in Groups" below)

### Premium Assistance
Persons who remit premiums on a direct basis and wish to apply for premium-free coverage or premium assistance on the basis of income, may use the application form which will be supplied for this purpose as an insert with premium notices mailed in December, January and February next.

### Persons in Groups
Persons enrolled in groups who qualify for premium-free coverage or premium assistance will be reported to us by the group. Groups will be fully informed about this in the near future.

### New Identification Cards
The combined medical-hospital insurance plan will be known as the Ontario Health Insurance Plan. New health insurance identification cards will be supplied in advance of April 1st.

### IMPORTANT
Participation in the Ontario Health Insurance Plan will be based on each resident's present Ontario Hospital Insurance number and billing system. Anyone who is not now registered for Ontario Hospital Insurance should obtain an application from a bank, a hospital, or the Commission and register without delay in order to be insured on or before April 1, 1972.

Questions should be directed to:

Ontario Health Insurance Commission,
2195 Yonge Street, Toronto 7, Ontario

---

## INTRODUCING...

## YOUR NEW COMBINED GOVERNMENT PLAN

•

### AN OUTLINE OF REVISED GOVERNMENT POLICY

On Sept. 13, William Davis, Prime Minister of Ontario, announced important reforms in the premium system of financing hospital and medical insurance for Ontario residents. The new policy consists of four major changes: abolition of premiums for all pensioners aged 65 and over, reduction in premium levels generally, improvement in premium assistance provisions, and replacement of the separate OHSIP and OHSC premiums with a single combined health insurance premium. This new reform policy will reduce premium collections by $127 million annually.

**ONTARIO HEALTH INSURANCE COMMISSION**

---

## NEW POLICY

### Free Health Insurance for Pensioners
... Effective Jan. 1, 1972, hospital and medical insurance premiums will be waived for all residents of Ontario 65 years of age and over.

### Lower Premium Levels
... Effective April 1, 1972, the total health insurance premium will be reduced to $11 per month ($132 per year) for single persons and $22 per month ($264 per year) for couples and families. This represents a saving of $4.80 per year for single persons, $9.60 per year for couples and $45.00 per year for families, as compared with the present OHSIP-OHSC combined premium levels.

### Improved Premium Assistance
... Effective April 1, 1972, all single persons and families with no taxable income will be eligible for 100 per cent assistance on the new health combined premium. At present, such full premium assistance for low-income families and individuals is available only in respect of the OHSIP premium, not the OHSC premium.

... Effective April 1, 1972 eligibility for 50 per cent premium assistance will be broadened to include all single persons with taxable income under $1000 and all couples and families with taxable income under $2000. At present, partial premium assistance is available only in respect of the OHSIP premium and only up to taxable income levels of $500 for single persons, $1000 for couples and $1300 for families.

### New Combined Health Insurance Premium
... Effective April 1, 1972, the separate OHSIP and OHSC premiums will be combined into a single new health premium.

## QUESTIONS & ANSWERS

*Q. Why has the government introduced major changes in the present system of health insurance premiums?*
*A.* The reforms have been introduced in order to improve the equity and efficiency of health insurance financing. The new system will be fairer to low-income families and pensioners; it will treat subscribers uniformly both for hospital and medical coverage; and it will be cheaper to administer both for the government and for employers.

*Q. How will the government finance the $127 million reduction in premium revenues?*
*A.* The revenue loss resulting from the reform of health premiums will be accommodated within the general provincial budget.

*Q. Why are Ontario's health insurance premiums higher than in other provinces like Manitoba?*
*A.* There are a number of reasons. Under the national average cost-sharing formulas, the federal government pays a lower proportion of Ontario's hospital and medical costs than of other province's costs; Ontario's insured health services and treatment facilities are generally superior; other provinces, like Manitoba, finance their health insurance programs through higher income taxes or sales taxes in place of greater reliance on premiums.

*Q. Will the new health insurance premiums be increased in future years?*
*A.* Health insurance premiums in Ontario have not been increased for over three years, even though costs have steadily risen, in order to reduce the regressive impact of premium financing on low-income families. The government intends to continue this policy of holding down premium levels and shifting a larger share of health financing onto the general provincial tax structure.

*Q. What will happen under the new premium system to the health premium contribution paid by employers?*
*A.* Employers will be expected to maintain at least the same level of premium contributions on behalf of employees under the new system as they are paying under the existing system. Any dollar saving to the employers as a result of the lower premiums are to be passed on to the employees as, for example, in the form of a higher employer share of the new health premium, in the form of equivalent fringe benefits, or in the form of higher wages.

*Q. Under the new premium system, what proportion of premiums will be paid by individuals as opposed to employers?*
*A.* The proportion of total premiums paid by individuals will decline from 52% to 40% whereas the share paid by employers will increase from 48% to 60%. For example, the combined annual premium for a family is presently $309.00 compared with the new rate of $264.00. Therefore, if an employer is presently paying 50% of the premium, the individual share will decline from $154.50 to $109.50 or $9.12 per month.

*Q. Will persons removed from the income tax rolls in 1972 as a result of income tax reforms be eligible for full premium assistance after April 1, 1972?*
*A.* Yes. Eligibility for premium assistance is presently based on taxable income for the previous year. However, as of April 1, 1972 this will be changed to ensure that persons removed from the tax rolls in 1972 as a result of income tax reforms also benefit in 1972 from Ontario's reform of health premiums.

*Q. How many Ontario residents will get free health insurance coverage or pay partial premiums under the new premium system?*
*A.* Over 1½ million persons will be entitled to premium-free health insurance: 460,000 welfare recipients, 640,000 old age pensioners, and some 440,000 persons with no taxable income. In addition, some 400,000 persons will be insured at half premiums through the more generous criteria for partial premium assistance.

*Q. Will wives and eligible dependents of pensioners qualify for free coverage after January 1, 1972, even if they are not yet 65 years old?*
*A.* Yes. If such an insured person has an eligible dependent who is under 65 years old, this dependent will qualify for premium-free coverage as well.

*Q. If I am aged 65 or over and have already paid premiums to cover benefits after January 1, 1972, will there be a refund?*
*A.* Yes. If you pay your Hospital Insurance premiums on a direct basis, you will soon receive a premium exemption application to fill out. Your refund should be mailed within four weeks after this application is completed and returned to us. Any refundable OHSIP premiums will be sent to you separately.

*Q. When will the new combined health premium replace the present separate OHSIP and OHSC premiums?*
*A.* Conversion to the combined premium billing system will become effective for the benefit period commencing April 1, 1972.

*Q. Will the new health premiums of $11 and $22 cover nursing home benefits?*
*A.* Ontario plans to expand its health insurance program to cover nursing homes and home care services, effective April 1, 1972. To help finance this new insured benefit a charge of $3.50 a day will be levied on subscribers who use nursing home services. This fee of $3.50 a day will be over and above the regular health premium of $11 or $22 levied on all subscribers.

employer to form a group when he has more than 15 employees. Employee groups of more than 5 but less than 15 persons may, on application, form a mandatory group. The premiums for pay-direct participants are slightly different in that they are paid quarterly (every three months) at the rate of $33 for a single person, and $66 for a family. A family premium would cover the husband, his wife, and all unmarried, unemployed children up to the age of 18, and children of 18 and over who are financially dependent upon the parents because of

## WAITING PERIOD

| Condition* | Waiting Period |
|---|---|
| 1. No insurance (resident of Ontario) | The first day of the third month following the date application and premium are received. |
| 2. No insurance (immigrant) | The first of the month following receipt of application and premium (if application is made within 3 months of landing—if not, item 1 applies). |
| 3. Group to Pay-Direct | Continuous coverage, providing application is made together with Form 104). (See Form 104 and Application for Non-Group Enrollment.) |
| 4. Pay-Direct to Group | Continuous coverage. (The employer must be given the pay-direct OHIP number.) |
| 5. Group to Group | Continuous coverage (old employer must supply Form 104) |
| 6. Full-paying to part- or nonpaying | Will vary from case to case. (any premiums paid beyond date of acceptance for NP or PP will be refunded.) |
| 7. No insurance to PP or NP | The first of the third month following receipt of application. |
| 8. Group to PP or NP (direct) | No waiting period (Form 104 must be supplied). |
| 9. Group to PP or NP (in group) | The first of the third month following receipt of application (premium will be refunded if overpaid). |
| 10. Group or PD to NP if age 65 or over by January 31st, 1972 | Effective January 1st, 1972. |
| 11. Group or PD to NP because of reaching age 65 | The first of the month in which a member becomes age 65. |
| 12. No insurance, but age 65 or over | No waiting period. (Coverage may be back-dated to January 1st, 1972 or the first of the month in which a member became age 65, if applicant is a resident.) |
| 13. Over age 65 but nonresident | Full payment until 12 months of residence, then premium free, effective immediately. |
| 14. Contract holder over age 65 (deceased). | No waiting period. Spouse or dependents (under age 65) must apply for PD at full pay, unless eligible for premium assistance because of taxable income. |
| 15. Uninsured to Group | First day of third month following date of hire. |
| 16. Pay-Direct or nongroup | First day of the third month following the date the application is received by OHIP. Landed immigrants, persons 65 years of age or over, and people coming of age may warrant earlier effective date. (See Figure, *Application for Non-Group Enrollment.*) |

Note: Any lapse in premium or in notification of circumstances could result in a waiting period of 3 months.

*Code: PP—partial payment; NP—no payment; PD—pay direct.

ISSUED BY INSURED GROUPS IN COMPLIANCE WITH THE HEALTH INSURANCE COMMISSION ACT

# ONTARIO HEALTH INSURANCE COMMISSION

2195 YONGE STREET, TORONTO 295, ONTARIO

## CERTIFICATE OF PAYMENT · FORM 104

### USE THIS FORM TO CONTINUE YOUR INSURANCE

**①** WE CERTIFY THAT THE PAID-UP BENEFIT MONTH CURRENTLY PROVIDED FOR THIS PERSON THROUGH OUR GROUP ENDS AT ➤

| HEALTH INSURANCE NUMBER | SURNAME | INITIALS | SUPPLEMENTARY ✱ CODE | 12.01. A. M. |
|---|---|---|---|---|
| | | | | DAY | MO. | YEAR |
| ACCURACY IMPORTANT (8 FIGURES) | PLEASE TYPE OR PRINT CLEARLY | | | 1 |

GROUP NAME | GROUP NO. | DATE THIS FORM ISSUED

SIGNATURE OF GROUP OFFICIAL

SEE OVER ✱

**②** INSURED PERSON TO COMPLETE THIS SECTION (SEE ② OVER)

PLEASE PRINT CLEARLY

PLEASE ✓ IN PROPER BOXES

ADDRESS

OF

INSURED ✱ — P.O. BOX, RURAL ROUTE OR STREET ADDRESS

NAME OF CITY OR TOWN

✱ IF RURAL ROUTE OR GENERAL DELIVERY ENTER GIVEN NAME HERE (E.G. TOM, MARY, PETE SR, ETC.)

MR.

MRS.

MISS

SINGLE NO ELIGIBLE DEPENDENTS

FAMILY ONE OR MORE ELIGIBLE DEPENDENTS

DATE ............ SIGNATURE ............

✱ SEMI-PRIVATE SUPPLEMENT

IF YOU ARE NOW REGISTERED FOR SEMI-PRIVATE INSURANCE THROUGH THE COMMISSION, BUT DO NOT WISH TO CONTINUE IT, PLACE A CROSS (X) THROUGH THE SUPPLEMENTARY CODE PANEL ABOVE.

**FOR OFFICE USE ONLY**

| CAT. CODE | EFFECTIVE DATE | REV. DATE |
|---|---|---|
| | DAY | MO. | YR. | |

YOU MAY BE ELIGIBLE FOR PREMIUM ASSISTANCE OR PREMIUM EXEMPTION: IF SO, PLEASE PROVIDE DETAILS IN SECTION ③ OR ④ BELOW.

**③** ARE YOU ELIGIBLE FOR PREMIUM ASSISTANCE?

IF YOU HAVE BEEN A RESIDENT OF ONTARIO FOR THE PAST 12 MONTHS AND YOUR ESTIMATED TAXABLE INCOME FOR THE CURRENT YEAR WILL BE $1,000.00 OR LESS AS A SINGLE PERSON OR $2,000.00 OR LESS (INCLUDING INCOME OF SPOUSE) AS A FAMILY WITH ONE OR MORE DEPENDENTS, CHECK HERE ☐ SO THAT WE MAY SEND YOU AN APPLICATION FOR PREMIUM ASSISTANCE. (SEE ③ OVER)

DATE ............ SIGNATURE ............

**④** ARE YOU OR YOUR SPOUSE AGE 65 OR OVER?

IF SO, PLEASE SIGN AND DATE THE FOLLOWING STATEMENT: I HAVE BEEN A RESIDENT OF ONTARIO FOR THE PAST 12 MONTHS AND I REQUEST EXEMPTION FROM PAYMENT OF PREMIUMS BECAUSE MY AGE OR THE AGE OF MY SPOUSE IS 65 OR OVER. (SEE ④ OVER)

DATE BORN
MONTH | YEAR

SIGNATURE ............ DATE ............

**IMPORTANT:** IF YOU ARE PRESENTLY PAYING FOR SEMI-PRIVATE HOSPITAL COVERAGE AND IF YOU ARE APPROVED FOR PREMIUM FREE INSURANCE AS A RESULT OF COMPLETING SECTION ④, YOU WILL BE CONTACTED DIRECTLY BY THE PRIVATE INSURER REGARDING CONTINUATION OF YOUR SEMI-PRIVATE COVERAGE.

TO KEEP INSURED, FOLLOW CAREFULLY THE INSTRUCTIONS ON THE BACK OF THIS FORM

# CERTIFICATE OF PAYMENT-FORM 104-INSTRUCTIONS

**①** TO BE COMPLETED BY THE EMPLOYER OR COLLECTOR

When a person ceases to remit premiums through your group, you must immediately give him one of these forms with Section ① on the face of the Certificate completed so that he may take the necessary action to continue his insurance.

✱ NOTE: The date to be entered under the arrow is the first day of the month following the BENEFIT MONTH covered by your last deduction or payment for this person, e.g. if the last premium paid through your group for this person covers the benefit month of December **1968**, you should enter 1-1-69.

When a person transfers to your group from another group, he must give you the Certificate of Payment issued by his previous group (with Section ① and ② completed). Attach it to the Group Reconciliation Form (103) on which he is reported by you as a TRansfer-in.

**②** TO BE COMPLETED BY THE INSURED PERSON

To keep continuously insured YOU MUST TAKE IMMEDIATE ACTION as indicated below:

If you join an insured group without delay complete Section ② of the Certificate on the face of this form and give it to your new employer or collector immediately. He will then remit premiums on your behalf as required by, and subject to, Commission Regulations.

✱ NOTE: If the wife cannot remit premiums through a group but the husband can, the husband MUST use this form to begin payments through his group in his name.

If you do not immediately join an insured group, complete Section ② of the Certificate on the face of this form and send without delay to Ontario Health Insurance Commission, Toronto 295. It is not necessary to include payment. A premium notice will be sent to the address you provide, so that you may keep insured on a Pay-Direct basis.

**③** ARE YOU ELIGIBLE FOR PREMIUM ASSISTANCE?

PERSONS REQUESTING PREMIUM ASSISTANCE APPLICATION WILL ALSO BE SENT A PREMIUM NOTICE REQUESTING PAYMENT. IF PREMIUM ASSISTANCE IS APPROVED PREMIUMS PAID BEYOND THE EFFECTIVE DATE OF PREMIUM ASSISTANCE WILL BE REFUNDED.

**④** ARE YOU OR YOUR SPOUSE AGE 65 OR OVER?

INSURANCE MAY BE TRANSFERRED TO OLDER SPOUSE TO QUALIFY FOR PREMIUM FREE-COVERAGE. THIS MAY BE ARRANGED BY CHANGING INITIALS TO THAT OF THE OLDER SPOUSE ON THE FRONT OF THIS FORM. ALSO ENTER MONTH AND YEAR OF BIRTH (OLDER SPOUSE) IN DATE BORN PANEL ON FRONT OF FORM.

**IMPORTANT:** IF YOU ARE PRESENTLY PAYING FOR SEMI-PRIVATE HOSPITAL COVERAGE AND IF YOU ARE APPROVED FOR PREMIUM FREE INSURANCE AS A RESULT OF COMPLETING SECTION ④, YOU WILL BE CONTACTED DIRECTLY BY THE PRIVATE INSURER REGARDING CONTINUATION OF YOUR SEMI-PRIVATE COVERAGE.

THERE IS A PENALTY FOR MISUSE OF THIS FORM

physical or mental infirmity, or who are still attending a school, college, or university as full-time students. Any person who has an eligible dependent will pay the family premium.

Premium assistance is possible when people are in financial difficulty. Assistance can be temporary or it can go on for quite awhile. There are special forms for applying for premium assistance that will be shown at the end of this section. Extended health care benefits are available and refer to care received in a nursing home, or in a home for the aged by sick people who require skilled nursing service, or for regular medical care in an institution other than a hospital. Premium assistance or temporary assistance is dependent on the income of the individual entering the home.

## Types of Coverage

1. Single = one person on the contract.
2. Family = contract holder plus one or more dependents.
Dependents are:
1. Spouse.
2. Children under age 21 (unmarried and not employed) financially dependent on the contract holder.
3. Common law spouse.

| Current Coverage | Requested Coverage and Effective Date |
|---|---|
| Single and single | Family: First of third month following date of marriage.<br>A. Both insurance numbers must be quoted on application.<br>B. Both 104 forms must accompany the application, if group coverage.<br>Note: Correct mailing address must be supplied. |
| Single and family | Family: First of month following marriage.<br>Note: Any overpaid premium will be refunded on the single contract. |
| Family and family | Family: First of month following marriage.<br>Note: Overpaid premium will be refunded on one of the contracts. |
| Single and under-age dependent | Family: First of month following marrage.<br>Note: Premium overpaid on behalf of dependent can be refunded on request. |
| Single new parent | Family: Effective date of birth of baby.<br>Note: 90 days free coverage for infant. |
| Family to Single (death of holder or dependent) | Continuous coverage effect first of month following death.<br>Note: Survivor must notify OHIP if name of contract holder is to be changed. Overpaid premium will be refunded. |
| Under-age dependent to Single | A. First of month following twenty-first birthday. (Automatic deletion of dependent from parents' contract. Three months' premium are required with application unless qualified for premium assistance.)<br>B. Continuous coverage. (Coverage through group will start first of third month following date of hire.) |

## WHEN COVERAGE BEGINS

Coverage begins on the first day of the third month following the date your application is received by OHIP. However, applications for persons becoming aged twenty-one (formerly covered by parent) residents, aged sixty-five or older, new residents and landed immigrants, may warrant earlier effective dates, depending on individual circumstances.

## YOUR IDENTIFICATION CARD

Once enrolled, you will be supplied with an Ontario Health Insurance Identification Card to carry in your purse or wallet. It should be presented to the hospital, physician or practitioner each time insured services are required. ALWAYS QUOTE YOUR HEALTH INSURANCE NUMBER WHEN WRITING OR TELEPHONING THE PLAN.

## CHANGES AFFECTING YOUR COVERAGE

As a Non-Group participant it is important that you notify the Plan if:

- you change your address
- your marital status changes
- your eligible dependent turns age 21 or marries
- you or your spouse turn age 65
- you are enrolled as Single and acquire an eligible dependent

**If you (or your spouse) become employed where there is an insured group,** you must transfer your insurance to the group. To do so, give your employer your Ontario Health Insurance Number.

## FOR FURTHER INFORMATION

Contact your local Ontario Health Insurance Commission office or write to:

**ONTARIO HEALTH INSURANCE COMMISSION**
2195 YONGE STREET
TORONTO 295, ONTARIO

FORM 105 (1/72)

## APPLICATION
### FOR
## NON-GROUP
## ENROLMENT

### PROTECTION
### AGAINST THE COST OF

- Hospital Care
- Physicians' Services
- Practitioners' Services

*You are eligible for Non-Group Enrolment if you are a resident of Ontario not employed where there is an insured group.*

---

**THE PLAN** Ontario Health Insurance is a comprehensive Government-sponsored plan of health insurance for the people of Ontario. It provides a wide scope of benefits for medical and hospital services plus additional benefits for the services of certain health practitioners. This is the only plan of basic health insurance available to Ontario residents and all residents are entitled to participate. Tourists, transients and visitors to Ontario are not eligible.

## BRIEF OUTLINE OF BENEFITS

The following is only a concise description of benefits available under the Plan. More details are available on request.

## HOSPITAL CARE

The Plan pays for hospital care which is medically necessary in the treatment of an insured patient in a standard (public) ward of an approved hospital. It also covers a broad range of hospital out-patient services plus medically-prescribed physiotherapy in private non-hospital facilities approved by the Commission.

## AMBULANCE SERVICE

Essential and medically-necessary ambulance service is a benefit of the Plan but the insured person is required to pay a small portion of the cost of each trip.

## MEDICAL SERVICES

Benefits are provided for medically-necessary physicians' services received at home, in a doctor's office or in hospital. This includes the services of general practitioners and specialists. Payments are made at the rate of 90% of the Ontario Medical Association Schedule of Fees (1971).

## OTHER SERVICES

Specified dental surgery performed in hospital is covered up to 90% of the Ontario Dental Association Schedule of Fees (1969) . . . Eye examinations by refraction by an optometrist to determine the need for glasses: $10.00 per person . . . Chiropractic, Osteopathic and Chiropody (Podiatry) services: up to $100.00, plus $25.00 for radiographic examinations, per person, for each of these three types of services. The dollar maximums quoted above apply to the twelve-month period beginning July 1, each year.

## CARE OUTSIDE ONTARIO

Insured physicians' and practitioners' services received outside Ontario are covered to the same extent they would be paid for in Ontario. The amount payable for hospital care is determined by the Commission on the basis of the medical need to obtain the care outside Ontario.

## SERVICES NOT COVERED

Any hospital charges for private or semi-private accommodation;

Hospital visits solely for the administration of drugs;

Dental care, in hospital, which is normally provided in the dentist's office; Fees for dental services other than specified;

Eyeglasses, special appliances;

Private duty nursing fees;

Drugs, vaccines, biological serum or extracts or their synthetic substitutes (except when provided in hospital); Drugs taken home from the hospital;

Transportation charges other than approved ambulance service;

Medical examinations required for applications for employment or the continuance of employment, life insurance, schools, camps or recreation;

Payment for any health service other than those provided by approved hospitals or the physicians and practitioners specified in this brochure.

---

**PREMIUM RATES . . .**

The premiums are $11.00 a month for the single person and $22.00 a month for the family. Pay-Direct participants, however, pay quarterly i.e., $33.00 single and $66.00 family every three months. The family premium covers husband, wife and all unmarried, unemployed children under the age of twenty-one, and children of twenty-one and over who are financially dependent because of physical or mental infirmity. Any person who has an eligible dependent pays the family premium.

---

*See Sections 7 and 8 of the application regarding free coverage for residents aged 65 or over and premium assistance.*

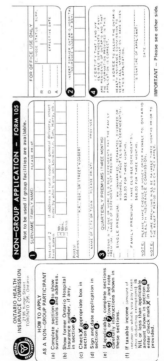

4. Children over age 21 if mentally or physically infirm.
5. Grandchildren, adopted children or foster children, if financially dependent on contract holder.

Changes in Types of Coverage: OHIP must be notified within 30 days of the change date.

## Groups

A group may be formed with 6 to 14 employees. Every employer with 15 or more employees is required by the Ontario Hospital Insurance Commission Act to form a group. Once a group has been formed all eligible employees must be included.

Payroll deductions are made to pay the monthly premiums. The employer may pay or contribute to the employee's premium. The amount contributed by the employer will depend on the existing employer/employee agreement. (See page 21 of the OHI Manual.)

When an employee is enrolled in a group, he will be assigned a group number. This number will appear on his identification card, along with his OHIP number.

Groups are supplied with the following forms,* which are used to up-date members and remittance.

**Form 102.** Group Remittance Summary shows previous month's return and any additions or deletions for current month.

**Form 103.** Group Reconciliation Form gives detailed information on additions, deletions to the groups.

**Form 116.** Request for Refund. This gives detailed information about any request for refunds which were not legally payable.

**OHI-1.** Request for premium exemption for group members aged 65 or over.

**Form 108.** Request for exemption. To be completed by employee for premium exemption.

**Form 104.** Certificate of Payment. To be completed and submitted to OHIP with form 102 (Group Remittance Summary Advice) before taking any credit. (See *Certificate of Payment, Form 104.*)

Pay-direct members of OHSC are issued the following forms with their premium notice:

**OHI 3.** Exemption Form. I.B.M. computer card to be completed by member and returned to OHSC, if age is over 65.

**OHI 10.** Letter to member, with instructions to complete the OHI 4 card.

**OHI 4.** Sent with OHI-10 letter to members, following OHI 3.

Application for a Premium Assistance Form is forwarded to all OHSC pay-direct members. Application is made on Form 519 (1/72) and is shown here.

Application for Temporary Assistance is made on Form E539 (2/72), shown on opposite page.

---

*Three forms only are shown as examples, as OHIP will supply any forms upon request.

ONLY APPLICABLE IF YOUR TAXABLE INCOME
IS WITHIN LIMITS LISTED ON REVERSE SIDE

FOR OFFICE USE ONLY

## APPLICATION FOR PREMIUM ASSISTANCE

INSURANCE NUMBER

SUBSCRIBER'S SURNAME

INITIALS

FOR OFFICE USE ONLY

| CATE-GORY | STATUS P.A.A.S. |

SUPP. CODE

SEE NOTE (A)

GROUP NUMBER

SUBSCRIBER'S ADDRESS

HOW MANY PEOPLE ARE INSURED
UNDER THIS NUMBER?

ADULTS | DEPENDANTS

TELEPHONE NUMBER

OCCUPATION | DATE OF BIRTH | MARITAL STATUS

☐ MARRIED ☐ SEPARATED ☐ WIDOWED
☐ SINGLE ☐ DIVORCED ☐ OTHER

### DECLARATION OF INCOME

FOR OFFICE USE ONLY

ITEMS # 1 AND # 4 MUST BE COMPLETED.   IF APPLICABLE, COMPLETE ITEMS # 2 AND # 3.

| | YEAR | DOLLARS | CENTS |
|---|---|---|---|
| 1. TOTAL INCOME OF YOU AND YOUR SPOUSE FOR YEAR ENDING DECEMBER 31 LAST – SEE NOTE (B) . . . . . . . . | | | |
| 2. ESTIMATED INCREASE IN COMBINED INCOME FOR THE CURRENT YEAR – SEE NOTE (C) . . . . . . . . . . . | | | |
| 3. ESTIMATED TOTAL INCOME OF YOU AND YOUR SPOUSE FOR THE CURRENT YEAR . . . . . . . . . . . . . | | | |

4. ELIGIBLE DEPENDANTS FOR WHOM YOU CLAIM EXEMPTION FOR INCOME TAX PURPOSES –
SEE NOTE (D)

| WIFE/HUSBAND | | CHILDREN UNDER SIXTEEN | | CHILDREN AND ADULTS OVER SIXTEEN | |

I HEREBY APPLY FOR PREMIUM ASSISTANCE. I HAVE BEEN A RESIDENT OF ONTARIO FOR THE PAST
TWELVE MONTHS. I AGREE TO ALLOW THE ONTARIO HEALTH INSURANCE COMMISSION TO VERIFY
ALL STATEMENTS MADE BY ME ON THIS APPLICATION.

DATE | SIGNATURE OF SUBSCRIBER

THERE IS A PENALTY FOR KNOWINGLY FILING FALSE INFORMATION.

NOTES:
THE FOLLOWING SHOULD BE READ AND USED AS A GUIDE WHEN COMPLETING YOUR
APPLICATION FOR PREMIUM ASSISTANCE:

(A)   IT IS IMPORTANT THAT YOU ENTER YOUR ONTARIO HEALTH INSURANCE NUMBER. ENTER YOUR SUPPLEMENTARY CODE IF YOU HAVE SUPPLEMENTARY COVERAGE. YOU WILL FIND THESE NUMBERS ON YOUR ONTARIO HEALTH INSURANCE CERTIFICATE.

IF YOU ARE A GROUP SUBSCRIBER, PLEASE ENTER YOUR GROUP NUMBER. A GROUP SUBSCRIBER MUST WAIT FOR OUR ACKNOWLEDGEMENT AND CONFIRMATION OF PREMIUM ASSISTANCE BEFORE EXEMPTING HIS/HER SELF FROM HIS/HER GROUP.

IF YOU ARE NOT ENROLLED FOR ONTARIO HEALTH INSURANCE, AND YOU ARE NOT EMPLOYED WHERE THERE IS AN OHIP GROUP, PLEASE COMPLETE AND RETURN WITH THIS APPLICATION, AN APPLICATION FOR NON GROUP ENROLMENT. THESE APPLICATIONS ARE AVAILABLE AT OHIP OFFICES, HOSPITALS, AND CHARTERED BANKS THROUGHOUT THE PROVINCE.

(B)   TOTAL INCOME IS YOUR GROSS INCOME BEFORE DEDUCTIONS, OR IF YOU ARE MARRIED, THE COMBINED INCOME OF YOU AND YOUR WIFE/HUSBAND.

(C)   IF YOU HAVE SINGLE COVERAGE AND ANTICIPATE AN INCREASE IN THE CURRENT YEAR OF MORE THAN $500.00 IN YOUR TOTAL INCOME, ENTER THIS ESTIMATED INCREASE IN ITEM 2. IF YOU HAVE FAMILY COVERAGE AND ANTICIPATE AN INCREASE IN THE CURRENT YEAR OF MORE THAN $850.00

IN YOUR COMBINED TOTAL INCOME, ENTER THIS ESTIMATED INCREASE IN ITEM 2. IF YOU ANTICIPATE AN INCREASE OF LESS THAN $500.00 A YEAR (SINGLE COVERAGE) OR LESS THAN $850.00 A YEAR (FAMILY COVERAGE), LEAVE ITEMS 2 AND 3 BLANK.

(D)   INCLUDE HERE ALL PERSONS FOR WHOM YOU AND YOUR WIFE OR HUSBAND CLAIM PERSONAL EXEMPTION FOR INCOME TAX PURPOSES.

(E)   WE WILL ASSUME THAT, IN ACCORDANCE WITH ANY NEW TAX REFORMS, YOU ARE ENTITLED TO NORMAL EXEMPTIONS FOR SINGLE OR MARRIED STATUS, DEPENDANTS, UNEMPLOYMENT INSURANCE, EMPLOYMENT EXPENSES, CANADA PENSION PLAN CONTRIBUTIONS, ETC. ON THIS BASIS WE WILL ESTIMATE YOUR TAXABLE INCOME FOR THE CURRENT YEAR FOR PREMIUM ASSISTANCE PURPOSES.

HOWEVER, IF YOU HAVE ANY OTHER SIGNIFICANT ALLOWABLE EXEMPTIONS SUCH AS CHILD CARE, REGISTERED PENSION, HIGH MEDICATION COSTS, ETC., PLEASE LIST THEM BELOW OR ATTACH SEPARATELY AND WE WILL TAKE THEM INTO CONSIDERATION WHEN ASSESSING YOUR TAXABLE INCOME.

# Semi-Private Hospital Coverage

Semiprivate coverage for premium-exempt persons are now billed directly by the semiprivate carrier, e.g., Blue Cross (a sample form is shown), Cumba, and H.M.C. (Hospital Medical Care).

Those persons now applying for semiprivate coverage through pay-direct or a group will continue to be billed with their regular OHIP billing.

**APPLICATION FOR TEMPORARY ASSISTANCE**

| INSURANCE NUMBER | SURNAME | INITIALS | DATE OF BIRTH |
|---|---|---|---|
| | | | DAY  MONTH  YEAR |

MARITAL STATUS
- [ ] MARRIED
- [ ] SEPARATED
- [ ] SINGLE
- [ ] WIDOWED
- [ ] DIVORCED
- [ ] OTHER

ADDRESS

NUMBER OF DEPENDENTS
(SPOUSE & CHILDREN)

TELEPHONE NUMBER

USUAL OCCUPATION

ARE YOU PRESENTLY EMPLOYED?
- [ ] YES
- [ ] NO

### STUDENTS ONLY

NAME AND ADDRESS OF SCHOOL

DATE COURSE COMMENCED
DAY  MONTH  YEAR

EXPECTED DATE COURSE COMPLETED
DAY  MONTH  YEAR

| DECLARATION OF INCOME | | DECLARATION OF LIQUID ASSETS | |
|---|---|---|---|
| LIST YOUR PRESENT MONTHLY INCOME INCLUDING THE INCOME OF YOUR SPOUSE AND DEPENDENT CHILDREN | | LIST ALL YOUR LIQUID ASSETS AND THOSE OF YOUR SPOUSE AND DEPENDENT CHILDREN | |
| WAGES & SALARY (SELF) | $ | CASH | $ |
| WAGES & SALARY (SPOUSE) | | BANK DEPOSITS | |
| WORKMAN'S COMPENSATION | | CREDIT UNION DEPOSITS | |
| PENSIONS | | SAVINGS BONDS | |
| U. I. C. BENEFITS | | OTHER BONDS & SECURITIES | |
| SUPPLEMENTARY UNEMPLOYMENT OR SICK BENEFITS | | OTHER (SPECIFY) | |
| GRANTS, BURSARIES OR SCHOLARSHIPS | | | |
| MANPOWER TRAINING ALLOWANCE | | | |
| OTHER (SPECIFY) | | | |
| | | | |
| TOTAL | $ | TOTAL | $ |

### CONDITIONS

I AM THE APPLICANT NAMED IN THIS APPLICATION.

ALL STATEMENTS IN THIS APPLICATION ARE TRUE TO THE BEST OF MY KNOWLEDGE AND NO INFORMATION HAS BEEN CONCEALED OR OMITTED.

MY FINANCIAL POSITION IS SUCH THAT I AM UNABLE TO CONTINUE ALL OR ANY PORTION OF THE SUBSCRIPTION FOR MY PRESENT COVERAGE OR I AM UNABLE TO PURCHASE COVERAGE.

I AGREE TO ALLOW THE ONTARIO HEALTH INSURANCE COMMISSION TO VERIFY ALL STATEMENTS MADE BY ME ON THIS APPLICATION.

I AGREE THAT ANY STATEMENT MISREPRESENTED ON THIS APPLICATION WILL AUTOMATICALLY FORFEIT MY RIGHT TO PRESENT ASSISTANCE FROM THE ONTARIO HEALTH INSURANCE COMMISSION, AND THAT THE COMMISSION RESERVES THE RIGHT TO RECOVER ANY PORTION OF THE SUBSCRIPTION PAID ON MY BEHALF.

I AM TEMPORARILY UNABLE TO PAY THE REQUIRED PREMIUMS AS A RESULT OF (PLACE X IN APPROPRIATE BOX) —
- [ ] UNEMPLOYMENT
- [ ] ILLNESS
- [ ] DISABILITY
- [ ] FINANCIAL HARDSHIP

SIGNATURE                                         DATE

REMEMBER TO ENCLOSE YOUR PREMIUM NOTICE WITH THIS APPLICATION.

ANY OTHER RELEVANT INFORMATION PERTAINING TO FINANCIAL CIRCUMSTANCES ?

| FOR OFFICE USE ONLY | | | | | | | | |
|---|---|---|---|---|---|---|---|---|
| T.I. | I.A. | I.E. | T.A. | A.A. | A.E. | FROM | TO | STN. |

Ontario residents have a Government Health Insurance Plan to cover basic health needs . . . but that's not always enough. Blue Cross covers the extra cost of semi-private hospital care.

The Blue Cross semi-private hospital plan is designed to complement basic government hospital insurance. As a convenience for you and the hospital, the hospital will bill the semi-private care directly to Blue Cross.

## Certificates

If you are under the age of 65 years, the coverage will be handled through the Ontario Health Insurance Commission and you will receive a certificate from them showing the number "33" under the supplementary column of this certificate. The premiums for the Blue Cross semi-private coverage will be included with the premiums for your Ontario Health Insurance and one combined payment will cover both premiums.

If you are age 65 or over, the application will be handled in the Blue Cross office and you will receive a separate certificate from Ontario Blue Cross which must be shown at the hospital in order to have semi-private care billed to Blue Cross. The billing for the semi-private premiums will come to you direct from Blue Cross and is to be paid directly to the Blue Cross office at Ferrand Drive, Don Mills, Ontario.

## Pays extra costs

Blue Cross makes direct payment to the hospital for the extra cost of semi-private accommodation up to a maximum of $5.50 per day . . . when your standard ward charges are paid by the Ontario Health Insurance Commission. Your Blue Cross "pay-direct" plan is flexible. You can even occupy private accommodation and Blue Cross will pay up to the semi-private level, to a maximum of $5.50 per day.

## No limit

Unlimited days semi-private coverage in public active-treatment or public convalescent hospital accommodation to coincide with the number of days available under Ontario Health Insurance.

## Good away from home

Coverage outside Ontario up to the cost of comparable semi-private accommodation in Ontario – when standard ward charges are paid by the Ontario Health Insurance Commission.

## No overlap

The Blue Cross "supplementary" plan for hospital care is specially designed to enable persons with Ontario Health Insurance to prepay the additional cost of semi-private accommodation. Because of this, there is no possible overlapping of benefits or premiums with the provincial standard ward plan.

## Chronic care

Blue Cross provides up to $3.00 per day for a maximum of 120 days per benefit year for semi-private accommodation occupied in public chronic hospitals and chronic wing facilities in public hospitals.

Note: This plan does not cover accommodation in TB sanatoria, mental hospitals or nursing homes.

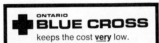

**ONTARIO**
## BLUE CROSS
keeps the cost **very** low.

In keeping with the concept of Blue Cross non-profit operation, the quarterly rates, if you are under 65 years of age and billed by the Ontario Health Insurance Commission, are:

SINGLE **$3.00**     FAMILY **$6.00**

in addition to your Ontario Health Insurance premiums.

If you are age 65 or over, billing will be made directly from the Blue Cross office on a semi-annual basis. The semi-annual amount requested will be:

SINGLE **$6.00**     FAMILY **$12.00**

*As you can see from the above, the monthly rates for Blue Cross semi-private coverage are Single $1.00 per month and Family $2.00 per month. However, they must be billed on a quarterly or semi-annual basis in order to cut the cost of administration.

*Just complete this request for Blue Cross semi-private hospital care coverage and mail it today in an envelope addressed to Ontario Blue Cross, Ferrand Drive, Don Mills, Ontario.*

INITIALS

SURNAME _____ PLEASE PRINT CLEARLY

ADDRESS _____ PLEASE PRINT CLEARLY

CITY _____ PLEASE PRINT CLEARLY   OHIC NUMBER

☐ I am under 65 years of age and would like to add Blue Cross semi-private hospital care to my Ontario Health Insurance Plan.   ☐ I want single coverage.   ☐ I want family coverage.

☐ I am 65 years of age or over and would like to have semi-private hospital care through the Blue Cross pay-direct plan.

Signature _____

Please do not send any payment with this application.

### HOW TO ENROL

Simply complete the attached application form and mail to: Ontario Blue Cross, Ferrand Drive, Don Mills, Ontario. Your Blue Cross coverage will become effective on the benefit date specified in your first combined premium notice from the Commission, or if you are 65 years of age or over, the coverage will be effective on the first day of the fifth month following receipt of the application in the Blue Cross office.

**Please do not send any payment with this application.**

---

Coverage such as Blue Cross may be arranged by an employer on a group basis and when this is done Form 104 will show code number "33" in the box with the asterisk to the top right of the form.

Immigrants coming into Canada obviously must acquire coverage for medical expenses as soon as possible when the province to which they emigrate does not have immediate coverage, such as in Nova Scotia. All the plans delineate how this can be done. H.M.C. is an example of a carrier having a bridging plan to insure people during the waiting period before joining the Provincial Plan, where there is one, as in New Brunswick or British Columbia. The Hospital Medical Care form shows the amount of this insurance for each province. People coming to Canada for a holiday may and should have coverage for medical expenses while here, for misfortune could mean disastrous results financially for the uninsured. The enrollment card for H.M.C. for immigrants and visitors is shown.

A typical plan for those on holiday is that offered by Blue Cross. The coverage can be for a single person or a family, and for 21, 42, or 63 days, at a cost of $10, $18, or $26 for a single person, and $20, $36, or $52 for a family. The benefits and the type of coverage these amounts pay for is shown in the Figure shown on the following page. The form shown is for Ontario but Blue Cross coverage for vacationers or visitors to Canada can be had for any part of the Dominion.

---

**IMPORTANT!**

YOU are required to be a resident of the province of your destination for various periods before you are eligible for the provincial Hospital Medical Services Plans. This waiting period is usually three months; H M C is designed to insure you and/or your family during this period.

## FACTS AND INFORMATION
### ON PROVINCIAL HOSPITAL AND MEDICAL SERVICE PLANS AND H M C RATES
Visitors see front panel for rates

### NEWFOUNDLAND — IMMIGRANTS
Waiting period for Provincial Plans

| HOSPITAL | MEDICAL |
|---|---|
| none | none |
| SINGLE ——— | FAMILY ——— |

Visitors are not eligible for the Provincial plans

### PRINCE EDWARD IS. — IMMIGRANTS
Waiting period for Provincial Plans

| HOSPITAL | MEDICAL |
|---|---|
| none | none |
| SINGLE ——— | FAMILY ——— |

Visitors are not eligible for the Provincial plans

### NOVA SCOTIA — IMMIGRANTS
Waiting period for Provincial Plans

| HOSPITAL | MEDICAL |
|---|---|
| 3 months | 3 months |

Premiums for insured period

| SINGLE $38.00 | FAMILY $91.00 |
|---|---|

All single applicants over age 65 — $44.00
Visitors are not eligible for the Provincial plans

### NEW BRUNSWICK — IMMIGRANTS
Waiting period for Provincial Plans

| HOSPITAL | MEDICAL |
|---|---|
| 3 months | 3 months |

Premiums for insured period

| SINGLE $38.00 | FAMILY $91.00 |
|---|---|

All single applicants over age 65 — $44.00
Visitors are not eligible for the Provincial plans

### QUEBEC — IMMIGRANTS
Waiting period for Provincial Plans

| HOSPITAL | MEDICAL |
|---|---|
| 3 months | none |

Premiums for insured period

| SINGLE $25.50 | FAMILY $53.50 |
|---|---|

All single applicants over age 65 — $30.00
Visitors are not eligible for the Provincial plans

### ONTARIO — IMMIGRANTS
Waiting period for Provincial Plans

| HOSPITAL | MEDICAL |
|---|---|
| 3 months | none |

Premiums for insured period

| SINGLE $25.50 | FAMILY $53.50 |
|---|---|

All single applicants over age 65 — $30.00
Visitors are not eligible for the Provincial plans

### MANITOBA — IMMIGRANTS
Waiting period for Provincial Plans

| HOSPITAL | MEDICAL |
|---|---|
| none | none |
| SINGLE ——— | FAMILY ——— |

Visitors are not eligible for the Provincial plans

### SASKATCHEWAN — IMMIGRANTS
Immigrants and discharged Members of the Canadian Forces
No waiting period for Provincial Plans

#### SPECIAL RESIDENTS
FROM THE CONTINENTAL UNITED STATES OF AMERICA
1. Returning Canadian citizens   2. Returning Residents
3. Certain persons in Canada in connection with their trade or profession who hold Non-Immigrant Arrival-Departure Cards
4. A person in Canada who holds a Student Entry Certificate
Coverage is provided on completion of the three month period following the date of entry to the province.

| HOSPITAL | MEDICAL |
|---|---|
| 3 months | 3 months |

Premiums for insured period

| SINGLE $38.00 | FAMILY $91.00 |
|---|---|

All single applicants over age 65 — $44.00
Visitors are not eligible for the Provincial plans

### ALBERTA — IMMIGRANTS
Waiting period for Provincial Plans

| HOSPITAL | MEDICAL |
|---|---|
| none | none |
| SINGLE ——— | FAMILY ——— |

Visitors are not eligible for the Provincial plans

### BRITISH COLUMBIA — IMMIGRANTS
Waiting period for Provincial Plans

| HOSPITAL | MEDICAL |
|---|---|
| 3 months | 1st day of the 2nd month |

Premiums for insured period

| SINGLE $38.00 | FAMILY $91.00 |
|---|---|

All single applicants over age 65 — $44.00
Visitors are not eligible for the Provincial plans
NEW ARRIVALS COVERED IN THEIR COUNTRY OF ORIGIN
ENQUIRE IMMEDIATELY WITH THE B.C. MEDICAL PLAN

### NORTH WEST TERR. & YUKON — IMMIGRANTS
Waiting period for Provincial Plans

| HOSPITAL | MEDICAL |
|---|---|
| 3 months | 3 months |

Premiums for insured period

| SINGLE $38.00 | FAMILY $91.00 |
|---|---|

All single applicants over age 65 — $44.00
Visitors are not eligible for the Provincial plans

## HOSPITAL MEDICAL CARE
700 Bay St.  •  Telephone 367-0440
Underwritten by
Mutual of Omaha Insurance Company
TORONTO, CANADA

---

## ENROLMENT INSTRUCTIONS

1. Complete the Enrolment Form. Be sure to sign.

2. Fill in the bank authorization your personal cheque or money order.

3. If you use your own cheque, or money order please staple to this form.

4. Please detach and mail in self-folding self-addressed envelope, just fold where indicated and seal, no postage required.

Note: Acceptance of applications made more than 45 days after arrival in Canada will be at the option of the Company.

HOSPITAL MEDICAL CARE PROGRAMME

### INSURANCE ENROLMENT CARD
### HOSPITAL MEDICAL CARE

Date ...............

Immigrant ☐
Visitor ☐
Returning Canadian ☐ ...............                    **Age** ......

First    (Please Print Name)    Last

Address: ...............
(Temporary)          (Street)          (City)          (Province)

Address: ...............
(Permanent)          (Street)          (City)          (Province)

Country of Origin and Address: ...............

Plan I—Hospital and Medical ☐    Single ☐    Family ☐

Plan II—Hospital Only ☐    Single ☐    Family ☐

Life Ins. Beneficiary ...............    Relationship ...............
Amt. Enclosed $ ...............

Enclosed is my signed Bank Authorization or Money Order.

**Arrival date must be filled in.**    Important  Arrival Date ......

Signed: ...............    Phone Number: ......
Applicant or Sponsor

**—If renewal please quote #** ...............

**BENEFITS: HOSPITAL**

1. Hospital care in government approved active treatment hospitals at regular daily rates up to a maximum of $60.00 (Sixty Dollars) per day and to a limit of 30 (Thirty) days. Hospitals in Canada charge all inclusive daily rates. The payment rate set on this agreement is average.

2. Out-patient and emergency care in hospital to a limit of $500.00 during the life of the agreement.

3. The cost of a local ambulance, at prevailing rates, to the nearest hospital for emergency treatment.

**BENEFITS: MEDICAL-SURGICAL**

1. Medical-Surgical *In-patient Hospital* Care for a period of 30 (Thirty) days with payment up to the current Ontario Medical Association General Practice Schedule of Fees.

2. Medical-Surgical *Out-patient and Emergency Hospital Care* with payment up to the current Ontario Medical Association General Practice Schedule of Fees, to a maximum of $500.00 during the term of the agreement.

3. Services in a private laboratory or clinic for tests or x-rays as ordered by a medical doctor up to a maximum of $60.00 during the term of the agreement.

**LIMITATIONS:**

1. Hospital and Medical-surgical care will be paid only if rendered in Public Hospitals for active treatment.

2. Medical-surgical coverage will be provided only for patients in hospital (except as provided for out-patient and emergency hospital care and in private laboratories or clinics) up to the current Ontario-Medical Association General Practice Schedule of Fees.

3. Maternity cases or confinements in hospital for childbirth are not covered.

4. Benefits under this agreement are not covered if the patient is entitled to receive same from any government agency or department.

5. Benefits under this agreement are not available for tooth extractions, dental care, cosmetic surgery or plastic surgery.

6. Benefits are not available under this agreement if the patient has come to Canada for the purpose of receiving hospital or medical-surgical care or treatment.

7. No benefits are available beyond the boundaries of Canada or the continental United States of America. (See terms of agreement re limitation on benefits paid in the United States.)

**Terms of the Agreement**

1. The effective date of the agreement shall be the date the application and premium are received in the Blue Cross office in Don Mills, Ontario, or the date of the visitor's arrival in Canada, if the application and premium are received before arrival.

2. All applications must be accompanied by the proper premium payment in Canadian currency in order to become effective.

3. Payment will be made by Blue Cross by cheque directly to the subscriber upon receipt of hospital accounts or physicians' accounts showing all necessary information, such as dates, diagnosis or other pertinent items; or accounts may be assigned to the Hospital or Physician by the patient and sent directly to Blue Cross. If assigned, accounts must state clearly "VISITORS' HEALTH COVERAGE" and be properly shown as assigned. Payment will be made by Blue Cross in Canadian currency.

4. The benefits are sold for terms of 21 days, 42 days and 63 days from the effective date of the agreement. If the patient covered under this agreement is admitted to hospital during that period, but not discharged from hospital until after the benefit period has expired, then the patient shall be covered until such discharge date provided always that the 30 days of benefit provided under the agreement have not been fully used before such discharge date, in which case benefits will be paid to the maximum 30 days.

5. Benefits under this agreement shall be provided in the United States of America only as it relates to incidental or circumstantial travel. Then this agreement is modified to provide for 15 (Fifteen) days hospital care up to a maximum of $120.00 (One Hundred and Twenty Dollars) per day in a participating hospital of any American Blue Cross Plan. All other terms of this agreement stay as written.

A general picture of OHIP coverage for Ontario follows, arranged in a style similar to that of the other provinces' plans. It is hoped that a closer examination of one province's plan will be helpful when considering those of other provinces, as the similarities are greater than the differences in nearly all cases.

*PROVINCE OF ONTARIO*

*Name of Plan:*      Ontario Health Insurance Plan (OHIP)

*Provincial Legislation:*      The Health Insurance Act, 1972.

*Effective Date:*      April 1, 1972.

*Administration and Method of Operation:*      The Minister of Health is responsible for the administration and operation of the Plan. The Ontario Health Insurance Plan performs functions necessary to determine eligibility and collection of premiums, approves and assesses claims for inspired health services, determines the amounts to be paid, and authorizes payment.

## PROVINCE OF ONTARIO (Continued)

*Method of Provincial*
*Financing:*

Monthly premiums: $11 single, and $22 for a family. Persons in receipt of social assistance are covered without application and without payment of a premium. Single persons having taxable income of not more than $1000 in the preceding taxation year are eligible for partial premium assistance of $5.50 per month; and an insured person with one dependent with a taxable income of not more than $2000 is eligible for partial premium assistance of $11 monthly. Temporary assistance may be granted during employment, illness, disability or financial hardship, upon application directly to OHIP, 2195 Yonge Street, Toronto.

*Utilization Fees:*
None.

*Insured Persons:*
Every person who is a resident of Ontario is entitled to become an insured person upon application and every dependent of an insured person is also an insured person. Coverage is *mandatory* for employees of an employer if their number totals *15 or more*. Employee groups of more than 5 but less than 15 persons may, upon application, form a mandatory group. Organizations having five or more members may nominate one member as a collector, and may then be designated as a collector's group.

*Date upon which Resident*
*becomes a Beneficiary:*

On October 1, 1969, for persons who applied *before* that date; otherwise, on the first day of the third month after eligibility, under a pay-direct application confirmed by OHIP, and after the first premium is paid, and, by administrative ruling, on the first day of the month following the month in which employment commenced, if entering a mandatory group.

*Insured Services:*
All services rendered by physicians that are medically required.

Twenty-four specified dental-surgical procedures, if performed in hospital by a dental surgeon;

Examination of the eyes, particularly by refraction, for the purpose of determining a need for corrective lenses. When the service is performed by an optometrist the amount payable is $10. OHIP also covers specified treatments by chiropodists, chiropractors, osteopaths, in nursing homes, and homes for the aged.

Chiropractic, osteopathic, and chiropody (podiatry) services will be paid up to $100, plus $25 for radiography examinations per person, for each of the three types of service. That is the total amount approved for any 12-month period, beginning July 1 of each year.

Homes for the aged and nursing homes are now covered under the OHIP Plan, under the "Extended Health Care" section. OHIP rates cover the major portion of cost. Nursing homes and homes for the aged must meet the required standards for facilities and services. All doctors are provided with a list of acceptable and participating nursing homes and homes for the aged. Persons who qualify pay about $5 per day and the plan pays the remainder. People must have been residents of Ontario, and registered in OHIP to qualify for extended health care. Where there is financial hardship, the Ministry of Health and Community

Effective April 1, 1972, Ontario residents insured under the Ontario Health Insurance Plan (who have been residents of Ontario for one year or longer) become eligible for the Extended Health Care benefit.

The prime purpose of this new benefit is to lift the bulk of the financial burden from insured residents who have a continuing medical need for institutional health care but do not require the facilities of a hospital. It is also designed to help provide a better balance for the health care system.

The Extended Health Care benefit is in addition to the broad scope of the Plan's usual insured services. The cost of this benefit is shareable between the Plan and the resident. Persons who qualify will be responsible for paying $3.50 a day and the Plan will pay the remainder of the Home's approved daily cost for *medically-necessary* services in standard ward accommodation. Any charges by the Home for preferred accommodation (semi-private and private) will be charged to the resident.

**WHAT IS "EXTENDED HEALTH CARE"?**
"Extended Health Care" refers to care received in a Nursing Home or Home for the Aged by a sick person who requires skilled nursing service and regular medical supervision in an institution other than a hospital.

**WHO WILL QUALIFY FOR THIS BENEFIT?**
Nursing Homes and Homes for the Aged provide two basic categories of service:

1. Institutional "living" accommodation for people needing assistance with the normal acts of daily life.

2. Institutional care for persons with conditions which do not require hospital care but do make it necessary for them to receive regular skilled nursing service and regular supervision by a physician, usually on a long-term basis.

It is persons who come within category two (2) above, for whom the Extended Health Care benefit is designed. In other words, the benefit *does not apply to insured persons who are in a Nursing Home or Home for the Aged simply because they require living accommodation or because they are no longer physically or mentally capable of coping, unassisted, with day-to-day living.* Other provisions are made by Government to assist such residents who need financial support for this kind of "domiciliary" service, and information regarding this is available from the Ontario Ministry of Community and Social Services, Hepburn Block, Queen's Park, Toronto.

**HOW WILL IT WORK?**
Residents who are in Nursing Homes and Homes for the Aged as of April 1, 1972 will be medically assessed to determine whether or not they qualify for the Extended Health Care benefit. This assessment will begin throughout the Province prior to April 1. A person who qualifies will be eligible from April 1, until it is certified in medical reports that he or she no longer requires skilled nursing care and regular medical supervision. If and when this happens, the resident will be notified regarding the date the benefit will cease.

**AFTER APRIL 1, 1972**
An insured Ontario resident who seeks admission to a Nursing Home or Home for the Aged on or after April 1, 1972, will be medically assessed to assist the Plan to determine if he or she qualifies for the Extended Health Care benefit.

Where a resident of a Home does not qualify for the benefit as of April 1, 1972, but later becomes in need of constant skilled nursing service and medical supervision, the benefit will be made available upon approval by the Plan.

**WILL ALL NURSING HOMES BE APPROVED?**
All nursing homes licensed to provide extended care will be included in the program. To be licensed as a participating Nursing Home, the Home must meet the required standards of facilities and services.

The Extended Health Care benefit will be provided in licensed participating Nursing Homes and approved Homes for the Aged, including most municipal Homes for the Aged and many Homes for the Aged operated by charitable organizations.

Doctors will be provided with a list of participating Nursing Homes and Homes for the Aged.

*For further information, contact:*
**ONTARIO HEALTH INSURANCE COMMISSION**
**EXTENDED HEALTH CARE PROGRAM**
**2195 YONGE STREET**
**TORONTO 295, ONTARIO**

FORM G 617 (2/72)

## PROVINCE OF ONTARIO (Continued)

Social Services can be solicited for help. Virtually all circumstances can be taken care of; e.g., when a person *needs* private or semiprivate care and accommodation, and carries no Blue Cross, Hospital Medical Care, or so on, the Ministries mentioned should be approached as the problem can generally be solved by them. Further information can be obtained from the Ontario Health Insurance Commission, Extended Health Care Program, 2195 Yonge Street, Toronto. (See Figure, *Ontario Health Insurance Commission, Extended Health Care Program.*)

*Exclusions:* Services that a person is eligible for and entitled to under the Hospital Insurance and Diagnostic Services Act (Canada) or under any other Act of the Parliament of Canada, except the Medical Care Act (Canada) or under the Workmen's Compensation Act or under legislation of any other jurisdiction; cosmetic surgery unless medically required; expenses for traveling time or mileage; advice by telephone; court testimony, preparation of records, reports, certificates or communications; any service or examination for the purpose of an application for insurance or under a requirement for keeping insurance in force or for admission to school, college, university, camp or association, employment, passport, visa or other similar document, legal requirements or proceedings; laboratory or other diagnostic procedures provided as hospital services to the extent that these are covered under the Hospital Services Commission Act, and laboratory services and clinical pathology, except when ordered by a physician and performed under the direction of a physician; dental care (other than the dental surgical procedures specified in regulations), including

*PROVINCE OF ONTARIO* (Continued)

x-ray and anesthetist services; nursing services; ambulance services; dressing and case materials; use of operating, plaster or fracture rooms; drugs, vaccines, biological sera or extracts or their synthetic substitutes; eye glasses; special appliances; oxygen; physical therapy or other similar treatments.

*Out-of-Province Benefits:*

Payment for insured health services rendered by a physician or practitioner outside Ontario is at the same rate as for Ontario or may be adjusted by OHIP as a special emergency, in which case higher rates of payment may be considered.

*Extension of Coverage after Loss of Residence:*

If insured becomes resident of another province participating under the Medical Care Act (Canada): until his coverage under the plan in that province takes effect or after four months, whichever occurs first.

*Method and Scale of Payments to Physicians:*

Physicians who have opted *into* the plan usually bill OHIP directly and receive payment at the rate of 90 per cent of the OMA scale as full payment. The schedule used is the 1971 Scheule of Fees established by the Ontario Medical Association.

Those few doctors who opted out of the plan either bill the patient in full, whereupon the patient has the option either to pay the doctor at that time, or to wait until he receives his settlement from OHIP and then pay the doctor, or the doctor may forward a "pay subscriber" claim card and the patient pays the doctor's bill at his discretion.

*Provision for Extra-billing by Physicians:*

Where the physician or practitioner has *NOT* opted into the plan, and intends to charge more than the amount payable under the plan, he shall so advise the patient prior to rendering the service.

*Provision for Private Insurance Coverage:*

None. The Act provides that as of October 1, 1969, no person shall enter into or renew a contract of insurance for the payment of all or any part of the cost of insured health services performed in Ontario and received by any person eligible to become an insured person under the Act.

# WORKMEN'S COMPENSATION AND INSURANCE EXAMINATIONS

Workmen's Compensation claims can be made by a doctor or hospital on account card Form 92 if there is no lost time involved, or on the same card, along with a Doctor's First Report, pink Form 8, if the workman is going to be off work beyond the day of the accident. Compensation is paid for working days lost, providing the workman has suffered a personal injury as a result of an accident arising because of and in the course of his employment. For example, a workman who works Monday to Friday, and who is injured on Friday and able to return to work on Monday, would not be entitled to compensation, but if he

# INSTRUCTIONS FOR COMPLETING REPORTS AND ACCOUNT CARDS

### TREATMENT MEMORANDUM (FORM 156)

The purpose of this form is to identify the workman. As shown on the form, the accident will be reported by the employer. This form should not be sent to the board, but the fact that it has been received should be indicated on account cards for new claims.

**NOTE** When a workman presents himself for initial treatment without a treatment memorandum, an account card and or the Doctor's First Report should always be completed and mailed immediately. The workman should also be advised to have his employer send the Employer's Report of Accident to the Workmen's Compensation Board. A form has been developed to assist you in this respect emphasizing the fact that failure to have the report submitted could result in the account for services rendered being his responsibility. Supplies of this Form 516 are available on request.

Attention clinics and partnerships: Clinics and partnerships receive a supply of account cards for each specialist according to specialty within the group. Separate payee code numbers are assigned for each specialty as well as general practice. It is important that the treating doctor's proper card be used to ensure payment at the correct fee schedule.

### SOCIAL INSURANCE NUMBER

The inclusion of this number in the appropriate block on account cards and report forms will be of assistance in the correct association of your submissions with a workman's claim file.

### MEDICAL AID ACCOUNT ENQUIRY (FORM 178)

Due to lack of adequate information from an employer, treating agency or workman, there are occasions when a claim cannot be allowed without extensive enquiry. This may result in a delay in payment of accounts.

You will note that our reply to your enquiry will be provided on the reverse side of this form. This will ensure a prompt reply and will assist you in identifying the account in question.

It is important that you indicate your name and address in the space provided on the front of this form since this will be used for mailing purposes when returning your enquiry.

### DOCTOR'S FIRST REPORT (FORM 8)

This form should be completed in full and mailed as soon as possible when

(A) The workman will be totally or partially disabled beyond the day of accident.

(B) The diagnosis is hernia or ruptured intervertebral disc.

(C) A request is received from the Workmen's Compensation Board.

It is of extreme importance that this form be completed as soon as it is recognized that a case falls into categories (A) or (B). Perhaps a notation in your day book would serve as a reminder to your nurse or secretary that a report should be completed and mailed. When a report is requested category (C) it is because medical evidence is necessary to determine the workman's entitlement even though the workman was disabled less than three days.

### ACCOUNT CARD (FORM 92 FOR DOCTORS) (FORM 91 FOR DRUGLESS PRACTITIONERS)

The account card must be used to submit fees for all services including x-rays, etc. These accounts are for your exclusive use and should not be transferred to or used by any other practitioner as this will result in misdirection of payment. PLEASE DO NOT USE PAPER ACCOUNTS.

Payments are made twice monthly and you will receive a medical aid remittance statement with each cheque. This will show (1) settled accounts with appropriate codes explaining reason for adjustments, if any. (2) accounts that have been received and identified with a claim, but settlement is pending because of necessary enquiry regarding treatment or the workman's entitlement under the Act. If an account does not appear on a remittance statement within two months of submission, an enquiry may be made by submitting a form 178 (Medical Aid Account Enquiry) for each such account.

### X-RAY REPORT (FORM 104) AND X-RAY ACCOUNT CARD

The cards to be used for X-RAY ACCOUNTS ONLY are identified as such. The new X-Ray Report Form 104, must show the same information as the X-Ray Account Card. The report and card may be completed in one operation by using a carbon insert. The report and account must be clipped and submitted together. PLEASE DO NOT PIN OR STAPLE.

### IMPORTANT

Listing the CLAIM NUMBER, if available, and properly completing the section of the form containing the workman's and employer's names and addresses, diagnosis and date of accident is essential to identify the report with the established claim. In many cases your report will be the Board's first indication of the accident, and therefore, all of the above detail is necessary to set up a claim.

FORM 204 REV. 10-68

Form 204. Instructions for Reports and Account Cards.

TREATMENT MEMORANDUM

DOCTOR/HOSPITAL

MR.
MRS.      LAST NAME
MISS      | D | O | E |   |   |   |   |   |   |   |   |   |   |   |   |   |   |   |   |

FIRST NAME(S)
| R | I | C | H | A | R | D |   |   |   |   |   |   |   |   |   |   |   |   |   |

ADDRESS .1 Right Street, TORONTO, ONTARIO . . . . . . . . .

CLAIMS TO HAVE BEEN INJURED IN OUR EMPLOY ON

21st. October. . . . . . . . . . . . . . . . . . . . . . . . . . . . 19 . . . . .

AND REQUIRES MEDICAL AID.

WE ARE SENDING A REPORT TO THE WORKMEN'S COMPENSATION BOARD, ONTARIO.

FIRM . . . . . . . Black, White, Red & Green, Limited, . . . . . . . . . . .

ADDRESS . . . . . Mud Works, 1 Wrong Street, TORONTO, ONTARIO . . . . . .

OFFICIAL . . . . . A. W. Oman, S.R.N., of the above Works . . . .

---

THE WORKMAN HAS THE INITIAL CHOICE OF DOCTOR, BUT MAY NOT CHANGE DOCTORS WITHOUT PERMISSION OF THE WORKMEN'S COMPENSATION BOARD, ONTARIO.

---

DOCTOR – IF IT APPEARS THAT THE WORKMAN WILL BE DISABLED FROM EARNING FULL WAGES ON **ANY DAY BEYOND THE DAY OF ACCIDENT,** PLEASE SUBMIT A DOCTOR'S FIRST REPORT, FORM 8, TO THE WORKMEN'S COMPENSATION BOARD. DELAY IN COMPLETION WILL DELAY PAYMENT OF COMPENSATION. WHEN SUBMITTING YOUR ACCOUNT PLEASE INDICATE THAT YOU HAVE RECEIVED THIS FORM.

FORM 156
REV. 9. 68

Treatment memorandum.

were unable to return until Wednesday he would be entitled to two days compensation for Monday and Tuesday. In both cases medical expenses which are necessary would be paid. Compensation is paid on 75 per cent of the workman's salary, up to a maximum of $7000 per year. This money is tax-free. Compensation is not paid for the day of injury or the day the worker returns to work.

A patient arriving at the doctor's office or at the hospital for treatment under the Workmen's Compensation Act should have with him a Treatment Memorandum, filled in by the firm for which he works. As will be seen from the sample shown here, it contains the workman's name, his address, the date of the accident, the firm's name and address, and the signature of an official from the firm. If the worker does not have this form, he should be told to report this to his employer or it could result in the account for services-rendered being sent to him.

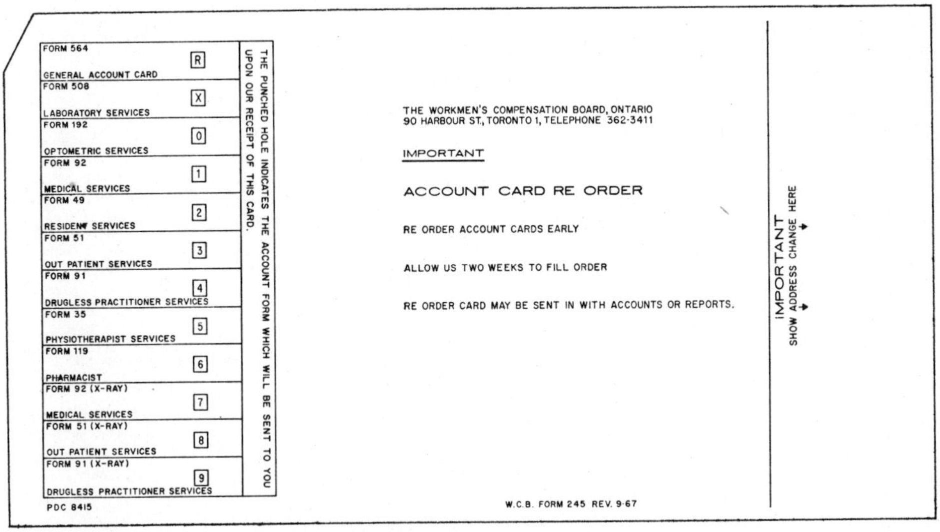

Reorder form for Account Cards.

The medical secretary should see that she has an adequate supply of all Workmen's Compensation Board (W.C.B.) forms by using the account card re-order form illustrated here.

A patient might be directed to a hospital or doctor if he's hurt while at work, or he might be told to go to his own doctor. In either case, where no lost time is involved, the doctor or hospital will use the Workmen's Compensation Board Card to submit the charge for treatment and claim for payment. The top of the card is self-explanatory. Very often the patient cannot remember his social insurance number, so this space must be left blank temporarily, and the patient requested to telephone in this number as soon as he is able. If he cannot do this, the number must be obtained from a member of his family or his place of employment. The claim number, located on the top right-hand side of the card, is the claim number the Board gives to this particular claim; it does not come from the doctor's office or the hospital. The doctor's account number identifies him to the W.C.B.

The medical assistant would not necessarily use a new file for each patient concerned with a W.C.B. claim. These claims, like life insurance examinations, may be one-time only calls, and she would probably find it more efficient to use one card for all W.C.B. claims, numbering them as suggested, and marking them off as the remittance statements and their accompanying checks arrive. The assistant has a notation of the appointment in her diary, and also in the daybook.

Life insurance examinations for insurance companies are billed by the doctor directly to the insurance company. The patient does not pay himself. This bill may be sent on an ordinary bill form, or it may be presented on an itemized form supplied for that purpose.

In all cases where life insurance examinations are to take place, the doctor is contacted by mail or telephone by the insurance company, and the appointment with the patient is made thereafter. Usually the company chooses a doctor

To ensure having forms always available, please complete and mail this order form to the Secretary of your Provincial Division (see addresses below).

## ORDER FORM

The Secretary,

(Provincial Medical Society or Division C. M. A.)

........................................................................................

Address ........................................................................................

........................................................................................

Please forward................pads of "Combined Form (CMHIA-1) for Accident & Sickness Claims" to the undersigned.

(Please print signature and full address)

................................................................................M.D.

........................................................................................

........................................................................................

Addresses—Secretaries of C.M.A. Divisions.

**British Columbia**—E. C. McCoy, M.D., 1807 W. 10th Ave., Vancouver 9, B.C.

**Alberta**—R. Woolstencroft, M.D., 9901-108th St., Edmonton, Alta.

**Saskatchewan**—E. H. Baergen, M.D., 932 Spadina Cres. E., Saskatoon, Sask.

**Manitoba**—Mr. R. P. H. Sprague, Second Floor, 201 Kennedy Street, Winnipeg 1, Manitoba

**Ontario**—Glenn I. Sawyer, M.D., 244 St. George St., Toronto 5, Ont.

**Quebec**—Mr. Guy Blouin, The Province of Quebec Medical Association, 1350 Sherbrooke St. West, Suite 1410, Montreal 25, P.Q.

**Nova Scotia**—C. J. W. Beckwith, M.D., Sir Charles Tupper Bldg., 15th Floor, Halifax, N.S.

**New Brunswick**—F. L. Whitehead, M.D., Suite 170, Courtenay Centre, Saint John, N.B.

**Prince Edward Island**—John Craig, M.D., 48 St. Clair Ave., Charlottetown, P.E.I.

**Newfoundland**—Mr. Gerald Lynch, O'Mara Martin Building, Rawlins Cross, St. John's, Nfld.

Order form.

with whom the person to be insured has had no former contact, for obvious reasons. If the insurance company contacts the doctor by telephone, the insurance company notifies the person to be examined and tells him of the appointment that has been made on his behalf; if the insurance company *writes* to the doctor, the doctor will contact the patient and make the appointment. An itemized form for the examination would most likely be filled in by the doctor while he conducted the examination, and the assistant would only need to check the form to see that it was correctly signed before sending it off for payment.

The card illustrated below, *Form 92, laceration of thumb,* shows that John Doe, aged 47, who lives at the address in Scarborough shown, and who is employed by A.B.C. Construction Ltd., lacerated his thumb on March 8th, 1974. He went to his own doctor (an office call) the next day, had treatment, and was told he might return to work. The charge was $5, which the Board will pay.

The next Form 92 illustrated, for an employee who stepped on a nail, indicates that John Doe was injured at work and sent with a Treatment Memoran-

Account Card Form 92 for an employee with laceration of the thumb.

dum to the doctor. In this instance time-off is involved and therefore compensation is required, so the doctor must also fill in a pink Form 8, which is illustrated on page 710.

In the latter case, Doe was injured on March 9th, 1974, and could not return to work. His return-to-work date was set for March 16th, 1974, or one week later. The 9th was a Thursday, and the 16th a Thursday, so Doe is entitled to four days compensatory pay as well as all of his medical expenses because he does not normally work on Saturday and Sunday. He will be off work for four calendar days only, that is, Friday, Monday, Tuesday, and Wednesday, and for these he is entitled to compensation.

As will have been seen, pink Form 8 (page 710), is very simple to fill in and will normally be attended to by the doctor. The assistant should see to it that the form is correct, and that the details at the bottom of the form are all completed, including the telephone number, and preferably all in type (except for the signature). Note that Form 8D2 is a similar form for skin diseases.

Account Card Form 92 for employee who stepped on nail.

FORM 8
REV. 1.68

Ⓔ

THE WORKMEN'S COMPENSATION BOARD, ONTARIO
90 HARBOUR STREET, TORONTO 1, TELEPHONE 362-3411

**DOCTOR'S FIRST REPORT**

CLAIM NO.

FIRM NO. – W.C.B. USE        RATE NO. – W.C.B.

| WORKMAN'S SURNAME – PLEASE PRINT | MR. | GIVEN OR CHRISTIAN NAMES |
|---|---|---|
| D O E | MRS. MISS | J O H N |

WORKMAN'S ADDRESS    1 Pennyfarthing Street, Sudbury, Ontario.        SOCIAL INSURANCE NO.

EMPLOYER'S NAME    Smith Construction, Limited    ADDRESS  1 Right Street, Sudbury, Ontario.

| DOCTOR – PLEASE COMPLETE IN FULL AND MAIL AS SOON AS POSSIBLE WHEN: | NOTE |
|---|---|
| 1 THE WORKMAN WILL BE TOTALLY OR PARTIALLY DISABLED BEYOND THE DAY OF ACCIDENT. —OR— 2. THE DIAGNOSIS IS HERNIA OR RUPTURED INTERVERTEBRAL DISC —OR— 3. A REQUEST IS RECEIVED FROM THE WORKMEN'S COMPENSATION BOARD | A. USE THE REVERSE OF THIS FORM WHEN NECESSARY. B. THE INFORMATION ON THIS FORM IS USED IN DETERMINING A WORKMAN'S ENTITLEMENT TO COMPENSATION. YOUR DELAY CAN HOLD UP PAYMENT. C. DO NOT USE AS A FORMAL CONSULTATION REPORT. D. SUPPLIES OF THIS FORM PROVIDED ON REQUEST. PLEASE KEEP A SUFFICIENT STOCK ON HAND. |

1  DATE OF ACCIDENT    March 9th    19--    DATE OF YOUR FIRST TREATMENT  March 9th,    19 --

2  WHO RENDERED FIRST TREATMENT?  Myself    WHEN? March 9th,    19 --

3  WORKMAN'S HISTORY OF INJURY    He states that he stepped on a nail

4  DESCRIBE FULLY THE INJURY WHEN FIRST EXAMINED. SPECIFY RIGHT OR LEFT.    Deep puncture wound right foot

ARE DENTAL SERVICES REQUIRED?  YES ☐  NO ☒

5  DIAGNOSIS    As above

IS PERMANENT DISABILITY PROBABLE?  YES ☐  NO ☒

6  DESCRIBE COMPLICATIONS, IF ANY.

7  WAS THIS INJURY SUFFICIENT TO DISABLE THE WORKMAN FROM HIS REGULAR WORK?  yes
→ IF SO, FOR HOW LONG? _____
→ ON WHAT DATE WILL HE BE FIT FOR HIS REGULAR WORK?  R.T.W. March 16th,  19--

8  IF HE IS PHYSICALLY CAPABLE OF UNDERTAKING SUITABLE WORK, GIVE DATE FIRST ABLE.    19

9  TREATMENT, INCLUDING ANY OPERATIVE PROCEDURE AND DATE.    Tetanus toxoid - dry bandage

| W.C.B. USE ONLY | | | |
|---|---|---|---|
| STATUS | INJURY | INJURY | CLAIMS OFFICER |

IS TREATMENT COMPLETED?  YES ☒  NO ☐

10  INDICATE PRIOR HISTORY OF SIMILAR CONDITION AND ANY PHYSICAL DEFECT.

11  INDICATE ANY PROPOSED PHYSIOTHERAPY – PRIOR AUTHORITY REQUIRED UNLESS GIVEN AT A CENTRE APPROVED BY THE BOARD.

12  IF HOSPITALIZED, NAME AND ADDRESS OF HOSPITAL    IF APPLICABLE, NAME OF SPECIALIST

DOCTOR'S NAME – PLEASE PRINT    R. A. Herriott,

ADDRESS    Sudbury, Ontario.    PHONE  284-7863

DOCTOR'S SIGNATURE  Herriott's signature here

DATE  March 10th, 19--

Form 8 for employee entitled to compensation.

The claim number that appears at the top right hand corner of the W.C.B. cards and forms is given by the W.C.B. This is a seven-digit number preceded by a letter, such as "A" "C" or "M." It is not essential that the assistant know what these letters stand for; they are an internal identifier for W.C.B. use. Since the numbers are part of the claim number they should be used in all correspondence. The terminal digit of the claim number identifies the section to which this claim belongs, e.g., A-7894123, belongs to Section 3. If the assistant must telephone the W.C.B. regarding any matter, she should use the full claim number and tell the operator her problem so she can relay the call to the proper place.

Legally, all W.C.B. claims are continuing claims; that is, if an injury that apparently had healed becomes troublesome at a later time, the patient is entitled to further treatment. Obviously the chore of filing this information is enormous and, in fact, microfilm is used by the Board a great deal. Almost all medical-aid claims are microfilmed after four months.

Once the W.C.B. receives a Form 92 requesting payment, it prepares a Medical Aid Remittance Form (page 714), on which it accounts for the payment it will make or has made. The claim number is the seven-digit number referred to earlier, followed by the name of the doctor making the claim, and the doctor's account number with the W.C.B. The next item is the adjustment code, and it is followed by a column showing the amount asked for or submitted, and the final column shows the amount the W.C.B. paid. **Any diversity in these figures is accounted for.** For instance, suppose the amount submitted was $50, the amount the Board paid was $40, and the adjustment code was given as 80. The assistant should turn the statement over and look at 80, and the discrepancy will be explained. Invariably the amount claimed has been adjusted to conform with the scale established by the W.C.B.

Payment is made easier if the doctor's accounts are all numbered. These numbers can go in the column that carries the doctor's account number with the W.C.B., on both the remittance statement and on Form 92. The assistant's job is made much easier by this system. She can see at a glance which accounts have been paid because she can check off the corresponding number on the patients' cards.

A radiologist uses a Form 92 which indicates that this is an x-ray account. His report goes on a card which is stamped "X-ray Account Only," but is otherwise the same as all other 92's. Instead of a pink Form 8 or any other written report, the radiologist sends his report on the Radiological Report Form shown. Again, the Form is self-explanatory, and the only parts of it that would normally concern the assistant are the top and bottom sections, which are familiar; the body part x-rayed and the findings will appear as a note from the doctor that the assistant will type in the places provided.

Two scales of fees are involved here; one for the specialist (the W.C.B. never objects to an opinion being requested), and one for the radiologist. The same forms are used by both the specialist and the radiologist when seeking payment of a claim.

Form 26 is a progress report, as is Form 41, and the *Board* will send these to a doctor or to a workman, respectively, when it requires either to be completed. Often a workman will ask the doctor's assistant to fill in his "41" form and she should endeavor to help in this matter. Sometimes a specialist or a consultant will not use Form 26 but will instead write a letter, stating the patient's present condition and the prognosis. Usually the doctor himself, if he does use a "26," will complete it, and all his assistant need do is to make sure that the date, signature, and address are legible, and if not, type them in UNDERNEATH the originals. The expression "chicken scratch" is frequently used to describe a doctor's writing, so the assistant should be sure that the W.C.B. can read it.

THE WORKMEN'S COMPENSATION ACT, ONTARIO

FORM 8D2
REV. 12, 66

## DOCTOR'S REPORT ON SKIN DISEASE

|  | DATE OF DISABILITY | CLAIM NUMBER |
|--|--|--|

WORKMAN'S NAME AND ADDRESS

EMPLOYER'S NAME AND ADDRESS

DOCTOR'S NAME AND ADDRESS

THE FOLLOWING REPORT MUST BE COMPLETED AND SENT BY THE DOCTOR TO THE WORKMEN'S COMPENSATION BOARD, 90 HARBOUR STREET, TORONTO 1.

**HISTORY**

1. FROM WHOM WAS THE HISTORY OBTAINED? WORKMAN ☐ EMPLOYER ☐ OTHER ...................

2. WAS ANY HISTORY OBTAINED OF PREVIOUS SKIN DISEASE, ASTHMA, HAY FEVER OR FOOD ALLERGY? NO ☐ IF YES, GIVE DETAILS.

3. DESCRIBE THE NATURE OF THE WORKMAN'S PARTICULAR JOB.

4. HOW LONG HAD HE BEEN EMPLOYED AT THIS JOB?

5. LIST POSSIBLE CAUSAL AGENTS.

6. IS THE PLACE OF WORK :— HOT ☐ HUMID ☐ WET ☐ DUSTY ☐ POORLY VENTILATED ☐ SATISFACTORY ☐

7. WHEN DID THE CONDITION FIRST APPEAR? GIVE THE PATIENT'S DESCRIPTION OF EARLY LESIONS.

WERE THE PALMS FIRST AFFECTED?

8. LIST PARTS AFFECTED IN ORDER OF INVOLVEMENT.

**EXAMINATION**

1. WAS THE ENTIRE BODY, INCLUDING THE FEET, EXAMINED? YES ☐ NO ☐

2. INDICATE TYPE OF SKIN :— FAIR ☐ INTERMEDIATE ☐ DARK ☐
   THIN ☐ " " ☐ COARSE ☐
   DRY ☐ " " ☐ OILY ☐

3. DESCRIBE LESIONS UNDER THE FOLLOWING HEADINGS :—
   ACUTE ☐ ERYTHEMA ☐ WEEPING ☐
   SUB–ACUTE ☐ VESICLES ☐ SCALING ☐
   CHRONIC ☐ CRUSTING ☐ EXCORIATIONS ☐

4. DEGREE OF INVOLVEMENT :— MINOR ☐ MODERATE ☐ SEVERE ☐

5. IS PYOGENIC INFECTION PRESENT? YES ☐ NO ☐
   IF YES, INDICATE WHETHER : PRIMARY ☐ SECONDARY ☐ PUSTULES ☐ FURUNCLES ☐
   LYMPHANGITIS ☐ FEVER AND MALAISE ☐

6. IS FUNGUS INFECTION PRESENT? YES ☐ NO ☐
   WERE SCRAPINGS TAKEN FOR EXAMINATION OR CULTURE? YES ☐ NO ☐
   IF YES, WHAT WERE THE FINDINGS?

PLEASE COMPLETE AND SIGN THE OTHER SIDE

Form 8D2. Report on skin diseases.

*(Illustration continued on opposite page.)*

7 ON THE DIAGRAM SHOWN, PLEASE SHADE ALL AREAS OF SKIN ERUPTION.

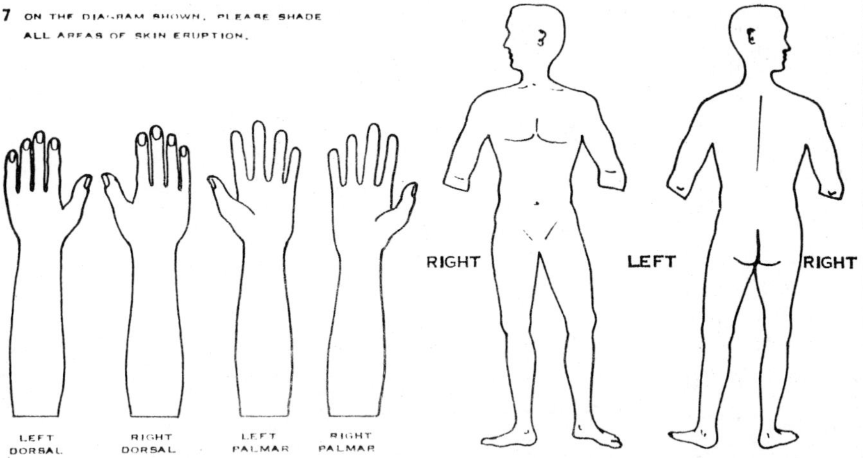


**DIAGNOSIS**

1 WHAT IS YOUR DIAGNOSIS ?

2 DO YOU CONSIDER THE CONDITION WAS CAUSED BY :–
A) A PRIMARY IRRITANT ? YES ☐ NO ☐ B) A SENSITIZER ? YES ☐ NO ☐
IF THE LATTER, WHAT EVIDENCE IS THERE OF SPECIFIC SENSITIVITY ?

3 DO YOU BELIEVE THE CONDITION IS OCCUPATIONAL ? YES ☐ NO ☐

4 STATE YOUR REASONS FOR SO BELIEVING.

**TREATMENT**

1 TOPICAL (LIST ALL MEDICATIONS)

2 SYSTEMIC (LIST ALL MEDICATIONS)

3 IS THE PATIENT'S CO-OPERATION GOOD ? ☐ FAIR ? ☐ POOR ? ☐

**CONCLUSIONS/RECOMMENDATIONS**

1 IS THE PATIENT AT WORK ☐ AT HOME ☐ IN HOSPITAL ☐ HOSPITAL NAME..........................

2 IS THE WORKMAN FIT FOR HIS USUAL WORK ? YES ☐ NO ☐ IF YES, FROM WHAT DATE ?..................
B) IF NOT, HOW LONG HAVE YOU ADVISED HIM TO STAY OFF ?........................................
C) IF FIT FOR OTHER OR MODIFIED WORK, STATE TYPE AND DATE ................ FROM ...............
D) WILL A CHANGE OF OCCUPATION BE NECCESSARY ? YES ☐ NO ☐
E) IF YES, PERMANENTLY ☐ TEMPORARILY ☐ (STATE PERIOD)..........................................

3 DOES THERE APPEAR TO BE A DERMATOLOGICAL HAZARD IN THE EMPLOYMENT THAT SHOULD BE LOOKED INTO ? YES ☐ NO ☐

ANY ADDITIONAL COMMENTS.

DATE OF INITIAL EXAMINATION.........................19.......  DATE REPORT COMPLETED.........................19.........

DATE OF LAST EXAMINATION.........................19........  DOCTOR'S SIGNATURE.........................................

(Form 8D2. Reverse side of report.)

THE WORKMEN'S COMPENSATION ACT. ONTARIO
**MEDICAL AID REMITTANCE STATEMENT**

(F.)

*NOTICE* - IF ACCOUNTS NOT PAID,
PLEASE **DO NOT RESUBMIT**.
IF ACCOUNT DOES NOT APPEAR ON
REMITTANCE STATEMENT WITHIN TWO
MONTHS OF SUBMISSION, PLEASE
SUBMIT **FORM 178** 'MEDICAL AID
INQUIRY' FOR EACH ACCOUNT.

| CLAIM NO. | NAME OF CLAIMANT | PAYEE ACCT. NO. | ADJ. CODE | AMOUNT BILLED | AMOUNT PAID |
|---|---|---|---|---|---|
| "A","C" "R" 8643152 | John Doe | 12345 (D.12)* | 80 | $50.00 | $40.00 |

*D.12 is number secretary gave Doe's claim so
that she might easily identify it in case of
a query over payment.

12345 is number W.C.B. gave to the doctor so
that it could identify his claims every time
he sent one.

SEE REVERSE SIDE FOR ADJUSTMENT CODES

**KEY TO ADJUSTMENT CODES**

*REFERS TO ITEMS OF GENERAL PROVISIONS OF THE FEE SCHEDULE.
(A "CR" SUFFIX TO AN ITEM DENOTES A DEDUCTION FROM YOUR ACCOUNT. AN ADJUSTMENT CODE WILL EXPLAIN THE REASON.)

11. PROFESSIONAL FEE ADJUSTED TO SCHEDULE.
12. DETENTION FEES REDUCED OR DELETED. SEE PARA. 13*
13. FEE FOR SUPPORTIVE OR CONVALESCENT CARE DELETED. SEE PARA. 5*
14. SEE DEFINITION RE CLASSIFICATION OF CONSULTATION, GENERAL, SPECIFIC OR PARTIAL ASSESSMENT. SEE PARA. 21*
15. PORTION OF FEE FOR AFTERCARE PAID TO DOCTOR RENDERING SERVICE. SEE PARA. 5*
16. PAYMENT BASED ON FEE FOR SIMILAR SERVICE.
17. NO ALLOWANCE FOR CONCURRENT TREATMENT. SEE PARA. 10*
18. PAYMENT FOR AFTERCARE INCLUDED IN SURGICAL FEE. SEE PARA. 3*
19. PAYMENT FOR PRE-OPERATIVE CONSULTATION AND/OR EXAMINATION INCLUDED IN SURGICAL FEE. SEE PARA. 21(E)*
20. FATAL CASE. ACCOUNT ADJUSTED AS PER PARA. 14*
21. PAID AT GENERAL PRACTICE RATES.
22. ASSISTANT'S FEE ADJUSTED OR DELETED. SEE PARA. 8*
23. PROFESSIONAL FEE ADJUSTED ACCORDING TO PARA. 19*
24. A COMBINATION OF CODES 11 AND 18.
25. THIS PORTION OF SCHEDULED FEE PAID FOR AFTERCARE. 11.*
26. SEE SPECIAL LETTER.
29. ERROR-IN ADDITION.
30. PHYSIOTHERAPY TREATMENT NOT IN ACCORDANCE WITH REGULATIONS. SEE PARA. 17*
31. TREATMENT BEYOND 17 DAYS NOT AUTHORIZED, BALANCE REJECTED.
32. CHARGE FOR CLINIC TREATMENT FACILITIES ADJUSTED.
33. MILEAGE CHARGE ADJUSTED OR NOT ALLOWED. SEE PARA. 11*
34. ACCOUNT SUBMITTED LATE. SEE PARA. 12*
35. ASSESSED AT YOUR REQUEST.
36. AMOUNT SHOWN PAID AS A RESULT OF APPEAL.
40. CLAIM NOT ALLOWED, WORKMAN HAS NO ENTITLEMENT UNDER ACT FOR COST OF SERVICE.
41. CLAIM NOT ALLOWED, PAYMENT LIMITED TO AMOUNT SHOWN.
42. ACCOUNT IS DUPLICATE OF PART OR ALL OF PREVIOUSLY RECEIVED ACCOUNT.
43. CHARGE REJECTED. NOT PART OF WORKMEN'S ENTITLEMENT UNDER THE ACT.
44. UNAUTHORIZED CHANGE OF PRACTITIONERS. SEE MEDICAL HANDBOOK, PAGES 69 AND 70.

45. PAYMENT CANNOT BE CONSIDERED AS WORKMAN HAS NOT ELECTED TO CLAIM COMPENSATION.
46. PAYMENT CANNOT BE CONSIDERED AS MEDICAL REPORT OUTSTANDING. RESUBMIT ACCOUNT WITH REPORT.
47. PAYMENT CANNOT BE CONSIDERED AS WORKMAN HAS NOT ANSWERED CORRESPONDENCE.
48. ACCOUNT REJECTED. SHOULD BE PAID BY EMPLOYER.
49. OCULO VISUAL ASSESSMENT NOT PART OF WORKMAN'S ENTITLEMENT UNDER THE ACT.
50. CHARGES INCLUDED IN PER DIEM RATE OR OUTPATIENT FLAT RATE.
51. WORKMAN HAS NO ENTITLEMENT FOR PRIVATE ACCOMMODATION - ACCOUNT PAID AT SEMI-PRIVATE RATE.
52. OUT-PATIENT CHARGES ADJUSTED TO ESTABLISHED RATE.
53. YEAR END SETTLEMENT ON PREVIOUSLY PAID PRIOR YEAR DAYS.
54. NO PAYMENT OF OUTPATIENT CHARGE FOR FOLLOW-UP VISIT WHEN HOSPITAL FACILITIES NOT REQUIRED.
60. CHARGE FOR DRUGS AND/OR DRESSINGS ADJUSTED TO SCHEDULE. SEE PARA. 20*
61. UNABLE TO PAY FOR DRUGS AND/OR DRESSINGS AS NAME, SIZE, STRENGTH, QUANTITY, ETC. NOT SPECIFIED.
62. CHARGES FOR DRUGS REQUIRING PRIOR AUTHORITY DELETED. SEE PARA. 20*
63. CHARGES FOR DRUGS OR DRESSINGS INCLUDED IN PROFESSIONAL FEE. SEE PARA. 20*
64. A COMBINATION OF CODES 60 AND 61.
65. A COMBINATION OF CODES 60 AND 62.
66. A COMBINATION OF CODES 60 AND 63.
67. A COMBINATION OF CODES 11 AND 60.
68. A COMBINATION OF CODES 11 AND 61.
69. A COMBINATION OF CODES 11 AND 63.
70. AMOUNT DEDUCTED. THIS ACCOUNT HAS BEEN PAID TWICE.
71. AMOUNT DEDUCTED. PAYMENT PROCESSED IN YOUR FAVOUR IN ERROR.
72. AMOUNT DEDUCTED. ACCOUNT PAID IN ERROR-CLAIM NOT ALLOWED.
73. AMOUNT DEDUCTED. ACCOUNT PAID IN ERROR - CLAIM NOT YET ALLOWED.
74. AMOUNT DEDUCTED AT YOUR REQUEST.
80. X-RAY ADJUSTED TO AGREE WITH SCHEDULE.
81. X-RAY ADJUSTED BECAUSE OF INADEQUATE EXAMINATION.
82. X-RAY ADJUSTED DUE TO POOR QUALITY OF FILM.
83. X-RAY ADJUSTED DUE TO LATE SUBMISSION.

Medical Aid Remittance Form.

The form shown here as No. 10 6.65 should be filled out by the doctor, as is Form 43 Rev. 12.65. The first, a pink form, is used in the case of the death of a workman, and is the doctor's report of death. The second is used in the case of disability occurring, and is a doctor's special report. It is white and delineates exactly the extent of disability. Both forms have a reverse side, which is shown here, and where necessary the assistant must make sure that both sides of the form are correctly filled out, signed, and dated.

*(Text continued on page 722.)*

| WORKMAN'S SURNAME (PLEASE PRINT) | | | | | | | | | | | | | GIVEN OR CHRISTIAN NAMES | | CLAIM NO. | |
|---|---|

D O E — John Albert

WORKMAN'S ADDRESS IN FULL / SOCIAL INSURANCE NO. / AGE / FIRM NO.

1 Right Street, Ottawa, Ontario — 435-408-760 — 49

EMPLOYER'S NAME AND ADDRESS / RATE NO.

Wacky Construction, Limited  4 Wrong Street, Ottawa

DIAGNOSIS

Sub-dural haematoma, result of fall from construction

ACCIDENT DATE (NOT DATE TREATED) — DAY 1 MONTH 4 YEAR 19-- — DR'S ACCOUNT NO. 12345

| TREATMENT DATE | WHERE SEEN | TREATMENT (USE BACK OF FORM IF NECESSARY) | AMOUNT BILLED |
|---|---|---|---|
| DAY 1 MON 4 YEAR -- | H | Description of X-rays performed, and diagnosis | 50 00 |

Radiologist's name and address

| FIRST DATE | LAST DATE | SFR | INJ | TCA | ADJ CODE | TOTAL IF ITEMS ON BOTH SIDES | 50 00 |
|---|---|---|---|---|---|---|---|
| DAY MON YEAR | DAY MON YEAR | | | | | FOR W.C.B. USE | |

DOCTOR'S SIGNATURE

PDC 8303

APPROVAL

92

Form 92 for radiologist's use.

| WORKMAN'S SURNAME (PLEASE PRINT) | | | | | | | | GIVEN OR CHRISTIAN NAMES | CLAIM NO. |
|---|---|

D O E — John Albert

WORKMAN'S ADDRESS IN FULL / SOCIAL INSURANCE NO. / AGE / FIRM NO.

1 Right Street, Ottawa — 435-408-760 — 49

EMPLOYER'S NAME AND ADDRESS / RATE NO.

Wacky Construction Limited, 4 Wrong Street, Ottawa

FORM 104
REV. 5.67

ACCIDENT DATE (NOT DATE SEEN) — DAY 1 MONTH 4 YEAR 19-- — ACCOUNT NO. 12345

### THE WORKMEN'S COMPENSATION BOARD, ONTARIO
## RADIOLOGICAL REPORT

REQUIREMENTS — THAT THE RADIOGRAPHS, THE REPORTS OF
RADIOLOGICAL FINDINGS AND DIAGNOSIS, WITH THE ACCOUNT
CARD FOR RADIOLOGICAL CHARGES ONLY, BE FORWARDED AS
A SINGLE SUBMISSION WITHIN 14 DAYS OF EXAMINATION TO
THE BOARD AT 90 HARBOUR STREET, TORONTO 1, ONTARIO.

| OUT PATIENT | IN PATIENT | DATE OF ADMISSION | DATE X-RAY TAKEN | ORIGINAL EXAM | REPEAT EXAM | FILM NO. |
|---|---|---|---|---|---|---|
| ☐ | X | 1 4 19 -- | 1 4 19-- | X | ☐ | C. 567 |

ATTENDING DOCTOR'S FULL NAME
Patient's doctor's name

NAME AND ADDRESS OF X-RAY LABORATORY

NAME OF RADIOLOGIST OR MEDICAL PRACTITIONER
Radiologist's name

Radiologist's name and address

PART X-RAYED   Description of X-rays taken

RADIOLOGICAL FINDINGS AND DIAGNOSIS (USE BACK OF FORM IF NECESSARY)

Radiologist's opinion after reading the X-rays

(Fees will be according to scale set down by W.C.B.
and will depend on whether made by a specialist or
a radiologist.)

Signature of radiologist

IF NECESSARY, USE BACK OF FORM

SIGNATURE OF RADIOLOGIST OR MEDICAL PRACTITIONER

W.C.B. COMMENT

Radiologist's report.

| **THE WORKMEN'S COMPENSATION BOARD, ONTARIO** | **DOCTOR'S PROGRESS** |
|---|---|
| 90 HARBOUR STREET, TORONTO 1, TELEPHONE 362-3411 ● AREA CODE 416 | **REPORT** |

MAILING ADDRESS

## MESSAGE TO DOCTOR

*PLEASE COMPLETE AND RETURN
THIS FORM PROMPTLY AS FURTHER
COMPENSATION CAN NOT BE PAID
UNTIL IT IS RECEIVED.*

### PLEASE COMPLETE THIS PORTION IN FULL

1. DATE OF EXAMINATION ON WHICH
   REPORT IS BASED.                                    WHEN WILL WORKMAN BE SEEN AGAIN?

2. HOW MUCH LONGER WILL WORKMAN BE DISABLED?

3. DESCRIBE PHYSICAL FINDING WHEN EXAMINED.

### PLEASE GIVE DETAILS TO QUESTIONS ANSWERED "YES"

4. ANY TREATMENT SINCE LAST REPORT?                    NO    YES

5. ANY FACTORS DELAYING RECOVERY?                      NO    YES

6. WILL ANY PERMANENT DISABILITY RESULT
   FROM THE INJURY?                                    NO    YES

7. AT TIME OF EXAMINATION COULD HE:

   (A) DO HIS USUAL WORK?                              NO    YES    DATE

   (B) DO PART TIME OR SUITABLE WORK?                  NO    YES    DATE

8. IS HE HOSPITALIZED?                                 NO    YES

9. (A) IS HE RECEIVING PHYSIOTHERAPY?                  NO    YES

   (B) WOULD TREATMENT AT THE BOARD'S
       REHABILITATION CENTRE BE
       BENEFICIAL?                                     NO    YES

   (C) CAN HE TRAVEL ALONE?                            NO    YES

10. HAS HE BEEN EXAMINED BY A CERTIFIED                NO    YES    WHO
    SPECIALIST?                                                     WHEN

| DATE | DOCTOR'S SIGNATURE | ADDRESS | REV. 4.70 **26** |

Progress report.

## THE WORKMEN'S COMPENSATION BOARD, ONTARIO ▮ WORKMAN'S PROGRESS REPORT
90 HARBOUR STREET, TORONTO 1, TELEPHONE 362-3411 • AREA CODE 416

MAILING ADDRESS

CLAIM NO.

ACCIDENT DATE          FIRM NO.        RATE NO.

AGE          SOCIAL INSURANCE NO.

AREA OF INJURY

### MESSAGE TO WORKMAN

PLEASE COMPLETE **ONLY** THE SECTION OF THIS FORM THAT APPLIES TO YOU.

RETURN THE FORM PROMPTLY SO FURTHER CONSIDERATION MAY BE GIVEN YOUR CLAIM.

IF THERE IS A DOCTOR'S REPORT FORM ATTACHED PLEASE TAKE IT TO YOUR DOCTOR FOR COMPLETION.

## ARE YOU WORKING?

NO

PLACE A CHEQUE MARK (√) IN THE BOX THAT APPLIES TO YOU. COMPLETE **ONLY** THE SECTION THAT IS THE SAME COLOUR AS THE BOX YOU CHECKED.

YES

IS YOUR ADDRESS DIFFERENT FROM THE ONE SHOWN ABOVE?  NO  YES — IF YES, SHOW NEW ADDRESS

DID YOUR DOCTOR SAY YOU COULD GO TO WORK?  NO  YES — IF YES, SHOW DATE YOU CAN GO

YOUR DOCTOR'S NAME

DATE YOU LAST SAW HIM

IS IT NECESSARY FOR YOU TO TRAVEL TO ANOTHER CITY OR TOWN TO SEE YOUR DOCTOR?  NO  YES

DID YOU WORK BETWEEN FIRST LAY-OFF AND NOW?  NO  YES — IF YES, SHOW DATES  FROM    TO

YOUR SIGNATURE          TODAY'S DATE

**IMPORTANT** - KEEP IN TOUCH WITH YOUR EMPLOYER ABOUT RETURNING TO WORK

IS YOUR ADDRESS DIFFERENT FROM THE ONE SHOWN ABOVE?  NO  YES — IF YES, SHOW NEW ADDRESS

IS YOUR EMPLOYER DIFFERENT FROM THE ONE SHOWN ABOVE?  NO  YES — IF YES, SHOW NEW EMPLOYER

DATE YOU RETURNED TO WORK

DO YOU HAVE A REDUCTION IN WAGES CAUSED BY THE INJURY?  NO  YES

DID YOU WORK BETWEEN DATE OF FIRST LAY-OFF AND LATEST RETURN TO WORK DATE?  NO  YES — IF YES, SHOW DATES  FROM    TO

YOUR SIGNATURE          TODAY'S DATE          REV. 11/68 **41**

AUTOMATED BUSINESS FORMS LTD.

Progress report.

THE WORKMEN'S COMPENSATION ACT, ONTARIO

FORM 10 6.65

DOCTOR'S REPORT OF DEATH

CLAIM NUMBER

DEAR DOCTOR

PLEASE COMPLETE THIS REPORT FULLY AND RETURN IT TO US AS SOON AS POSSIBLE.

THE WORKMEN'S COMPENSATION BOARD,
90 HARBOUR STREET, TORONTO 1, ONT.
EMPIRE 2 3411

DECEASED NAME AND ADDRESS

DOCTOR'S NAME AND ADDRESS

AGE AT TIME OF DEATH

1  (A) DATE OF ACCIDENT................19......
   (B) DATE OF DEATH................19

2  (A) PLACE OF ACCIDENT.........PROVINCE OF.......
       HOSPITAL OR
   (B) PLACE OF DEATH (CITY OR TOWN).  STREET ADDRESS

3  (A) WHO RENDERED FIRST TREATMENT?

4  (A) DATE OF YOUR FIRST VISIT?
   (B) PLACE OF YOUR FIRST VISIT?

5  STATE NATURE, EXTENT AND REGION OF INJURY

6  DESCRIBE CONDITION FOUND ON FIRST VISIT

7  DESCRIBE BRIEFLY SUBSEQUENT SYMPTOMS AND COURSE

8  DESCRIBE ANY COMPLICATIONS AND GIVE DATE OF DEVELOPMENT

9  DESCRIBE TREATMENT

CAUSE OF DEATH

|  | | APPROXIMATE INTERVAL BETWEEN ONSET AND DEATH |
|---|---|---|
| 10 | (1) IMMEDIATE CAUSE—STATE THE DISEASE, INJURY OR COMPLICATION WHICH CAUSED DEATH,NOT THE MODE OF DYING,SUCH AS HEART FAILURE,ASPHYXIA,ASTHENIA ETC. (A) ...... | |
| | DUE TO | |
| | MORBID CONDITIONS, IF ANY, GIVING RISE TO IMMEDIATE CAUSE (STATE IN ORDER BACKWARDS FROM IMMEDIATE CAUSE), (B) ...... | |
| | DUE TO | |
| | (C) ...... | |
| | (2) OTHER MORBID CONDITIONS (IF IMPORTANT) CONTRIBUTING TO DEATH BUT NOT CAUSALLY RELATED TO IMMEDIATE CAUSE ...... | |

PLEASE COMPLETE THE OTHER SIDE ALSO

| 11 | IF A CORONER'S INQUEST WAS HELD,GIVE CORONER'S NAME AND ADDRESS ...... |
|---|---|
| 12 | (A) IF A POST MORTEM WAS PERFORMED, BY WHOM? ...... |
| | (B) POST MORTEM FINDINGS (IF KNOWN) ...... |

.......... DATE .......... 19 .......... SIGNATURE OF ATTENDING DOCTOR

ADDITIONAL INFORMATION WHICH MAY BE OF ASSISTANCE IN CONSIDERING THE MERITS OF THE CLAIM MAY BE WRITTEN BELOW.

Form 10 6.65 Report of death.

THE WORKMEN'S COMPENSATION BOARD, ONTARIO
90 HARBOUR ST., TORONTO 1, TELEPHONE 362-3411

FORM 43   REV. 12.65

## DOCTOR'S SPECIAL REPORT

DOCTOR —
PLEASE EXAMINE THIS WORKMAN AND COM-
PLETE THIS REPORT FOR THE BOARD.

MAILING ADDRESS

1. OF WHAT DOES THE WORKMAN COMPLAIN?

2. DESCRIBE FULLY ANY PHYSICAL IMPAIRMENT RESULTING FROM THE ACCIDENT (SHORTENING, DEFORMITY, LIMITATION OF MOVEMENT, IMPAIRMENT OF VISION, SCARRING ETC.,) INDICATE WHETHER RIGHT OR LEFT SIDE.

**FOR LACK OF MOVEMENT AND AMPUTATIONS PLEASE COMPLETE THE CHART ON THE BACK**

3. WHAT TREATMENT, IF ANY, DO YOU SUGGEST?

4. WHAT IMPROVEMENT, IF ANY, DO YOU EXPECT?

5. DESCRIBE ANY PRE-EXISTING PHYSICAL IMPAIRMENT.

**FOR EYE CASES ALSO COMPLETE BELOW**

6. WAS THE INJURED EYE PREVIOUSLY NORMAL? IF NOT, GIVE DETAILS. WERE GLASSES WORN?

MARK ON THE CHARTS BELOW THE SITE AND EXTENT OF ANY LESIONS PRESENT. PLEASE INDICATE THE VISUAL ACUITY FOR BOTH EYES.

7.
BEFORE
CORRECTION _____

AFTER
CORRECTION _____

CORRECTING
LENS _____

**RIGHT EYE**

BEFORE
CORRECTION _____

AFTER
CORRECTION _____

CORRECTING
LENS _____

**LEFT EYE**

8. ARE GLASSES NEEDED BECAUSE OF THE ACCIDENT?   YES ☐   NO ☐   HAVE THEY BEEN PROVIDED?   YES ☐   NO ☐

DOCTOR'S SIGNATURE _____

**43**

DATE OF EXAM _____

ADDRESS _____

Report of disability.

*(Illustration continued on opposite page.)*

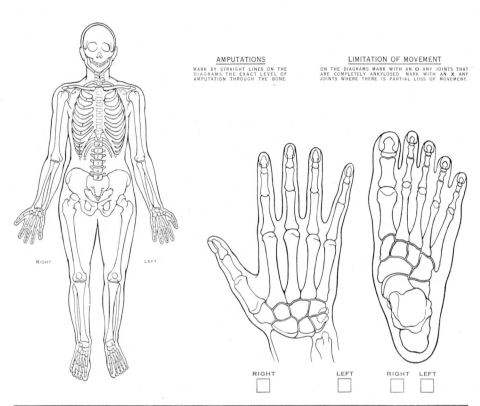

AMPUTATIONS

MARK BY STRAIGHT LINES ON THE
DIAGRAMS THE EXACT LEVEL OF
AMPUTATION THROUGH THE BONE.

LIMITATION OF MOVEMENT

ON THE DIAGRAMS MARK WITH AN O ANY JOINTS THAT
ARE COMPLETELY ANKYLOSED. MARK WITH AN X ANY
JOINTS WHERE THERE IS PARTIAL LOSS OF MOVEMENT.

RIGHT    LEFT

RIGHT    LEFT    RIGHT    LEFT

## FOR HAND CASES ALSO COMPLETE BELOW

DESCRIBE ANY PRE-EXISTING DEFECTS IN THE RIGHT HAND

DESCRIBE ANY PRE-EXISTING DEFECTS IN THE LEFT HAND

### FLEXION AND EXTENSION OF IMPAIRED
### FINGERS AND THUMBS

IN THE TABLE OPPOSITE, SHOW, IN DEGREES, THE
ANGLE OF UTMOST ACTIVE FLEXION. ALSO SHOW,
IN DEGREES, THE LACK OF EXTENSION. IN BOTH
CASES THE MEASUREMENT SHOULD BE MADE FROM A
STRAIGHT LINE, AS SHOWN IN THE ILLUSTRATION.
E.G. IF THE FINGER SHOWN BELOW WERE ANKYLOSED,
BOTH THE ANGLE OF UTMOST FLEXION AND THE
ANGLE DENOTING LACK OF EXTENSION WOULD BE 15°

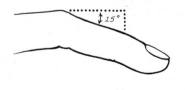

| THUMB | | PROX | DISTAL | |
|---|---|---|---|---|
| ANGLE OF UTMOST FLEXION | | | | |
| LACK OF EXTENSION | | | | |
| WHAT IS THE CONDITION OF ADDUCTION? | | | | |
| WHAT IS THE CONDITION OF ABDUCTION? | | | | |
| (THESE MAY BE DESCRIBED IN FRACTIONS OR PERCENTAGES) | | | | |

| FINGERS | | PROX | 2ND | DIS AL |
|---|---|---|---|---|
| INDEX | ANGLE OF UTMOST FLEXION | | | |
| | LACK OF EXTENSION | | | |
| MIDDLE | ANGLE OF UTMOST FLEXION | | | |
| | LACK OF EXTENSION | | | |
| RING | ANGLE OF UTMOST FLEXION | | | |
| | LACK OF EXTENSION | | | |
| SMALL | ANGLE OF UTMOST FLEXION | | | |
| | LACK OF EXTENSION | | | |

Report of disability.

MEDICAL AID ACCOUNT INQUIRY                                SEE BACK OF FORM FOR REPLY ➤➤→

| LAST NAME | | | | | | | | | | | | FIRST NAME(S) | CLAIM NUMBER |

PATIENT'S FULL ADDRESS                                                  ACCIDENT DATE - NOT TREATMENT DATE

EMPLOYER'S NAME AND ADDRESS                                             SOCIAL INSURANCE NO.

NATURE OF INJURY                                                        DATE OF SERVICES

| PAYEE CODE NO. | ACCOUNT NO. | NATURE OF SERVICES |
| | | |

| | PROFESSIONAL | ☐ | HOSPITALIZATION |

**ENTER YOUR NAME AND ADDRESS FOR RETURN**  ☐ EMERGENCY    ☐ X-RAY
**MAILING PURPOSES**  ▼    ▼                 ☐ PHYSIOTHERAPY  ☐ DRUGS

REASON FOR FOLLOW UP

☐ ACCOUNT FILED PAYMENT NOT RECEIVED

☐ BALANCE OF $_____ STILL OWING

☐ OTHER (SPECIFY)

SEND TO

THE WORKMEN'S COMPENSATION BOARD
90 HARBOUR ST., TORONTO 1, ONTARIO

FORM
**178**
REV.6.67

PAYMENT OF MEDICAL AID ACCOUNTS IS MADE ONCE MONTHLY  PLEASE ALLOW SUFFICIENT TIME FOR PROCESSING

THE WORKMEN'S COMPENSATION BOARD, ONTARIO
90 HARBOUR STREET, TORONTO 1   TELEPHONE 362-3411

**IN REPLY TO YOUR INQUIRY**

1 ☐ PAYMENT APPEARS ON OUR
     REMITTANCE STATEMENT DATED          19    ITEM NO.    PAGE NO.    AMOUNTS $

2 ☐ PAYMENT WILL BE INCLUDED ON NEXT REMITTANCE STATEMENT

3 ☐ WE DO NOT HAVE YOUR ACCOUNT.  PLEASE RESUBMIT

4 ☐ UNABLE TO PAY ACCOUNT.  CLAIM NOT YET ADJUDICATED.

5 ☐ WORKMAN HAS NO ENTITLEMENT UNDER ACT FOR COST OF SERVICES.

6 ☐ X-RAY FILMS NOT RECEIVED. PLEASE SUBMIT ON FORM 104 WITH FILMS.

7 ☐ ACCOUNT ADJUSTED FROM $            TO $            SEE ADJUSTMENT CODE NO.

8 ☐

Form 178.   Request for claim payment.

If the medical assistant has any doubt about acceding to a patient's request for "special" treatment, she should ask herself "is preferential treatment medically NECESSARY?". If the answer still is not clear, she should further ask herself "would the patient have this kind of attention if he were paying for it?". The Board pays for "all necessary and reasonable" medical expenses, and a good assistant will soon learn to discern which claim is valid and which is not. A taxi may be necessary and essential for a woman of 65, but it is unnecessary for a young man or woman of 20, each having the same injury.

Finally, even with the best of attention and care an occasional claim will not be paid. Invariably this will happen because the claim card or form has not been filled out properly by the payee, and it is then necessary to send in Form 178, illustrated here to ask that the claim be paid. The back of Form 178 is used for the Board's reply.

Form 178 calls for all the details which would have appeared on the original claim, including the patient's name and address, the accident date and the treatment date, the employer's name and address, the nature of the injury, the payee's code number, the number of the account, the nature of the service, and the reason for the follow-up. The form is sent to the Workmen's Compensation Board, which will reply on the reverse side of the form. If the W.C.B. cannot trace the account, they will request that it be resubmitted, or if they need more information, they will request it. If the W.C.B. finds that the workman has no claim number (in which case the doctor must request payment from the patient) they will ask for any x-ray films they may need, or will pay the account at a later date, perhaps adjusting the amount claimed, and indicate the adjustment code number.

Only when Form 178 has been sent and replied to should an account be resubmitted. To do so without first carrying out this procedure would probably delay payment of the account.

## BIBLIOGRAPHY

Pollock. *The Law of Partnership.* 15 Ed. Gower (Ed.) London, Stevens and Sons, Ltd., 1953.

Smyth, J. E. and Soberman, D. A. *The Law and Business Administration in Canada.* 2nd Ed. Toronto, Prentice-Hall of Canada, Ltd., 1968, pp. 522–538.

Underhill. *The Principles of the Law and Partnership.* 7th Ed. Hesbeth (Ed.) Butterworth and Co., Ltd., 1958.

# INDEX

Page numbers in *italics* indicate illustrations.
Page numbers followed by a t indicate a table.

Syringe (*Continued*)
disposable, carton for, *452*
cutting device for, *452*
filling of, 420
from an ampule, 422
removing substances from, 451
reusable, 451
sterilization of, 453
stuck, opening of, 452, *453*
types of tips on, 458
Syrup, 392
Systemic drugs, 402, 414–419
oral route for, 414
Systolic pressure, 527

Table surfaces, cleaning of, 312
Tablets, types of, 391
Tachypnea, 525
Tax identification number, 276
application form for, *278*
Tax record, guidelines for retaining, 183
Telegraph services, 118–119
Telephone, effective use of, 99–119
special equipment for, 117
Telephone answering services, 113
automatic, 114
operator-answered, 113
Telephone calls, answering of, 102
charging for, 190
complaints about care or fees, 111
conference calls, 117
direct distance dialing, 116
from angry callers, 111
from family and friends, 111
from other physicians, 110
from unidentified callers, 111
incoming, 100
screening of, 103
long distance, 116
office procedure form for, *108*
outgoing, 115
requests for information, 110
second calls, 104
termination of, 104
third party requests for information, 110
transferring of, 104
troublesome, 110
wrong numbers, 117
Telephone dictation, 118
Telephone message, information required in, 105
memorandum for, 106
recording of, 105
taking action on, 107
transmitting of, 105
Telephone numbers, organization of, 115
Telephone technique, 99–119
administrative matters and, 109
appointments for new patients and, 107
assistance, offer of, 103
assistance with insurance and, 109
diction in, guide to, 101
for incoming calls, 100
for prescription refills, 110
for referral to physician, 110

Telephone technique (*Continued*)
for troublesome calls, 111, 112
examples of, 113
identification of caller in, 102
inquiries about bills and, 109
personality in, 99
receiving laboratory reports and, 109
reports from hospitals and, 109
reports from patient and, 109, 110
requests for house calls, 112
rules for, 100, 105
salutations, use of, 102
scheduling appointments by, 82
return visits and, 109
when caller must hold the line, 103
Teller, definition of, 229
Temperature, axillary, 523
charting of, *520*
groin, 523
measurement of, 519
recording of, 522
rectal, 522
Temporary file, organization of, 179
Termination conversion, definition of, 302
Tests, Coomb's, 502
for skin sensitivity, 368
Huhner, 596
light and accommodation, 619
Marshal-Marchetti, 595
Rubin's, 595
Schick, 381
tuberculin, 381
Tetanus, 367
Therapy, physical, 539–551. See also *Physical therapy.*
Thermal death point, 467
Thermometers, 522
electronic, 523, *524*
Thiamin (vitamin $B_1$), 341
Thigh, injections in, 418
Third class mail, 124
Third party liability, 197
Thoracic medicine, sterilization problems in, 485
Thorax, movement of, Color Plate 6
Throat, administering drugs to, 413
Throat cultures, technique for taking, 373
Thrush, 507
Thumb forceps, *435*, 436
Thyroxine iodine test, 503
Tickler file, 179
Tincture(s), 392, 411
Tissue forceps, *435*, 436
Toenail, resection of, 598
Tonometers, 446, *447*, 619, *620*
Tooth, structure of, Color Plate 9
Topical drugs, 402, 410–414
Tort, 66
Touch-tone telephone, 118
Towel clamps, 433, *433*
Trade names of drugs, 386
Tranquilizers, 397t, 401
Transcription, skills of, 133
Transmittal of Wage and Tax Statements, 282, *283*
Transportation arrangements for meetings, 155